REVIEW
OF
ORTHOPAEDICS

REVIEW
OF
ORTHOPAEDICS

MARK D. MILLER, M.D.

Major, US Air Force Medical Corps;
Clinical Assistant Professor of Surgery
Uniformed Services University of The Health Sciences
F. Edward Hébert School of Medicine
Bethesda, Maryland;
Department of Orthopaedic Surgery
Wilford Hall USAF Medical Center
Lackland Air Force Base
San Antonio, Texas

W.B. SAUNDERS COMPANY

A Division of Harcourt Brace & Company

Philadelphia / London / Toronto / Montreal / Sydney / Tokyo

W.B. SAUNDERS COMPANY
A Division of
Harcourt Brace & Company

The Curtis Center
Independence Square West
Philadelphia, Pennsylvania 19106

Library of Congress Cataloging-in-Publication Data

Review of orthopaedics / [edited by] Mark D. Miller.
     p.   cm.
   ISBN 0-7216-4553-4
   1. Orthopedics.   I. Miller, Mark D.
   [DNLM: 1. Bone Diseases. 2. Joint Diseases. WE 200 R454]
  RD731.R44 1992
  617.3–dc20
  DNLM/DLC
  for Library of Congress   92-7547
                                              CIP

Review of Orthopaedics   ISBN 0-7216-4553-4

Printed in Mexico.

Last digit is the print number: 9   8   7   6   5   4   3

I dedicate this book to my devoted wife who understood my obsession, my children who suffered through the ceaseless hours of writing and editing it, and my parents who taught me the value of persistence.

I also gratefully acknowledge and dedicate this book to the editors for sharing their experience and expertise, and to all orthopaedic residents, past, present, and future.

Consulting Editors

* Contributions made while assigned to Wilford Hall USAF Medical Center, Lackland AFB, San Antonio, Texas

Consulting Associate Editors

Foreword

Dr. Mark Miller is an active duty Air Force officer and is a product of the Wilford Hall USAF Medical Center Orthopaedic Residency program in San Antonio, Texas. He has carefully reviewed orthopaedic textbooks, lecture notes, Academy publications, examinations, journals, and review course notes to compile the manuscript, and he utilized a select panel of orthopaedic surgeons to review and edit it. This book is of value not only to residents who are studying for intraining examinations and certifying examinations but also for practicing orthopaedists to help them review and study for the Orthopaedic Self-Assessment Examination and any future recertification examination.

CHARLES A. ROCKWOOD, JR.

Acknowledgments

It is impossible to recognize every person that in some way contributed to this book, but I would be remiss not to mention a few of the key "behind the scenes" people. First and foremost I must mention my wife Brenda who spent countless hours helping with organizing, reorganizing, word processing, and using her computer wizardry in preparation of the manuscript and illustrations. Next I should recognize the outstanding talents of Allen B. Tyler, whose quality medical illustrations speak for themselves. I wish to also thank the residents and staff of the Department of Orthopaedic Surgery at Wilford Hall USAF Medical Center. In addition to the staff selected as editors for individual sections, I appreciate the many comments and support from the entire department. I must again recognize the outstanding group of editors who were willing to take time out of their busy schedules to add the key element of experience to the text. I also appreciate the interest and support of Dr. Norman Rich, Professor and Chairman of the Department of Surgery at the Uniformed Services University, F. Edward Hébert School of Medicine. Finally, I am grateful to the editors at W.B. Saunders Company for their interest in this project and for "fine-tuning" the manuscript.

Preface

The writer does the most, who gives the reader the most knowledge and takes from him the least time.

C.C. Colton *Lacon*, Preface

This book was created to fill an important void in the existing orthopaedic literature. Although there exists a large number of quality texts of operative orthopaedics, musculoskeletal basic science, and the various sub-specialties, nowhere is there an essential "core" of orthopaedic knowledge. This book attempts to provide this core by distilling the existing orthopaedic textbooks, journal articles, review courses, intraining examinations, self assessment guides, and specialty examinations into one resource.

REVIEW OF ORTHOPAEDICS has been extensively edited by two groups of consultants: First by a cadre of younger orthopaedic surgeons who have recently finished residency and fellowship training and successfully completed their boards, and second by an impressive assemblage of senior surgeons who have added a vital element of experience to the text.

It is my intention that this book will serve as a review for intraining and board examinations, and also as a curriculum guide for orthopaedic residency training programs.

MARK D. MILLER, M.D.

Contents

CHAPTER 1

Pediatric Orthopaedics

I. Embryology—Beginning at day 12 after conception, the **primitive streak** appears and, beginning caudally, ectodermal cells migrate between endoderm and ectoderm to form the **mesoderm**. **Mesenchyme** comes from mesoderm and gives rise to connective tissues, muscles, vessels, blood cells, and the GU system. Between days 15 and 21, the **notochord** is formed at the cranial end of the primitive streak as ectoderm forms a primitive knot that becomes a blastopore and eventually differentiates into the notochord (Fig. 1–1). **Neural crest** cells also differentiate at this time and later form the peripheral nervous system (**PNS**), autonomic nervous system (**ANS**), and Schwann cells. **Somites** are formed from mesoderm, line both sides of the notochord, and eventually total 42–44 pairs. Each somite develops into a lateral dermatome, a medial myotome, and a ventral sclerotome forming skin, muscle, and skeletal elements, respectively (Fig. 1–2). **Limb buds** develop between 4 and 6 weeks (Fig. 1–3) and quickly form the upper extremity, with pronated forearms that then rotate externally. A few days later the lower extremity forms and eventually rotates internally. Although finger rays are present at 7 weeks, the hand continues to differentiate until week 13 (Fig. 1–4). The median artery, which initially supplies the hand, evolves at about 6 weeks. **Bone** is formed through mesenchymal aggregation into a cartilage model that is systematically replaced by bone (except for a few bones that are formed without a cartilage model through intramembranous ossification—skull, scapula). **Primary centers of ossification** appear in the diaphyses of bones between 7 and 12 weeks. Most secondary centers of ossification (except the distal femur) are not present until after birth.

II. Bone Dysplasias (Dwarfs)

A. Introduction—According to Rubin, **dysplasia** refers to deformities caused by intrinsic bone disturbance (e.g., achondroplasia); **dystrophy** alludes to deformities caused by metabolic or nutritional deficiencies (e.g., mucopolysaccharidoses); and **dysostosis** is the term used when there are underlying mesodermal or ectodermal abnormalities (e.g., diastrophic dysplasia). Histologic changes common to all dysplasias include horizontal orientation of primary trabeculae adjacent to the physis. **Proportionate** dwarfism includes diastrophic dysplasia, cleidocranial dysplasia, and the mucopolysaccharidoses. **Disproportionate** dwarf-

ing conditions are also sometimes referred to as short-limb (achondroplasia, metaphyseal chondrodysplasias) or short-trunk (Kneist syndrome, spondyloepiphyseal dysplasia) varieties. Dysplasias can also be characterized based on the area of growth affected (Fig. 1–5).

B. Achondroplasia
 1. Introduction and Etiology—Achondroplasia is an autosomal dominant (AD) (with 80% spontaneous mutation), disproportionate, short-limbed form of dwarfism caused by abnormal enchondral bone formation (defect in proliferative zone). It is a quantitative and not a qualitative cartilage defect. Enchondral growth is much more affected than appositional growth. It may be associated with late childbirth (after 36 yo).
 2. Signs and Symptoms—Clinical features include a normal trunk and short limbs, affecting proximal segments less than distal (rhizomelia). Typically, these patients will have prominent foreheads, button noses, small nasal bridges, trident hands (inability to approximate extended middle and ring fingers), thoracolumbar kyphosis (the most common spinal deformity), lumbar stenosis (short pedicles with decreased interpedicular distances), radial head subluxation, and hypotonia. Involved children typically have normal intelligence but delayed walking and other motor milestones. Although sitting height may be normal, standing height is in the lower 3%. Radiographs show narrowing of the interpedicular distance L1–S1, T12/L1 wedging, generalized posterior vertebral scalloping, delayed appearance of growth plates, and broad, short iliac wings ("champagne glass" pelvic outlet). Achondroplasia may also be associated with radial and tibial bowing (fibula and ulna less affected), coxa valga, genu varum (with disproportionately long fibula), and metaphyseal flaring with "inverted V"–shaped distal femoral physis. Symptoms are usually related to root or cord compression. This can occur at any level, including the foramen magnum (which may cause episodes of apnea).
 3. Treatment—Nonoperative treatment should include weight loss (typically a problem), bracing, and exercises (unpredictable). Surgical options include decompression and fusion for severe

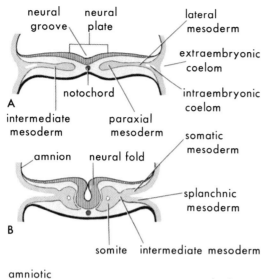

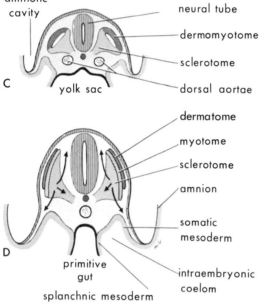

FIGURE 1–1. Formation of the neural tube (*A–D*, 18, 22, 26, and 28 days' gestation, respectively). (From Moore, K.L.: The Developing Human. Philadelphia, W.B. Saunders Company, 1982; reprinted by permission.)

kyphosis (most will correct spontaneously but anterior decompression and strut grafting and posterior fusion without instrumentation are indicated for kyphosis >60 degrees); multilevel decompression for stenosis (recommended for interpedicular distances of <20 mm at L1 and <16 mm at L5), and fibular epiphysiodesis and/or tibial osteotomies for genu varum. Limb lengthening procedures are controversial. Preoperative pulmonary evaluation is required because of associated respiratory problems.

C. Spondyloepiphyseal Dysplasia—Three forms are generally recognized.
   1. Congenita form—Short-trunked dwarfism associated with primary involvement of the vertebra (beaking) and epiphyseal centers (affects the proliferative zone), clinical heterogenicity, and variable inheritance patterns. The clinical and radiographic differences are frequently age related and not distinguishable at birth. Delayed appearance of epiphysis, platyspondyly, scoliosis, odontoid hypoplasia, coxa vara, and genu valgum are common. Patients should also be screened for associated retinal disorders.
   2. Tarda form—These patients typically have later manifestations of the disorder, which affects primarily the spine and larger joints. Affected children often are susceptible to premature osteoarthritis (osteotomies may be helpful) and scoliosis (treated like idiopathic scoliosis).
   3. Pseudoachondroplastic Dysplasia—Although considered separately in some classifications, this disorder, which has an autosomal dominant inheritance pattern, is clinically similar in appearance to achondroplasia but affected children will have normal facies. Radiographs demonstrate metaphyseal flaring and delayed epiphyseal ossification. Orthopaedic manifestations of the disorder include cervical instability and significant lower extremity bowing.

D. Chondrodysplasia Punctata—Characterized by multiple punctate calcifications seen on radiographs in infancy. The AD (Conrads-Hünermann) form has a wide variation of clinical expression. The severe autosomal recessive (AR) rhizomelic form is usually fatal in the first year of life. Ophthalmologic disorders and spinal deformities are common.

E. Kneist Syndrome—AD, short-limbed, short-trunked, disproportionate dwarfism with joint stiffness/contractures, scoliosis, kyphosis, dumbbell-shaped femora, and hypoplastic pelvis and spine. May be related to an abnormality of cartilage proteoglycan metabolism, and physes may have a characteristic "Swiss cheese" appearance histologically. Radiographs show osteoporosis and platyspondyly or hypoplasia. Respiratory problems and cleft palate are common; associated retinal detachment requires ophthalmology consult. Early therapy for joint contractures is required. Reconstructive procedures may be required for early hip degenerative arthritis.

F. Metaphyseal Chondrodysplasia—Heterogeneous group of disorders characterized by metaphyseal changes of tubular bones with normal epiphyses. The physis (proliferative and hypertrophic zones) actually appears histologically to be more affected than the metaphysis, hence the term metaphyseal dysostoses has fallen out of favor. Several types are recognized, including the following:
   1. Jansen-(Rare) AD, retarded, short-limbed dwarf with wide eyes, monkey-like stance, and hypercalcemia.
   2. Schmid-AD, short-limbed dwarf not diagnosed until older, with stunting of growth and bowing of legs. Often confused with rickets but has normal labs.
   3. McKusick—AR, cartilage-hair dysplasia (hypoplasia of cartilage and small diameter of hair) seen more commonly in the Amish population. Atlantoaxial instability is common and requires flexion-extension radiographs for proper evaluation.

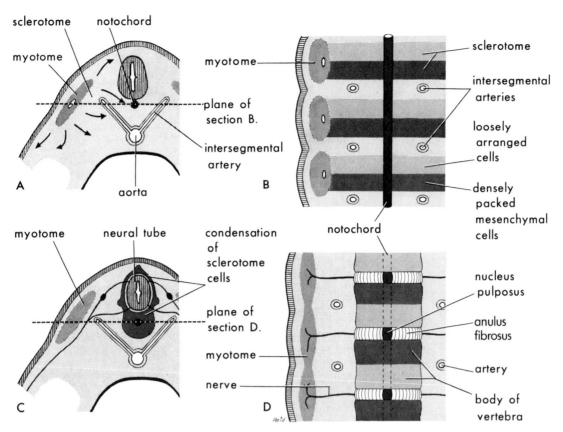

FIGURE 1–2. Further development of the axial skeleton. *A* and *B*, Transverse and frontal sections, respectively, of 4-week embryo. *C* and *D*, Similar sections of 5-week embryo. Note that the vertebral body forms from the cranial and caudal halves of two successive sclerotome masses. (From Moore, K.L.: The Developing Human. Philadelphia, W.B. Saunders Company, 1982; reprinted by permission.)

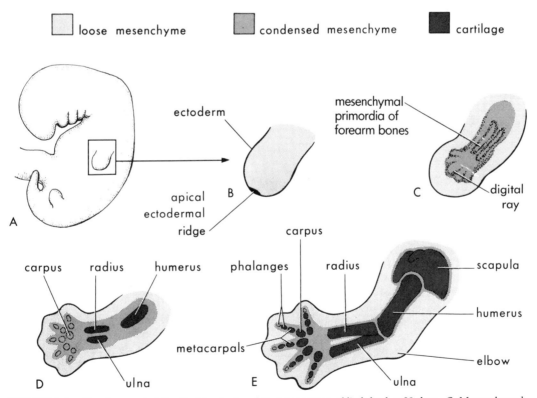

FIGURE 1–3. Development of the limb bud. *A* and *B*, Appearance of limb bud at 28 days. *C*, Mesenchymal primordium at 33 days. *D* and *E*, Further development at 6 weeks. (From Moore, K.L.: The Developing Human. Philadelphia, W.B. Saunders Company, 1982; reprinted by permission.)

3

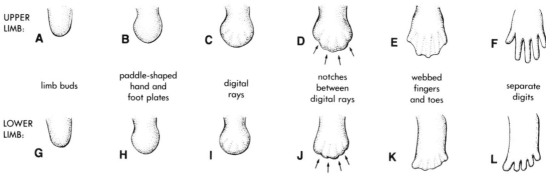

FIGURE 1–4. Development of the hands and feet. *A–F*, Development of the hand (4–8 weeks). *G–L*, Development of the foot (4½–8½ weeks). (From Moore, K.L.: The Developing Human. Philadelphia, W.B. Saunders Company, 1982; reprinted by permission.)

G. Multiple Epiphyseal Dysplasia—Short-limbed disproportionate dwarfing often not manifested until age 5–14. A milder form (Ribbing) and a more severe form (Fairbank) exist. The disorder is characterized by irregular and/or delayed ossification present at multiple epiphyses. Short, stunted metacarpals/metatarsals, irregular femora (mimics Legg-Calvé-Perthes disease, but it is bilateral and symmetric, is not associated with metaphyseal cysts, and often has early acetabular changes), abnormal ossification (tibial "slant sign" and flattened femoral condyles), T12/L1 notching and deformed ring apophysis, valgus knees (consider

early osteotomy), waddling gait; and early hip arthritis are common.

H. Dysplasia Epiphysealis Hemimelica (Trevor's Disease)—Essentially an osteochondroma that causes half of the epiphysis (usually the medial half) to enlarge (with an irregular mass), usually at the knee. Partial excision of the prominent overgrowth (if symptomatic), and later osteotomies, may be required.

I. Progressive Diaphyseal Dysplasia (Camurati-Engelmann Disease)—Autosomal dominant inheritance; affected children are often "late walkers" (be-

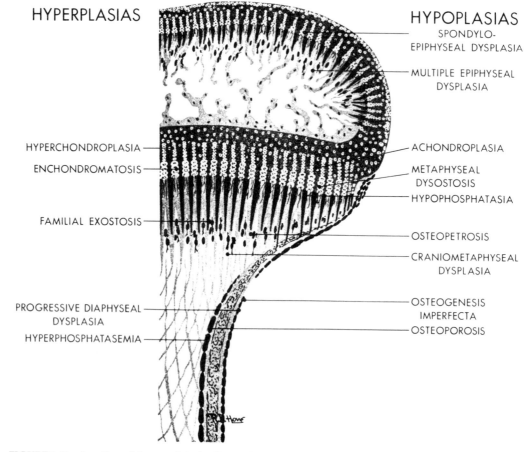

FIGURE 1–5. Location of abnormalities leading to dysplasias. (From Rubin, P.: Dynamic Classification of Bone Dysplasias. Chicago, Year Book Medical Publishers, 1964; reprinted by permission.)

TABLE 1–1. MAIN TYPES OF MUCOPOLYSACCHARIDOSIS

Syndrome	Inher[a]	Intel[b]	Cornea	Urinary Excretion	Other
I Hurler's	AR	MR	Cloudy	Dermatan/heparan sulfate	Worst prognosis
II Hunter's	XR	MR	Clear	Dermatan/heparan sulfate	
III Sanfilippo's	AR	MR	Clear	Heparan sulfate	Nl until 2 yo
IV Morquio's	AR	Nl	Cloudy	Keratan sulfate	**Most common**

[a] Inheritance: AR, autosomal recessive; XR, sex-lined recessive.
[b] Intelligence: MR, mental retardation; Nl, normal.

cause of associated muscle weakness), with symmetric cortical thickening of long bones. Radiographs demonstrate widened, fusiform diaphyses with increased bone formation and sclerosis. The tibia, femur, and humerus are most often affected (in that order), affecting only the diaphyseal portion of bone. Symptomatic treatment includes salicylates, nonsteroidal anti-inflammatory drugs (NSAIDs), and steroids for refractory cases.

J. Mucopolysaccharidosis—Proportionate dwarfism caused by accumulation of mucopolysaccharides (MPS) from a hydrolase enzyme deficiency. MPS consist of glycosaminoglycans attached to a link protein with a hyaluronic acid core (see Chapter 2, Basic Sciences). Diagnosis is based on finding complex sugars in the urine. Bony changes include thickened skull, wide ribs, anterior beaking of vertebrate, wide flat pelvis, coxa valga with unossified femoral heads, and bullet-shaped metacarpals. Four main types include Hurler's, Hunter's, Sanfilippo's, and Morquio's (Table 1–1). C1–C2 instability (odontoid hypoplasia) seen with Morquio's may present with myelopathy, which requires decompression and cervical fusion (proximal tibial bone graft is favored over iliac crest graft because of the unavailability of cancellous bone between the two tables of the ilium).

K. Diastrophic Dysplasia—Autosomal recessive, severe, short-limbed dwarfism associated with a disorder of type II collagen in the physis. This "twisted" dwarf classically has a cleft palate, severe joint contractures (esp. hip and knees), cauliflower ears, hitchhiker thumb, rigid clubfeet, midthoracic kyphoscoliosis, cervical kyphosis (re-

quires immediate treatment with neurologic sequela), thoracolumbar kyphoscoliosis, spina bifida occulta, and atlantoaxial instability. Wide release of clubfeet, osteotomies for contractures, and spinal fusion are often required.

L. Cleidocranial Dysplasia (Dysostosis)—Autosomal dominant proportionate dwarfism that affects bones formed intramembranously. Patients present with dwarfism (or stunted growth) with absent clavicle(s), delayed skull suture closure, coxa vara (consider intertrochanteric osteotomy if varus is <100 degrees), delayed ossification of the pubis, and wormian-type bone.

M. Dysplasias Associated with Neoplasms—Includes multiple hereditary exostosis (osteochondromatosis), fibrous dysplasia, Ollier's disease (enchondromatosis), and Maffucci's syndrome (enchondromatosis and hemangiomas). These entities are discussed in Chapter 7, Orthopaedic Pathology.

N. Dysplasia Summary—The various types of dysplasia are summarized in Table 1–2.

III. Chromosomal and Teratologic Disorders

A. Down Syndrome (Trisomy 21)—Most common chromosomal abnormality; its incidence increases with advanced maternal age. Usually associated with increased growth, ligament laxity, hypotonia, mental impairment, heart disease (50%), endocrine disorders (hypothyroidism and diabetes), and premature aging. Orthopaedic problems include spinal abnormalities (atlantoaxial instability, scoliosis, spondylolisthesis); hip instability (open reduction ± osteotomy usually required); slipped capital femoral epiphysis, patella dislocation; and

TABLE 1–2. TYPES OF DYSPLASIA

Dysplasia	Type[a]	Inher[b]	Zone[c]	Clinical Findings	Radiographic Features
Achondroplasia	Dis	AD/SM	Epi	Facies, spine abnormalities	Stenosis, leg bowing
SED[d] (Congenita)	Dis	AD	Epi	Cleft palate, lordosis	Platyspondyly
SED (pseudoachondroplastic)	Dis	AD/AR	Epi	Normal facies	Fragmented epiphysis
SED (tarda)	Dis	XR	Epi	Kyphosis, hip pain	Hip dysplasia, thick vertebrae
Chondrodysplasia punctate	Dis	AD	Phy	Flat facies	Stippled epiphyses
Kneist	Dis	AD	Phy	Retinal detachment, scoliosis	Dumbell femora
Metaphyseal chondrodysplasia	Dis	AD/AR	Met	Wide eyes, leg bowing	Bowed legs
Multiple epiphyseal	Dis	AD	Epi	Late—waddling gait	Irregular epiphyseal ossification
Dysplasia epiphysealis hemimelica	Dis	—	Met	Bowed legs	Hemi-enlarged epiphysis
Diaphyseal	Dis	AD	Dia	Delayed walking	Symmetric cortical thickening
Mucopolysaccharidosis	Pro	AD/XR	Hyp	Cornea, sugars, AAI	Thick bone, Bullet metacarpals
Diastrophic	Pro	AR	Phy	Palate, ear, thumb	Kyphoscoliosis
Cleidocranial dysostasis	Pro	AR	Met	Absent clavicles	Delayed physeal closure

[a] Type: Dis, disproportionate; Pro, proportionate.
[b] Inheritance: AD, autosomal dominant; AR, autosomal recessive; SM, spontaneous mutation; XR, sex-linked recessive.
[c] Zone: Epi, epiphyseal; Phy, physical; Met, metaphyseal; Dia, diaphyseal; Hyp, hypophyseal.
[d] Spondyloepiphyseal dysplasia.

asymptomatic planovalgus feet. Atlantoaxial instability is evaluated with flexion-extension radiographs of the C-spine. Asymptomatic children with instability should be restricted from contact sports, diving, and gymnastics. Atlantoaxial fusion has an extremely high complication rate and is usually reserved for patients with neurologic compromise (often with >7 mm of instability demonstrated on flexion-extension views). Preoperative cardiac evaluation is essential.

B. Turner's Syndrome—45-XO females with short stature, sexual infantilism, web neck, and cubitus valgus. Hormonal therapy can exacerbate scoliosis. Genu valgum and shortening of the fourth and fifth metacarpals usually require no treatment. Malignant hyperthermia is common with anesthetics.

C. Noonan's Syndrome—Short stature, web neck, and cubitus valgus deformities in boys with normal sexual genotypes. Increased risk for malignant hyperthermia with anesthetics.

D. Prader-Willi Syndrome—Chromosome 15 abnormality causing a floppy, hypotonic infant who becomes an intellectually impaired, obese adult with an insatiable appetite. Growth retardation, hip dysplasia, hypoplastic genitalia, and scoliosis are common.

E. Menkes' Syndrome—X-linked recessive disorder of copper transport affecting bone growth and causing characteristic "kinky" hair. May be differentiated from occipital horn syndrome (which also affects copper transport) by the characteristic bony projections from the occiput of the skull in that disorder.

F. Rett's Syndrome—Progressive impairment and stereotaxic abnormal hand movements characterizes this disorder. It is seen in girls at 6–12 months of age who present with developmental delay much like cerebral palsy. Affected children typically have scoliosis with a C-shaped curve and spasticity. Affected boys have an X chromosome locus.

G. Teratogens
   1. Fetal Alcohol Syndrome—Maternal alcoholism can cause growth disturbances, CNS dysfunction, dysmorphic facies, hip dislocation, C-spine vertebral and upper extremity fusions, congenital scoliosis, and myelodysplasia.
   2. Maternal Diabetes—May lead to heart defects, sacral agenesis and anencephaly. Careful management of pregnant diabetics is essential.
   3. Other teratogens, including drugs (e.g., aminopterin, phenytoin, thalidomide), trace metals, maternal conditions, infections, and intrauterine factors, may also lead to orthopaedic manifestations in affected children.

IV. Hematopoietic Disorders

A. Gaucher's Disease—Aberrant autosomal recessive lysosomal storage disease (also known as familial splenic anemia) characterized by accumulation of cerebroside in cells of the reticuloendothelial system (RES). Commonly seen in children of Jewish descent, it is associated with osteopenia, metaphyseal enlargement (failure of remodeling), femoral head necrosis (head-within-head deformity) moth-eaten trabeculae, patchy sclerosis, and "Er-

lenmeyer flask" distal femora. Affected patients may complain of bone pain, and occasionally experience a "bone crisis" (similar to sickle cell anemia). Bleeding abnormalities are also common. Histologic exam demonstrates characteristic lipid-laden histiocytes. Treatment is basically supportive; new enzyme therapies may be beneficial in the future.

B. Niemann-Pick Disease—Caused by accumulation of phospholipid in RES cells. Seen commonly in Eastern European Jews. Marrow expansion and cortical thinning are common in long bones; coxa valga is also seen.

C. Sickle Cell Anemia—Sickle cell disease (affects 1% of blacks) is more severe but less common than sickle cell trait (8% prevalence). Crises usually begin at age 2–3 and may lead to characteristic bone infarctions. Growth retardation/skeletal immaturity; osteonecrosis of femoral and humeral heads; osteomyelitis (often in diaphysis); septic arthritis (probably best treated with a third-generation cephalosporin; some studies have demonstrated *Salmonella* to be the most common organism); and dactylitis (acute hand/foot swelling) are all common. Aspiration and culture are necessary to differentiate infarction from osteomyelitis. Radiographs commonly show osteoporosis and cortical thinning. Preoperative oxygenation and exchange transfusion are helpful for affected patients requiring surgery.

D. Thalassemia—Similar to sickle cell anemia in presentation. More common in people of Mediterranean descent. Common symptoms include bone pain and leg ulceration. Radiographs show osteoporosis and distorted trabeculae.

E. Hemophilia—Sex-linked recessive (XR) disorder with decreased factor VIII (hemophilia A) or factor IX (hemophilia B), associated with bleeding episodes and skeletal/joint sequelae. Can be mild (5–25% of factor present), moderate (1–5% available), or marked (<1% of factor present). Hemarthrosis presents with painful swelling and decreased range of motion of affected joints. Deep intramuscular bleeding is also common and can lead to the formation of a pseudotumor (blood cyst), which can occur in soft tissue or bone. Ultrasound can help to diagnose bleeding into muscles (most commonly in the lower extremity). Intramuscular hematomas can lead to compression of adjacent nerves (e.g., an iliacus hematoma may cause a femoral nerve paralysis, and may mimic a bleed into the hip joint). Factor levels should be elevated to at least 25% following major bleeding episodes. Radiographic findings in hemophilia include squaring of the patellas and condyles and generalized osteoporosis. Cartilage atrophy from enzymatic matrix degeneration is frequent. Therapy includes fracture management, contracture release, osteotomies, synovectomy (prevents recurrent hemarthrosis; radiation synovectomy is sometimes done), and total joint arthroplasty. Mild to moderate hemophilia A can be treated with desmopressin (DDAVP). Factor VIII levels should approach 100% before surgery and should be maintained at >50% for 1 week postoperatively. Tourniquets can be used, vessels should be ligated rather than cauterized, and rigid fixation of fractures will decrease postoperative bleeding. **Antibody inhibitors** are present in 4–20% of hemophiliacs and **are a relative contraindication to surgery**. Large levels of factor VIII or Autoplex (activated prothrombin) are required to offset these inhibitors. Because of the amount of blood component therapy required in the treatment of this disorder, a large percentage of hemophiliacs are HIV positive. The incidence of this in the older hemophiliac population (before donor screening and newer component treatment) approaches 100%.

F. Leukemia—The most common malignancy of childhood. Causes demineralization of bones and septic arthritic and occasional lytic lesions. Radiolucent "leukemia" lines may be seen in the metaphyses of affected bones in older children. Management of leukemia includes chemotherapy.

G. Acquired Immunodeficiency Syndrome (AIDS)—Caused by HIV. Children born with AIDS are becoming more common in neonatal units, and supportive care is indicated. Protection for surgeons with patients at risk (IV drug abusers, homosexuals, hemophiliacs, etc.) is essential (see Chapter 2, Basic Sciences, Part 7: Orthopaedic Infections).

V. Metabolic Disease/Arthritides (see also Chapter 2, Basic Sciences)

A. Rickets (Osteomalacia in adult)—Decrease in calcium ± phosphorus affecting mineralization at the epiphyses of long bones. Classically, brittle bones with **physeal cupping/widening**, bowing of long bones, transverse radiolucent (Looser's) lines, ligamentous laxity, flattening of the skull, enlargement of costal cartilages (rachitic rosary), and dorsal kyphosis (cat back) characterize this disorder. There are several varieties of rickets based on the underlying abnormality (GI, kidney, diet, end organ, etc.). This is discussed in detail in Chapter 2, Basic Sciences. Histologically, **widened osteoid seams** and "Swiss cheese" trabeculae are characteristic in bone; at the growth plate there is gross distortion of the maturation zone (enlarged and distorted) and a poorly defined zone of provisional calcification.

B. Osteogenesis Imperfecta—Defect in collagen (procollagen to type I collagen sequence and abnormal cross-linking) leading to decreased collagen secretion, bone fragility (brittle "wormian" bone), short stature, scoliosis, tooth defects, hearing defects, and ligamentous laxity. Four types have been identified (Sillence), although the disorder is probably best considered as a continuum with different inheritance patterns and severity.

Type	Inher	Sclerae	Features
I	AD	Blue	Preschool age (tarda), hearing loss (A = teeth involved, B = teeth not affected)
II	AR	Blue	Lethal; concertina femur, beaded ribs
III	AR	Nl	Fractures at birth; progressive, short stature
IV	AD	Nl	Milder form, normal hearing (A = teeth involved, B = teeth not affected)

Histologically, increased diameter of haversian canals and osteocyte lacunae, increased numbers of cells, and replicated cement lines are seen. Fractures are common and initial healing is normal, but bone typically does not remodel. Spinal deformities, including scoliosis (50%, bracing ineffective, fuse at 50 degrees), and compression fractures occur. Goal in treatment is fracture management and long-term rehabilitation. Bracing is indicated for most problems. Sofield osteotomies ("shish kebab" bone with telescoping intramedullary rods) are sometimes required.

C. Idiopathic Juvenile Osteoporosis—A rare, self-limited disorder that appears at ages 8–14 with osteopenia, growth arrest, and bone and joint pain. Serum calcium and phosphorous levels are normal. Typically, there is spontaneous resolution 2–4 years after onset of puberty. One must differentiate this disorder from other causes of osteopenia (e.g., osteogenesis imperfecta, malignancy, and Cushing's disease).

D. Osteopetrosis—Failure of osteoclastic and chondroclastic resorption, probably secondary to a defect in the thymus leading to dense bone, "rugger jersey" spine, marble bone, and "Erlenmeyer flask" proximal humerus/distal femur. Milder form is autosomal dominant, "malignant" form is autosomal recessive. Bone marrow transplant may be helpful in treatment of the malignant form (see Chapter 2, Basic Sciences).

E. Infantile Cortical Hyperostosis (Caffey's disease)—Soft tissue swelling and bony cortical thickening (esp. jaw and ulna) that follows a febrile illness in 0–9-week-old. Radiographs show characteristic periosteal reaction. This disorder may be differentiated from trauma (and child abuse) based on single bone involvement in the latter. A similar presentation may occur in older children (>6 months) with hypervitaminosis A. Caffey's disease, however, does not have bleeding gums, fissures at the corners of the mouth, and liver enzyme abnormalities associated with hypervitaminosis A. Infection, scurvy, and progressive diaphyseal dysplasia may also be in the differential diagnosis for all-age children.

F. Connective Tissue Syndromes—A heterogeneous group of disorders with a broad spectrum of features; however, several generalizations may be made.

1. Marfan's Syndrome—AD disorder of collagen synthesis (possibly the α_1 subunit) associated with arachnodactyly, long slender "seida" fingers, pectus deformities, scoliosis, cardiac (valvular) abnormalities, and ocular findings (superior lens dislocation). Other abnormalities may include dural ectasia and meningocele. Joint laxity is treated conservatively; scoliosis and spondylolisthesis are treated aggressively. Protrusio acetabuli can be treated with early triradiate cartilage fusion.

2. Ehlers-Danlos Syndrome—AD disorder with hyperextensibility of "cigarette paper" skin, joint hypermobility and dislocation, soft tissue/bony fragility, and soft tissue calcification. Failure of other supporting connective tissue can lead to vascular and visceral tears as well. Types II and III (of XI) are most common and least

disabling. Treatment consists of physical therapy, orthotics, and arthrodesis (soft tissue procedures fail).

3. Homocystinuria—AR inborn error of methionine metabolism (decreased enzyme cystathionine β-synthase). Accumulation of the intermediate metabolite homocysteine in the production of the amino acid cysteine can lead to osteoporosis, a marfanoid-like habitus (but with stiff joints), and inferior lens dislocation. Diagnosis is made by demonstrating increased homocystine in urine (cyanide-nitroprusside test). This disorder is differentiated from Marfan's syndrome based on the direction of lens dislocation and the presence of osteoporosis in homocystinuria. Spontaneous thrombotic episodes can be initiated by minor procedures, anesthesia, and surgery. CNS effects including mental retardation and seizures are also common in this disorder. Early treatment with vitamin B$_6$ and a decreased methionine diet is often successful.

G. Juvenile Rheumatoid Arthritis (JRA)—Persistent noninfectious arthritis lasting more than 6 weeks to 3 months after other possible etiologies have been ruled out. In order to confirm the diagnosis one of the following is required: rash, presence of rheumatoid factor, iridocyclitis, cervical spine involvement, pericarditis, tenosynovitis, intermittent fever, or morning stiffness. JRA affects girls more than boys and commonly involves the wrist (flexed and ulnar deviated) and hand (fingers extended, swollen, and radially deviated). Cervical spine involvement can lead to kyphosis, facet ankylosis, and atlantoaxial subluxation. Lower extremity problems include flexion contractures (hip and knee flexed, ankle dorsiflexed), subluxation, and other deformities (hip protrusio, valgus knees, and equinovarus feet). Five types of JRA are usually identified (Schaller) (see Table 1–3). Synovial proliferation leads to joint destruction (chondrolysis) and soft tissue destruction. Radiographs can show rarefaction of juxta-articular bone. Therapy includes night splinting, salicylates, and, rarely, synovectomy (for chronic swelling refractory to medical management). Arthrodesis and arthroplasty may be required for severe JRA.

H. Ankylosing Spondylitis—Typically affects adolescent males with asymmetric lower extremity large joint arthritis and heel pain ± eye symptoms; hip and back pain may develop later. Diagnosis is confirmed with HLA-B27 antigen test, and radiographs showing bilateral and symmetric sacroiliac erosion and late vertebral changes. Control of back muscle spasms, NSAIDs, and physical therapy are the mainstays of treatment.

I. Acute Rheumatic Fever—Autoimmune process affecting children 5–15 yo that follows an untreated streptococcal infection by 2–4 weeks. Can present with migratory arthritis, fever, carditis, subcutaneous nodules, and **erythema marginatum** (pink rash on trunk and extremities but not face, ± history of strep infection). The Jones criteria are used for diagnosis (see Chapter 2, Basic Sciences). Treatment includes salicylates and appropriate antibiotics.

VI. Birth Injuries

A. Brachial Plexus Palsy—Decreasing in severity as a result of better obstetric management, but still 2:1000 births have injury associated with stretching or contusion of the brachial plexus. Occurs more commonly with larger babies, shoulder dystocia, forceps delivery, breech position, and prolonged labor. Three types are commonly recognized:

Type	Roots	Deficit	Prognosis
Erb-Duchenne	C5,6	Deltoid, cuff, elbow flexors, wrist & hand dorsiflexors; "waiter's tip" deformity	Best
Total Plexus	C5–T1	Sensory and motor; flaccid arm	Worst
Klumpke	C8–T1	Wrist flexors, intrinsics; Horner	Poor

The key to therapy is maintaining passive range of motion and awaiting return of motor function (up to 18 months). Up to 90 + % will eventually resolve without intervention. However, **lack of biceps function 3 months after injury** carries a poor prognosis and **is an indication for surgery** (nerve grafting). Late surgery (4 yo) is required to obtain functional motion. Options include releasing contractures (Fairbanks), latissimus and teres major transfer to the shoulder external rotators (L'Episcopo), tendon transfers for elbow flexion (Clarke's pectoral transfer and Steindler's flexorplasty), proximal humerus rotational osteotomy (Wickstrom), and microsurgery (grafting or possibly intercostal transfer).

B. Torticollis—Congenital deformity resulting from contracture of the sternocleidomastoid muscle and associated with other "molding disorders" such as

TABLE 1–3. TYPES OF JUVENILE RHEUMATOID ARTHRITIS

Type	%	Joints	ANA[a]	RF[b]	Systemic Sx	Progress
Systemic—Still's	25	Many	–	–	Fever, rash, organomegaly	25%
Polyarticular/RF –	15	Many	1/3	–	Mild fever	30%
Polyarticular/RF +	15	Many	1/3	+	Mild	25%
Pauciarticular I (F)	30	Large	+	–	Iridocyclitis[c]	15%
Pauciarticular II (M)	15	Large	–	–	HLA-B27 +, spondylitis	15%

[a] Antinuclear antibodies.
[b] Rheumatoid factor
[c] Slit lamp exam is important to identify iridocyclitis, which is seen early in the pauciarticular form.

hip dysplasia and metatarsus adductus (up to 20% association with hip dysplasia). Differential diagnosis includes cervical spine anomalies and ophthalmologic disorders that may require the child to tilt their head to see normally. Birth trauma, occlusion of venous flow, or a hematoma results in fibrosis of the muscle and a palpable mass noted within the first 4 weeks of life. Most (90%) will respond to passive stretching within the first year. Surgery (resection of the distal fibers of the muscle) may be required if torticollis persists beyond the first year. Torticollis may also be associated with congenital atlanto-occipital abnormalities.

C. Congenital Pseudarthrosis of the Clavicle—May be confused with a fracture of the clavicle but involves the middle third of the right clavicle, does not have associated fracture callus, and is nonpainful at birth. Surgical repair should be considered for pain and sometimes cosmesis.

VII. Cerebral Palsy (CP)

A. Introduction—Nonprogressive neuromuscular disorder with onset before 2 yo resulting from injury to the immature brain. Etiology includes perinatal infections (TORCH), prematurity (most common), anoxic injuries, head injuries, and meningitis. Children may present with numerous orthopaedic problems. Commonly, immobility leads to joint contractures that, if uncorrected, can progress to cartilage deformity and joint dysplasia.

B. Classification—CP can be classified based on physiology (according to the movement disorder) or topography (according to geographic distribution).

1. Physiologic Classification
   a. Spasticity—Characterized by increased muscle tone and hyperreflexia, with slow, restricted movements (because of co-contraction of agonist and antagonists). This form of CP is the most common and is most amenable to operative intervention.
   b. Athetosis—Characterized by constant succession of slow, writhing, involuntary movements, this form of CP is less common and more difficult to treat.
   c. Ataxia—Characterized by an inability to coordinate muscles for voluntary movement, resulting in an unbalanced, wide-based gait. Also less amenable to orthopaedic treatment.
   d. Mixed—Typically involves a combination of spasticity and athetosis with total body involvement.

2. Topographic Classification
   a. Hemiplegia—Involves the upper and lower extremity on the same side, usually with spasticity. These children often develop early "handedness." All children with hemiplegia will be able to walk, regardless of treatment.
   b. Diplegia—Patients have more extensive involvement of the lower extremity than the upper extremity. Most diplegics will eventually walk. IQ may be normal, strabismus is common.
   c. Totally involved—These children have extensive involvement, low IQ, and high mortality and are usually nonambulators.

C. Orthopaedic Assessment—Based on thorough birth and developmental history taking, and examination. A patient's locomotor profile is based on the persistence of primitive reflexes; the presence of two or more usually means the child will be a nonambulator. Commonly tested reflexes include Moro (startle) and parachute reflexes, which normally disappear at 4–5 months of age. Surgery is best reserved for the child over 3 yo with spastic CP, good intelligence, and voluntary motor control. Muscle imbalance yields later bony changes; therefore, the general surgical plan is to perform soft tissue procedures early and, if necessary, bony procedures later. Selective dorsal root rhizotomy is a neurosurgical procedure that is gaining enthusiasm in the treatment of CP. This treatment, indicated only for spastic CP, includes resection of dorsal rootlets not exhibiting a myographic or clinical response upon stimulation. It may help reduce spasticity and complement orthopaedic management of this type of CP. Discussion of specific disorders follows. Discussion of hand disorders is included in Chapter 5, Hand.

D. Gait disorders—Probably the most common problem seen by the orthopaedist. In diplegics, gait is typically characterized by a crouched gait, toe walking, and flexed knees. Hemiplegics usually present with toe walking only. Dynamic EMGs and motion lab analysis can often be helpful (and may become essential). Lengthening of continuously active muscles and transfer of muscles out of phase is often helpful. Timing and indications for surgeries require experience and skill because surgeries often should be done in tandem to best correct the problem (e.g., often heel cord lengthening alone may exacerbate a crouched gait). In general, surgery is typically accomplished in the 4–5-yo age group, and a few generalized guidelines are given in Table 1–4.

E. Spinal disorders—Most commonly involve scoliosis, which can be severe, especially with a spastic quadriplegic, and is associated with increased pseudoarthrosis if treated with conventional therapy. Treatment is tailored to the needs of the patient. Custom-molded seat inserts allow better positioning but do not prevent curve progression. Anterior and posterior fusion or segmental instrumentation is favored in patients who can no longer sit properly. Fusion to the sacrum is required with a fixed pelvic obliquity (e.g., with Luque rods to the pelvis—Galveston technique). Kyphosis is also common and may require fusion and instrumentation.

F. Hip subluxation/dislocation—Spastic hip usually requires both a bony and a soft tissue procedure; both hips are done with soft tissue procedures. Characterized by four stages:

1. Hip at Risk—This is the only exception to the general rule of avoiding surgery in CP the first 3 years of life. Abduction <45 degrees with partial uncovering of the normal head on radiographs. May benefit from adductor release ± neurectomy of anterior branch of obturator nerve.

2. Hip Subluxation—Best treated with adductor tenotomy in children with abduction of <20 degrees ± psoas release/recession. Femoral or pel-

TABLE 1–4. SURGICAL OPTIONS FOR GAIT DISORDERS

PROBLEM	DIAGNOSIS	SURGICAL OPTIONS
Hip flexion	Contraction (Thomas)	Psoas tenotomy or recession
Spastic hip	Decreased abduction/ uncovered head	Adductor release, osteotomy (late)
Hip adduction	Scissoring gait	Adductor release
Femoral anteversion	Prone internal rotation decreased	Osteotomy, VDRO, Hamstring lengthening
Knee flexion	Contraction, increased popliteal angle	Hamstring lengthening, rectus transfer
Knee hypertension	Recurvatum	Rectus femoris lengthening
Stiff leg gait	EMG—hamstring, quadriceps continuous, passive knee flexion decreased with hip extension	Distal rectus transfer to hamstrings
Talipes equinus	Toe walking	Achilles lengthening, Achilles transfer
Talipes varus	Standing position	Split ant. or post. tibialis transfer (based on EMG findings)
Talipes valgus	Standing position	Peroneal lengthening, Grice subtalar fusion
Hallux valgus	Exam/radiographs	Osteotomy, MTP fusion

vic osteotomies may be considered for later cases with femoral anteversion or acetabular dysplasia.

3. Spastic Dislocation—Acute dislocations (rare) may benefit from open reduction, femoral shortening, varus derotation osteotomy, and Chiari osteotomy. Late dislocations may best be left out or treated with a Shanz abduction osteotomy. Varus derotational osteotomies are often successful, usually in 8–10-year-olds with femoral anteversion and hip dislocation/subluxation.

4. Windswept hips—Characterized by abduction of one hip and adduction of the contralateral hip. Treatment is best directed at attempting to abduct the adducted hip with bracing or tenotomies. Associated scoliosis is treated similarly to idiopathic scoliosis.

G. Knee Abnormalities—Usually includes flexion contractures and decreased range of motion. Hamstring lengthening is often helpful (may sometimes increase lumbar lordosis). Rectus transfer (to the gracilis) allows better knee function and foot clearance in the swing phase of gait.

H. Foot and Ankle Abnormalities—Common in CP, and gait and dynamic electromyographic evaluation is often helpful.

1. Equinovalgus foot—More common in spastic diplegia. Caused by spastic peroneals, contracted heel cords, and ligamentous laxity. Peroneus brevis lengthening is often helpful to cor-

rect moderate valgus. Subtalar arthrodesis is reserved for severe valgus deformities.

2. Equinovarus foot—More common in spastic hemiplegia, and is caused by overpull of the posterior and/or anterior tibialis tendons. Lengthening of the posterior tibialis is rarely indicated because of recurrence and development of a calcaneovalgus foot. Likewise, transfer of an entire muscle (posterior or anterior tibialis) is rarely recommended. **Split muscle transfers are helpful**, however, in certain circumstances, especially **when the affected muscle is spastic in both stance and swing phases** of gait. The split posterior tibialis transfer (rerouting half of the tendon dorsally to the peroneus brevis) is used in cases with spasticity of the muscle, flexible varus foot, and weak peroneals. Complications include decreased foot dorsiflexion. Split anterior tibialis transfer (rerouting half of its tendon posteriorly to the cuboid) is used in patients with spasticity of the muscle and a flexible varus deformity. Complications of this procedure include overcorrection. Most recently, combined split anterior tibial tendon transfer and intramuscular lengthening of the posterior tibial tendon (Barnes and Herring) has been recommended for dynamic varus of the hindfoot and adduction of the forefoot in both stance and swing phases of gait.

VIII. Neuromuscular Disorders

A. Arthrogrypotic Syndromes

1. Arthrogryposis Multiplex Congenita (Amyoplasia)—Nonprogressive disorder of multiple etiologies with multiple congenitally rigid joints, believed to be caused by oliogohydramnios and any condition limiting fetal movement. This disorder, which can be myopathic, neuropathic, or mixed, is associated with loss of anterior horn cells and other neural elements in the spinal cord, possibly secondary to an in utero viral infection. Evaluation should include neurologic studies, enzyme tests, and muscle biopsy (at 3–4 months). Affected patients typically have normal facies, normal intelligence, multiple joint contractures, and no visceral abnormalities. Upper extremity involvement usually includes adduction and internal rotation of the humerus, elbow extension and wrist flexion, and ulnar deviation. In the lower extremity, rigid clubfeet, hip dislocation, and knee contractures are common. The spine may be involved with characteristic "C-shaped" (neuromuscular) scoliosis. Fractures are also common (25%). Treatment includes soft tissue releases (especially hamstrings), open reduction of unilateral hip dislocation, aggressive surgical treatment of clubfeet (often requiring talectomy), and attempts at achieving ambulation. Knee contractures should be corrected before hip reduction in order to maintain reduction. Upper extremity treatment consists of passive stretching, serial casts for elbow contractures, and possibly osteotomies after 4 years of age to allow independent eating.

2. Larsen's Syndrome—Similar to arthrogryposis in clinical appearance, but joints are less

rigid. The disorder primarily is associated with multiple joint dislocations (including bilateral congenital knee dislocations), abnormal (flattened) facies, scoliosis, and cervical kyphosis.

3. Distal Arthrogryposis Syndrome—Autosomal dominant disorder that predominately affects the hands and feet. Ulnarly deviated fingers (at MCP joints), MCP and PIP flexion contractures, and adducted thumbs with web space thickening are common. Clubfeet and vertical talus are common in the feet.

4. Multiple Pterygium Syndrome—Autosomal recessive disorder characterized by cutaneous flexor surface webs, congenital vertical talus, and scoliosis.

B. Myelodysplasia

1. Introduction—Disorder of spinal cord development/closure or secondary rupture of developing cord secondary to hydrocephalus (two theories are proposed for etiology). Includes spina bifida occulta (defect in vertebral arch with confined cord and meninges); meningocele (sac without neural elements protruding through defect); myelomeningocele (spina bifida) (with protrusion of sac with neural elements); and rachischisis (neural elements exposed without any covering). Can be diagnosed in utero (increased α-fetoprotein), with high-risk infant (usually with a positive family history). Muscle imbalance and intrauterine positioning frequently lead to hip dislocations, knee hyperextension, and clubfeet. Function is primarily related to level of the defect and other associated congenital abnormalities. **Sudden changes in function (rapid increase of scoliotic curvature, spasticity, and new neurologic deficit) can be associated with tethered cord, hydrocephalus (most common), and hydromyelia** (increased fluid in the central canal of cord), among other defects. Head CT (70% of myelodysplastics have hydrocephalus) and myelogram or spinal MRI are required. **Fractures are also common in myelodysplasia,** most often about the knee and hip in the 3–7-yo age group, and frequently can only be diagnosed by noting **redness, warmth, and swelling.** Treatment is conservative (avoid disuse). Fractures usually heal with abundant callus. Myelodysplasia level is based on the lowest functioning level. L4 is a key level because quadriceps can function and allow community ambulation.

2. Treatment principles—Careful observation of patients with myelodysplasia is important.

Several myelodysplasia "milestones" have been developed to asses their progress:

Age	Function	Treatment
4–6 mo	Head control	Positioning
6–10 mo	Sitting	Supports/orthotics
10–12 mo	Prone mobility	Prone board
12–15 mo	Upright stance	Standing orthosis
15–18 mo	Upright mobility	Trunk/extremity orthosis

Treatment utilizes a team approach to allow maximum function consistent with the patient's level and other abnormalities and as normal a development as possible. Proper use of orthotics is essential in myelodysplasia. Determination of ambulation potential is based on the level of the deficit. Surgery in myelodysplasia focuses on balancing of muscles and correction of deformities. Myelodysplasia levels are important to recognize (Table 1–5).

3. Hip Problems—Hip dislocation occurs frequently in myelodysplastics because of paralysis of the abductors and extensors with unopposed hip flexors and abductors. **Hip dislocation is most common at the L3–L4 level.** Treatment of hip dislocation is controversial, but in general, containment is only essential in patients with functioning quadriceps. The aim of hip surgery is to maintain range of motion and achieve full hip extension. Containment is a secondary concern. Treatment of hip dislocation is based on level of defect: if L2 or higher, leave both hips symmetric; if L4 or lower (and neurologically stable), reduce hips and perform a varus or Pemberton osteotomy to avoid future leg length discrepancy or pelvic obliquity. The role for posterior iliopsoas muscle transfer has not been well established.

4. Knee Problems—Usually includes quadriceps weakness (usually treated with KAFOs). Flexion deformities (associated with hip flexion deformities, calcaneovalgus feet, and tethered cord) are not important in wheelchair-bound patients but can be treated with hamstring release and posterior capsular release. Recurvatum (associated with clubfeet and hip dislocation) is rarely a problem and can be treated early with serial casting and KAFOs. Tenotomies (quadriceps lengthening) are sometimes required. Valgus deformities are usually not a problem. Sometimes, iliotibial band release or late osteotomies may be needed.

TABLE 1–5. CHARACTERISTICS OF MYELODYSPLASIA LEVELS

Level	Hip	Knee	Feet	Orthosis	Ambulation
L1	External rotation/flexed	—	Equinovarus	HKAFO	Nonfunctional
L2	Adduction/flexed	Flexed	Equinovarus	HKAFO	Nonfunctional
L3	Adduction/flexed	Recurvatum	Equinovarus	KAFO	Household
L4	Adduction/flexed	Extended	Cavovarus	AFO	Household +
L5	Flexed	Limited flexion	Calcaneal valgus	AFO	Community
S1			Foot deformities	Shoes	Near normal

5. Ankle and Foot Deformities—Affected patients may present with a valgus foot. Total-contact AFOs often are helpful, but clubfoot release, tendon release (posterior tibialis, anterior tibialis, Achilles), and other procedures may be required. Triple arthrodesis should be avoided in most myelodysplastics and is used only for severe deformities with sensate feet. Ankle valgus (resulting from a disparity in fibular versus tibial growth) is addressed by tibial osteotomy or hemiephysiodesis (older patients) if the fibula is shortened, or Achilles tendon tenodesis to the fibula (younger patients). For severe rotational deformities distal tibia osteotomy may be required, but is associated with a high complication rate. Subtalar angular deformities may be corrected with fusion, and calcaneus deformity by an anterolateral release. Subtalar procedures in general should be avoided and AP radiographs of the ankle should be carefully reviewed to rule out more common involvement of this joint.
6. Spine Problems—Scoliosis can result from the spine disorder itself (and is treated like congenital scoliosis) or may be paralytic in nature. Attempts at bracing (TLSO) may fail and require subcutaneous rodding for very young children and fusion later. **Rapid curve progression** can be associated with hydrocephalus or a **tethered cord**, which may manifest as lower extremity spasticity (MRI is helpful in evaluation of these children). Segmental Luque sublaminar wiring with fixation to the pelvis (Galveston technique) or to the front of the sacrum (Dunn technique), usually preceded by anterior release and fusion, is often required in curves >60 degrees. Kyphosis in myelodysplasia is an extremely difficult problem. Resection of the kyphosis with local fusion (Lindseth) or fusion to the pelvis is required in some cases. This should be delayed as long as possible to prevent recurrence.
7. Pelvic obliquity can occur in myelodysplasia as a result of prolonged unilateral hip contractures or scoliosis. Custom seat cushions, TLSO, spinal fusion, and ultimately, pelvic osteotomies may be required for treatment.

C. Myopathies (Muscular Dystrophies)—Noninflammatory inherited disorders with progressive muscle weakness. Treatment focuses on physical therapy, orthotics, genetic counseling, and surgery for severe problems (includes tibialis posterior transfers, release of flexion contractures, and early fusion for neuromuscular scoliosis). Fusion (often T2–sacrum) should be done earlier than in idiopathic scoliosis (often at 25 degrees of curvature) before pulmonary status deteriorates. Several types of muscular dystrophy are classified based on their inheritance pattern:

1. **Duchenne's**—Sex-linked recessive abnormality of young males with clumsy walking, decreased motor skills, lumbar lordosis, calf pseudohypertrophy, +Gowers (rises by walking the hands up the legs to compensate for gluteus maximus and quadriceps weakness), and **markedly elevated CPK**. Hip extensors are typically the first muscle group affected.

Muscle biopsy shows foci of necrosis and connective tissue infiltration. Treatment is based on keeping the patient ambulatory as long as possible. KAFO bracing and release of contractures are important. These children usually die of cardiorespiratory complications before age 20. Differential diagnosis includes **Becker's** dystrophy (also sex-linked recessive) often seen in a 7-yo, red-green color blind male with a similar picture but less severe.
2. **Fascioscapulohumeral**—Autosomal dominant disorder typically seen in a 6–20-yo with facial muscle abnormalities, normal CPK, and winging of the scapula (stabilize with scapulathoracic fusion).
3. **Limb-Girdle**—Autosomal recessive disorder (10–30-yo with pelvic or shoulder girdle involvement and decreased CPK values).
4. Other—**Gower's** (distal involvement, high incidence in Sweden); **ocular, occulopharyngeal** (high incidence in French-Canadians).

D. Myotonic Myopathies—AD disorders with inability of muscles to relax after contractures. Three basic types:
1. Myotonia Congenita (Thomsen's)—widespread involvement, no weakness, increased hypertrophy.
2. Dystrophic Myotonia (Steinert's)—small gonads, heart disease, low IQ, distal/lower extremity involvement, "dive bomber" EMG.
3. Paramyotonia Congenita (Eulenburg's)—symptoms develop with exposure to cold, especially in the hands (symptoms often respond to quinine therapy).

E. Congenital Myopathies—Nonprogressive AD disorders that present as a "floppy baby." Hypotonia is predominately in the pelvic and shoulder girdles. Muscle biopsy histochemical analysis required for differentiation of four types.

F. Polymyositis, Dermatomyositis—characterized by a febrile illness that may be acute or insidious. Females predominate and typically have photosensitivity, increased CPK and ESR values. Muscles are tender, brawny, and indurated. Biopsy demonstrates the pathognomonic inflammatory response.

G. Hereditary Neuropathies—Disorders that are associated with multiple CNS lesions include the following:
1. Friedreich's Ataxia—Spinal cerebellar degenerative disease with onset before 10 yo. Presents with staggering, wide-based gait, cavus foot (treated with plantar release ± metatarsal and calcaneal osteotomies early, and triple arthrodesis late), and scoliosis (treated much like idiopathic scoliosis but patients may not tolerate bracing). **Involves motor and sensory defects**.
2. Charcot-Marie-Tooth Disease (Peroneal Muscular Atrophy)—Autosomal dominant motor-sensory demyelinating neuropathy. Two forms are described, a hypertrophic form with onset in the second decade of life, and a neuronal form with onset in the third or fourth decade, but with more extensive foot involvement. Cavus feet (often requiring posterior tibialis

tendon transfer early and triple arthrodesis for fixed deformities) and progressive lower extremity weakness and atrophy ("stork legs") are common. Decreased motor nerve conduction velocities are helpful in making the diagnosis. **Involves motor defects only**.

3. Déjérine-Sottas Disease—Autosomal recessive hypertrophic neuropathy of infancy. Delayed ambulation, pes cavus foot, foot drop, stocking glove dysesthesia, and spinal deformities are common.

4. Riley-Day Syndrome (Dysautonomia)—One of five inherited (AR) sensory and autonomic neuropathies. This disease is found only in patients of Ashkenazic Jewish ancestry. Clinical presentation includes dysphagia, alacrima, pneumonia, excessive sweating, postural hypotension, and sensory loss.

H. Myasthenia Gravis—Chronic disease with insidious development of easy muscle fatigability caused by competitive inhibition of acetylcholine receptors at motor end plate. Treatment consists of an acetylcholinesterase or thymectomy.

I. Anterior Horn Cell Disorders

1. Poliomyelitis—Viral destruction of anterior horn cells in the spinal cord and brain stem motor nuclei; has all but disappeared in the U.S. after vaccine was developed. Many surgical procedures still used were developed for treatment of polio. The hallmark of polio is muscle weakness with normal sensation.

2. Spinal Muscle Atrophy (Werdnig-Hoffmann Disease)—Autosomal recessive loss of anterior horn cells from the spinal cord. Often associated with a progressive scoliosis that is best treated surgically before curves reach 50 degrees. Patients have symmetric paresis with more involvement of the lower extremity and proximal muscles. Four types of spinal muscle atrophy (Table 1–6) are commonly recognized (Evans and Drennan) but it probably represents a spectrum of a single disease.

J. Acute Idiopathic Postinfectious Polyneuropathy **(Guillain-Barré Syndrome)**—Symmetric ascending motor paresis caused by demyelination following viral infection. **CSF protein typically elevated**. Usually self-limited, better prognosis with acute form.

K. Overgrowth Syndromes

1. Proteus Syndrome—Overgrowth of hands and feet with bizarre facial disfigurement, scoliosis, genu valgum, hemangiomas, lipomas, and nevi.

2. Klippel-Trenaunay Syndrome—Overgrowth caused by underlying AV malformations. Associated with cutaneous hemangiomas and varicosities. Severely hypertrophied extremities often require amputation.

3. Hemihypertrophy—Can be caused by various syndromes, but most are idiopathic. This disorder is often associated with renal abnormalities (esp. Wilms' tumor). Management of associated leg length discrepancy is discussed below.

IX. Pediatric Spine

A. Idiopathic Scoliosis

1. Introduction—Lateral deviation and rotation of the spine without an identifiable cause, but may be related to a proprioception disorder. Most patients have a positive family history, but there is variable expressivity. The curve description is characterized by its apex. Right thoracic curves, with apex at T7 or T8, are the most common, followed by double major (right thoracic and left lumbar), left lumbar, and right lumbar curves, in that order. In adolescents, **left thoracic curves** are extremely rare, and **evaluation of the spinal cord by MRI** is suggested to rule out cord abnormalities. The adolescent form of idiopathic scoliosis is the most common, but one also sees the infantile form (left thoracic curve seen in England that may be related to supine positioning of neonates) and juvenile form (right thoracic with earlier onset than adolescent form). Curve progression is more likely with greater curve magnitudes (>20 degrees), younger age (<12 yo), and lesser Risser stage (0–1) at presentation. About 75% of immature patients with curves 20–30 degrees will progress at least 5 degrees. Severe curves (>90 degrees) may be associated with cardiopulmonary dysfunction, early death, pain, and a decreased self-image.

2. Diagnosis—Patients are often referred via school screening (benefit debated). Physical findings include shoulder or pelvic asymmetry, spinal curvature, and asymmetric rib hump (seen with forward bending). Careful neurologic examination to detect spinal cord pathology is important (especially with left thoracic curves). Standing posteroanterior radiographs are obtained and curves are measured based upon the Cobb method (measured perpendicular to end plate of most tilted [end] vertebra) (Fig. 1–6). Typically there is hypokyphosis of the apical vertebrae. Inclusion of the iliac crest

TABLE 1–6. TYPES OF SPINAL MUSCLE ATROPHY

Type	Onset	Ambulation	Scoliosis First Decade	Survival	Comments
I[a]	Birth	None	60+°	0–10 yo	Severe respiratory involvement
II	6 mos	None	50°	>35 yo	Have head control
III	1 yr	Orthotics	20°	>45 yo	Fusion for scoliosis
IV[b]	Child	Can run	Variable	>55 yo	Loose ambulation by mid-30s

[a] Werdnig-Hoffman disease.
[b] Kugelberg-Welander disease.

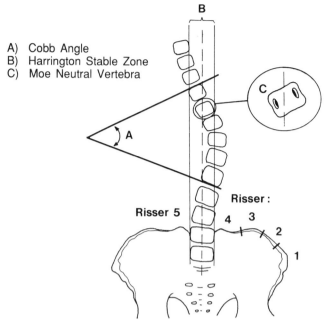

A) Cobb Angle
B) Harrington Stable Zone
C) Moe Neutral Vertebra

FIGURE 1–6. Composite illustration of measurements in idiopathic scoliosis. Note Cobb angle (*A*), Harrington's stable zone (*B*), stable vertebrae (*C*) and Risser staging.

on radiographs allows determination of skeletal maturity (based on ossification of the iliac crest apophysis and graded 0–5 [Risser stage]). A lateral radiograph to assess for spondylolisthesis is often recommended.

3. Treatment is based on the maturity of the patient (Risser stage and presence of menarche), degree of curve, and curve progression. Treatment options include observation, bracing, and surgery. Bracing only helps to halt curve progression and will not improve cosmetic appearance. The Milwaukee brace is used for some curves, but most often the TLSO is used for curves with apex below T7. Patients with thoracic lordosis or hypokyphosis are not candidates for bracing. Part-time brace wear appears to be as effective as the traditional 23-hour/day regimen. Night-time bracing (Charleston brace) is under investigation. Electrical stimulation of the convex paraspinal muscles has largely been abandoned due to lack of proven efficacy. Surgical options include instrumentation without fusion for infantile and juvenile forms of scoliosis and a variety of methods for adolescent

idiopathic scoliosis. Posterior fusion and instrumentation with Harrington distraction rods has been the gold standard. Sublaminar wiring (Luque) offers excellent fixation but carries a greater risk of neurologic injury. The Drummond technique of spinous process wiring provides improved fixation without increased risk of neurologic sequelae. Cotrel-Dobousset and TSRH implants allow for segmental fixation and rotational correction, and do not require long-term immobilization. They are expensive, however, and their superiority to standard systems remains to be demonstrated in long-term follow-up studies. Dwyer or Zielke anterior instrumentation is useful in selected lumbar or thoracolumbar curves. Anterior instrumentation may result in more correction and save lower fusion levels, but may be associated with higher pseudarthrosis rates and an uncosmetic scar. Rib resection is usually successful in patients with unacceptably prominent rib humps. The following general treatment guidelines apply:

Curve	Progression	Risser	Therapy
0–25°	—	Immature	Serial observation
25–30°	5–10°	Immature	Brace
30–40°	—	Immature	Brace
>40°	—	Immature	Surgery
>50°	—	Mature	Surgery (young adults)

4. Fusion Levels—Successful surgery is based, among other considerations, on picking appropriate fusion levels. Several methods have been developed to select correct levels. Harrington recommended fusion one level above and two levels below the end vertebrae if these levels fell within the **stable zone** (within parallel lines drawn vertically up from the lumbosacral facet joints). Moe recommends fusion to the **neutral vertebra** (without rotation—pedicles symmetric) (Fig. 1–6). It is virtually never necessary to fuse to the pelvis in adolescent idiopathic scoliosis. Cochran identified a markedly **increased incidence of late low back pain with fusion to L5,** and some increase with fusion to L4; every attempt, therefore, should be made to stop the fusion at L3 or above. King identified five patterns and treatment options (Table 1–7; Fig. 1–7).

TABLE 1–7. PATTERNS OF IDIOPATHIC SCOLIOSIS AND TREATMENT OPTIONS (AFTER KING)

Type	Definition	Flexibility (Flexion-Extension)	Treatment
I	S-shaped thoracolumbar curve, crosses midline	Lumbar < thoracic (or lumbar curve larger)	Fuse lumbar and thoracic vertebrae
II	S-shaped thoracolumbar curve, crosses midline	Lumbar > thoracic (and thoracic curve larger)	Fuse thoracic vertebrae[a]
III	Thoracic curve, lumbar vertebrae do not cross midline	Lumbar vertebrae highly flexible	Fuse thoracic vertebrae
IV	Long thoracic curve	L4 tilts to thoracic curve	Fuse through L4
V	Double thoracic curve	T1 tilts to upper curve	Fuse through T2

[a] Recent experience with lumbar curves greated than 50° suggests that large lumbar curves should be included in the fusion for rotational correction.

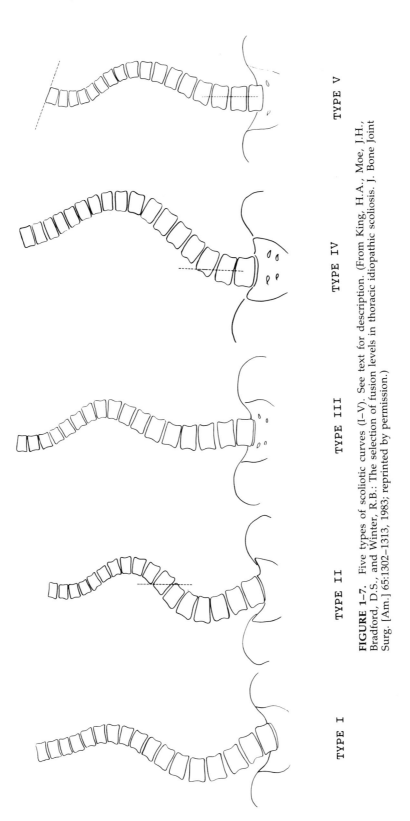

TYPE I   TYPE II   TYPE III   TYPE IV   TYPE V

FIGURE 1–7. Five types of scoliotic curves (I–V). See text for description. (From King, H.A., Moe, J.H., Bradford, D.S., and Winter, R.B.: The selection of fusion levels in thoracic idiopathic scoliosis. J. Bone Joint Surg. [Am.] 65:1302–1313, 1983; reprinted by permission.)

5. Complications—The most disastrous complication of spinal surgery is a neurologic deficit that was not present preoperatively. Successful surgical intervention is based on careful technique (intraoperative monitoring [SSEP] ± wake-up test and clonus tests are helpful). Attempting excessive correction or placement of sublaminar wires is associated with increased risk of neurologic damage. Minimizing blood loss and the use of autologous blood is important to avoid transfusion-associated problems. Surgical complications can include pseudarthrosis (1–2%), wound infection (1–2%), and implant failure (early hook cutout and late rod breakage). Late rod breakage frequently signifies a failure of fusion. An asymptomatic pseudarthrosis (no pain or loss of curve correction) should be observed only, because the results of late repair do not differ from those performed early. Use of a compression implant facilitates pseudarthrosis repair. Creation of a "flat back syndrome," or early fatiguability and pain from loss of lumbar lordosis, can be minimized with rod contouring and with effective use of compression and distraction devices. Treatment of this condition requires posterior closing wedge osteotomies and the results appear to be improved, with maintenance of correction, if anterior release and fusion precede the posterior osteotomies.

6. Infantile Idiopathic Scoliosis—Presents at age 2 months to 3 years with left-sided thoracic scoliosis, male predominance, plagiocephaly (skull flattening), and other congenital defects. Most cases have been reported from Great Britain. The rib-vertebra angle difference (RVAD) (Mehta) of the apical vertebra (>20 degrees) and overlap of the apical vertebral body and rib (Phase II) are associated with increased likelihood of progression. Treatment is as follows:

Curve	Progression	RVAD	Treatment
<25°	—	<20°	Serial observation
25–35°	10°	20–25°	Cast/brace
>35°	>10°		Neuro/MRI workup, instrumentation without fusion or combined ant. and post. fusion

7. Juvenile Idiopathic Scoliosis—Scoliosis in 3–10 year olds is similar in presentation and treatment to adolescent scoliosis. A high risk of curve progression is seen. Fusion should be delayed until the onset of the adolescent growth spurt if possible. The use of spinal instrumentation without fusion (as in infantile scoliosis) may facilitate this.

B. Neuromuscular Scoliosis—Many children with neuromuscular disorders develop scoliosis or other spinal deformities. In general, neuromuscular curves are longer, involve more vertebrae, and are less likely to have compensatory curves than in idiopathic scoliosis. Additionally, neuromuscular curves progress more rapidly and may progress after maturity. These curves may be associated with pelvic obliquity, bony deformities, and cervical involvement, again separating them from idiopathic curves. Pulmonary complications are also more frequent, including decreased pulmonary function, pneumonia, and atelectasis. Curve progression in patients who are already wheelchair bound may make them bedridden. Orthotic use is limited (best for ambulatory patients with CP and an idiopathic-type curve) and Milwaukee braces are contraindicated (pressure sores). Fusion is often required early, and frequently involves more levels than in idiopathic curves. Fusion to the pelvis may be required for fixed pelvic obliquity, and the Galveston technique of pelvic fixation (bending the caudal end of the rods from the lamina of S1 to pass into the posterosuperior iliac spine and between the tables of the ilium just anterior to the sciatic notch) appears to be beneficial. The goal of treatment is stability and balance, and curve correction is limited. Patients with upper motor neuron disease (usually CP) may be initially treated with custom seat orthotics and usually require fusion for curve progression beyond 50 degrees. Severely involved children require fusion to the sacrum and may require both anterior and posterior procedures. Posterior fusion alone is associated with increased pseudarthrosis rates and development of the "crankshaft phenomenon." Lower motor neuron disease (polio and spinal muscle atrophy) is treated with orthotics initially. Failing this, instrumentation without fusion is carried out in young children (<10 yo) with fusion reserved for older children (girls >12 and boys >14 yo). Severe curves require early correction, usually with Luque instrumentation. Myopathic disease (muscular dystrophy) often results in rapidly progressive, severe scoliosis and markedly decreased pulmonary function soon after the child is wheelchair bound. Bracing is not recommended, and fusion (with Luque instrumentation) is usually done for >25-degree curves in patients with adequate pulmonary function to allow sitting and prolong their limited lifespan. Acute curve progression or changes in neurologic status should be aggressively investigated with spinal MRI to rule out tethering of the spinal cord.

C. Congenital Spine Disorders—Due to a developmental defect in the formation of the mesenchymal anlage at the 4th–6th week of development. Three basic types of defects: **failure of segmentation** (typically results in vertebral bar), **failure of formation** (due to lack of material, may result in a hemivertebrae), and **mixed**. Tomography is helpful in defining the vertebral anomalies (Fig. 1–8). MRI of the spine should be obtained prior to any surgery to assess for intraspinal anomalies. Associated anomalies include GU (25%), cardiac (10%), and dysraphism (25%, usually diastematomyelia [cleft in spine]). Renal ultrasound is used to rule out associated kidney abnormalities.

1. Congenital Scoliosis—Most common congenital spine disorder. The worst prognosis (most likely to progress) is seen with a unilateral unsegmented bar with a contralateral hemivertebra. Best prognosis is with a block vertebra (bilateral failure of segmentation). **A unilateral unsegmented bar is a common disorder and is**

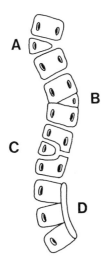

FIGURE 1–8. Composite illustration demonstrating vertebral anomalies leading to congenital scoliosis. *A,* Fully segmented hemivertebra. *B,* Unsegmented hemivertebra. *C,* Incarcerated hemivertebra. *D,* Unilateral unsegmented bar.

likely to progress. An incarcerated hemivertebra (within the lateral margins of the vertebrae above and below) has a better prognosis than an unincarcerated hemivertebra. A fully segmented hemivertebra is free with normal disc spaces on both sides, whereas an unsegmented hemivertebra is fused above and below (Fig. 1–8). **Unilateral unsegmented bars should be treated operatively at the outset;** other deformities should demonstrate progression before surgical options are considered. Bracing may be effective for compensatory curves or for smaller, supple curves above and below a vertebral anomaly, but is ineffective in controlling congenital curves. Anterior and posterior hemivertebrae excision has been reported to be associated with increased risk of neurologic deficit, but may be indicated for hemivertebrae with increasing curves and imbalance, particularly lumbosacral vertebrae. Convex anterior and posterior hemiepiphysiodesis/arthrodesis is safer, but may be less effective in correcting imbalance. Posterior fusion, either with or without instrumentation, is the mainstay of treatment for most progressive curves, but in younger patients (girls <10 and boys <12) bending or rotation of the fused spine from continued anterior spinal growth ("crankshaft phenomenon") is common and anterior/posterior fusion may be required.

2. Congenital Kyphosis—May be secondary to failure of formation (type I), failure of segmentation (type II), or mixed (type III) abnormalities, with **failure of formation (type I [which is also the most common]) having the worst prognosis** for progression (95% progress) and neurologic involvement of all spinal deformities. Type I congenital kyphosis is also the most likely to result in paraplegia (neurofibromatosis

is second). The presence of congenital kyphosis secondary to a hemivertebra is an indication for surgery. Posterior fusion is favored in young children (<5 yo) with curves less than 55 degrees; combined anterior and posterior fusion is reserved for older children or more severe curves; and anterior vertebrectomy, spinal cord decompression; and fusion followed by posterior fusion are indicated for curves involving a neurologic deficit. A type II congenital kyphosis can be observed to document progression, but progressive curves should be fused posteriorly.

D. Neurofibromatosis—Autosomal dominant disorder of neural crest cells often associated with neoplasia and skeletal abnormalities. Two of the following seven findings are necessary to establish the diagnosis:

DIAGNOSTIC CRITERIA	REQUIREMENTS
At least 6 café-au-lait spots	>5 mm (prepubital), >15 mm (mature)
Neurofibromas	2 or more (or 1 plexiform type)
Axillary/inguinal freckles	Multiple
Osseous lesion	Sphenoid dysplasia, cortical thinning
Optic glioma	Presence
Lish nodules	2 or more iris lesions by slit lamp exam
Family history	First-degree relative with neurofibromatosis

The spine is the most common site of skeletal involvement in neurofibromatosis, and careful scrutiny of radiographs for vertebral scalloping, **enlarged foramina,** penciling of the transverse processes or ribs, severe apical rotation, or a paraspinal mass may demonstrate this disorder in come cases otherwise thought to be idiopathic. Spinal deformity secondary to neurofibromatosis is characteristically kyphoscoliosis in the thoracic spine with dystrophic skeletal changes, but nondystrophic scoliosis (without kyphosis) and cervical spine deformity may be seen. Nondystrophic scoliosis is treated as appropriate for idiopathic scoliosis, but in dystrophic deformities, nonoperative treatment of any progressive curve >20 degrees is futile. Surgical treatment consists of posterior fusion with instrumentation for cases without significant kyphosis (<50 degrees), and combined anterior fusion with strut grafting and posterior fusion/instrumentation for cases with more severe kyphosis. Neurologic involvement is common in neurofibromatosis and may be caused by the deformity itself, an intraspinal tumor, a soft tissue mass, or dural ectasia. Anterior decompression and strut grafting followed by posterior fusion is required in these cases. Because of a high pseudarthrosis rate, some authors recommend routine augmentation of the posterior fusion mass at 6 months.

E. Other Spinal Abnormalities
1. Diastematomyelia—Fibrous, cartilaginous, or osseous bar creating a longitudinal cleft in the

spinal cord. Usually occurs in the lumbar spine and can lead to tethering of the cord with associated neurologic defects. Intrapedicular widening on plain radiographs is suggestive, and myelo-CT or MRI is necessary to fully define the pathology. A diastematomyelia must be resected prior to correction of a spinal deformity, but if otherwise asymptomatic and without neurologic sequelae, it may be observed.

2. Sacral Agenesis—Partial or complete absence of the sacrum and lower lumbar spine. Highly associated with maternal diabetes, it is often accompanied by GI, GU, and cardiovascular abnormalities. Clinically, children have a prominent lower L-spine and atrophic lower extremities, and may sit in a "Buddha" position. Motor impairment is at the level of the agenesis, but sensory innervation is largely spared. Management may include amputation or spinal-pelvic fusion.

F. Low Back Pain—In children, complaints of back pain and especially painful scoliosis should be taken seriously. Acute back pain can be associated with discitis (presents with refusal to move the spine or walk, increased ESR, and disc space narrowing [late]); osteomyelitis (systemic illness, leukocytosis); and occasionally herniated nucleus pulposis (HNP) (which presents as sciatica *and* back pain in older children, and may require operative intervention). Spondylolysis is common in athletic injuries, and conservative treatment is usually adequate. Painful scoliosis can often signify a tumor (especially osteoid osteoma) or spinal cord anomaly. Technetium bone scanning is an excellent screening modality in the child or adolescent with back pain. Further specificity in a still unclear clinical setting may be garnered from CT scanning (spondylolysis, HNP), or MRI (infection, HNP).

G. Kyphosis
1. Congenital Kyphosis—Discussed in Section C, Congenital Spine Disorders.
2. Scheuermann's Disease—Classic definition is increased thoracic kyphosis (>45 degrees) with **5 degrees** or more **wedging at three sequential vertebrae**. Other radiographic findings include disc narrowing, end plate irregularities, spondylolysis (30–50%), scoliosis (33%), and Schmorl's nodes (Sörenson). Scheuermann's is more common in males, and typically presents in adolescents with poor posture and occasionally aching pain. Physical examination characteristically shows hyperkyphosis that does not reverse on attempts at hyperextension, and tight hamstrings. Neurologic sequelae secondary to disc herniation or extradural spinal cysts are rare, but have been reported. Treatment consists of bracing (Milwaukee) for a progressive curve in a patient with 1 year or more of skeletal growth remaining. Bracing may effect 5–10 degrees of permanent curve correction, but is less effective for kyphosis of >74 degrees. In the skeletally mature symptomatic patient with severe kyphosis (>65 degrees) surgical correction may be indicated. Posterior fusion with compression instrumentation is the treatment of choice, preceded by anterior release and interbody fusion for curves not correcting to 55

degrees or less on hyperextension. Lumbar Scheuermann's is less common than thoracic, but may cause back pain on a mechanical basis (more common in athletes and laborers). The pain is usually self-limited. There is an increased incidence of spondylolisthesis with Scheuermann's kyphosis.

3. Postural Round Back—Also associated with kyphosis but does not have vertebral body changes. Forward bending demonstrates kyphosis but there is no sharp angulation as in Scheuermann's. Correction with backward bending and prone hyperextension is typical. Treatment includes a hyperextension exercise program. Occasionally bracing is required, but surgery is rarely indicated.

4. Other causes of Kyphosis—Include trauma, infections, spondylitis, bone dysplasias (mucopolysaccharidosis), and neoplasms. Additionally, postlaminectomy kyphosis can be severe and requires anterior and posterior fusion early. Performance of total laminectomies in immature patients without stabilization is contraindicated.

H. Cervical Spine Disorders—Many different disorders:
1. Klippel-Feil Syndrome—Multiple fused cervical segments due to a failure of normal segmentation of the cervical somites at 3–8 weeks' gestation. Often associated with congenital scoliosis, renal disease (aplasia) (33%), synkinesis (mirror motions), Sprengel's deformity, congenital heart disease, brain stem abnormalities, or congenital cervical stenosis. The classic triad of a low posterior hairline, short "web" neck, and decreased cervical range of motion is seen in less than 50% of cases. Most therapy is conservative, but chronic pain or myelopathy associated with instability may require surgical treatment. Affected children should avoid collision sports.

2. AtlantoAxial instability
   a. AP instability—Associated with Down syndrome (trisomy 21), JRA, various osteochondrodystrophies, os odontoideum, and other abnormalities. In patients with Down with a normal neurologic exam, simple avoidance of contact sports is appropriate, but with myelopathy or >10 mm of subluxation on flexion-extension films, spinal fusion is indicated (high complication rate). An Atlanto Dens Interval (ADI) of >5 mm should be treated with activity restriction in the absence of myelopathy.
   b. Rotatory Atlantoaxial subluxation—May present with torticollis; can be caused by retropharyngeal inflammation (Grisel's disease). This is probably caused by secondary ligamentous laxity and is best treated with traction and bracing early. Late diagnosis may require C1–C2 fusion. Traumatic atlantoaxial subluxation can present as torticollis. This can be treated initially with a soft collar for up to 1 week. If symptoms persist past this point, cervical traction should be initiated. If discovered late (>1 month), then fusion may be required. Rotatory atlantoaxial

subluxation can also be caused by rheumatoid arthritis, ankylosing spondylitis, Down syndrome, congenital anomalies, and cervical tumors. CT can be helpful in evaluating this disorder.

3. Os Odontoideum—Previously thought to be due to a failure of fusion of the base of the odontoid, which appears like a type II odontoid fracture. Recent evidence suggest that this may represent a traumatic process. Therapy is conservative unless instability (>3 mm translation on flexion-extension radiographs) is present, which will require posterior C1–C2 fusion.

4. Pseudosubluxation of the Cervical Spine—Subluxation of C2 on C3 (and occasionally C3 on C4) of up to 40% or 4 mm can be normal in children <8 yo because of the orientation of the facets. Rapid resolution of pain, relatively minor trauma, lack of anterior swelling, continued alignment of the posterior interspinous distances and the posterior cervical line (Schwisk) on radiographs, and reduction of the subluxation with neck extension help to differentiate this from more serious disorders.

5. Intervertebral Disc Calcification Syndrome—Pain, decreased range of motion, low-grade fevers, increased ESR, and radiographic disc calcification (within the annulus) without erosion characterize this disorder, which usually involves the C-spine. Conservative treatment is indicated for this self-limited condition.

6. Basilar impression/invagination—Bony deformity at the base of the skull causes cephalad migration of the odontoid into the foramen magnum. Symptoms of weakness, parasthesias, and hydrocephalus may result. Treatment is often operative and may include transoral resection of the dens, occipital laminectomy, and occipitocervical fusion and wiring.

X. Upper Extremity Problems (See Also Chapter 5, Hand)

A. Sprengel's Deformity—Undescended scapula often associated with winging, hypoplasia, and omovertebral connections (30%). It is the most common anomaly of the shoulder. Affected scapulae are usually small, relatively wide, and medially rotated. Increased association with Klippel-Feil syndrome, kidney disease, scoliosis, and diastematomyelia exists. Surgery for cosmetic or functional deformities (decreased abduction) includes spinous process release (Woodward) or detachment and movement of the scapula (Schrock, Green). Surgery is best done in the 3–8-year-old.

B. Congenital Pseudarthrosis of the Clavicle—Failure of union of the medial and lateral ossification centers of the right clavicle. Etiology may be related to pulsations of the underlying subclavian artery. Presents as an enlarging, painless, nontender mass. Radiographs show rounded sclerotic bone at the pseudarthrosis site. Surgery (open reduction–internal fixation with bone grafting) is controversial, but is indicated for unacceptable cosmetic deformities or with significant functional symptoms (mobility of the fragments and winging of the scapula).

C. Deltoid Fibrotic Bands—Short fibrous bands replace the deltoid muscle and cause abduction contractures at the shoulder, with elevation and winging of the scapula when the arms are adducted. Surgical resection of these bands is often required.

XI. Lower Extremity Problems

A. Introduction—Lower extremity problems that are best considered as a whole are presented in this section in order to provide a basis for understanding and comparison.

B. Rotational Problems of the Lower Extremities—Include femoral anteversion, tibial torsion, and metatarsus adductus. All of these problems may be a result of intrauterine positioning and commonly present with an intoeing gait. These deformities are usually bilateral, and the clinician should be wary of asymmetric findings. Evaluation should include the measurements noted in Table 1–8 and illustrated in Figure 1–9.

1. Metatarsus Adductus—Forefoot is adducted at the tarsal-metatarsal joint. **Usually seen in the first year.** May be associated with hip dysplasia (10–15%). Approximately 85% will resolve spontaneously; others respond to passive stretch and casting and rarely require tarsal-metatarsal release or metatarsal osteotomies. Rigidity and heel valgus should be sought out and require treatment with casting early.

2. Tibial Torsion—Most common cause of intoeing. Usually **seen during the second year** of life and can be associated with metatarsus adductus. It is often bilateral (L>R), and may actually be secondary to excessive medial ligamentous tightness. Medial rotation of the tibia at the knee causes the intoeing gait. Usually improves with growth. Denis Browne night splinting can be used if symptoms persist, but its efficacy is questionable. Operative correction is seldom necessary except in severe cases, which are addressed with a supramalleolar osteotomy.

3. Femoral Anteversion—Internal rotation of the femur **seen in 3–6-year-olds**. Increased medial rotation and decreased lateral rotation noted on exam of child with an intoeing gait with patellas

TABLE 1–8. EVALUATION OF ROTATIONAL PROBLEMS OF THE LOWER EXTREMITIES

MEASUREMENT	TECHNIQUE	NORMAL VALUES	SIGNIFICANCE
Foot-progression angle	Foot vs. straight line	−5° to +20°	Nonspecific rotation
Medial rotation	Prone hip ROM	20–60°	>70°, femoral anteversion
Lateral rotation	Prone hip ROM	30–60°	<20°, femoral anteversion
Thigh-foot angle	Knee bent—foot up	0° to +20°	<−10°, tibial torsion
Foot lateral border	Convex, medial crease	Straight, flexible	Metatarsus adductus

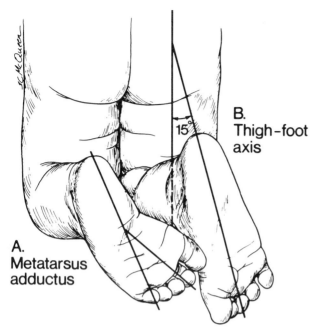

FIGURE 1–9. *A,* Deviation of the forefoot in metatarsus adductus. *B,* Note also normal thigh-foot angle (15 degrees); negative thigh-foot angles (<10 degrees) are seen in tibial torsion. (From Fitch, R.D.: Introduction to pediatric orthopedics. In Sabiston's Essentials of Surgery, Sabiston, D.C., Jr., ed. Philadelphia, W.B. Saunders, 1987; reprinted by permission.)

medially rotated. Children with this problem classically sit in the "W" position. If associated with tibial torsion, femoral anteversion may lead to patellofemoral problems. This disorder usually spontaneously corrects by age 10, but in older child with <10 degrees of medial rotation, femoral derotational osteotomy (intertrochanteric best) may be considered for cosmesis.

XII. Hip and Femur

    A. Developmental Dysplasia of the Hip (DDH)

        1. Introduction—Previously called congenital dysplasia of the hip (CDH), this disorder represents abnormal development or dislocation of the hip secondary to capsular laxity and mechanical factors (e.g., intrauterine positioning). Decreased intrauterine space explains the increased incidence of (DDH) in first-born children and with oligohydraminosis. It is commonly associated with other "packaging problems" such as torticollis (20%) and metatarsus adductus (10%), and is partially characterized by increased amounts of type III collagen. DDH is seen most commonly the left hip (67%) in females (85%) with positive family history (20+%), increased maternal estrogens, and breech births (30–50%). This disorder includes the spectrum of complete dislocation, subluxation, instability, and hip dysplasia. The teratologic form is most severe and usually requires surgery early. If left untreated, muscles about the hip contract and the acetabulum becomes flatter (dysplastic) and filled with fibro-fatty debris (pulvinar). The capsule and labrum become redundant and the head may be trapped by the iliopsoas tendon

(causing an "hourglass" constriction) or may block reduction (inverted limbus), and an abnormal femoral head and "false acetabulum" develop. Three phases are commonly recognized: (1) dislocated (Ortolani +), (2) dislocatable (Barlow +), and (3) subluxatable (Barlow suggestive).

        2. Diagnosis—Early diagnosis is possible with Ortolani test (elevation and abduction of femur relocates a dislocated hip) and Barlow test (adduction and depression of femur dislocates a dislocatable hip). Later diagnosis is made with asymmetry of legs (demonstrated with patient supine with feet together and knees flexed—Allis or Galeazzi test [knee on affected side will be lower]); decreased abduction; positive Trendelenburg stance; and accentuation of skin folds on the affected side. Repeat examination, especially in the infant, is important because irritability can distort the exam. Radiographs may be helpful in the older child (>3 months), and measurement of the acetabular index (normally <30 degrees), Perkins line (normally the ossific nucleus is medial to this line), and evaluation of Shenton's line are useful (Fig. 1–10). Later, delayed ossification of the femoral head on the affected side may be seen. Ultrasound is also useful in making the diagnosis and in evaluating reduction, especially in younger children prior to ossification of the femoral head, but it is operator dependent. Arthrography is helpful following closed reduction to determine concentric reduction (<6 mm widening).

        3. Treatment—Treatment is based on achieving and maintaining early "concentric reduction" in order to prevent future degenerative joint disease. Specific therapy is based on the child's age and includes the Pavlic harness, which is designed to hold infants (<6 months) reduced in about 100 degrees of flexion and mild abduction (The "human position" [Salter]). Reduction should be confirmed by radiographs or ultrasound after placement in the harness and the

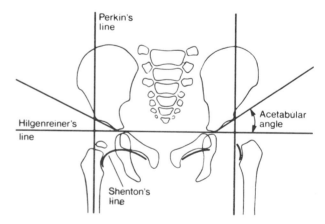

FIGURE 1–10. Common measurements used in evaluation of congenital dysplasia of the hip. Note delayed ossification, disruption of Shenton's line, and increased acetabular angle (index) on the left (dislocation) hip. (From Fitch, R.D.: Introduction to pediatric orthopedics. In Sabiston's Essentials of Surgery, Sabiston, D.C., Jr., ed. Philadelphia, W.B. Saunders, 1987; reprinted by permission.)

brace adjusted accordingly. The position of the hip should be within the "safe zone" of Ramsey (between maximum adduction before redislocation and excessive abduction causing high risk of avascular necrosis [impingement of the posterosuperior branch of the medial femoral circumflex artery]). Patients with a narrow safe zone should be considered for an adductor tenotomy. The child is placed in the harness and radiographs or ultrasound is obtained to assess reduction. If unsatisfactory, the harness is adjusted (usually by increasing the amount of flexion), and the study is repeated. A stable reduction must be demonstrated in the harness early (within 2–4 weeks). Treatment continues until the hip is reduced and stable. Weaning of the harness is generally done over a period twice as long as the treatment. Children between 6 and 18 months and younger infants in whom Pavlic treatment fails will need closed reduction. Prereduction traction is controversial. An arthrogram is usually done at the time of closed reduction to check for a medial dye pool of ≤5 mm. The arthrogram may show an inverted limbus or an hourglass constriction of the capsule indicating an incomplete reduction. Alternatively, ultrasound can be used in the operating room to assess the results of closed reduction. Casting after reduction for at least 4 months should be done and followed by nighttime bracing. Open reduction is reserved for 12–18-month-olds who fail closed reduction, have an obstructed limbus, or have an unstable safe zone; and for 18-month-old to 6-year-old children initially. This is usually done through an anterior approach (less risk to the medial femoral circumflex artery) and may include capsulorraphy, adductor tenotomy, or perhaps femoral shortening. Risks associated with both open and closed reductions include osteonecrosis (from direct vascular injury or impingement). The following treatment guidelines are appropriate:

SITUATION	FINDINGS	TREATMENT
Newborn:		
Dislocated	+ Ortolani test	Pavlic harness
Dislocatable	+ Barlow test	Pavlic harness
Subluxatable	Barlow test rides up edge	Supportive/Pavlic harness
<6 mo:		
Dislocatable/ reducible	+ Ortolani test	Pavlic harness
Unreducible	− Ortolani test	Pavlic harness → traction, closed reduction
>6 mo:		
Unreducible	− Ortolani test	Traction and closed reduction
Failed closed reduction	>5 mm medial dye pool	Open reduction
>3 yr:		
Dislocated	Trendelenburg gait, leg asymmetry (Allis test)	Open reduction, shortening ± pelvic osteotomy

4. Osteotomies—Osteotomies may be required in toddlers and school age children. Osteotomies

are required for instability, failure of acetabular development, or progressive femoral head subluxation after reduction. Osteotomies should only be done after congruent reduction, satisfactory range of motion, and reasonable femoral sphericity is achieved by closed or open methods. Discovery after 8 yo (and younger in patients with bilateral DDH) may not necessitate reduction because the acetabulum has no chance of remodeling. However, it may be indicated in conjunction with salvage procedures. The choice of femoral vs. pelvic osteotomy is sometimes a matter of the surgeon's choice. Some surgeons prefer to do pelvic osteotomies after age 4 and femoral osteotomies prior to this age. In general, pelvic osteotomies should be done when severe dysplasia is accompanied by significant radiographic changes on the acetabular side (i.e., increased acetabular index, failure of lateral acetabular ossification, etc.); whereas changes on the femoral side (e.g., marked anteversion) are best treated by femoral osteotomies. The following are common reconstructive osteotomies (Fig. 1–11):

OSTEOTOMY	PROCEDURE	REQUIREMENT
Femoral	Intertrochanteric osteotomy (VDRO)	Concentric reduction
Salter	Innominate osteotomy, open wedge	Concentric reduction
Steel	Salter + osteotomy of both ramii	Concentric reduction
Sutherland	Salter + pubic osteotomy	Concentric reduction
Dial	Periacetabular	Surgeon's experience
Pemberton	Through acetabulum roof, medial displacement distally	Concentric reduction
Chiari	Through ilium above acetabulum; makes roof	Salvage procedure

The varus derotational osteotomy (VDRO) is indicated for DDH with associated coxa valga that reduces with abduction and medial rotation. Salter osteotomies may be required in patients with instability after reduction or persistent acetabular dysplasia. It is not recommended on patients with bilateral DDH because it will uncover the opposite hip. The **Salter osteotomy may lengthen** the affected **leg** up to 1 cm. The Steel (triple) innominate osteotomy is favored in older children because their symphysis pubis does not rotate as well. Pemberton osteotomies are often favored in paralytic dislocations and patients with posterior acetabular deficiency. This osteotomy is more versatile, and is often recommended for DDH, but it is technically difficult. The Dial osteotomy is technically difficult and rarely used. The Chiari or Shelf osteotomy is recommended in cases with inadequate femoral head coverage, and is a salvage procedure. The **Chiari osteotomy will shorten the affected leg** and requires periarticular soft tissue metaplasia for success. Other procedures include greater trochanteric advancement in a person

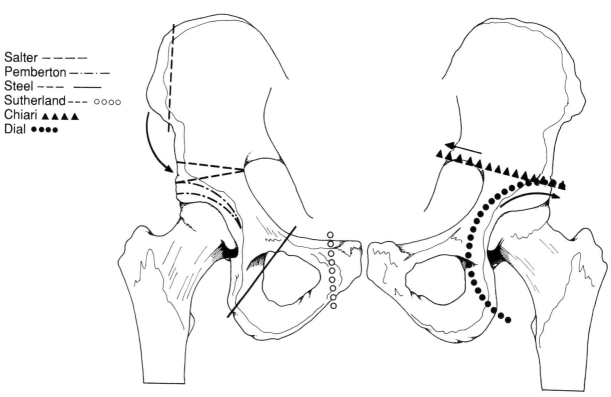

Salter — — — —
Pemberton —·—·—
Steel — — — ——
Sutherland — — — ○○○○
Chiari ▲▲▲▲
Dial ●●●●

FIGURE 1–11. Common pelvic osteotomies in the treatment of developmental dysplasia of the hip.

>8 yo with greater trochanteric overgrowth. This may present with weak abductors, thigh pain, and Trendelenburg gait in a patient with a short femoral neck on radiographs.

B. Congenital Coxa Vara—Decreased neck-shaft angle from defect in ossification of the femoral neck. It is bilateral in ⅓ to ½ of cases. Coxa vara can be congenital (noted at birth and differentiated from DDH by MRI), developmental (AD—progressive), or acquired (trauma, LCP, slipped capital femoral epiphysis, etc.). May present with a waddling gait (bilateral) or a painless limp (unilateral). Radiographs classically demonstrate a triangular ossification defect in the inferomedial femoral neck in developmental coxa vara. Evaluation of Hilgenreiner's epiphyseal angle (the angle between Hilgenreiner's line and a line through the proximal femoral physis) is the key to treatment. An angle of <45 degrees will spontaneously correct, whereas an angle of >60 degrees (and a neck-shaft angle of < 110 degrees) will usually require surgery. Proximal femoral (valgus) ± derotation osteotomy (Pauwel) is indicated for a neck-shaft angle <90 degrees, a vertically oriented physeal plate, or progressive deformities, or with significant gait abnormalities.

C. Legg-Calvé-Perthes Disease (Coxa Plana)—Noninflammatory, self-limited deformity of the weight-bearing surface of the femur probably secondary to a vascular insult leading to osteonecrosis of the proximal femoral epiphysis. Usually seen in a 4–8-yo boy with delayed skeletal maturity. There is an increased incidence with a positive family history, low birth weight, and abnormal birth presen-

tation. Symptoms include pain (**often knee pain!**), effusion (from synovitis) and limp. Decreased hip ROM (especially abduction and internal rotation) and a Trendelenburg stance are also common. **Age is the key to prognosis; presentation after 8 yo represents a poor prognosis.** Up to 12% of cases are bilateral but will be at different stages and are asymmetric (vs. multiple epiphyseal dysplasia). Differential diagnosis includes septic arthritis, blood dyscrasias, hypothyroidism, and epiphyseal dysplasia. Bony necrosis is followed by revascularization and resorption via creeping substitution that eventually allows remodeling and fragmentation. Radiographic findings vary with the stage of disease, but include cessation of growth of the ossific nucleus, medial joint space widening, and development of a "crescent sign" representing subchondral fracture. Four radiographic stages (Waldenström) are usually described based on the appearance of the capital femoral epiphysis:

STAGE	CHARACTERISTICS
Initial	Physeal irregularity, metaphyseal blurring, radiolucencies
Fragmentation	Radiolucencies and radiodensities
Reossification	Normal density returns
Healed	Residual deformity

Caterall has defined four stages based on the amount of femoral involvement (seen as the crescent sign). This has been simplified by Salter and Thompson based on whether the lateral margin of the capital femoral epiphysis (CFE) is involved (Fig. 1–12):

Caterall	Salter and Thompson	Location	Prognosis
I	A	Anterior (seen on lateral view)	Good
II	A	Anterior and partial lateral	Good
III	B	Anterior and lateral margin	Poor
IV	B	Throughout CFE dome	Poor

The crescent sign represents a pathologic fracture of the resorbing femoral head and is best seen on a frog-leg view of the pelvis. Bone scan and MRI may help identify early involvement, but does not correlate with the extent of involvement. Newer, magnified bone scans may help identify the revascularization pattern. Maintaining the sphericity of the femoral head is the most important factor in achieving a good result. Use of circular templates (Mose) is helpful in evaluation this. Early hip degenerative joint disease (DJD) results from aspherical femoral heads. Poor prognosis is associated with older children (>8 yo), female sex, advanced stages (with lateral margin of the CFE involved), loss of containment, and decreased hip range of motion (decreased abduction). Radiographic findings associated with poor prognosis (Caterall's "head at risk" signs) include: (1) lateral calcification, (2) Gage's sign (V-shaped defect laterally), (3) lateral subluxation, (4) metaphyseal cysts, and (5) horizontal growth plate. Treatment for stages III and IV is based on **first obtaining range of motion (usually with bed rest and traction) and then containment (with an abduction brace** such as the Scottish Rite brace **or surgery).** Bracing should continue until the increased density on radiographs disappears, representing the end of the fragmentation stage (usually 1 year after onset of symptoms). Some recommend continuing bracing until new bone is seen on the anterolateral portion of the femoral head. Advanced flattening of the femoral head can make it "noncontainable." Because abduction results in hinging and subluxation, bracing at this stage is not effective. Treatment options include Chiari osteotomy, cheilectomy (of the femoral head prominence) and valgus osteotomy (a newer technique with some promise). Distal transfer of the greater trochanter is occasionally required to offset overgrowth of the greater trochanter (which is not affected and continues to grow).

D. Slipped Capital Femoral Epiphysis—Disorder of the proximal femoral epiphysis of the femur seen in puberty caused by weakness of the perichondral

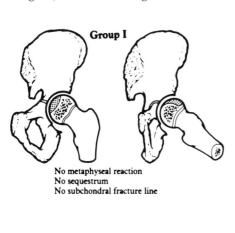

Group I

No metaphyseal reaction
No sequestrum
No subchondral fracture line

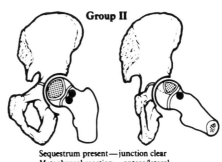

Group II

Sequestrum present—junction clear
Metaphyseal reaction—antero/lateral
Subchondral fracture line—anterior half

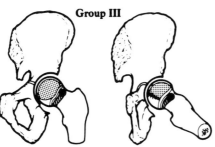

Group III

Sequestrum — large — junction sclerotic
Metaphyseal reaction — diffuse antero/lateral area
Subchondral fracture line — posterior half

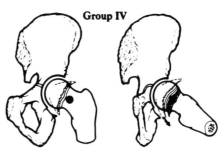

Group IV

Whole head involvement
Metaphyseal reaction — central or diffuse
Posterior remodelling

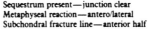
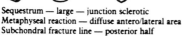

FIGURE 1–12. The Catterall classification of Legg-Calvé-Perthes disease. Note significant involvement of the lateral margin of the capital femoral epiphysis in groups III and IV (Salter and Thompson "B"). (From Fitch, R.D.: Introduction to pediatric orthopedics. In Sabiston's Essentials of Surgery, Sabiston, D.C., Jr., ed. Philadelphia, W.B. Saunders, 1987; reprinted by permission.)

ring and slip through the hypertrophic zone of the growth plate. The femoral head remains in the acetabulum and the neck displaces anteriorly and externally rotates. Slipped CFE is seen commonly in black obese adolescent boys with a positive family history. Up to 25% of cases are bilateral. May be associated with hormonal changes in younger children, hypothyroidism, or advanced renal disease. May present with a coxalgic, externally rotated gait, decreased ROM (esp internal rotation), thigh atrophy, and hip or knee pain. Symptoms vary with acuteness of the slip:

Slip	Duration of Sx	Symptoms
Acute	<3 Weeks	Prodrome of knee pain
Chronic	>3 Weeks	Insidious onset
Acute on chronic		Acute pain with old slipped CFE

Radiographs show the slip, which is classified based upon the percentage of slip: grade I, 0–33%; grade II, 33–50%; and grade III, >50%. In mild cases, the loss of the lateral overhang of the femoral ossific nucleus (Klein's line) and blurring of the proximal femoral metaphysis may be all that is seen on the AP film. If seen acutely (within 3 weeks) then limited closed reduction and pinning is indicated. Later, recommended therapy is pinning in situ, or epiphysiodesis if deformity is severe in a heavy patient. **Forceful reduction** before pinning **is never indicated**. Pin placement can be percutaneous with one pin. The pin should be placed anteriorly on the femoral neck, ending in the central portion of the femoral head. Prophylactic pinning of the opposite hip is no longer recommended. Intertrochanteric (Kramer) or subtrochanteric (Southwick) osteotomies may be required with severe slips to increase ROM in patients that do not have adequate remodeling and have limited flexion (<90 degrees). Complications from the disorder itself or therapy include chondrolysis (narrowed joint space and decreased motion seen; treatment includes traction, NSAIDs, and physical therapy); osteonecrosis (can result from traction and manipulation, especially with acute slips; also can be a result of superior screw placement; treatment is partial weight bearing and observation); and perhaps DJD (pistol grip deformity of proximal femur).

E. Proximal Femoral Focal Deficiency (PFFD)—A developmental defect of the proximal femur recognizable at birth. Clinically, patients with PFFD have a short, bulky thigh that is flexed, abducted, and externally rotated. PFFD can be associated with coxa vara or fibular hemimelia (50%). Congenital knee ligamentous laxity and contracture are also common. Treatment must be individualized based on leg length discrepancy, adequacy of proximal musculature, femoral rotation, and proximal joint stability. The percentage of shortening is constant over growth and allows an assessment of final outcome. Four groups exist (Fig. 1–13); these can be subdivided into two categories based on the requirement for amputation: Aitken classes A and B have a femoral head present (and may be treated with limb lengthening procedures), whereas classes C and D do not (usually require amputation or ankle disarticulation with knee fusion (or Van Nes rotationplasty—with a stable ankle and patient and parent acceptance).

F. Leg length Discrepancy (LLD)—There can be many causes of leg length discrepancy, including congenital disorders (hemihypertrophy dysplasias, PFFD, DDH, etc.), paralytic disorders (spasticity, polio, etc.), infection (pyogenic disruption of the growth plate), tumors, and trauma. Long-term problems associated with LLD include inefficient gait, equinus contractures of the ankle, postural scoliosis, and low back pain. The discrepancy must be measured accurately (with blocks of set height under affected side, scanogram, etc.), and can be tracked with the Green Anderson or Mosely graph (with serial leg-length films or CT scanograms and bone age determinations). In general, projected discrepancies at maturity of <2 cm are treated with shoe lifts and other nonoperative means; 2–5-cm differences can be treated with epiphysiodesis of the unaffected side (usually done percutaneously with the aid of a C-arm [or shortening at maturity]); and discrepancies of >5 cm with lengthening. Using standard techniques, distraction of 1 mm/day is typical. The Ilizarov principles, including metaphyseal corticotomy (preserving the medullary canal and blood supply) followed by gradual lengthening, can achieve even greater lengths. Physeal distraction with the technique of chondrodiastasis allows limb lengthening without corticotomies or osteotomies. This procedure must be done near skeletal maturity because the physis almost always fuses following limb lengthening. Gross estimates of LLD can be made using the following assumption of growth per year up to age 16 in boys and 14 in girls: distal femur, 3/8th inch/year; proximal tibia, 2/8th inch/yr; and proximal femur, 1/8th inch/year. However, use of the Mosely data gives more accurate data.

G. Lower Extremity Inflammation and Infection (see also Chapter 2, Basic Sciences, Part 7: Orthopaedic Infections)

1. Transient Synovitis—Most common cause of painful hips in childhood; however, it is a diagnosis of exclusion. Can be related to viral infection, allergic reaction, or trauma; however, etiology is unknown. Onset can be acute or insidious. Symptoms, which are self-limited, include voluntary limitation of motion and muscle spasm. Rule out septic hip with aspiration (especially in children with fever, leukocytosis, or elevated ESR), then observe in Buck's traction for 24–48 hours.

2. Osteomyelitis—More common in children due to rich metaphyseal blood supply and thick periosteum. Most common organism is *Staph. aureus* (except in neonates, in whom **group B strep is more common**). *H. influenzae* is also common in 6-month-olds to 4-year-olds. A history of trauma is common and may predispose children to osteomyelitis. Osteomyelitis in children usually begins through hematogenous seeding of a bony metaphysis in the small arterioles that bend just below the physis, where blood flow is sluggish and there is poor phagocytosis, cre-

TYPE		FEMORAL HEAD	ACETABULUM	FEMORAL SEGMENT	RELATIONSHIP AMONG COMPONENTS OF FEMUR AND ACETABULUM AT SKELETAL MATURITY
A	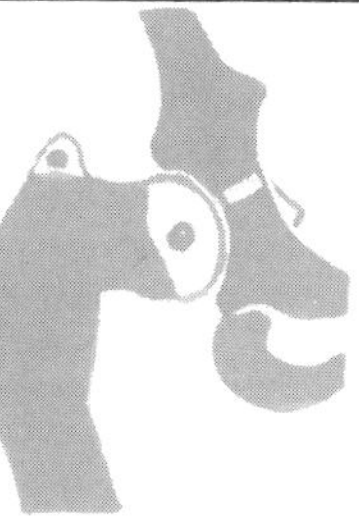	Present	Normal	Short	Bony connection between components of femur Femoral head in acetabulum Subtrochanteric varus angulation, often with pseudarthrosis
B	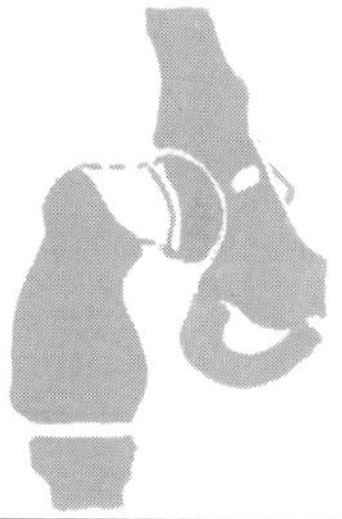	Present	Adequate or moderately dysplastic	Short, usually proximal bony tuft	No osseous connection between head and shaft Femoral head in acetabulum
C	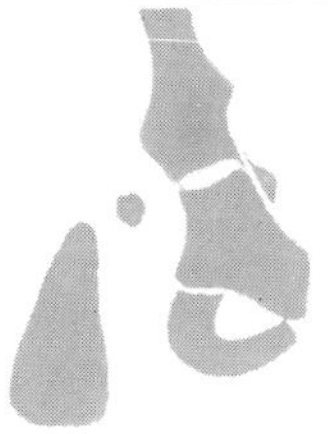	Absent or represented by ossicle	Severely dysplastic	Short, usually proximally tapered	May be osseous connection between shaft and proximal ossicle No articular relation between femur and acetabulum
D	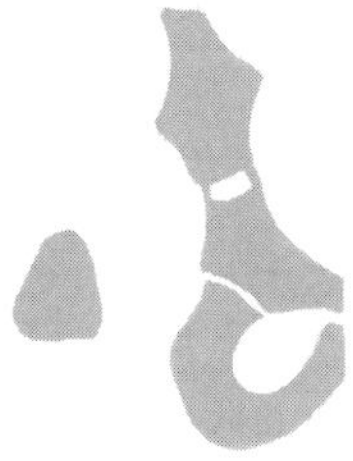	Absent	Absent Obturator foramen enlarged Pelvis squared in bilateral cases	Short, deformed	(none)

FIGURE 1–13. Aitken classification of proximal femoral focal deficiency. Note lack of femoral head in types C and D. (From Tachdjian, M.O.: Pediatric Orthopaedics, 2nd ed. Philadelphia, W.B. Saunders, 1990; reprinted by permission.)

ating a bone abscess (Fig. 1–14). Pus lifts the thick periosteum and puts pressure on the cortex, causing coagulation. Cortical bone may die and become a sequestrum. Finally, subperiosteal new bone forms around the dead sequestrum, forming an involucrum. Chronic bone abscesses may become surrounded by thick, fibrous tissue and sclerotic bone (Brodie's abscess). Clinically, the child presents with a fever (which may not be present) and a tender, warm, sometimes swollen area over a long bone metaphysis. Although labs may be helpful (blood cultures, WBC, ESR), and studies are also useful (x-rays with only soft tissue swelling early, metaphyseal rarefaction late; technetium bone scan and gallium scan), the definitive diagnosis is made with aspiration (50% positive cultures). IV antibiotics (usually a third-generation cephalosporin [e.g., cefotaxime {Claforan}] in neonates and a first-generation cephalosporin [e.g., Ce-

fazolin {Ancef}] in older children; followed by antibiotics specific for organisms cultured) are the best initial treatment if osteomyelitis is caught early with no radiographic changes and rapid response to treatment. Later, with no response to antibiotics, or with frank pus on aspiration or in the face of a sequestered abscess (not accessible by antibiotics), operative drainage and débridement are required. Specimens should be sent to pathology as well as for culture. The wound can be closed over a drain. IV antibiotics can be changed to appropriate po antibiotics after a good response to treatment (usually at 7–10 days) and with sensitive oral antibiotics. Antibiotics should be continued until the ESR returns to normal.

3. Septic Arthritis—Can develop from osteomyelitis (especially in neonates, in whom transphyseal vessels allow proximal spread into the joint) in joints with an intra-articular metaphysis (hip

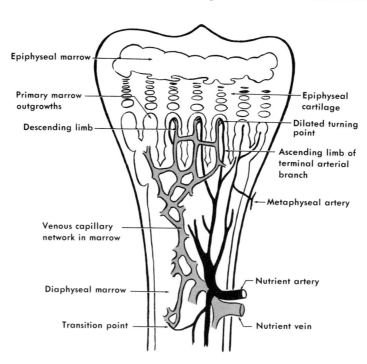

Epiphyseal marrow

Primary marrow outgrowths

Descending limb

Epiphyseal cartilage

Dilated turning point

Ascending limb of terminal arterial branch

Metaphyseal artery

Venous capillary network in marrow

Diaphyseal marrow

Nutrient artery

Transition point

Nutrient vein

FIGURE 1–14. Illustration of metaphysical sinusoids where sluggish blood flow increases susceptibility to osteomyelitis. (From Tachdjian, M.O.: Pediatric Orthopaedics, 2nd ed. Philadelphia, W.B. Saunders, 1990; reprinted by permission.)

and shoulder); or can be from hematogenous spread of infection. Because pus is chondrolytic, septic arthritis in children is an acute surgical emergency. Organisms vary with age:

Age	Common Organisms	Empiric Antibiotics
<12 mo	Staph, Group B Strep	First-generation cephalosporin
6 mo–5 yr	Staph, H. influenzae	Second- or third-generation cephalosporin
5–12 yr	S. aureus	First-generation cephalosporin
12–18 yr	S. aureus, N. gonorrhoeae	Oxacillin/Cephalosporin

Symptoms of decreased ROM and severe pain with passive motion may be accompanied by systemic symptoms of infection. Patients with gonorrhea septic arthritis usually have a preceding migratory polyarthralgia small red papules, and multiple joint involvement. This organism typically elicits less WBC response (50K vs. >100K in other septic arthritides) and usually does not require surgical drainage. Large doses of penicillin are required to treat this organism. Radiographs may show widened joint space or even dislocation. Joint fluid aspirate shows high WBC count, a glucose level 50 mg/dl less than serum levels, and, in cases with gram-positive cocci or gram-negative rods, a high lactic acid level. Ultrasound can be helpful to identify the presence of an effusion. Aspiration should be followed by incision and drain-

age if necessary (especially in the hip, culture of synovium is also recommended). Spinal tap should be considered in a septic joint caused by H. influenzae because of increased incidence of meningitis. This may not be necessary with selection of an antibiotic that is known to cross the blood-brain barrier. IV antibiotics are changed to specific oral antibiotics after a good response to treatment is seen and only in reliable patients/parents and good drug tolerance. Prognosis is usually good except in younger patients, associated osteomyelitis, and in the hip joint.

XIII. Knee and Leg

A. Genu Varum/Valgum—Normally genu varum (bowed legs) evolves naturally to genu valgum (knocked knees) by age 2½, with a gradual transition to physiologic valgus by age 4. Observation of gait is important in evaluating patients to determine if there is a thrust at the onset of weight bearing. This indicates weak restraints and connotes an increased likelihood of progression.

1. Genu Varum (Bowed Legs)—Normal in children <2 yo. Radiographs in physiologic bowing typically show flaring of the tibia and femur in a symmetric fashion. Pathologic conditions that can cause genu varum include osteogenesis imperfecta, osteochondromas, trauma, various dysplasias, and most commonly, Blount's disease. **Blount's disease** (tibia varum) differs from physiologic genu varum because it is caused by a disorder of the posterior medial tibial physis. Affected children are most commonly black obese males. Radiographs may show a metaphyseal-diaphyseal angle of >11 degrees early

(this angle is formed by lines between the metaphyseal beaks and the perpendicular to the longitudinal axis of the tibia). The epiphyseal-metaphyseal angle is also useful (Fig. 1–15). The infantile form of Blount's disease (most common) is usually bilateral, and is associated with internal tibial torsion. Adolescent Blount's is less severe and predominately unilateral. Treatment is based on age and stage of disease (Lagenshold I–VI with VI characterized by a metaphyseal-epiphyseal bony bridge):

AGE	STAGE	TREATMENT
<18 mo	I–II	None
18–24 mo	I–II	A frame/Blount brace (night)
2–3 yr	I–II	Modified locked KAFO
3–8 yr	III–V	Valgus rotational osteotomy
7–8 yr	VI	Resection of bony bridge

2. Genu Valgum (Knock Knees)—Up to 15 degrees at the knee is common in 2–6-yo children. Pathologic genu valgum may be associated with renal osteodystrophy (most common cause if bilateral), tumors (e.g., osteochondromas), infections (may stimulate proximal asymmetric tibial growth), trauma, etc. With larger amounts of genu valgum, night bracing may be appropriate. Consider surgery (at the site of the deformity) only in >10-year-olds with >10 cm between medial malleoli or >15–20 degrees of valgus. Hemiepiphysiodesis of the medial side is effective prior to the end of growth for severe deformities.

B. Tibial Bowing—Three types based on apex of curve:

1. Posteromedial—Physiologic bowing usually

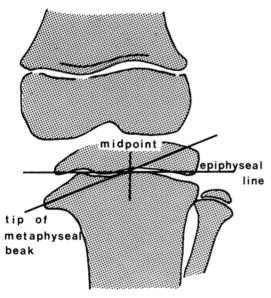

FIGURE 1–15. Blount's disease and measurement of the epiphyseal-metaphyseal angle. (From Tachdjian, M.O.: Pediatric Orthopaedics, 2nd ed. Philadelphia, W.B. Saunders, 1990; reprinted by permission.)

seen before 18 months at the junction of the middle and distal thirds of the tibia. May be the result of abnormal intrauterine positioning. It is commonly associated with calcaneovalgus feet and tight anterior structures. Spontaneous correction is the rule, but follow to evaluate late leg length discrepancy. Late contralateral epiphysiodesis may be required due to an average LLD of 3–4 cm. Tibial osteotomies are not indicated.

2. Anteriomedial Tibial bowing—Typically caused by fibular hemimelia. A congenital longitudinal deficiency of the fibula, it is the most common long bone deficiency and **the most common skeletal deformity in the leg**. It is usually associated with anteriomedial bowing. It is often accompanied by ankle instability, equinovarus foot (± absent lateral rays), tarsal coalition, and femoral shortening. Classically has skin dimpling seen over the tibia. Significant leg length discrepancy often results from this disorder. Hemimelia can be intercalary, which involves the whole bone (absent fibula), or terminal. Fibular hemimelia is frequently associated with femoral abnormalities like coxa vara and PFFD. Treatment varies from a simple shoe lift or bracing to Syme amputation. Amputation is usually done at about 10 months. For less severe cases lengthening and reconstruction of the mortise (Gruca) may be an alternative. This procedure should include resection of the fibular anlage to avoid future foot problems.

3. Anterolateral Tibial Bowing—Congenital pseudarthrosis of the tibia is the most common cause of anterolateral bowing. It is often accompanied by neurofibromatosis (50%—but only 10% of patients with neurofibromatosis have this disorder). Classification (Boyd) is based on bowing, presence of cystic changes, sclerosis, or dysplasia. Dysplasia and cystic changes are most common. Early treatment with total contact brace to protect from fractures, intramedullary fixation with excision of hamartomatous tissue, and autogenous bone grafting (osteosynthesis) for nonhealing fractures. Vascularized fibular graft or Ilizarov methods should be considered if this fails. Osteotomies and electrical stimulation alone are contraindicated. Amputation (Symes) and prosthetic fitting are indicated after two or three failed surgical attempts.

4. Other Lower Limb Deficiencies—Include tibial hemimelia, an autosomal dominant disorder that is a congenital longitudinal deficiency of the tibia. Much less common than fibular hemimelia, and is often associated with other bony abnormalities (especially lobster-claw hand). Clinically, the extremity is shortened and anterolaterally bowed with a prominent fibular head and equinovarus foot, with the sole of the foot facing the perineum. Treatment may include Symes or a below-knee amputation. Severe deformities with an absent tibia require knee disarticulation. Fibular transposition (Brown) has been unsuccessful, especially with absent quadriceps function and absent proximal tibias.

C. Osteochondritis Dissecans—Intra-articular lesion usually of the knee with disorderly enchondral ossification of epiphyseal growth. Common in 10–15-year-olds and can affect many joints, especially the knee and elbow (capitellum). The lesion is thought to be secondary to trauma, ischemia, or abnormal epiphyseal ossification. The lateral intercondylar portion of the medial femoral condyle of the knee is most frequently involved (seen best on notch view). Classified into three categories based on age of appearance (Pappas):

Category	Age Group	Prognosis	Treatment
I	0–adolescence	Excellent	Rest, immobilize
II	Teenage children	Intermediate	Rest, arthroscopy of large defects
III	20 +, closed physis	Poor; fragments/defects	Operative

Symptoms include activity-related pain, localized tenderness, stiffness and swelling ± mechanical symptoms. Radiographs should include the tunnel (notch) view to evaluate the condyles. Differential diagnosis includes anomalous ossification centers. Surgical therapy includes drilling with multiple holes, fixation of large fragments, and bone grafting of large lesions in patients with closed physes. Commonly treated arthroscopically. Poorer prognosis is associated with lesions in the lateral femoral condyle and patella.

Arthroscopic Classification and Treatment of Osteochondritis Dissecans (After Guhl)

Classification	Treatment
1. Intact lesion	K wire drilling
2. Early-separated lesion	In situ pinning
3. Partially detached lesion ⎫	Debridement of base
4. Salvagable loose body ⎬	and reduction and pinning
5. Unsalvagable loose body	Removal and debridement of base

D. Osgood-Schlatter Disease—Osteochondritis or fatigue failure of the tibial tubercle apophysis due to stress from the extensor mechanism in a growing child. Radiographs may show irregularity and fragmentation of the tibial tubercle. Usually self-limited; late excision of separate ossicles is occasionally required.

E. Discoid Meniscus—Abnormal development of the lateral meniscus leads to the formation of a disc-shaped (or hypertrophic) rather than the normal crescent-shaped meniscus. Typically, radiographs will demonstrate widening of the cartilage space on the affected side (up to 11 mm). If symptomatic and torn, it can be arthroscopically débrided.

XIV. Feet (Fig. 1–16)

A. Clubfoot (Congenital Talipes Equinovarus)—Forefoot adduction and hindfoot varus with the calcaneus inverted under the equinus talus. Talar neck deformity (medial and plantar deviation) with medial rotation of the calcaneus and medial displacement of the navicular and cuboid occurs. Clubfoot is more common in males, and half are bilateral. It is associated with shortened/contracted muscles (intrinsics, plantar flexors, and invertors),

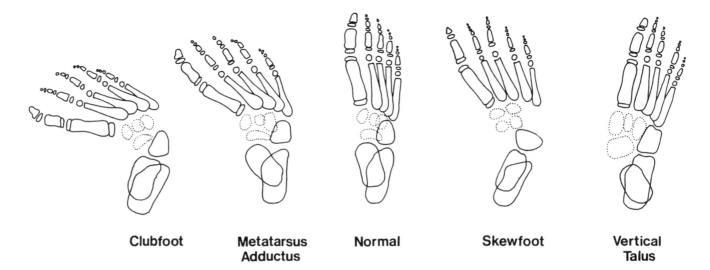

Clubfoot   **Metatarsus Adductus**   **Normal**   **Skewfoot**   **Vertical Talus**

FIGURE 1–16. AP view of common childhood foot disorders. Note; *A,* Varus position of hindfoot adducted forefoot in clubfoot; *B,* Normal hindfoot and adducted forefoot in cMTA; *C,* Normal foot; *D,* Valgus hindfoot (with increased talocalcaneal angle), and adducted forefoot in skewfoot, and; *E,* Increased talocalcaneal angle and lateral deviation of the calcaneus in congenital vertical talus.

joint capsules, ligaments, and fascia that lead to the associated deformities. Can be associated with hand anomalies (Streeter's dysplasia and congenital bands), diastrophic dwarfism, arthrogryposis, and myelomeningocele. Radiographs should include the **dorsiflexed lateral** view (Turco)—talus-calcaneus angle >35 degrees is normal; a smaller angle with a flat talar head is seen with clubfoot. On the AP view a talus-calcaneus (Kite) angle of 20–40 degrees is normal (<20 degrees seen with clubfoot); negative talus–first metatarsal angle without clubfoot (normally 0–20 degrees) (Fig. 1–17). "Parallelism" of the calcaneus and talus is seen on both views. In true (rigid) clubfoot (refractory to casting with a midfoot crease and a small heel) only 10–15% will respond to serial manipulation and casting. Nevertheless, 3 months of casting is the recommended therapy for children initially, and it will facilitate later surgery. Failing this, surgical subtalar and posterior capsular release with tendon lengthening (Turco) (posteromedial release with attention also to posterolateral corner) is favored, usually at 3–9 months. The following structures are addressed:

STRUCTURE	PROCEDURE
Achilles tendon	Z-lengthening
Calcaneal fibular ligament	Release
Post. talofibular ligament	Release
Post. tibialis tendon	Z-lengthening
Subtalar capsule	Release
Superficial deltoid	Release
Fibulocalcaneal ligament	Partial release
Tibiotalar, subtalar capsule	Complete release
Talonavicular tibionavicular (pseudo)	Release

The posterior tibial artery must be carefully protected. Often the dorsalis pedis artery is insufficient. Casting for several months is usually required postoperatively. In older patients (3–10 yo), medial opening or lateral column shortening osteotomies or cubital decancelization is recommended. For children who present with refractory clubfoot late (8–10 yo), triple arthrodesis is the only procedure possible to eliminate associated pain. Triple arthrodesis is contraindicated in patients with insensate feet because it causes a rigid foot that may lead to ulceration. Talectomy may be a better procedure in these patients.

B. Forefoot Adduction (Fig. 1–16)
1. Metatarsus Adductus (MTA) (see Section XI: Lower Extremity Problems, B: Rotational Problems of the Lower Extremities, above)—Adduction of the forefoot commonly associated with DDH. Four types have been identified (Berg):

TYPE	FEATURES
Simple MTA	MTA
Complex MTA	MTA + lateral shift of midfoot
Skew foot	MTA + valgus hindfoot
Complex skew foot	MTA, lateral shift, valgus hindfoot

If peroneal stimulation corrects MTA then it will usually respond to stretching. Otherwise, manipulation and casting may be required. Surgery in refractory cases (usually those with medial creases) includes abductor hallucis longus recession (for atavistic great toe), tarsometatarsal release, or metatarsal osteotomies (favored by most), after a trial of observation.
2. Medial Deviation of the Talar Neck—Benign disorder of the foot that generally corrects spontaneously.

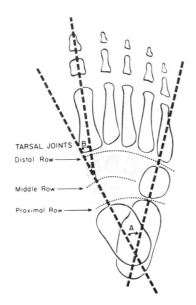

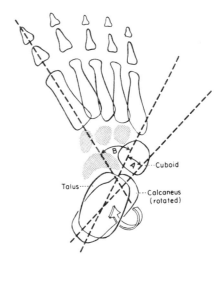

FIGURE 1–17. Radiographic evaluation of club feet. Note "parallelism" of the talus and calcaneus with a talus-calcaneus angle (*A*) of <20 degrees and negative talus–first metatarsal angle (*B*) on the clubfoot side. (From Simons G.W.: Analytical radiography of club feet. J. Bone Joint Surg [Br.] 59:485–489, 1974; reprinted by permission.)

3. Serpentine ("Z") Foot (Complex Skew Foot)—Associated with residual tarsometatarsal adductus, tarsonavicular lateral subluxation, and hindfoot valgus. No good therapy or surgical option is available. Realignment of tarsal bones should be accompanied by subtalar arthrodesis ± metatarsal osteotomies later.

C. Pes Cavus—Cavus deformity of the foot (elevated longitudinal arch) due to fixed plantar flexion of the forefoot. There are four basic types of pes cavus:

TYPE	FOREFOOT	HINDFOOT	RADIOGRAPHS
Simple	Balanced	Neutral	
Cavovarus	Plantar flexed	Varus	Decreased talus-
Calcaneus	Fixed equinus	Calcaneus	calcaneus
Equinocavus	Equinus	Equinus	angle

Pes cavus is commonly associated with neurologic disorders including polio, CP, Friedreich's ataxia, and Charcot-Marie-Tooth disease; full neurologic workup is mandatory. Lateral block test (Coleman) (lift placed under lateral foot) assesses hindfoot flexibility of the cavovarus foot (flexible feet correct to normal). Nonoperative management is rarely successful. Surgery includes plantar release, first (or multiple) metatarsal osteotomy, tendon transfers, and, if lateral block test shows an abnormality, a calcaneal osteotomy. Triple arthrodesis is reserved for rigid deformities in patients at maturity.

D. Pes Calcaneovalgus
1. Congenital Vertical Talus (Rocker-Bottom foot)—Irreducible dorsal dislocation of the navicular on the talus with a fixed talocalcaneonavicular complex. Clinically, the talar head is prominent medially, the sole is convex, the forefoot is abducted and dorsiflexed, and the hindfoot is in equinovalgus. Patients may demonstrate a "peg-leg" gait (awkward gait with limited forefoot pushoff). It is a common cause of rigid flatfoot, which can be isolated or can occur with chromosomal abnormalities, myeloarthropathies, and neurologic disorders. **Plantar flexed lateral radiographs** show that a line along the long axis of the talus passes below the metatarsal-cuneiform axis (tarsal–first metatarsal angle >60 degrees [normally 0–20 degrees dorsal tilt], calcaneus–first metatarsal angle >20 degrees) (Fig. 1–18). AP radiographs show a talus-calcaneus angle of >40 degrees (normally 20–40 degrees). Differential diagnosis includes oblique talus (corrects with plantar flexion), tarsal coalition, and paralytic pes valgus. Three months of corrective casting (foot plantar flexed and inverted) or manipulative stretching is tried initially. Surgery at 6–12 months consists of soft tissue release/lengthening. Late treatment includes subtalar arthrodesis (2½–6 yo) and triple arthrodesis (>6 yo).
2. Oblique Talus—Talonavicular subluxation that reduces with plantar flexion of the foot. Treatment is observation and sometimes UCBL shoe inserts.

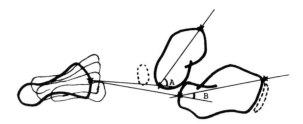

FIGURE 1–18. Plantar-flexed lateral radiographic features in congenital vertical talus. *A*, Talar axis–metatarsal base angle (normally 3 ± 6 degrees). *B*, Calcaneal axis–metatarsal base angle (normally −9 ± 5 degrees). Both angles are increased in congenital vertical talus. (From Hamanishi, C.: Congenital vertical talus. J. Pediatr. Orthop. 4:319, 1984; reprinted by permission.)

E. Tarsal Coalition—AD disorder of mesenchymal segmentation lending to fusion of tarsal bones and rigid flatfoot. Most commonly involve talocalcaneal or calcaneonavicular tarsal bones and is the leading cause of peroneal spastic flatfoot. Symptoms, which appear at the age of 8–12 years for calcaneonavicular coalitions and 12–16 years for talocalaneal coalitions, may include calf pain and flatfoot with limited subtalar motion. Coalition or synostosis can be osseous, cartilaginous, or fibrous. **Calcaneonavicular coalition is most common** and is best **seen on special oblique x-rays (Slomann)**. Lateral radiographs may show elongation of the anterior process of the calcaneus ("anteater" sign). Talocalcaneal coalition may be suggested by talar beaking on lateral views (does not signify degenerative joint disease) or an irregular middle calcaneal facet on Harris axial view. **The best study for talocalcaneal coalition is a CT scan.** Early surgery in symptomatic cases involving <50% of the middle facet in talocalcaneal conditions to resect a bar (with soft tissue interposition) will avoid later requirement for a triple arthrodesis, but observation is reasonable for asymptomatic bars in younger children. A trial of immobilization is recommended for older symptomatic patients. Older patients may do well with selective talonavicular and calcaneal cuboid fusion for talocalcaneal coalition and bar resection for calcaneonavicular coalition. Advanced cases require triple arthrodesis.

F. Calcaneal Valgus Foot—Newborn condition associated with intrauterine positioning. Common in firstborn children. Presents with a dorsiflexed hindfoot with eversion and abduction of the hindfoot that is passively correctable to neutral. Treatment is passive stretching and observation.

G. Juvenile Bunions—Often are bilateral and associated with a familial incidence. This disorder is less common and usually less symptomatic than the adult counterpart. May be associated with ligamentous laxity and a long first ray. Usually found in adolescent females. Wide shoes and arch supports help early. Surgery is considered with an intermetatarsal angle >10 degrees (metatarsus primus varus) and a hallux valgus angle >20 degrees. Distal metatarsal procedures are often more successful than proximal ones. Metatarsus primus varus may require osteotomy and distal capsular reefing. Complications include overcorrection and hallux varus. Recurrence is frequent (>50%), especially if only soft tissue procedures are done, and it is best to wait until maturity to reoperate.

H. Köhler's Disease—Osteonecrosis of the tarsal navicular, usually presents at about 5 yo. Pain caused by repetitive trauma to the maturing epiphysis. Radiographs characteristically show sclerosis of the navicular. Symptoms usually resolve spontaneously with activity restriction ± immobilization.

I. Flexible Pes Planus—Foot is flat only when standing and not with toe walking or with foot hanging. Frequently familial and almost always bilateral. Commonly associated with minor lower extremity rotational problems and generalized ligamentous laxity. Symptoms including aching midfoot or pretibial pain can occur. Lateral radiographic findings mimic those seen in vertical talus, but a plantarflexed lateral view demonstrates that a line along the long axis of the talus passes above the metatarsal-cuneiform axis. Treatment is observation only, not special shoewear. Sometimes soft arch supports are helpful but not corrective. Thorough evaluation should be completed to rule out tight heel cords (treated with stretching and occasional Achilles tendon lengthening) and decreased subtalar motion (consider coalition). UCBL heel cups are sometimes indicated in advanced cases with pain (symptomatic treatment only). Calcaneal osteotomy or select fusions may provide pain relief at the expense of inversion/eversion in adolescents with disabling pain refractory to every means of conservative treatment. The following radiographic views may be helpful:

VIEW	ASSESSMENT
Standing AP	Talar head coverage, talus-calcaneus angle
Standing lateral	Calcaneal/talar equinus, talus-calcaneus angle
Obliques	To rule out coalition

J. Habitual Toe Walker—Contracture of Achilles tendon. Usually responds to serial casting, sometimes requires lengthening of the Achilles tendon.

K. Accessory Navicular—Can be a normal variant seen in up to 12% of the population. Commonly associated with flat feet. Symptoms usually include medial arch pain with overuse. Symptoms usually abate with activity restriction and/or immobilization. External oblique radiographic views are often helpful in diagnosis. Most cases respond spontaneously, occasionally, excision of the accessory bone can correct symptoms (but not flatfoot) in most patients.

L. Ball-and-Socket Ankle—Abnormal formation with a spherical talus (ball) and a cup-shaped tibio fibular articulation (socket). It usually requires no treatment, but should be recognized because of high association with tarsal coalition (50%), absent lateral rays (50%), and leg length discrepancies.

M. Congenital Toe Disorders

1. Syndactyly—Fusion of the soft tissues (simple) and sometimes bone (complex) of the toes. Simple syndactyly usually does not require treatment; complex syndactyly is treated as it is in the hand.

2. Polydactyly (Extra digits)—May be autosomal dominant and usually involves the lateral ray in patients with a positive family history. Treatment usually includes ablation of the supranumerary digit and any bony protrusion of the common metatarsal (typically the border digit is excised—not the best formed). The procedure is usually done at age 9–12 months, but some rudimentary digits can be ligated in the newborn nursery.

3. Oligodactyly—Congenital absence of the toes. May be associated with more proximal dysgenesis (i.e., fibular hemimelia) and tarsal coalition. The disorder usually does not require treatment.

4. Atavistic Great Toe (Congenital Hallux Varus)—Great toe adduction deformity that is often associated with supranumerary toes. Must be differentiated from metatarsus adductus. Usually the deformity occurs at the MTP joint and also includes a short, thick first metatarsal and a firm band (the abductor hallucis muscle) that may be responsible for the disorder. Surgery, which is sometimes required, includes release of the abductor muscle.

5. Overlapping Toe—The fifth toe overlaps the fourth (usually bilaterally) and may cause problems with shoewear. Initial treatment includes passive stretching and buddy taping. Surgical options include extensor tenotomy, dorsal capsulotomy, and syndactylization to the fourth toe (McFarland).

6. Underlapping Toe (Congenital Curly Toe)—Usually occurs at the lateral three toes and is rarely symptomatic. Surgery (flexor tenotomies) is infrequently indicated.

SELECTED BIBLIOGRAPHY

Adelaar, R.S., Williams, R.M., and Gould, J.S.: Congenital convex pes valgus: Results of an early comprehensive release and a review of congenital vertical talus at Richmond Crippled Children's Hospital and the University of Alabama in Birmingham. Foot Ankle 1:62–73, 1980.

Albright, J.A., and Miller, E.A.: Osteogenesis imperfecta (Editorial Comment). Clin. Orthop. 159:2, 1981.

Ali, M.S., and Hooper, G.: Congenital pseudarthrosis of the ulna due to neurofibromatosis. J. Bone Joint Surg. [Br.] 64:600–602, 1982.

Allen, B.L., Jr., and Ferguson, R.L.: The Galveston technique of pelvic fixation with Luque-rod instrumentation of the spine. Spine 9:388–394, 1984.

Barnes, M.J., and Herring, J.A.: Combined-split anterior tibial-tendon transfer and intramuscular lengthening of the posterior tibial tendon. J. Bone Joint Surg. [Am.] 73:734–738, 1991.

Bassett, G.S.: Lower-extremity abnormalities in dwarfing conditions. Instr. Course Lect. 39:389–397, 1990.

Bassett, G.S.: Orthopaedic aspects of skeletal dysplasias. Instr. Course Lect. 39:381–387, 1990.

Beals, R.K., and Rolfe, B.: Current concepts review. VATER association. A unifying concept of multiple anomalies. J. Bone Joint Surg. [Am.] 71:440, 1989.

Beaty, J.H.: Legg-Calvé-Perthes disease: Diagnostic and prognostic techniques. Instr. Course Lect. 38:291–296, 1989.

Beaty, J.H., and Canale, S.T.: Current concepts review. Orthopaedic aspects of myelomeningocele. J. Bone Joint Surg. [Am.] 72:626, 1990.

Berg, E.F.: A reappraisal of metatarsus adductus and skewfoot. J. Bone Joint Surg. 68A:1185, 1986.

Berkeley, M.E., Dickson, J.H., Cain, T.E., and Donovan, M.M.: Surgical therapy for congenital dislocation of the hip in patients who are twelve to thirty-six months old. J. Bone Joint Surg. [Am.] 66:412–420, 1984.

Bethem, D., Winter, R.B., Lutter, L., Moe, J.H., Bradford, D.S., Lonstein, J.E., and Langer, L.O.: Spinal disorders of dwarfism. J. Bone Joint Surg. [Am.] 63:1412–1425, 1981.

Bialik, V., Fishman, J., Katzir, J., et al.: Clinical assessment of hip instability in the newborn by an orthopedic surgeon and a pediatrician. J. Pediatr. Orthop. 6:703–705, 1986.

Bialik, V., Reuveni, A., Pery, M., et al.: Ultrasonography in developmental displacement of the hip: A critical analysis of our results. J. Pediatr. Orthop. 9:154–156, 1989.

Bleck, E.E.: Current concepts review. Management of the lower extremities in children who have cerebral palsy. J. Bone Joint Surg. [Am.] 72:140, 1990.

Bleck, E.E.: Metatarsus adductus: Classification and relationship to outcomes of treatment. J. Pediatr. Orthop. 3:2–9, 1983.

Bleck, E.E.: Orthopedic Management of Cerebral Palsy. Philadelphia, J.B. Lippincott, 1987.

Boal, D.K., and Schwenkter, E.P.: The infant hip: Assessment with real-time US. Radiology 157:667–672, 1985.

Boyd, H.B.: Pathology and natural history of congenital pseudarthrosis of the tibia. Clin. Orthop. 166:5–13, 1982.

Boyer, D.W., Mickelson, M.R., and Ponseti, I.V.: Slipped capital femoral epiphysis: Long-term follow-up study of 121 patients. J. Bone Joint Surg. [Am.] 63:85–95, 1981.

Bradford, D.S., Ahmed, K.B., Moe, J.H., Winter, R.B., and Lonstein, J.E.: The surgical management of patients with Scheuermann's disease: A review of twenty-four cases managed by combined anterior and posterior spine fusion. J. Bone Joint Surg. [Am.] 62:705–712, 1980.

Bradford, D.S., and Hensinger, R.M., eds.: The Pediatric Spine. New York, Thieme-Stratton, 1985.

Bradford, D.S., Lonstein, J.E., Ogilvie, J.W., and Winter, R.B., Eds.: Moe's Textbook of Scoliosis and Other Spinal Deformities, 2nd Ed. Philadelphia, W.B. Saunders Co., 1987.

Brown, F.W., and Pohnert, W.H.: Construction of a knee joint in meromelia tibia (congenital absence of the tibia). A 15 year follow-up study. J. Bone Joint Surg. 54A:1333, 1972.

Canale, S.T.: Problems and complications of slipped capital femoral epiphysis. Instr. Course Lect. 38:281–290, 1989.

Canale, S.T., Griffin, D.W., and Hubbard, C.N.: Congenital muscular torticollis. A long-term follow-up. J. Bone Joint Surg. [Am.] 64:810–816, 1982.

Canale, S.T., Harkness, R.M., Thomas, P.A., et al.: Does aspiration of bones and joints affect results of later bone scanning? J. Pediatr. Orthop. 5:23–26, 1985.

Carr, W.A., Moe, H.H., Winter, R.B., and Lonstein, J.E.: Treatment of idiopathic scoliosis in the Milwaukee brace. J. Bone Joint Surg. [Am.] 62:599–612, 1980.

Carroll, N.C.: Assessment and management of the lower extremity in myelodysplasia. Orthop. Clin. North Am. 18:709–724, 1987.

Carson, W.G., Lovell, W.W., and Whitesides, T.E., Jr.: Congenital elevation of the scapula. Surgical correction by the Woodward procedure. J. Bone Joint Surg. [Am.] 62:1199–1207, 1981.

Castelein, R.M., and Sauter, A.J.M.: Ultrasound screening for congenital dysplasia of the hip in newborns: Its value. J. Pediatr. Orthop. 8:666–670, 1988.

Catterall, A.: Legg-Calvé-Perthes Disease. Instr. Course Lect. 38:297–303, 1989.

Catterall, A.: Legg-Calvé-Perthes syndrome. Clin. Orthop. 158:41–52, 1981.

Certner, J.M., and Root, L.: Osteogenesis imperfecta. Orthop. Clin. North Am. 21:151–162, 1990.

Chambers, R.B., Cook, T.M., and Cowell, H.R.: Surgical reconstruction for calcaneonavicular coalition. Evaluation of function and gait. J. Bone Joint Surg. [Am.] 64:829–836, 1982.

Chiari, K.: Medial displacement osteotomy of the pelvis. Clin. Orthop. 98:55–71, 1974.

Christensen, F., Soballe, K., Ejsted, R., et al.: The Catterall classification of Perthes' disease: An assessment of reliability. J. Bone Joint Surg. [Br.] 68:614–615, 1986.

Clarke, N.M.P., Clegg, J., and Al-Chalabi, A.N.: Ultrasound screening of hips at risk for CDH: Failure to reduce the incidence of late cases. J. Bone Joint Surg. [Br.] 71:9–12, 1989.

Coleman, S.S.: Complex Foot Deformities in Children. Philadelphia, Lea & Febiger, 1983.

Coleman, S.S., and Chestnut, W.J.: A simple test for hindfoot flexibility in the cavovarus foot. Clin. Orthop. 123:60–62, 1977.

Cowell, H.R.: The management of club foot (Editorial). J. Bone Joint Surg. [Am.] 67:991–992, 1985.

Crawford, A.H.: The role of osteotomy in the treatment of slipped capital femoral epiphysis. Instr. Course Lect. 38:273–280, 1989.

Crawford, A.H., Jr., and Bagamery, N.: Osseous manifestations of neurofibromatosis in childhood. J. Pediatr. Orthop. 6:72–88, 1986.

Crawford, A.H., Marxen, J.L., and Osterfeld, D.L.: The Cincinnati incision: A comprehensive approach for surgical procedures of the foot and ankle in childhood. J. Bone Joint Surg. [Am.] 64:1355–1358, 1982.

Cummings, R.J., and Lovell, W.W.: Current concepts review: Operative treatment of congenital idiopathic club foot. J. Bone Joint Surg. [Am.] 70:1108, 1988.

Daoud, A., and Saighi-Bouaouina, A.: Treatment of sequestra, pseudarthroses, and defects in the long bones of children who have chronic hematogenous osteomyelitis. J. Bone Joint Surg. [Am.] 71:1448–1468, 1989.

Dawe, C., Wynne-Davies, R., and Fulford, G.E.: Clinical variation in dyschondrosteosis: A report on 13 individuals in 8 families. J. Bone Joint Surg. [Br.] 64:377–381, 1982.

Dee, R., Mango, E., and Hurst, L.C.: Principles of Orthopaedic Practice. New York, McGraw-Hill Book Co., 1989.

Dell, P.C., and Sheppard, J.E.: Thrombocytopenia, absent radius syndrome: Report of two siblings and review of the hematologic and genetic features. Clin. Orthop. 162:129–134, 1982.

Denis, F.: Cotrel-Dubousset instrumentation in the treatment of idiopathic scoliosis. Orthop. Clin. North Am. 19:291–311, 1988.

Dickhaut, S.C., and DeLee, J.C.: The discoid lateral-meniscus syndrome. J. Bone Joint Surg. [Am.] 64:1068–1073, 1982.

Dickson, J.H., Erwin, W.D., and Rossi, D.: Harrington instrumentation and arthrodesis for idiopathic scoliosis. A twenty-one-year follow-up. J. Bone Joint Surg. [Am.] 72:678, 1990.

Diggs, L.W.: Bone and joint lesions in sickle-cell disease. Clin. Orthop. 52:119–143, 1967.

Drummond, D.S., Moreau, M., and Cruess, R.L.: The results and complications of surgery for the paralytic hip and spine in myelomeningocele. J. Bone Joint Surg. [Br.] 62:49–53, 1980.

Engler, G.L.: Preoperative and intraoperative considerations in adolescent idiopathic scoliosis. Instr. Course Lect. 38:137–141, 1989.

Epps, C.H., Jr.: Current concept review: Proximal femoral focal deficiency. J. Bone Joint Surg. [Am.] 65:867–870, 1983.

Epps, C.H., Jr., and Schneider, P.L.: Treatment of hemimelias of the lower extremity. Long-term results. J. Bone Joint Surg. [Am.] 71:273, 1989.

Evans, G.A., Drennan, J.C., and Russman, B.S.: Functional classification and orthopaedic management of spinal muscular atrophy. J. Bone Joint Surg. [Br.] 63:516–622, 1981.

Fabry, F., and Meire, E.: Septic arthritis of the hip in children: Poor results after late and inadequate treatment. J. Pediatr. Orthop. 3:461–466, 1983.

Fackler, C.D.: Nonsurgical treatment of Legg-Calvé-Perthes disease. Instr. Course Lect. 38:305–308, 1989.

Ferguson, R.L., and Allen, B.L., Jr.: Considerations in the treatment of cerebral palsy patients with spinal deformities. Orthop. Clin. North Am. 19:419–425, 1988.

Fielding, J.W., Hensing, R.N., and Hawkins, R.J.: Os odontoideum. J. Bone Joint Surg. [Am.] 62:376–383, 1980.

Finsterbush, A., and Pogrund, H.: The hypermobility syndrome. Clin. Orthop. 168:124–127, 1982.

Fitch, R.D.: Introduction to pediatric orthopedics. In Sabiston's Essentials of Surgery, Sabiston, D.C., Jr., ed. Philadelphia, W.B. Saunders, 1987.

Gage, J.R., and Winter, R.B.: Avascular necrosis of the capital femoral epiphysis as a complication of closed reduction of congenital dislocation of the hip: A critical review of twenty years experiences at Gillette Children's Hospital. J. Bone Joint Surg. [Am.] 54:373–388, 1972.

Galpin, R.D., Roach, J.W., Wenger, D.R., et al.: One-stage treatment of congenital dislocation of the hip in older children, including femoral shortening. J. Bone Joint Surg. [Am.] 71:734, 1989.

Goldberg, M.J.: The Dysmorphic Child: An Orthopedic Perspective. New York, Raven Press, 1987.

Green, N.E., and Edwards, K.: Bone and joint infections in children. Orthop. Clin. North Am. 18:555–576, 1987.

Green, W.T.: The surgical correction of congenital elevation of the scapula (Sprengel's deformity). J. Bone Joint Surg. [Am]:149, 1957.

Guhl, J.: Osteochondritis dissecans in Shahriaree, H, Ed.: O'Connors Textbook of Arthroscopic Surgery. Philadelphia, J.B. Lippincott, 1984.

Hamanishi, C.: Congenital vertical talus: Classification with 69 cases and new measurement system. J. Pediatr. Orthop. 4:318–326, 1984.

Hayashi, L.K., Yamaga, H., Ida, K., and Miura, T.: Arthroscopic meniscectomy for discoid lateral meniscus in children. J. Bone Joint Surg. [Am.] 70:1348, 1988.

Hensinger, R.N., DeVito, P.D., and Ragsdale, C.G.: Changes in the cervical spine in juvenile rheumatoid arthritis. J. Bone Joint Surg. [Am.] 68:189–199, 1986.

Herndon, W.A., Knauer, S., Sullivan, J.A., et al.: Management of septic arthritis in children. J. Pediatr. Orthop. 6:576–578, 1986.

Herring, J.A.: Legg-Calvé-Perthes disease: A review of current knowledge. Instr. Course Lect. 38:309–315, 1989.

Hoffer, M.M., Feiwell, E., Perry, R., et al.: Functional ambulation in patients with myelomeningocele. J. Bone Joint Surg. [Am.] 55:137–148, 1973.

Insall, J.: Current concepts review: Patellar pain. J. Bone Joint Surg. [Am.] 64:147–152, 1982.

Iwasaki, K.: Treatment of congenital dislocation of the hip by the Pavlik harness: Mechanisms of reduction and usage. J. Bone Joint Surg. [Am.] 65:760–767, 1983.

Jackson, M.A., and Nelson, J.D.: Etiology and medical management of acute suppurative bone and joint infections in pediatric patients. J. Pediatr. Orthop. 2:313–323, 1982.

Jacobs, R.F., Adelman, L., Sack, C.M., et al.: Management of Pseudomonas osteochondritis complicating puncture wounds of the foot. Pediatrics 69:432–435, 1982.

Jacobsen, S.T., Crawford, A.H., Millar, E.A., and Steel, H.H.: The Syme amputation in patients with congenital pseudarthrosis of the tibia. J. Bone Joint Surg. [Am.] 65:533–537, 1983.

Jahss, M.H.: Evaluation of the cavus foot for orthopedic treatment. Clin. Orthop. 181:52–63, 1983.

Jones, K.L., and Robinson, L.K.: An approach to the child with structural defects. J. Pediatr. Orthop. 3:238–244, 1983.

Kalamchi, A., and McFarland, R., III: The Pavlik harness: Results in patients over 3 months of age. J. Pediatr. Orthop. 2:3–8, 1982.

Keller, R.B.: Nonoperative treatment of adolescent idiopathic scoliosis. Instr. Course Lect. 38:129–135, 1989.

King, H.A., Moe, J.H., Bradford, D.S., and Winter, R.B.: The selection of fusion levels in thoracic idiopathic scoliosis. J. Bone Joint Surg. [Am.] 65:1302–1313, 1983.

King, H., Moe, J., Bradford, D., and Winter, R.: Selection of fusion levels in thoracic idiopathic scoliosis. Orthop. Trans. 5:25, 1981.

Kling, T.F., Jr., and Hensinger, R.N.: Angular and torsional deformities of the lower limbs in children. Clin. Orthop. 176:136–147, 1983.

Koop, S.E., Winter, R.B., and Lonstein, J.E.: The surgical treatment of instability of the upper part of the cervical spine in children and adolescents. J. Bone Joint Surg. [Am.] 66:403–411, 1984.

Kopits, S.E.: Orthopedic complications of dwarfism. Clin. Orthop. 114:153–179, 1976.

Kostuik, J.P.: Current concepts review. Operative treatment of idiopathic scoliosis. J. Bone Joint Surg. [Am.] 72:1108, 1990.

Koval, K.J., Lehman, W.B., Rose, D., et al.: Treatment of slipped capital femoral epiphysis with a cannulated-screw technique. J. Bone Joint Surg. [Am.] 71:1370, 1989.

Kurz, L.T., Mubarak, S.J., Schultz, P., Park, S.M., and Leach, J.: Correlation of scoliosis and pulmonary function in Duchenne muscular dystrophy. J. Pediatr. Orthop. 3:347–353, 1983.

Langenskiold, A.: Tibia vara: Osteochondrosis of deformans tibae: Blount's disease. Clin. Orthop. 158:77–82, 1981.

Leibovic, S.J., Ehrlich, M.G., and Zaleske, D.J.: Sprengel deformity. J. Bone Joint Surg. [Am.] 72:192, 1990.

Lewin, J.S., Rosenfield, N.S., Hoffer, P.B., et al.: Acute osteomyelitis in children: Combined Tc-99m and Ga-67 imaging. Radiology 158:795–804, 1986.

Lonstein, J.E.: Adolescent idiopathic scoliosis: Screening and diagnosis. Instr. Course Lect. 38:105–113, 1989.

Lonstein, J.E., and Beck, K.: Hip dislocation and subluxation in cerebral palsy. J. Pediatr. Orthop. 6:521–526, 1986.

Lonstein, J.E., Bjorklunk, S., Wanninger, M.H., and Nelson, R.P.: Voluntary school screening for scoliosis in Minnesota. J. Bone Joint Surg. [Am.] 64:481–488, 1982.

Lonstein, J.E., and Carlson, J.M.: The prediction of curve progression in untreated idiopathic scoliosis during growth. J. Bone Joint Surg. [Am.] 66:1061–1071, 1984.

Lonstein, J.E., and Carlson, J.M.: Prognostication in idiopathic scoliosis. Orthop. Trans. 5:22, 1981.

Lowe, T.G.: Current concepts review. Scheuermann disease. J. Bone Joint Surg. [Am.] 72:940, 1990.

Luque, E.R.: Segmental spinal instrumentation for correction of scoliosis. Clin. Orthop. 163:192–198, 1982.

Maldague, B., and Malghem, J.: Dynamic radiologic patterns of Paget's disease of bone. Clin. Orthop. 217:126–151, 1987.

Mankin, H.J.: Rickets, osteomalacia, and renal osteodystrophy: An update. Orthop. Clin. North Am. 21:81–96, 1990.

Mazur, J.M., Shurtleff, D., Menelaus, M., et al.: Orthopaedic management of high-level spina bifida. Early walking compared with early use of a wheelchair. J. Bone Joint Surg. [Am.] 71:56, 1989.

McAndrew, M.P., and Weinstein, S.L.: A long-term follow-up of Legg-Calvé-Perthes disease. J. Bone Joint Surg. [Am.] 66:860–869, 1984.

McFarland, B.: Congenital deformaties of the spine and limbs in Platt, H., Ed.: Modern Trends in Orthopedics. New York, P.B. Hoeber, 1950, p. 107.

McKay, D.W.: New concept of and approach to clubfoot treatment: Section I—Principles and morbid anatomy. J. Pediatr. Orthop. 2:347–356, 1982.

McKusick, V.A.: Heritable Disorders of Connective Tissue, 4th ed. St. Louis, C.V. Mosby Company, 1972.

McMaster, M.J., and Ohtsuka, K.: The natural history of congenital scoliosis: A study of two hundred and fifty-one patients. J. Bone Joint Surg. [Am.] 64:1128–1147, 1982.

Mehta, M.H.: The rib-vertebra angle in the early diagnosis between resolving and progressive infantile scoliosis. J. Bone Joint Surg. 54B:230, 1973.

Mielke, C.H., Lonstein, J.E., Denis, F., et al.: Surgical treatment of adolescent idiopathic scoliosis: A comparative analysis. J. Bone Joint Surg. [Am.] 71:1170–1177, 1989.

Miller, J.A.A., Nachemson, A.L., and Schultz, A.B.: Effectiveness of braces in mild idiopathic scoliosis. Spine 9:632–635, 1984.

Montgomery, S., and Hall, J.: Congenital kyphosis: Surgical treatment at Boston Children's Hospital. Orthop. Trans. 5:25, 1981.

Moore, K.L.: The Developing Human. Philadelphia, W.B. Saunders Company, 1982.

Morrissy, R.T.: Principles of in situ fixation in chronic slipped capital femoral epiphysis. Instr. Course Lect. 38:257–262, 1989.

Morrissy, Raymond T., ed. Lovell & Winter's Pediatric Orthopaedics, 3rd ed. Philadelphia, J.B. Lippincott Co., 1990.

Morrissy, R.T.: A symposium: Congenital pseudarthrosis. Clin. Orthop. 166:1–61, 1982.

Moseley, C.F.: Assessment and prediction in leg-length discrepancy. Instr. Course Lect. 38:325–330, 1989.

Mose, K.: Legg-Calvé Perthes disease: A comparison among three methods of conservative treatment. Arhus Universitets Fortuget, 1964.

Moses, J.M., Flatt, E.E., and Cooper, R.R.: Annular constricting bands. J. Bone Joint Surg. [Am.] 61:562–565, 1979.

Olney, B.W., and Asher, M.A.: Excision of symptomatic coalition of the middle facet of the talocalcaneal joint. J. Bone Joint Surg. [Am.] 69:539–544, 1987.

Oppenheim, W., Smith, C., and Christie, W.: Congenital vertical talus. Foot Ankle 5:198–204, 1985.

Orthopaedic Knowledge Update Home Study Syllabus I, II, and III. Chicago: American Academy of Orthopaedic Surgeons, 1984, 1987, 1990.

Paley, D.: Current techniques of limb lengthening. J. Pediatr. Orthop. 8:73–92, 1988.

Pang, D., and Wilberger, J.E., Jr.: Spinal cord injury without radiographic abnormalities in children. J. Neurosurg. 57:114–129, 1982.

Poppas, A.M.: Osteochondrosis dissecans. Clin. Orthop. 158:59–69, 1981.

Paterson, D.: Congenital pseudarthrosis of the tibia. Clin. Orthop. 247:44–54, 1989.

Peterson, H.A.: Skewfoot (forefoot adduction with heel valgus). J. Pediatr. Orthop. 6:24–30, 1986.

Price, C.T.: Metaphyseal and physeal lengthening. Instr. Course Lect. 38:331–336, 1989.

Pueschel, S.M., Herndon, J.H., Gelch, M.M., Senft, K.E., Scola, F.H., and Goldberg, M.J.: Symptomatic atlantoaxial subluxation in persons with Down syndrome. J. Pediatr. Orthop. 4:682–688, 1984.

Quinlan, W.R., Brady, P.G., and Regan, B.F.: Congenital pseudarthrosis of the clavicle. Acta Orthop. Scand. 51:489–492, 1980.

Ramsey, P.L., Lasser, S., and MacEwen, G.D.:Congenital dislocation of the hip: Use of the Pavlik harness in the child during the first six months of life. J. Bone Joint Surg. [Am.] 58:1000–1004, 1976.

Rees, D., Jones, M.W., Owen, R., et al.: Scoliosis surgery in the Prader-Willi syndrome. J. Bone Joint Surg. [Br.] 71:685–688, 1989.

Rennie, A.M.: The inheritance of slipped upper femoral epiphysis. J. Bone Joint Surg. [Br.] 64:180–184, 1982.

Richardson, E.G., and Rambach, B.E.: Proximal femoral focal deficiency: A clinical appraisal. South. Med. J. 72:166–173, 1979.

Rubin, P.: Dynamic Classification of Bone Dysplasias. Chicago, Year Book Medical Publishers, 1964.

Salter, R.B., Hansson, G., and Thompson, G.H.: Innominate osteotomy in the management of residual congenital subluxation of the hip in young adults. Clin. Orthop. 182:53–68, 1984.

Schaller, J.G.: Chronic arthritis in children: Juvenile rheumatoid arthritis. Clin. Orthop. 182:79–89, 1984.

Schoenecker, P.L., Capelli, A.M., Millar, E.A., et al.: Congenital longitudinal deficiency of the tibia. J. Bone Joint Surg. [Am.] 71:278, 1989.

Schoenecker, P.L., Meade, W.C., Pierron, R.L., et al.: Blount's disease: A retrospective review and recommendations for treatment. J. Pediatr. Orthop. 5:181–186, 1985.

Schrock, R.D.: Congenital abnormalities at the cervicothoracic level. AADS Instr. Course Lect. 6, 1949.

Scoles, P.V., and Quinn, T.P.: Intervertebral discitis in children and adolescents. Clin. Orthop. 162:31–36, 1982.

Segal, L.S., Drummond D.S., Zanott, R.M., Ecker, M.L., and Mubanik, S.J.: Complications of posterior arthrodesis of the cervical spine in patients who have Down syndrome. J. Bone Joint Surg. [Am] 73:1547–1554, 1991.

Shapiro, F.: Consequences of an osteogenesis imperfecta diagnosis for survival and ambulation. J. Pediatr. Orthop. 5:456–462, 1985.

Shapiro, F., and Bresnan, M.J.: Orthopaedic management of childhood neuromuscular disease. Part II: Peripheral neuropathies, Friedreich's ataxia, and arthrogryposis multiplex congenita. J. Bone Joint Surg. [Am.] 64:949–953, 1982.

Sillence, D.O.: Osteogenesis imperfecta: An expanding panorama of variance. Clin. Orthop. 159:11, 1981.

Simons, G.W.: Analytical radiography of club feet. J. Bone Joint Surg. [Br.] 59:485–489, 1974.

Simons, G.W.: A comparative evaluation of the current methods for open reduction of the congenitally displaced hip. Orthop. Clin. North Am. 11:161–181, 1980.

Simons, G.W.: Complete subtalar release in club feet: Part I. A preliminary report. Part II. Comparison with less extensive procedures. J. Bone Joint Surg. [Am.] 67:1044–1065, 1985.

Smith, A.D., Koreska, J., and Moseley, C.F.: Progression of scoliosis in Duchenne muscular dystrophy. J. Bone Joint Surg. [Am.] 71:1066–1074, 1989.

Sofield, H.A., and Miller, E.A.: Fragmentation realignment, and intramedullary rod fixation of deformities of the long bones in children. J. Bone Joint Surg. 41A:1371, 1959.

Sörenson, K.H.: Scheuermann's Juvenile Kyphosis. Copenhagen, Munksgaard, 1964.

Southwick, W.O.: Compression fixation after biplane intertrochanteric osteotomy for slipped capital femoral epiphysis. J. Bone Joint Surg. [Am] 55:1218, 1973.

Staheli, L.T., Clawson, D.K., and Hubbard, D.D.: Medial femoral torsion: Experience with operative treatment. Clin. Orthop. 146:222–225, 1980.

Staheli, L.T., Coleman, S.S., Hensinger, R.N., et al.: Congenital hip dysplasia. Instr. Course Lect. 33:350–363, 1984.

Staheli, L.T., Corbett, M., Wyss, C., et al.: Lower-extremity rotational problems in children: Normal values to guide management. J. Bone Joint Surg. [Am.] 67:39–47, 1985.

Stanescur, V., Stanescur, R., and Maroteaux, P.: Pathogenic mechanisms in osteochondrodysplasias. J. Bone Joint Surg. [Am.] 66:817–836, 1984.

Steele, H.H.: Triple osteotomy of the innominate bone. J. Bone Joint Surg. [Am.] 55:343–350, 1973.

Stromqvist, B., and Sunden, G.: CDH diagnosed at 2 to 12 months of age. J. Pediatr. Orthop. 9:208–212, 1989.

Sutherland, D.H., and Greenfield, R.: Double innominate osteotomy. J. Bone Joint Surg. [Am.] 59:1082–1091, 1977.

Suzuki, S., and Yamamuro, T.: Avascular necrosis in patients treated with the Pavlik harness for congenital dislocation of the hip. J. Bone Joint Surg. [Am.] 72:181, 1990.

Swanson, A.B.: A classification for congenital limb malformation. J. Hand Surg. 1:8–22, 1976.

Tachdjian, M.O.: Pediatric Orthopaedics, 2nd ed. Philadelphia, W.B. Saunders, 1990.

Tetzlaff, T.R., McCracken, G.H., Jr., and Nelson, J.D.: Oral antibiotic therapy for skeletal infections of children: II. Therapy of osteomyelitis and arthritis. J. Pediatr. 92:485–490, 1978.

Thompson, G.H.: Arthrogryposis multiplex congenita (Editorial). Clin. Orthop. 194:2–3, 1985.

Tolo, V.T.: Spinal deformity in short-stature syndromes. Instr. Course Lect. 39: 381–387, 1990.

Tolo, V.T.: Surgical treatment of adolescent idiopathic scoliosis. Instr. Course Lect. 38:143–156, 1989.

Tredwell, S.J., and Davis, L.A.: Prospective study of congenital dislocation of the hip. J. Pediatr. Orthop. 9:386–390, 1989.

Turco, V.J.: Resistant congenital club foot—One-stage posteromedial release with internal fixation: A follow-up report of a 15-year experience. J. Bone Joint Surg. [Am.] 61:805–814, 1979.

Victoria-Diaz, A., and Victoria-Diaz, J.: Pathogenesis of idiopathic club foot. Clin. Orthop. 185:14–24, 1984.

Viere, R.G., Birch, J.F., Herring, J.A., et al.: Use of the Pavlik harness in congenital dislocation of the hip. An analysis of failures of treatment. J. Bone Joint Surg. [Am.] 72:238, 1990.

Woodard, J.W.: Congenital elevation of the scapula, correction by release and transplanation of muscle origins. J. Bone Joint Surg. [Am] 43:219, 1961.

Weiner, D.S.: Bone graft epiphysiodesis in the treatment of slipped capital femoral epiphysis. Instr. Course Lect. 38:263–272, 1989.

Weinstein, S.L.: Adolescent idiopathic scoliosis: prevalence and natural history. Instr. Course Lect. 38:115–128, 1989.

Weinstein, S.L.: Indiopathic scoliosis: Natural history. Spine 11:780–783, 1986.

Weinstein, S.L., and Ponseti, I.V.: Curve progression in indiopathic scoliosis. J. Bone Joint Surg. [Am.] 65:447–455, 1983.

Winter, R.B., and Lonstein, J.E.: Adult idiopathic scoliosis treated with Luque or Harrington rods and subluminar wiring. J. Bone Joint Surg. [Am.] 71:1308, 1989.

Winter, R.B., Lonstein, J.E., Drogt, J., et al.: The effectiveness of bracing in the nonoperative treatment of idiopathic scoliosis. Spine 11:790–791, 1986.

Winter, R.B., Moe, J.H., Bradford, D.S., Lonstein, J.E., Pedras, C.V., and Weber, A.H.: Spine deformity in neurofibromatosis: A review of 102 patients. J. Bone Joint Surg. [Am.] 61:677–694, 1979.

Winter, R.B., Moe, J.H., and Lonstein, J.E.: The incidence of Klippel-Feil syndrome in patients with congenital scoliosis and kyphosis. Spine 9:363–366, 1984.

Winter, R.B., Moe, J.H., and Lonstein, J.E.: Posterior spinal arthrodesis for congenital scoliosis: An analysis of the cases of two hundred and ninety patients, five to nineteen years old. J. Bone Joint Surg. [Am.] 66:1188–1197, 1984.

Winter, R.B., Moe, J.H., and Lonstein, J.E.: The surgical treatment of congenital kyphosis. A review of 94 patients age 5 years or older, with 2 years or more follow-up in 77 patients. Spine 10:224–231, 1985.

Waldenström, J.: Der obere tuberkulöse cullumherd. Z. Orthop. Chir. 24:487, 1909.

Zinman, C., Wolfson, N., and Reis, N.D.: Osteochondritis dissecans of the dome of the talus. Computed tomography scanning in diagnosis and follow-up. J. Bone Joint Surg. [Am.] 70:1017, 1988.

Zionts, L.E., and MacEwen, G.D.: Treatment of congenital dislocation of the hip in children between the ages of one and three years. J. Bone Joint Surg. [Am.] 68:829–846, 1986.

CHAPTER 2

Basic Sciences

Part 1

Biomechanics

I. **Basic Definitions**

A. Biomechanics—The science of the action of forces, internal or external, on the living body.

B. Statics—The study of the action of forces on bodies at rest (in equilibrium).

C. Dynamics—The study of the motion of bodies and forces that produce the motion. There are three subtypes:

 1. Kinematics—The study of motion in terms of displacement, velocity, and acceleration without reference to the cause of the motion.

 2. Kinetics—Relates the action of forces on bodies to their resulting action.

 3. Kinesiology—The study of human movement/motion.

II. **Principal Quantities**

A. Basic Quantities—Described in the International System of units (SI), or metric system.

 1. Length—Meter (m)

 2. Mass—Amount of matter (kilogram [kg])

 3. Time—Second (s)

B. Derived Quantities (from Basic Quantities)

 1. Velocity—Time rate of change of displacement (m/s)

 2. Acceleration—Time rate of change of velocity (m/s^2)

 3. Force—Action of one body upon another (kg·m/s^2 [N])

III. **Newton's Laws**

A. First Law: Inertia—If a zero net external force acts on a body, the body will remain at rest or move uniformly. This allows us to do static analysis with the equation $\Sigma F = 0$ (the sum of the external forces applied to a body equals zero).

B. Second Law: Acceleration—$F = ma$ (the acceleration [a] of an object of mass m is directly proportional to the force applied to the object). Helps in dynamic analysis.

C. Third Law: Reactions—For every action there is an equal and opposite reaction. Leads to free body analysis.

IV. **Scalar and Vector Quantities**

A. Scalar Quantities—Have magnitude but no direction. Examples include volume, time, mass, and speed (not velocity).

B. Vector Quantities—Have magnitude and direction. Examples include force and velocity. Vectors have four characteristics: (1) magnitude (length of the vector); (2) direction (head of the vector); (3) point of application (tail of the vector); and (4) line of action (orientation of the vector). Vectors can be added, subtracted, and split into components (resolved) for analysis. The resultant of two vectors follows the principle of "parallelogram of forces."

V. **Free Body Analysis**—Uses forces, moments, and free body diagrams to analyze the action of forces on bodies.

A. Forces—A push or a pull causing external (acceleration) and internal (strain) effects. Forces can be split into their **components** (usually in the x and y directions) for easier analysis. Some elementary knowledge of trigonometry is helpful ($F_x = F \cos \theta$, $F_y = F \sin \theta$). Also, remember the following simple approximations:

$\sin 30° = \cos 60° \cong 0.5$
$\sin 45° = \cos 45° \cong 0.7$
$\sin 60° = \cos 30° \cong 0.9$

Representation of forces acting at a point is often an idealized situation, and actually is an integration of a distributed load over its applied area. The **resultant force** is represented as a single force equivalent to a system of forces acting on a body. The **equilibrant force** is of equal magnitude and opposite to the resultant force.

B. Moment—The rotational effect of a force on a body about a point (N·m). Any force acting at a distance from a point can produce a moment. The moment (or "torque") equals the force times the

37

perpendicular distance from a specified point (moment arm): $M = F \times d$.

C. Free Body Diagram (FBD)—Sketch of a body or portion thereof isolated from all other bodies and showing all forces acting upon it. Weight of objects acts through the center of gravity (CG). **The CG for the human body is just anterior to S2.**

D. Free Body Analysis—Can proceed after all forces are represented on the FBD; using the concept of equilibrium ($\Sigma F = 0$ and $\Sigma M = 0$), solve for unknowns. Assumes no change in motion, deformation, or friction. The following steps are used in analysis.
   1. Identify the system (objective, knowns, assumptions).
   2. Select a coordinate system.
   3. Isolate free bodies—FBD.
   4. Apply Newton's laws ($\Sigma F = 0$; $\Sigma M = 0$).
   5. Solve for unknowns.

E. Example—Calculate the biceps force necessary to suspend the weight of the forearm (20 N) with the elbow flexed to 90 degrees; assume biceps insertion is 5 cm distal to elbow and CG of forearm is 15 cm distal to elbow (Fig. 2–1). (Answer: 60 N.) Also solve for the joint force (J) (Fig. 2–1). (Answer: 40 N.)

VI. Other Important Basic Concepts

A. Work—Force acts on body to cause displacement. Work (W) = Force (only components parallel to the displacement) × Distance. Units: N·m [joules].

B. Energy—Ability to perform work (also joules). According to the Law of Conservation of Energy, energy is neither created or destroyed; it is transferred from one condition to another.

1. Potential Energy—Stored energy; the ability of a body to do work as a result of its position or configuration (strain energy).
2. Kinetic Energy—Energy than an object has due to its motion (velocity): $KE = \frac{1}{2} mv^2$.

C. Friction (f)—Resistance between two bodies when one slides over the other. Oriented opposite the applied force. When the applied force is $>f$, motion will begin.

D. Piezoelectricity—Electrical charge from deformation of crystalline structures when forces are applied. Concave (compression) side = electronegative, convex (tension) side = electropositive.

VII. Strength of Materials

A. Definition—A branch of mechanics that deals with relationships between externally applied loads and the resulting internal effects and deformations induced in the body subjected to these loads.
   1. Loads—Forces that act on a body (compression, tension, shear, torsion).
   2. Deformations—Temporary (elastic) or permanent (plastic) change in the shape of a body.
   3. Change in load produces change in deformation.

B. Stress—Intensity of internal force: **Stress = Force/Area.** Used to analyze the internal resistance of a body to a load. Helps in selection of materials. Can be compressive, tensile (a.k.a. normal; occurs in a direction perpendicular to applied force), or shear (occurs parallel to applied force). Stress has the units of N/m^2 (pascals [Pa]).

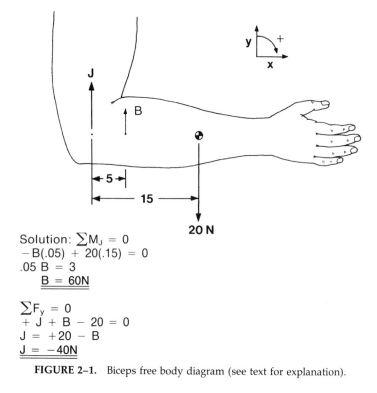

Solution: $\sum M_J = 0$
$-B(.05) + 20(.15) = 0$
$.05 B = 3$
$\underline{B = 60N}$

$\sum F_y = 0$
$+ J + B - 20 = 0$
$J = +20 - B$
$\underline{J = -40N}$

FIGURE 2–1. Biceps free body diagram (see text for explanation).

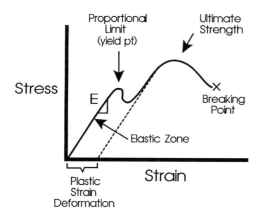

FIGURE 2–2. Stress-strain curve (see text for explanation).

C. Strain—Relative measure of the **deformation** of a body **as a result of loading**: Strain = change in Length/Original Length of an object. This can also be normal or shear. Strain is a proportion and therefore has no units.

D. Hooke's Law—Basically, stress is proportional to strain up to a limit (the proportional limit).

E. Young's Modulus (of Elasticity) (*E*)—A measure of the stiffness of a material or its ability to resist deformation: *E* = Stress/Strain (in elastic range of stress-strain curve it is the slope).

F. Stress-Strain Curve—Derived by axially loading a body and plotting stress vs. strain (Fig. 2–2).

   1. Proportional Limit (Yield Point)—Transition point from elastic to plastic range. Usually 0.2% strain in most metals.

   2. Ultimate Strength—Maximum strength obtained by material.

   3. Breaking Point—Point where the material fractures.

   4. Plastic Deformation—Change in length after removing load (before the breaking point) in the plastic range.

   5. Strain Energy—Area under the curve. Total Strain Energy = Recoverable Strain Energy (resilience) + Dissipated Strain Energy. A measure of the toughness of a material.

VIII. Materials versus Structures

A. Material—Related to a substance or element. Defined by mechanical properties (force, stress, strain) and rheologic properties (elasticity [ability to regain original shape], plasticity [permanent deformation], viscosity [resistance to flow or shear stress], and strength).

   1. Brittle materials (e.g., PMMA)—Exhibit a linear stress-strain curve up to the point of failure.

   2. Ductile materials (e.g., metal)—Undergo a large amount of plastic deformation prior to failure.

   3. Viscoelastic materials (e.g., bone and ligaments)—Exhibit stress-strain behavior that is time-rate dependent, and varies with the material. For example, in a bone-ligament interface, a slow rate of loading will result in an avulsion fracture of bone but a fast rate of loading will cause ligament failure.

   4. Isotropic materials—Possess the same mechanical properties in all directions.

   5. Anisotropic materials—Have mechanical properties that vary with the orientation of loading.

   6. Homogeneous materials—Have a uniform structure or composition throughout.

B. Structure—Related to both the material and shape of an object and its loading characteristics. A load deformation curve can be constructed similar to a stress-strain curve. The slope of the curve in the elastic range is referred to as the rigidity (vs. stiffness) of the structure. Bending rigidity is proportional to the base times the height cubed for a rectangular structure ($bh^3/12$), and is proportional to the radius to the fourth power for a cylinder (**torsional rigidity** $\propto \pi r^4/L$). This is closely related to the moment of inertia (*I*; resistance to bending), which is a function of the width and thickness of a structure; and the polar moment of inertia (*J*), which represents the resistance to torsion (twisting). The following equations use these concepts:

$$\sigma = my/I \tag{2–1}$$

$$\tau = Tr/J \tag{2–2}$$

IX. Orthopaedic Materials

A. Metals—Demonstrate stress-strain curves discussed in Section VII above. Other important concepts follow.

   1. Fatigue Failure—Occurs with repetitive loading cycles at stress below the ultimate tensile strength. Fatigue failure depends on the magnitude of the stress and number of cycles. If the stress is less than a predetermined amount of stress called the endurance limit, the material may be loaded cyclically an infinite number of times ($>10^6 \cdot$ cycles) without breaking. Above the endurance limit, the fatigue life of a material is expressed by the Stress (S) vs. number of loading cycles(n), or S-n, curve.

   2. Creep (a.k.a. Cold Flow)—Progressive deformation of metals over an extended period of time. If sudden stress followed by constant loading causes a material to continue to deform, then it demonstrates creep. This can produce a permanent deformity and may affect mechanical function (e.g., in a total joint arthroplasty [TJA]).

   3. Corrosion—Chemical dissolving of metals as may occur in the high-saline environment of the body. Several types of corrosion may occur:

Corrosion	Description
Galvanic	Dissimilar metals[a]; electrochemical destruction
Crevice	Occurs in fatigue cracks with low O_2 tension
Stress	Occurs in areas with high stress gradients
Fretting	From small movements abrading outside layer
Other	Includes inclusion, intergranular, and others

[a] Metals such as 316L stainless steel and Co-Cr-Mo will produce galvanic corrosion.

Corrosion can be decreased by using similar metals (e.g., with plates and screws), with proper design of implants, and with passivation (a thin layer that effectively separates the metal from the solution [e.g., stainless steel coating chromium oxide]).

4. Types of metals—Implants used in orthopaedics are typically made of 316L (L = low carbon) stainless steel (iron, chromium, and nickel), "supermetal" alloys (e.g., cobalt-chromium-molybdenum [65% Co, 35% Cr, 5% Mo] made with a special forging process), and titanium (Ti-6Al-4V). Each possesses a **different stiffness (E)** that will be compared with other materials below (Fig. 2–3). Problems associated with certain metals include stress shielding (increased with higher E metals); ion release (Co-Cr causes macrophage proliferation and synovial degeneration; Ti particulates may incite a histiocytic response); unknown association with neoplasms; and wear.

B. Nonmetals—Include polyethylenes, polymethyl methacrylate (PMMA—bone cement), silicone, and ceramics.

1. High-Density Polyethylene (HDP)—An ultra-high-molecular-weight polymer consisting of long chains of carbons used in weight-bearing components of TJAs. These materials are tough, ductile, resilient, and resistant to wear and exhibit low friction. Polyethylenes are viscoelastic and are susceptible to abrasion. They are also thermoplastic and may be altered by high-dose radiation. They are weaker than bone in tension and have a low E. Wear debris is associated with a histiocytic osteolytic response. Wear is increased with thinner (<5 mm), flatter, carbon fiber–reinforced polyethylene. Metal backing may help minimize plastic deformation of HDP (and loosening) but decreases its effective thickness (wear).

2. Poly-methyl-methacrelate (PMMA—bone cement)—Used for fixation (as a grout and not an adhesive) and load distribution for implants. It has poor tensile strength, is weaker than bone in compression, and has a low E. Reduction in the number of voids with insertion (vacuum, centrifugation, good technique) increases cement strength and decreases cracking. PMMA functions by mechanically interlocking with bone. **Insertion can lead to a precipitous drop in blood pressure**. Wear particles can incite a macrophage response that leads to loosening of prosthesis.

3. Silicones—Polymers used for replacement in non–weight-bearing joints. Their poor strength and wear capability are responsible for frequent synovitis with extended use.

4. Ceramics—A broad class of materials that contain metallic and nonmetallic elements bonded ionically in a highly oxidized state. Include biostable (inert) materials such as Al_2O_3 and bioactive (degradable) substances such as bioglass. They typically have a "high E," a high compressive strength, and a low tensile strength, are brittle, and have poor crack resistance characteristics. Their high conduciveness to tissue bonding is due to **high surface wetability and** high surface **tension**, which is also responsible for less friction and wear. Additionally, small grain size allows for an ultrasmooth finish and less friction. Calcium phosphates (e.g., hydroxyapatite) may have application as a coating (plasma sprayed) to allow increased strength of attachment and promote bone healing.

5. Other materials, such as polylactic acid–coated carbon, which serves as a biodegradable scaffolding, and newer polymer composites, some with carbon fiber reinforcement, are still investigational. Fabrication of these newer devices involves assembling "piles" of carbon fibers impregnated with matrix polymer (polysulfone or polyetheretherketone). Difficulties with abrasion and impact resis-

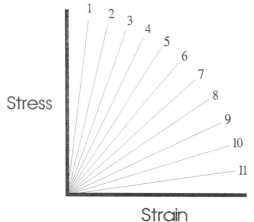

1. Al$_2$O$_3$ (ceramic)
2. Co-Cr-Mo (Alloy)
3. Stainless steel
4. Titanium
5. Cortical bone
6. Matrix polymers (PS, PEEK)
7. PMMA
8. Polyethylene
9. Cancellous bone
10. Tendon/ligament
11. Cartilage

Stress

Strain

Relative Values of Youngs Modulus
(Not to scale)

FIGURE 2–3. Comparison of Young's modulus (relative values; not to scale) for various orthopaedic materials.

tance, radiolucency, and manufacturing are still present.

C. Biomaterials—Possess certain unique characteristics including viscoelasticity (time dependent stress-strain behavior; discussed in Section VIII: Materials Versus Structures, A: Material), creep (discussed above), and stress relaxation (internal stresses decrease with time). They also are capable of self-adaptation and repair, and characteristics change with aging and sampling. Specific biomaterials are discussed below.

1. Bone—A composite of collagen and hydroxyapatite. Collagen has a low *E*, good tensile strength, and poor compressive strength. Calcium apatite is a stiff, brittle material with good compressive strength. The combination is an anisotropic material that resists many forces; it is **strongest in compression**, weakest in shear, and intermediate in tension. Cancellous is 25% as dense, 10% as stiff, and 500% as ductile as cortical bone. Bone is a dynamic material because of its ability for self-repair changes with aging (becomes stiffer and less ductile), and changes with prolonged immobilization (weaker).

2. Tendon—Strong in tension only; *E* is only 10% that of bone, but increases with slower loading. Fibers are oriented parallel. Demonstrates stress relaxation and creep.

3. Ligament—Fibers can be oriented parallel if it is required to resist major joint stress, or more randomly if it must resist forces from different directions. Stiffness = Force/Strain, as depicted on a force deformation graph (similar to *E* but does not consider the cross-sectional area). The bone-ligament complex will be softer (less stiff—decreased *E*) and have a lower yield point and tensile strength with prolonged immobilization. Bone resorption at the tendon insertion site also occurs.

4. Articular Cartilage—Contains 60% water, 25% collagen, and 15% proteoglycan. The ultimate tensile strength of cartilage is only 5% of bone, and *E* is 0.1% that of bone, nevertheless, because of its highly viscoelastic properties, it is well suited for compressive loading. Deformation and shift of water to/from cartilage is largely responsible for this.

D. Comparison of Common Orthopaedic Materials—Young's modulus of elasticity (*E*) for various orthopaedic materials is compared in Figure 2–3.

X. Orthopaedic Structures

A. Bone

1. Stress concentration effects, which occur at points of defects within the bone or implant-bone interface (stress risers), reduce overall strength with loading. Stress shielding by implants results in osteoporosis of adjacent bone due to lack of normal physiologic stresses. This occurs commonly under plates and at the femoral calcar in high-riding total hip arthroplasties. A hole of 20–30% of the bone diameter, regardless of whether it is filled with a screw, will reduce overall strength up to 50% and does not return to normal until 9–12 months following screw removal. Cortical defects can reduce strength 70% or more (less with oval defects due to less stress riser). Bone is anisotropic and viscoelastic. Cortical bone is excellent vs. torque; cancellous bone is good vs. compressive and shear forces.

2. Fracture—Type is based upon mechanism.
   a. Tension—By muscle pull, typically transverse, perpendicular to load and bone axis.
   b. Compression—By axial loading of cancellous bone.
   c. Shear—Commonly around joints; load parallel to bone surface, and fracture parallel to load.
   d. Bending—By eccentric loading or direct blows. Fracture begins on tension side and continues transversely/obliquely.
   e. Torsion—Shear and tensile stresses result in spiral fractures.

B. Ligaments and Tendons—These structures can sustain 5–10% tensile strain before failure (vs. bone, 1–4%). Tension rupture of fibers and shear failure between fibers commonly occurs. Most ligaments can undergo plastic strain to the point at which they cannot function effectively but are still in continuity. Soft tissue implants include stents, ligament augmentation devices, and scaffolding.

1. Stents—Internal splint devices. These include the Proplast Tendon Transfer Stabilizer using synthetic polymers, Gore-Tex Prosthetic ligaments, Xenotech (bovine tendon), and polyester implants. All are limited by not allowing adequate collagen ingrowth and eventually will fail.

2. Ligament augmentation devices (LADs) such as the Kennedy LAD (polypropylene yarn) and Dacron do allow some fibrous ingrowth, but use is limited.

3. Biodegradable Tissue Scaffolding—Allows immediate stability and long-term replacement with host tissue. Carbon fiber and polylactic acid (PLA)-coated carbon fiber devices have been used with limited success (slow ingrowth is improved with PLA coating).

C. Nonmetal Structures

1. Polyethylene—Used for acetabular cups and tibial trays. Newer ultrahigh-molecular-weight polyethylene (UHMWPE) has shown superior wear characteristics over high-density polyethylene (HDP).

2. PMMA—Weaker than bone, becomes weaker with antibiotic addition and porosity. Addition of carbon fibers may increase its strength.

D. Metal Implants

1. Screws—Characterized by pitch (distance between threads), lead (distance advanced in one revolution), root diameter (minimal/inner diameter ∝ tensile strength), and **outer diameter** (determines holding power [**pull-out strength**]).

2. Plates—Strength related to material and moment of inertia (thickness most important: rigidity ∝ t^3). Plates are most effective on the tension side. Types of plates include static compression (best in upper extremity; can be

stressed for compression), dynamic compression (e.g., tension band plate), neutralization (resists torsion), and buttress (protects bone graft). Stress concentration at open screw holes can lead to implant failure. **Serves best against tensile forces on plated side.** Blade plates provide increased resistance to torsional deformation in subtrochanteric fractures.

3. Intramedullary (IM) Nails—Require a high J to maximize torsional rigidity and strength. Reaming allows increased torsional resistance due to increased contact area and allows use of a larger nail with increased rigidity and strength. IM nails are better at resisting bending than rotational forces. Unslotted nails allow stronger fixation and less diameter, but at the expense of flexibility. Posterior starting points for femoral nails decrease hoop stresses and comminution of fractures.

4. External Fixators—**Increased rigidity with larger diameter pins** (most important), more pins, and placement of pins closer to the fracture site and in different planes. The rigidity of the frame itself is of secondary importance. The use of half pins may provide more secure fixation and lower incidence of pin loosening. Addition of a second bar in the same plane provides increased resistance to bending moments in the sagittal plane.

5. Total Hip Arthroplasty (THA)—Design has evolved to help reduce biomechanical constraints. Femoral components are designed for use with and without cement. Stem length is directly related to rigidity. Minimum compressive and tensile stresses in adjacent structures result from a design with a broad medial surface, a broader lateral surface, and a large moment of inertia. Femoral component design must account for rotational forces. Placement of the femoral component should be in neutral or slight valgus to decrease the moment arm, cement stress, and abductor length. Femoral head size should be a compromise between smaller (22-mm) components with decreased friction and torque but decreased ROM/stability, and larger (36-mm) components with increased friction and torque but increased ROM/stability. A 26- or 28-mm head seems to be ideal in most instances. Metal backing of acetabular components decreases the stress in cement and cancellous bone. Use of different metal alloys and titanium (with E closer to cortical bone) is being investigated. The use of Ti on weight-bearing surfaces may lead to fretting and blackening of soft tissues. UHMWPE serves as a "shock absorber" and should be at least 5 mm thick to prevent creep. Wear rate of UHMWPE in the acetabulum is about 0.1 mm/year. Other new concepts include computer design of THA stems, modularity, custom designs, and more flexible stems.

6. Total Knee Arthroplasty (TKA)—Design has evolved significantly after original design errors that did not take kinematics of the human knee into consideration (i.e., original hinge design). An appropriate compromise between total contact designs with excess stability (and less motion) but less wear and low-contact design with less stability and increased wear is being approached. Metal alloys are typically used.

7. Compression Hip Screws—Demonstrate loading characteristics superior to blade plates. Higher angled plates are subjected to lower bending loads but may be more difficult to insert. Sliding of the screw is proportional to the screw/side plate angle and the length of the screw in the barrel.

E. Implant Fixation—Three basic forms exist: interference fit, interlocking, and biologic.

1. Interlocking fit or mechanical or press fit components rely on the formation of a fibrous tissue interface. Loosening can occur if stability is not maintained and high-E substances are used (leading to increased bone resorption/remodeling).

2. Interlocking fit with PMMA as a grout, with a low E, allows a gradual transfer of stresses to bone. Aseptic loosening can occur over time. Careful technique with limiting of porosities and gaps and using a 3–5-mm thickness yields best results. Other improvements include low-viscosity cement, better bed preparation, plugging and pressurization, and better cement mixing.

3. Biologic fit or tissue ingrowth makes use of fiber-metal composites, void metal composites, or microbeads to create pore sizes of 40–400 μ (ideally 100–250 μ). Mechanical stability is required for ingrowth, which has been limited to 10–30% of the surface area. Problems include fiber/bead loosening, increased cost, proximal bone resorption (monocyte/macrophage mediated), corrosion, and decreased implant fatigue strength.

F. Bone-Implant Unit—The integrated unit is a composite structure that has shared properties. The more accurately the bone cross-section is reconstructed with metallic support, the better the loading characteristics. Plates should act as tension bands. Materials with increased E may result in bone resorption, whereas materials with decreased E may result in implant failure. Placement of implant initiates a race between bone healing and implant failure.

XI. Joint Biomechanics—General

A. Degrees of Freedom—Joint motion is described based upon rotation and translation in the x, y, and z directions. Therefore, six positions, or degrees of freedom, are used to describe motion. Fortunately, translations are usually relatively insignificant and can be safely ignored for most joints.

B. Joint Reaction Force (R)—The force generated within a joint in response to external forces (both intrinsic and extrinsic). Values correlate to predisposition to degenerative change.

C. Coupled Forces—Certain joints move in such a way that rotation about one axis is accompanied by an obligatory rotation about another axis, and these movements are coupled. For example, lateral bending of the spine is accompanied by axial rotation and these movements/forces are coupled.

D. Joint Congruence—Relates to the fit of two articular surfaces to each other, and is a necessary condition for joint motion. This can be evaluated radiographically. Movement out of a position of congruity causes increases in stresses in cartilage by allowing less contact area for distribution of the joint reaction force, predisposing the joint to degeneration.

E. Instant Centers—The point at which a joint rotates. In joints such as the knee, the location of the instant center changes during the arc of motion following a curved path. The instant center normally lies on a line perpendicular to the tangent to the joint surface at all points of contact. If the instant center lies on the joint surface, then pure rolling motion will occur. Pure sliding motion occurs with no angular change in position, and therefore has no instant center.

F. Friction and Lubrication—Resistance between two bodies when one slides over the other ($Ff = \mu N$). It is not a function of the contact area. Lubrication decreases the coefficient of friction between surfaces. Articular surfaces lubricated with synovial fluid have a coefficient of friction 10 times less than the best synthetic systems. Boundary and hydrostatic lubrication (discussed elsewhere) are largely responsible for this.

XII. Hip Biomechanics

A. Kinematics—

   1. Range of Motion:

Motion	Average Range	Functional Range
Flexion	115°	90° (120° squat)
Extension	30°	
Abduction	50°	20°
Adduction	30°	
Internal rotation (IR)	45°	0°
External rotation (ER)	45°	20°

   2. Instant Center—Simultaneous motion in all three planes for this ball-and-socket joint makes analysis impossible.

B. Kinetics—The joint reaction force (R) in the hip is three to six times body weight and is primarily due to contraction of muscles crossing the hip. This can be demonstrated with the free body diagram in Figure 2–4. With $A = 5$ and $B = 12.5$, using standard FBD analysis:

$$\Sigma MR = 0$$

$$-5 M_y + 12.5 W = 0 \qquad (2\text{–}3)$$

$$M_y = 2.5 W$$

$$\Sigma F_y = 0$$

$$-M_y - W + R_y = 0 \qquad (2\text{–}4)$$

$$R_y = 3.5 W$$

$$R = R_y/(\cos 30°) \qquad (2\text{–}5)$$

$$R = \underline{\underline{(\text{approx}) \ 4 W}}$$

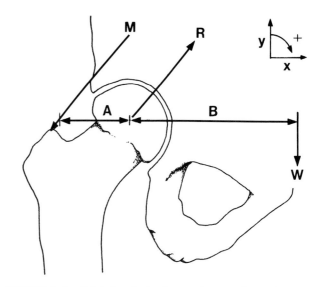

FIGURE 2–4. Pelvis free body diagram (see text for explanation).

One can see that an increase in the ratio of A/B (e.g., with medialization of the acetabulum or long-neck prosthesis, or lateralization of the greater trochanter) will decrease the joint reaction force. If $A = 7.5$ and $B = 10$, then R would equal approximately 2.3 W. R can also be reduced with shifting body weight over the hip (Trendelenburg gait), and with a cane in the contralateral hand (produces an additional moment—and can reduce R up to 60%!).

C. Other Considerations

   1. Stability—Largely based on intrinsic stability of deep-seated "ball-and-socket" design.
   2. Sourcil—Condensation of subchondral bone under the superomedial acetabulum. At this point R is maximal (Pauwels).
   3. Gothic Arch—Remodeled bone supporting the acetabular roof with the sourcil at its base (Bombelli).
   4. Neck-Shaft Angle—A varus angle results in decreased R and increased shear across the neck. A valgus angle creates increased R and decreased shear. Neutral or valgus is better for THA because PMMA resists shear poorly.
   5. Arthrodesis—**Position for hip arthrodesis should be 25–30 degrees of flexion and 0 degrees of abduction and rotation** (ER better than IR).

XIII. Knee Biomechanics

A. Kinematics

   1. Range of Motion—ROM of the knee ranges from +10 degrees of extension (recurvatum) to about 130 degrees of flexion. Functional ROM is from near full extension to about 90 degrees of flexion (117 degrees required for squatting and lifting). Rotation varies with flexion. At full extension, there is minimal rotation. At 90 degrees flexion, 45 degrees of external and 30 degrees of internal rotation are possible. Abduction/Adduction is essentially 0 degrees (a few degrees of passive motion is possible at 30 degrees of flexion normally).

Motion about the knee is a complex series of movements about a changing instant center of rotation (i.e., polycentric rotation).

2. Joint Motion—The instant centers, when plotted, describe a J-shaped curve about the femoral condyle. Flexion and extension of the knee involve both rolling and gliding motions. The femur internally rotates during the last 15 degrees of extension ("screw home" mechanism—related to size and convexity of medial femoral condyle [MFC] and musculature). Posterior rollback of the femur on the tibia during knee flexion increases maximum knee flexion. The axis of rotation of the intact knee is in the MFC. The patellofemoral joint is a sliding articulation (patella slides 7 cm caudally with full flexion), with an instant center near the posterior cortex above the condyles.

B. Kinetics—Extension is via the quadriceps mechanism, through the patellar apparatus; the hamstring muscles are primarily responsible for flexion at the knee.

1. Knee Stabilizers—Although bony contours have a role in knee stability, it is the *ligaments* and *muscles* of the knee that play the major role:

DIRECTION	STRUCTURES
Medial	Superficial MCL (1°), joint capsule, med. meniscus, ACL/PCL
Lateral	Joint capsule, IT band, LCL (mid), lat. meniscus, ACL/PCL (90°)
Anterior	ACL (1°), joint capsule
Posterior	PCL (1°), joint capsule; PCL tightens with IR
Rotatory	Combinations—MCL checks ER; ACL checks IR

The anterior cruciate ligament (ACL) typically is subjected to peak loads of 170 N in walking and up to 500 N with running. The ultimate strength of the ACL in young patients is about 1750 N. The ACL fails by serial tearing at 10–15% elongation.

2. Joint Forces
   a. Tibiofemoral—Joint surfaces in the knee are subjected to a **loading force equal to** three times the body weight in level walking, and up to **four times the body weight with walking steps**. Menisci help with load transmission (bear 1/3 to 1/2 of body weight), and removal of these structures increases contact stresses (up to four times load transfer to bone).
   b. Patellofemoral—The patella aids in knee extension by increasing the lever arm and in stress distribution. This joint has the thickest cartilage in the body because it must bear the most load—ranging from 1/2 W with normal walking to seven times W with squatting and jogging. Loads are proportional to the ratio of quadriceps force to knee flexion. The quadriceps provides an anterior subluxing force at 0–45-degree range of motion.

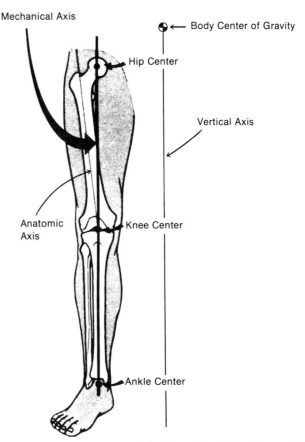

FIGURE 2–5. Knee axes. (Modified from Rohr, W.L.: Primary total knee arthroplasty. In Chapman's Operative Orthopaedics, p. 718. Philadelphia, J.B. Lippincott, 1988; reprinted by permission.)

3. Axes (Fig. 2–5):
   a. Mechanical Axis—Femoral head to center of ankle.
   b. Vertical Axis—From CG to ground.
   c. Anatomic Axis—Along shafts of femur and tibia.
   d. Relationships—Mechanical axis is 3 degrees valgus from vertical axis. Anatomic axis of femur is 6 degrees valgus from mechanical axis (9 degrees vs. vertical axis). Anatomic axis of tibia is 2–3 degrees varus from mechanical axis.
4. Arthrodesis—**0–7 degrees valgus; 10–15 degrees flexion**.

XIV. Ankle and Foot Biomechanics

A. Ankle
   1. Kinematics—Instant center is within the talus, lateral and posterior at the tips of the malleoli, and changes slightly with movement. The talus is described as forming a cone with the body and trochlea wider anteriorly and laterally. Therefore, the talus and fibula must externally rotate slightly with dorsiflexion. Ankle dorsiflexion and abduction are coupled movements in the ankle. Average ROM is dorsiflexion, 25 degrees; plantar flexion, 35 degrees; and rotation, 5 degrees.
   2. Kinetics—The tibiotalar articulation is the major weight-bearing surface of the ankle,

TABLE 2–1. ARCHES OF THE FOOT

ARCH	COMPONENTS	KEYSTONE	LIGAMENT SUPPORT	MUSCLE SUPPORT
Medial longitudinal	Calcaneus, talus, navicular, 3 cuneiforms, 1st–3rd metatarsals	Talus head	Spring (calcaneonavicular)	Tibialis post., flexor digitorum longus, flexor hallucis longus, adductor hallucis
Lateral longitudinal	Calcaneus, cuboid, 4th and 5th metatarsals		Plantar aponeurosis	Abductor digiti minimi, flexor digitorum brevis
Transverse	3 cuneiforms, cuboid, metatarsal bases			Peroneus longus, tibialis post., adductor hallucis (oblique)

supporting compressive forces up to five times body weight on level surfaces and shear (backward-to-forward) forces up to body weight. A large weight-bearing surface area allows for decreased stress (force/area) at this joint. The fibulotalar joint transmits about 1/6 of the force.

   3. Other Considerations—Stability is based on the shape of the articulation (mortise that is maintained by talar shape) and ligamentous support. The best stability is in dorsiflexion. A windlass action has been described in the ankle, where full dorsiflexion is limited by the plantar aponeurosis and further tension on the aponeurosis (e.g., with toe dorsiflexion) will cause the arch to rise. **Fusion should be in neutral or <5 degrees equinus with 5–10 degrees external rotation.**

  B. Subtalar Joint (Talus-Calcaneus-Navicular)—Axis of rotation is 42 degrees in the sagittal plane and 16 degrees in the transverse plane. Described as functioning like an oblique hinge. Its motions are also coupled with dorsiflexion, abduction, and eversion in one direction (pronation) and plantar flexion, adduction, and inversion (supination) in the other. Average ROM of pronation is 5 degrees; that of supination is about 20 degrees. Functional ROM is about 6 degrees.

  C. Transverse Tarsal Joint (talus-navicular, calcaneal-cuboid)—Motion is based on foot position with two axises of rotation (talonavicular and calcaneocuboid). With eversion of the foot (as in early stance phase), the two joints are parallel and ROM is permitted. With foot inversion (late stance), external rotation of the lower extremity causes the joints to no longer be parallel, and limited motion is allowed.

  D. Foot—Transmits about 1.2 times body weight with walking and three times body weight with running. Composed of three arches (Table 2–1). The second metatarsal (MT) Lisfranc joint is "key like" and stabilizes the second MT, allowing it to carry the most load with gait (first MT bears the most load while standing).

XV. Spine Biomechanics

  A. Kinematics—ROM varies with anatomic segment (Table 2–2). Analysis is based on the functional unit (**the motion segment = two vertebrae and their intervening soft tissues**). Six degrees of freedom exist about all three axes. Coupled motion is also demonstrated—especially with axial rotation and lateral bending. The instant center lies within the disc.

  B. Supporting Structures—Anteriorly includes the anterior longitudinal ligament, posterior longitudinal ligament, and vertebral discs. Posteriorly includes the intertransverse ligaments, capsular ligaments and facets, and ligamentum flavum (yellow ligament).

   1. Apophyseal joints—Resist torsion during axial loading, and the attached capsular ligaments resist flexion. Guide the motion of the motion segment. Direction of motion determined by the orientation of the facets of the apophyseal joint, which varies with each level. **In the C-spine, the facets are oriented 45 degrees to the transverse plane** and parallel to the frontal plane. In the **T-spine**, the **facets are oriented 60 degrees to the transverse plane** and 20 degrees to the frontal plane. In the **L-spine, the facets are oriented 90 degrees to the transverse plane** and 45 degrees to the frontal plane (i.e., they progressively tilt up [transverse plane] and in [frontal plane]).

  C. Kinetics

   1. The Disc—Behaves viscoelastically and demonstrates creep (deforms with time) and hysteresis (absorbs energy with repeated axial loads—and later decreases in function). Compressive stresses are highest in the nucleus pulposus and tensile stresses in the annulus fibrosus. Stiffness of the disc increases with increasing compressive load. With higher loads increased deformation and faster creep can be expected. Repeated torsional loading may separate the nucleus pulposus from the annulus and end plate and may force nuclear material out through an annular tear (which is produced by shear forces). Loads are increased with bending and torsional stresses.

TABLE 2–2. RANGE OF MOTION OF SPINAL SEGMENTS

LEVEL	FLEXION/ EXTENSION (°)	LATERAL BENDING (°)	ROTATION (°)	INSTANT CENTER
Occiput–C1	13	8	0	Skull, 2–3 cm above dens
C1–C2	10	0	45	Waist of odontoid
C2–C7	10–15	8–10	10	Vertebral body below
T-spine	5	6	8	Vertebra below/ disc centrum
L-spine	15–20	2–5	3–6	Disc annulus

2. The Vertebrae—Strength is related to the bone mineral content and size of the vertebrae (increased in the lumbar spine). Fatigue loading may lead to pars fractures. Compression fractures occur at the end plate.

XVI. Shoulder Biomechanics

A. Kinematics—The scapular plane is 30 degrees anterior to the coronal plane and is the preferred reference for ROM. Abduction of the shoulder requires external rotation of the humerus to prevent greater tuberosity impingement. With internal rotation contractures, patients cannot abduct past 120 degrees. Abduction is a result of glenohumeral motion (120 degrees) and scapulothoracic motion (60 degrees) in a 2:1 ratio. Movement at the acromioclavicular (AC) joint is responsible for the early part of scapulothoracic motion, and sternoclavicular (SC) movement is responsible for the later portion, with clavicular rotation along the long axis. Surface joint motion in the glenohumeral joint is a combination of rotation, rolling, and translation.

B. Kinetics—The following forces are important:

Motion	Muscle Forces	Comments
Glenohumeral		
Abduction	Deltoid, supraspinatus	Cuff depresses head (couple)
Adduction	Latissimus dorsi, pect. major, teres major	
Forward flexion	Pect. major, deltoid (ant.), biceps	
Extension	Latissimus dorsi	
IR	Subscapularis, teres major	
ER	Infraspinatus, teres minor, deltoid (post.)	
Scapular		
Rotation	Upper trapezoid, levator scapulae (ant.) serratus ant., lower trapezoid	Works through a force couple
Adduction	Trapezius, rhomboid, latissimus dorsi	
Abduction	Serratus ant., pectoralis minor	

The zero position (Saha)—165 degrees of abduction in the scapular plane—minimizes deforming forces about the shoulder. This is the ideal position for reduction of shoulder dislocations (or "fractures with traction"). Free body analysis of the deltoid force (Fig. 2–6) reveals the following:

$$\Sigma Mo = 0$$

$$3\,D - 0.05\,W\,(30) = 0 \qquad (2\text{–}6)$$

$$\underline{D = 0.5\,W}$$

C. Stability—Limited about the glenohumeral joint. The humeral head has a surface area larger than the glenoid (48 × 45 vs. 35 × 25). Bony stability is very limited and relies only on inclination (125

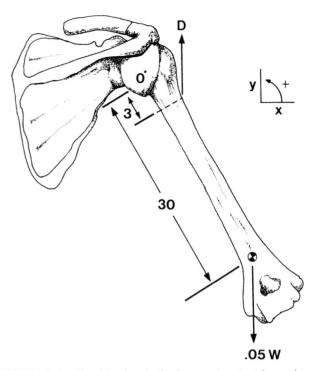

FIGURE 2–6. Shoulder free body diagram (see text for explanation).

degrees) and retroversion (25 degrees) of the humeral head and slight retrotilt of the glenoid. The ligaments (esp. middle and **inferior glenohumeral**) and rotator cuff are largely responsible for stability about the shoulder. **Position for fusion is 50 degrees** of true **abduction, 20 degrees of forward flexion, and 25 degrees of internal rotation. Avoid excessive external rotation**.

D. Other Joints—The AC joint allows scapular rotation (through the conoid and trapezoid ligaments) and scapular motion (through the AC joint itself). The SC joint allows clavicular protraction/retraction in a transverse plane (through the coracoclavicular ligament), clavicular elevation and depression in the frontal plane (also through the coracoclavicular ligament), and clavicular rotation around the longitudinal axis.

XVII. Elbow Biomechanics

A. Introduction—The elbow serves three functions: (1) serves as a component joint of the lever arm in positioning the hand; (2) is a fulcrum for the forearm lever; and (3) is a weight-bearing joint in patients using crutches.

B. Kinematics—Motion about the elbow includes flexion and extension (0–150 degrees with functional **ROM 30–130** degrees; axis of rotation is the center of the trochlea), and pronation and supination (P 80 degrees on S 85 degrees with **functional P and S of 50 degrees** each; axis is a line from the capitellum through the radial head and to the distal ulna [defines a cone]). The normal carrying angle (valgus angle at elbow) is 7 degrees for males and 13 degrees for females. This angle decreases with flexion.

C. Kinetics—The forces that act about the elbow have short lever arms and are relatively inefficient, resulting in large joint reaction forces and subjecting the elbow to degenerative changes. Flexion is primarily by the biceps, extension through the triceps, pronation with the pronators (teres and quadratus), and supination through the supinator. Static loads approach, and dynamic loads exceed, body weight. The FBD in Figure 2–7 demonstrates the inefficiency of elbow flexion:

$$\Sigma Mo = 0$$
$$-5\,B + 15\,W = 0 \qquad (2\text{–}7)$$
$$\underline{B = 3\,W}$$

Because the biceps inserts so close to the joint, it is relatively inefficient and must support three times the weight of the arm and any objects it holds.

D. Stability—Provided partially by articular congruity. Radial head provides about 30% of valgus stability and is more important in 0–30 degrees of flexion and pronation. The most stability of the elbow is medial, where the medial collateral ligament **(MCL) is the most important stabilizer (especially the anterior oblique fibers)**. Laterally, stability is provided by the lateral collateral ligament (LCL), anconeus, and joint capsule. Position of fusion for unilateral arthrodesis is about 90 degrees of flexion, for bilateral fusion, one elbow would be placed at 110 degrees of flexion (to reach mouth) and the other at 65 degrees of flexion (for hygiene needs). Fusion is difficult, and fortunately is rarely required.

E. Forearm—Seventeen percent of axial load is transmitted by the ulna. Line of center of rotation runs from the radial head to the distal ulna.

XVIII. Wrist and Hand Biomechanics

A. Wrist—Part of an intercalated link system.

1. Kinematics—Motion about the wrist includes flexion (65 degrees normal, 10 degrees functional), extension (55 degrees normal, 35 degrees functional), radial deviation (15 degrees normal, 10 degrees functional) and ulnar deviation (35 degrees normal, 15 degrees functional). Flexion and extension are primarily radiocarpal ($\frac{2}{3}$), but intercarpal movement is also important ($\frac{1}{3}$). Radial deviation is primarily due to intercarpal movement, whereas ulnar deviation relies on radiocarpal and intercarpal motion. The instant center for wrist motion is the head of the capitate, but is variable.

2. Columns—Three columns are described in the wrist (Taleisnik):

COLUMN	FUNCTION	COMMENTS
Central	Flexion-extension	Distal carpal row and lunate (link)
Medial	Rotation	Triquetrum
Lateral	Mobile	Scaphoid

3. Link System—The carpus makes up a system of three links in a chain (Gilford): radius-lunate-capitate. This allows for less motion to be required at each link, but adds to instability of the "chain." Stability, however, is enhanced by strong volar ligaments and the scaphoid, which bridges both carpal rows.

4. Relationships—Carpal collapse can be evaluated based on the ratio of carpal height/third metacarpal (MC) height (normally 0.54). Ulnar translation can be determined using the ratio of the ulna-to-capitate length/third MC height (normal is 0.30). The distal radius normally bears about 80% of the distal radioulnar joint load, and the distal ulna 20%. Ulnar load bearing can be increased with ulnar lengthening (e.g., in the treatment of Kienböck's disease), or decreased with ulnar shortening (e.g., for degenerative triangular fibrocartilage complex (TFCC) tears). Wrist arthrodesis is relatively common. A position of 10–20 degrees of dorsiflexion is good for unilateral fusion, and if bilateral fusion is necessary (avoid if possible), the other wrist should be fused in 0–10 degrees of palmar flexion.

B. Hand

1. Kinematics—ROM at the MCP joint includes 100 degrees of flexion and 60 degrees of abduction-adduction. PIP joints usually have about 110 degrees of flexion, and DIP joints 80 degrees.

2. Arches—The hand has two transverse arches (proximal ridge through the carpus and distal through the MC heads), and five longitudinal arches (through each of the rays).

3. Stability—MCP stability is provided by the volar plate and the collateral ligaments. The PIPs and DIPs rely more on joint congruity. Also there is a large ligament/articular surface ratio in these joints.

4. Other Concepts—The pulleys in the hand prevent bowstringing and decrease tendon excursion. Bowstringing increases the mo-

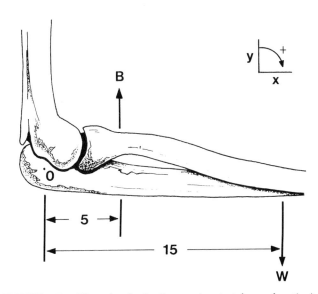

FIGURE 2–7. Elbow free body diagram (see text for explanation).

ment arm to the joint instant center. The sagittal bands allow extension at the MCP joint. With hyperextension at the MCPs, the intrinsics must function for PIP extension because the extensor tendon is lax. Normal grasp for males is 50 kg, and for females 25 kg (only 4 kg required for daily function). Normal pinch for males is 8 kg, and for females 4 kg (1 kg needed in day-to-day activities).

5. Kinetics—Joint loading with pinch is mostly the MCP, but because the MCPs have a larger surface area, the contact pressures (joint load/contact area) at the MCPs are less. The DIPs have the most contact pressures and subsequently develop the most degenerative change with time (Heberden nodes). Grasping contact pressures are less but focus on the MCPs; therefore patients with MCP arthritis frequently come from occupations requiring a lot of grasping activities. Compressive loads at the thumb with pinching include 3 kg at the interphalangeal (IP), 5 kg at the MCP, and 12 kg at the thumb CMC joint (an unstable joint), which leads to its frequent degeneration.

6. Arthrodesis—The following are recommended positions of flexion for fusion of joints in the hand:

JOINT	DEGREES OF FLEXION	OTHER FACTORS
MCP	20–30	
PIP	40–50	Less radial than ulnar
DIP	15–20	
Thumb CMC		MC in opposition
Thumb MCP	25	
Thumb IP	20	

Part 2

Orthopaedic Tissues

I. Bone

  A. Types—Normal bone is **lamellar**, immature or pathologic bone is **woven**. Woven bone is more random with more osteocytes, has increased turnover, and is weaker but more flexible than lamellar bone. Woven bone is not stress oriented. Mature, lamellar bone can be **cortical** or **cancellous**.

    1. Cortical Bone (a.k.a. Compact Bone) (Fig. 2–8)—Makes up 80% of the skeleton and is composed of tightly packed osteons or haversian systems that are connected by haversian (or Volkmann's) canals. These canals contain vessels, nerves, and osteoblasts. Interstitial lamellae lie between the osteons. Fibrils frequently connect lamellae but do not cross **cement lines** (where bone resorption stopped and new bone formation began). Cement lines also define the outer border of an osteon. Nutrition is via intraosseous circulation (canals and canaliculi **[cell processes of osteocytes]**). Cortical bone is characterized by a slow turnover rate, a high E, and *high* resistance to torsion and bending.

    2. Cancellous Bone (a.k.a. Spongy or Trabecular Bone)—Less dense and undergoes more remodeling according to lines of stress (Wolff's Law). It has a higher turnover rate and a smaller Young's modulus, but is more elastic than cortical bone.

  B. Cells

    1. Osteoblasts—Form bone. Derived from undifferentiated mesenchymal cell (stimulated by immobilization). These cells have increased endoplasmic reticulum, Golgi apparatus, and mitochondria in order to fulfill the cell's role in synthesis and secretion of matrix. More differentiated, metabolically active cells line bone surfaces and less active cells in "resting regions" or entrapped cells maintain the ionic milieu of bone. Disruption of the lining cell layer activates these cells.

    2. Osteocytes—Make up 90% of the cells in the mature skeleton and serve to maintain bone. These cells are former osteoblasts that are trapped within the newly formed matrix, which they help preserve. They have an increased nuclear-to-cytoplasm ratio with long interconnecting cytoplasmic processes, and are not as active as osteoblasts in matrix production. Osteocysts have an important role in the control of extracellular concentration of calcium and phosphorus and are directly stimulated by calcitonin and inhibited by parathyroid hormone (PTH).

    3. Osteoclasts—Resorb bone. These multinucleated, irregularly shaped giant cells originate from hematopoietic tissues (monocyte progenitors form giant cells by fusion), and possess a ruffled ("brush") border (plasma membrane enfoldings important in bone resorption) and a surrounding clear zone. Bone resorption, which occurs in depressions known as Howship's lacunae, is more rapid than bone formation; these two processes are linked ("coupled"). Osteoblasts are indirectly stimulated by PTH, vitamin D_3, PGE_2, thyroid hormone, and glucocorticoid and are inhibited by calcitonin.

    4. Osteoprogenitor Cells—Become osteoblasts. These local mesenchymal cells line haversian canals, endosteum, and periosteum, awaiting the stimulus to differentiate into osteoblasts.

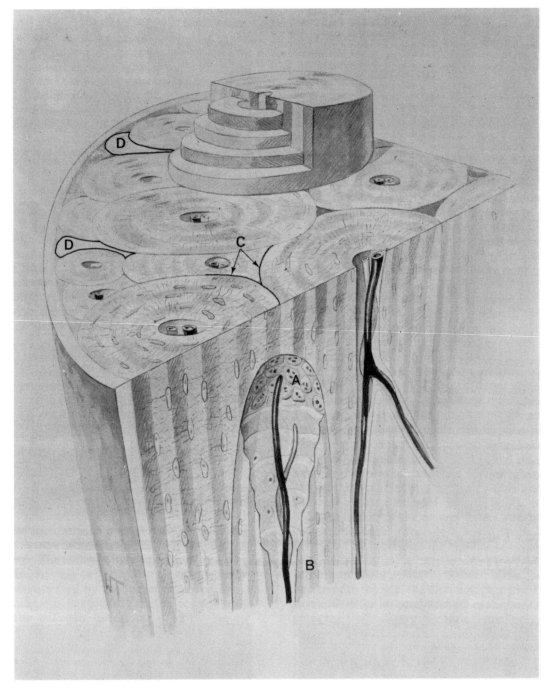

FIGURE 2–8. Segment demonstrating architecture of cortical bone. *A,* Cutting core of osteoclasts. *B,* Osteoblasts lay down new osteones. *C,* Cement lines. *D,* Interstitial lamellae. (From Owen, R., Goodfellow, J., and Bullough, P.: Scientific Foundations of Orthopaedics and Traumatology, p. 6. Philadelphia, W.B. Saunders, 1981; reprinted by permission.)

C. Matrix
  1. Organic Components—Make up 40% of the dry weight of bone.
    a. Collagen—Responsible for tensile strength. Makes up 90% of the matrix and is composed primarily of type I collagen (type I collagen accounts for 90% of all collagen in the body). Collagen structure consists of a triple helix of tropocollagen (two α_1 and one α_2 chains) that is quarter-staggered with hole zones (for calcification). Cross-linking decreases solubility and increases tensile strength of collagen.
    b. Proteoglycans—Partially responsible for compressive strength of bone, they actually inhibit mineralization. Composed of GAG-protein complexes discussed below in Section II: Cartilage.

c. Glycoproteins—such as osteonectin and fibronectin have a role in bone formation.
d. Phospholipids and Phosphoproteins—Promote mineralization. Osteocalcin attracts osteoclasts and is directly related to bone density.

2. Inorganic (Mineral) Components—Make up 60% of dry weight of bone.
    a. Calcium Hydroxyapatite (Ca_{10} $(PO_4)_6$ $(OH)_2$)—Responsible for compressive strength. Makes up most of the inorganic matrix, and is responsible for mineralization of the matrix. Primary mineralization is in the gaps in the collagen, secondary mineralization is on the periphery.
    b. Osteocalcium Phosphate (Brushite)—Makes up remaining inorganic matrix.

D. Bone Remodeling—Affected by mechanical function according to Wolff's Law. A genetically determined baseline level of bone may prevent complete loss of bone in paralyzed extremities. Removal of external stresses can lead to significant bone loss, but this can be reversed upon remobilization.

1. General—Bone remodels in response to stress and responds to piezoelectric charges (compression side is electronegative, stimulating osteoblasts; tension side is electropositive, stimulating osteoclasts).
2. Cortical Bone—Remodels by osteoclastic tunneling followed by layering of osteoblasts and successive deposition of layers of lamellae (after cement line has been laid down) until tunnel size has narrowed to the diameter of the osteonal central canal.
3. Trabecular Bone—Remodels by osteoclastic resorption (in Howship's lacunae) followed by osteoblastic laying down of new bone.

E. Surrounding Tissues
1. Periosteum—Connective tissue membrane that covers bone. It is more developed in children because of its role in deposition of cortical bone responsible for growth in bone diameter. The inner or cambium layer is loose, more vascular, and osteogenic; the outer fibrous layer is less cellular and contiguous with joint capsules.
2. Bone Marrow—Source of progenitor cells and controls inner diameter of bone.
    a. Red Marrow—Hematopoietic (40% water, 40% fat, 20% protein).
    b. Yellow Marrow—Inactive (15% water, 80% fat, 5% protein). Red marrow slowly transitions to yellow with age, beginning in the appendicular skeleton and later the axial skeleton.

F. Enchondral Bone Formation/Mineralization
1. Cartilage Model (Fig. 2–9)—Formed from mesenchymal anlage usually at 6 weeks. Vascular buds invade this model, bringing osteoprogenitor cells that differentiate into osteoblasts and form the primary centers of ossification at about 8 weeks. The cartilage model grows through appositional (width) and interstitial (length) growth. The marrow is formed by resorption of the central cancellous bone and invasion of myeloid precursor cells brought in by the capillary bud. Secondary centers of ossification develop at the bone ends, forming epiphyseal centers of ossification (growth plates), which are responsible for longitudinal growth of immature bones. Has a rich arterial supply composed of an epiphyseal artery (which terminates in the proliferative zone), metaphyseal nutrient arteries, and perichondrial arteries.

2. Physis—Two growth plates actually exist in immature long bones—a *horizontal* growth plate, the physis, and a *spherical* growth plate that allows growth of the epiphysis. The spherical growth plate has the same arrangement as the physis, but is less organized. Acromegaly and spondyloepiphyseal dysplasia affect physeal growth, multiple epiphyseal dysplasia dysplasia adversely affects growth in the epiphysis. Physeal cartilage is divided into zones based upon growth (Fig. 2–10).
    a. **Reserve Zone**—Cells store lipids, glycogen, and proteoglycan aggregates for later growth. Decreased O_2 tension occurs in this zone. Lysosomal storage disease (Gaucher's) and other diseases can affect this zone.
    b. **Proliferative Zone**—Longitudinal growth occurs with stacking of chondrocytes (top cell is the dividing "mother" cell). Increased O_2 tension, and increased proteoglycan in surrounding matrix (inhibits calcification). This zone functions in cellular proliferation and matrix production. Defects in this zone (chondrocyte proliferation and column formation) are seen in achondrodysplasia (does not affect intramembranous bone [width]).
    c. **Hypertrophic Zone**—Sometimes subdivided into three separate zones: maturation, degeneration, and provisional calcification. In the hypertrophic zone, cells increase five times in size, accumulate calcium in their mitochondria, and then die, releasing calcium from matrix vesicles. Osteoblasts, which migrate from sinusoidal vessels, use cartilage as a scaffolding for bone formation. Low O_2 tension and decreased proteoglycan aggregates aid in this process. This zone is widened in rickets, where little or no provisional calcification occurs. Enchondromas also originate in this zone. Mucopolysaccharide diseases also affect the zone, leading to chondrocyte degeneration (swollen, abnormal chondrocytes). **Physeal fractures are classically believed to occur through the zone of provisional calcification** (within the hypertrophic zone), but they probably traverse several zones.
3. Metaphysis—Adjacent to the physis, it expands with skeletal growth. Osteoblasts from osteoprogenitor cells line up on cartilage bars produced by physeal expansion. Primary spongiosa (calcified cartilage bars) is mineralized to form woven bone and remodeled to form secondary spongiosa and a "cutback zone" at the metaphysis. Cortical bone is made by remodeling of physeal (enchondral) and intramembranous bone in response to stress along periphery of growing long bones.
4. Periphery of the Physis—Composed of two elements:
    a. Groove of Ranvier—Supplies chondrocytes

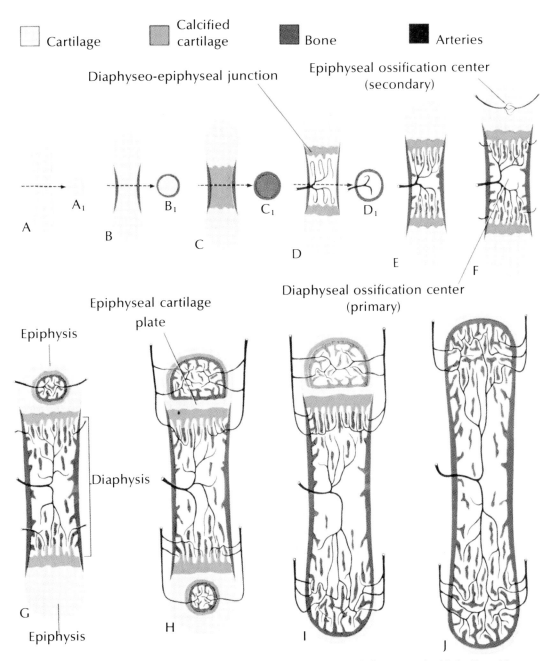

FIGURE 2–9. Enchondral ossification of long bones. Note that phases F–J often occur after birth. (From Moore, K.L.; The Developing Human, p. 346. Philadelphia, W.B. Saunders Company, 1982; reprinted by permission.)

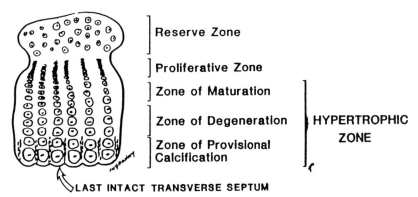

FIGURE 2–10. Physeal layers. (From Orthopaedic Science Syllabus, p. 11. Park Ridge, IL., American Academy of Orthopaedic Surgery, 1986; reprinted by permission.)

to the periphery of the growth plate for lateral growth (width).
   b. Perichondrial Ring of LaCroix—Dense fibrous tissue anchors and supports the physis.
5. Mineralization—Consists of seeding of collagen hole zones with calcium hydroxyapatite crystals through branching and accretion (crystal growth).

G. Intramembranous Ossification—Occurs without a cartilage model during embryonic life, usually in the flat bones (and clavicle, as well as providing growth in width for long bones). It is heralded by aggregation of mesenchymal cells into condensed layers or **membranes**. Cells adjacent to capillaries differentiate into osteoblasts and set up a center of ossification. This expands by appositional growth. Blastema bone is membranous bone formation that occurs in young children with amputations/resections, etc.

H. Bone Injury and Repair
   1. **Inflammation**—Bleeding from the fracture ends and soft tissue creates a hematoma, which provides a source of hematopoietic cells capable of secreting growth factors. Subsequently, granulation tissue forms around the fracture ends. Osteoblasts, from surrounding osteogenic precursor cells and/or fibroblasts, proliferate.
   2. **Repair**—Primary callus response occurs within 2 weeks. If the ends are not in continuity, bridging (soft) callus occurs (enchondral ossification). Another type of callus, medullary (hard) callus, supplements the bridging callus, and is slow and often late. The amount of callus is indirectly proportional to the amount of immobilization of the fracture. Primary cortical healing, which resembles normal remodeling, occurs with mechanical immobilization with near-anatomic reduction.
   3. **Remodeling**—This process begins during the middle of the repair phase and goes on long after the fracture has clinically healed (up to 7 years), and allows the bone to assume its normal configuration and shape based on the stresses it is exposed to (Wolff's Law). Throughout the process, woven bone formed in the repair phase is replaced with lamellar bone. Fracture healing is complete when there is repopulation of marrow.
   4. Fracture healing varies with the method of treatment. With closed treatment, "enchondral healing" with periosteal bridging callus occurs. With rigidly fixed fractures, direct osteonal or primary bone healing occurs without visible callus. Endocrine effects in fracture healing are also important.

Hormone	Effect	Mechanism
Cortisone	−	Decreased callus proliferation
Calcitonin	+?	Unknown
TH/PTH	+	Bone remodeling
Growth hormone	+	Increased callus volume

I. Bone Grafting—Allows a template (osteoconduction) for host osteoblasts and osteoclasts to function and may influence its own incorporation (osteoinduction). Commonly, autografts (from same person) or allografts (from another person) are used. Cancellous bone is commonly used in grafting nonunions, for cavitary defects, etc., because it is quickly remodeled and incorporated (via creeping substitution). Cortical bone is slower to turn over and is used for structural defects. Osteoarticular allografts are being increasingly used for tumor surgery and have the advantage that, when cryopreserved, up to 40–50% of chondrocytes can survive. Vascularized bone grafts, though technically difficult, allow quick union with preservation of most cells. Revascularized grafts are best in irradiated tissues and with large tissue defects. However, there is some donor site morbidity with the vascularized fibula graft. Nonvascular bone grafts are used more commonly. Bone grafts can be fresh (increased antigenicity); fresh frozen (preserves bone morphogenic protein [BMP], a 17,500-MW protein that promotes osteoinduction and preserves articular cartilage [40–50% of chondrocyte survive] with glycerol or DMSO preservation); freeze dried (lyophilized loses structural integrity and depletes BMP; commonly "croutons"); and bone matrix gelatin (BMG—digested source of BMP). Five stages of graft healing are recognized (Urist):

Stage	Activity
1—Inflammation	Chemotaxis stimulated by necrotic debris
2—Osteoblast Differentiation	From precursors
3—Osteoinduction	Osteoblast and osteoclasts function
4—Osteoconduction	New bone forms over scaffold
5—Remodeling	A process that continues for years

Cortical bone graft incorporates thorough slow remodeling of existing haversian systems via a process of resorption (which weakens the graft) followed by deposition of the new bone (restoring its strength). Resorption is confined to the osteon borders, and interstitial lamellae are preserved. Cancellous grafts are revascularized more quickly, and osteoblasts lay down new bone on old trabeculae, which are later remodeled ("creeping substitution"). All grafts must be harvested sterilely and donors must be screened for potentially transmissible diseases. Synthetic substitutes under investigation include hydroxyapatite (osteoconductive) and tricalcium phosphate (biodegradable), both of which encourage bone formation in nonstructural defects. Significant immunologic reactions are rare, and the need to match donor and host is not established.

II. Cartilage
A. Introduction—Cartilage can be one of several types. Growth plate (physeal) cartilage is discussed above, fibrocartilage is important in tendon and ligament insertion into bone (and in healing of articular cartilage), elastic cartilage is seen in tissues such as the trachea, fibroelastic cartilage makes up menisci, and finally, articular cartilage is critical in the function of joints, and will be the focus of this

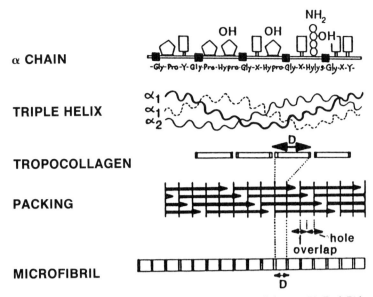

FIGURE 2–11. Collagen microstructure. (From Orthopaedic Science Syllabus, p. 73. Park Ridge, IL., American Academy of Orthopaedic Surgery, 1986; reprinted by permission.)

section. Articular cartilage functions in decreasing friction and in load distribution.

B. Articular Cartilage Composition

1. Water (65%)—Allows for deformation of cartilage surface in response to stress by shifting in and out of cartilage. Also responsible for nutrition and lubrication. Increased water content leads to increased permeability and decreased strength.

2. Collagen (15–20%) (Fig. 2–11)—Type II collagen allows for cartilaginous framework and **tensile** strength. Increased amounts of Gly, Lys-OH, Pro-OH, and hydrogen bonding are responsible for its unique characteristics. Small amounts of types I (superficial), IX, and XII collagen are also present.

3. Proteoglycans (10–15%) (Fig. 2–12)—Protein polysaccharides responsible for **compressive** strength. Composed of glycosaminoglycans (GAGs—disaccharide polymers). GAGs are bound to a hyaluronic acid core protein with **link proteins** (with increased amounts of keratin sulfate) that **stabilize the proteoglycan aggregates.** The proteogylcans, which have a half-life of 3 months, serve to trap and hold water.

4. Chondrocytes (5%)—Active in protein synthesis and possess a double effusion barrier. Produce collagen and proteoglycans and some enzymes for cartilage metabolism. Less active in the calcified zone. Deeper zones name decreased RER and increased intraplasmic filaments (degenerative products). Chondroblasts,

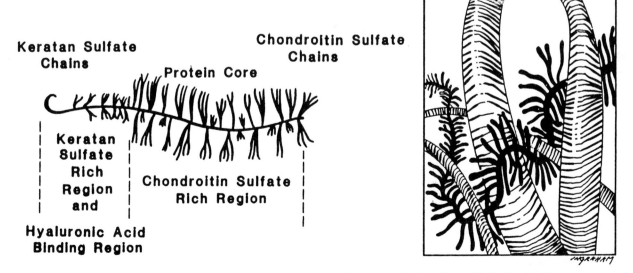

FIGURE 2–12. Cartilage microstructure. Note proteoglycans interspersed with collagen fibrils (inset). (From Orthopaedic Science Syllabus, p. 22. Park Ridge, IL., American Academy of Orthopaedic Surgery, 1986; reprinted by permission.)

TABLE 2–3. ARTICULAR CARTILAGE LAYERS

LAYER	WIDTH (μ)	CHARACTERISTIC	ORIENTATION	FUNCTION
Gliding zone	40	Decr. metabolic activity	Tangential	vs. shear
Transitional zone	500	Incr. metabolic activity	Oblique	vs. compression
Radial zone	1000	Incr. collagen size	Vertical	vs. compression
Tidemark	5	Undulating barrier	Tangential	vs. shear
Calcified zone	300	Hydroxyapatite crystals		Anchor

which are derived from undifferentiated mesenchymal cells (stimulated by motion), are later trapped in lacunae to become chondrocytes.

C. Articular Cartilage Layers—The various layers of articular cartilage are described in Table 2–3 and illustrated in Figure 2–13.

D. Other Factors—pH of cartilage is now usually 7.4— changes can disrupt the structure. Water content is critical to cartilage function:

WATER CONTENT	E (YOUNG'S MODULUS)	Permeability
Increased	Decreased	Increased
Decreased	Increased	Decreased

E. Articular Cartilage Aging—With aging, chondrocytes become larger, acquire increased lysosomal enzymes, and no longer reproduce. Collagen undergoes increased stiffness and decreased solubility with aging. Cartilage proteogylcans decrease in mass and size (decreased length of chondroitin sulfate chains) and change in proportion (decreased chondroitin sulfate, and **increased keratin sulfate**). Protein content increases while water content decreases. These changes decrease the elasticity of cartilage.

F. Articular Cartilage Healing—Deep lacerations below the tidemark that penetrate the underlying bone may heal with *fibrocartilage*, but this is not as durable as **hyaline** cartilage. Blunt trauma may in-

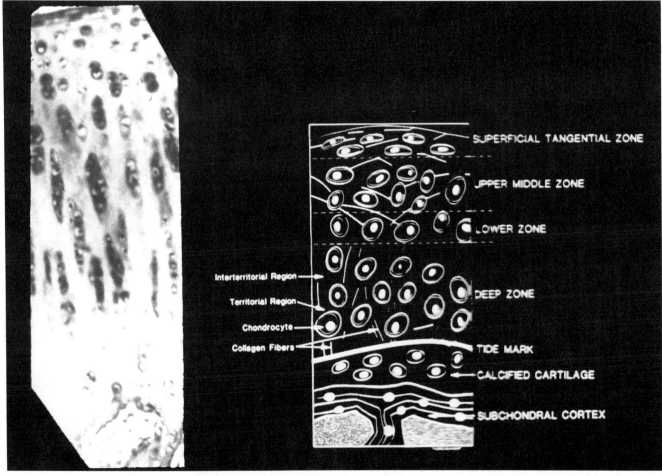

FIGURE 2–13. Cartilage zones. Note gliding zone (superficial tangential zone), transitional zone (upper zone), and radial zone (lower and deep zones) above the tide mark. (From Orthopaedic Science Syllabus, p. 20. Park Ridge, IL., American Academy of Orthopaedic Surgery, 1986; reprinted by permission.)

duce charges similar to osteoarthritis in cartilage. Continuous passive motion may have a positive effect on cartilage repair. Partial-thickness articular cartilage lacerations cause chondrocytes to proliferate.

III. Muscle

A. Noncontractile Elements (Fig. 2–14A)

1. Muscle Body—**Epimysium** surrounds individual muscle bundles, **perimysium** surrounds muscle fascicles, and **endomysium** surrounds individual fibers.

2. Myotendon Junction—the weak link in the muscle, **often the site of tears**, especially with eccentric contraction. Sarcolemma filaments interdigitate with basement membrane (type IV collagen), and the tendon tissue (type I collagen). Involution of muscle cells at this joint gives maximum surface area for attachment. Linking proteins and specialized membrane protein (vetroneotin) are also present.

3. Sarcoplasmic Reticulum—Stores calcium in intracellular membrane-bound channels, including T tubules (which go to each myofibril) and cisternae (small storage areas).

B. Contractile Elements (Fig. 2–14B)—Derived from myoblasts. Each **muscle** is composed of several muscle **bundles**, which in turn contain muscle **fibers** (the basic unit of contraction), which are made up of **myofibrils** (1–3 μ in diameter and 1–2 cm long), a collection of **sarcomeres.**

1. Sarcomere—Composed of thick and thin filaments in an intricate arrangement that allows fibers to slide past each other. Thick filaments are composed of **myosin**, thin filaments of **actin**. The thin filaments also have **troponin (C)** and **tropomycin** on their surface. The sarcomere is arranged into bands and zones as shown in Figure 2–15. Note that the H zone contains only thick (myosin) filaments and that the **I band is composed of solely thin (actin) filaments.** Thin filaments are attached to the Z line and extend across I bands, partially into the A band.

C. Action—Stimulus comes from the motor nerve and arrives at the motor end plate, releasing acetylcholine, which, in turn, depolarizes the sarcoplasmic reticulum, releasing calcium. Calcium binds to troponin (on the thin filaments), causing them to change the position of tropomycin (also on the thin filaments), and exposing the actin filament. Actin-myosin cross-bridges form and, with the breakdown of ATP, the thick and thin filaments slide past one another, contracting the muscle.

D. Types of Muscle Contraction—**Isotonic** contraction allows constant tension through a range of motion (using free weights). In **isometric** contraction, tension is generated but the muscle does not shorten. In a **concentric** contraction, the muscle shortens

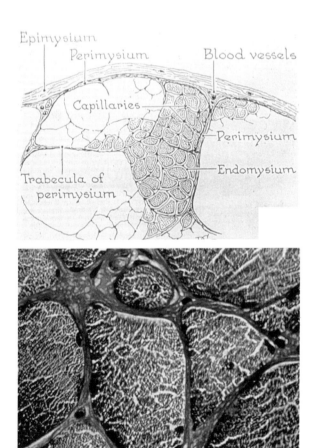

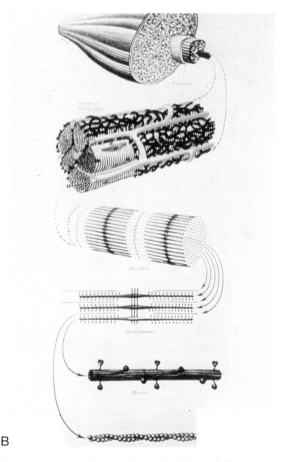

FIGURE 2–14. *A,* Muscle noncontractile elements. *B,* Muscle microstructure. (From Orthopaedic Science Syllabus, p. 27. Park Ridge, IL., American Academy of Orthopaedic Surgery, 1986; reprinted by permission.)

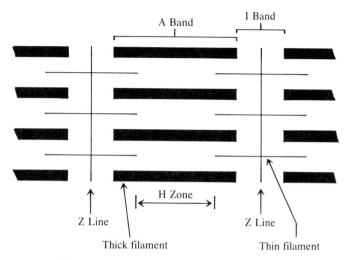

FIGURE 2–15. Bands and zones of a sarcomere.

and its tension is proportional to the externally applied load. In **eccentric** contraction, the muscle lengthens. **Isokinetic** contractions occur when maximal tension is generated in a muscle contracting at a constant speed over the full range of motion (not eccentric).

E. Types of Muscle Fibers—Include fast and slow twitch, and make up individual motor units (motor nerve and fibers innervated).

1. Slow Twitch (ST) (Type I; Oxidative) Fibers—**Aerobic**, and therefore have more mitochondria, enzymes, and triglycerides (energy source). They have low concentrations of glycogen and glycolytic enzymes (ATPase). A helpful way to remember: **slow red ox** (slow twitch fibers are slower, are typically more vascularized, and undergo aerobic oxidations). These fibers specialize in endurance activities. Slow twitch fibers are the first lost without rehabilitation.

2. Fast Twitch (FT) (Type II; Glycolytic) Fibers—Contract more quickly and their motor units are larger and stronger than ST fibers (increased ATPase). However, they do this at the expense of efficiency, and are **anaerobic.** Subtypes of type II fibers are based on myosin heavy chains.

3. Athletes and Training—The distribution of FT vs. ST fibers is genetically determined; however, different types of training can selectively improve these fibers. Endurance athletes typically have a higher percentage of ST fibers, whereas athletes participating in "strength"-type sports have more FT fibers. Training for endurance sports consists of decreased tension and increased repetitions, which will help increase the efficiency of the ST fibers and increase the numbers of mitochondria, capillary density, and oxidative capacity. Training for strength consists of increasing tension and decreasing repetition, which will lead to an increased number of myofibrils/fiber and hypertrophy of fast twitch fibers. Either form of training will slow the increase of the lactate in response to exercise. Oxygen consumption (VO_2) is an important consideration in athletic training.

4. Muscle injury—As noted earlier, most muscle strains (the most common sports injury) occur at the musculotendinous unit. Occurs most commonly with muscles crossing two joints (hamstring, gastrocnemius), with increased type II fibers with initial inflammation and later fibrosis. Muscle activation allows two times the energy absorption prior to failure. However, "bouncing" types of stretching are deleterious. Muscle soreness may result from eccentric muscle contractions and may be associated with changes in the I-line of the sarcomere. Tears in muscle typically heal with dense scarring. Surgical repair of clean lacerations in the midbelly of skeletal muscle usually results in minimal regeneration of muscle fibers distally, scar formation at the laceration, and recovery of about 1/2 of muscle strength. Denervation causes muscle atrophy and increased sensitivity to acetylcholine, causing spontaneous fibrillations at 2–4 weeks after damage to the motor axon.

5. Immobilization—Causes changes in the number of sarcomeres at the musculotendinous junction and acceleration of granulation tissue response in the injured muscle. Immobilization in lengthened positions decreases contractures and increases strength. Atrophy can be from disuse or altered nervous system recruitment. Electrical stimulation can help offset these effects.

IV. Synovium

A. Introduction—Synovium mediates the exchange of nutrients between the blood and joint fluid.

B. Tissues—Composed of vascularized connective tissue that lacks a basement membrane. Two cell types are present in synovium: **type A** cells, which are important in **phagocytosis;** and **type B** cells (fibroblast-like cells), which **produce synovial fluid.** Other undifferentiated cells have a reparative role. A third type of cell, type C, may exist as an intermediate cell type.

C. Synovial Fluid—Made up of proteinase, collagenases, hyaluronic acid, and prostaglandins, it is an ultrafiltrate of plasma added to fluid produced by the synovial membrane. It nourishes articular cartilage through diffusion, and lubricates via **hydrodynamic** (fluid separates the surfaces under load), **boundary** (slippery surfaces), **weeping** (fluid shift to loaded areas), and/or **boosted** (fluid entrapment) mechanisms. Lubricin, a glycoprotein, is the key lubricating component of synovial fluid. Analysis of synovial fluid in disease processes is important (discussed in Part 4: Arthritides, below).

V. Fibrous Tissues

A. Menisci—Broaden the contact area of synovial joints and are located in the AC, SC, glenohumeral, hip, and knee joints. These triangular semilunar structures are composed primarily of **type I collagen** with some type III, radially oriented, and linked with random fibers. They are composed of 75% water and only 2.5% proteoglycans. Only the outer 25% of menisci is vascularized; the remaining, acellular, portions depend upon diffusion for nutrition. Peripheral meniscal lesions can heal with fibrovascular scar formation.

B. Tendons (Fig. 2–16)—Dense, regularly arranged tissues that attach muscle to bone. Composed of fascicles (groups of collagen bundles) separated by endotenon, surrounded by epitenon, and enclosed within a paratenon or tendon sheath. Consist of fibroblasts that produce mostly **type I collagen** and are arranged in fascicles (composed of fibrils) with surrounding loose areolar tissue (peritenon). Insertion into bone is by way of transitional, calcified fibrocartilage (Sharpey's fibers), which helps dissipate stress. Although all tendons have some form of blood supply for nutrition, "vascular" tendons are surrounded by a vascular peritenon, whereas "avascular" tendons are nourished by vincula within tendon sheaths. Other sources of nutrition include synovial folds, periosteal attachments, and surrounding tissue. Tendinous structures tend to orient themselves along stress lines. Tendinous repair is initiated by fibroblasts that originate in the epitenon and macrophages that initiate healing and remodeling. Treatment of injuries affect their repair. Tendon healing occurs in large part through intrinsic capabilities. Tendon repairs are weakest at 7–10 days, they regain a majority of their original strength at 21–28 days and achieve maximum strength in 6 months. Early mobilization allows increased ROM but decreased strength. Immobilization leads to increased strength in the tendon substance, but at the expense of motion. Immobilization tends to decrease the strength at the tendon-bone interface.

C. Ligaments—Composed of type I collagen, these structures have a role in stability of joints. Their ultrastructure is similar to tendons, but the fibers are more variable and have higher elastin content. They also possess mechanoreceptors and free nerve endings that may have a role in stabilizing joints. Repair (in three phases as in bone) is benefited from normal stress and strain across the joint. Early repair is with type III collagen that is later converted to type I collagen. Avulsion of ligaments typically occurs between the unmineralized and mineralized fibrocartilage layers. Immobilization adversely affects the strength of repair. Exercise causes a decrease in the number but an increase in the size of collagen fibrils and leads to decreased stiffness.

D. Intervertebral Discs—Allow motion and stability of the spine. Composed of two components: the central nucleus pulposus (a hydrated gel with com-

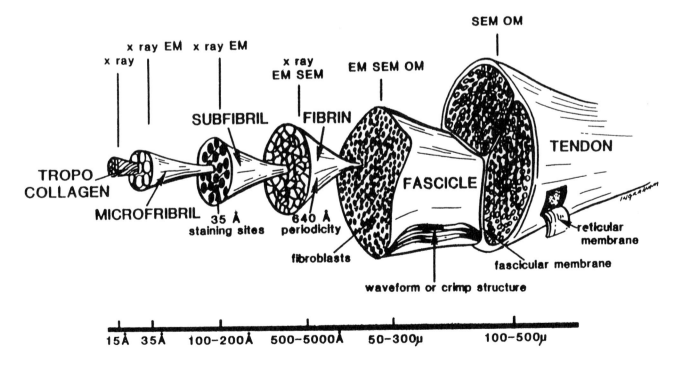

FIGURE 2–16. Tendon microstructure. (From Orthopaedic Science Syllabus, p. 35. Chicago, American Academy of Orthopaedic Surgery, 1986; reprinted by permission.)

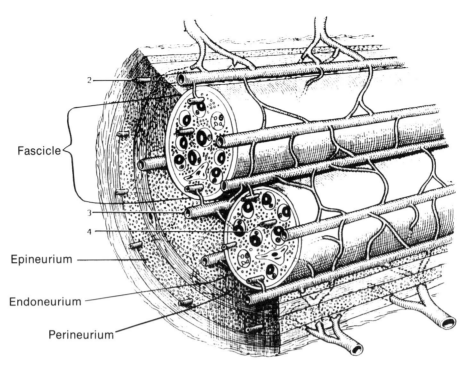

FIGURE 2–17. Peripheral nerve microstructure. Note microvascular structure: *1*, vessels of the nutrient artery; *2*, epineural system; *3*, interfascicular system; *4*, intrafascicular system. From Tubiana, R.: The Hand, p. 421. Philadelphia, W.B. Saunders, 1985; reprinted by permission.)

pressibility—high GAG/low collagen) and a surrounding annulus fibrosis (allows for extensibility and increased tensile strength—high collagen/low GAG). Composed of 85% water (decreased with age), proteoglycans (smaller and with more keratin sulfate than young cartilage), and **collagen types I and II (II inner, I outer)**.

VI. Nerves

   A. Peripheral Nerves

   1. Morphology (Fig. 2–17)—Individual nerve cells (neurons) are composed of a body with several afferent cytoplasmic extensions (dendrites) and one long efferent cytoplasmic extension (axon). Axons, coated with a fibrous tissue called endoneurium, are grouped into nerve bundles called fascicles that, in turn, are covered with connective tissue called perineurium. Peripheral nerves are composed of one (mono-), a few (oligo-), or several (poly-) fascicles and surrounding areolar connective tissue (epineurium) enclosed within an epineural sheath. The perineurium and endothelial cells of endoneurium make up the blood-nerve barrier.

   2. Nerve Fibers (Axons) (2–25 μ in Diameter)—Can be one of three types:

Type	Diam. (μ)	Myelination	Speed	Examples
A	10–20	Heavy	Fast	Touch
B	<3	Intermediate	Medium	ANS
C	<1.3	None	Slow	Pain

   3. Conduction—Most axons (portion of neurons that conducts impulses for long distances) are myelinated, with conduction occurring at gaps between Schwann cells (nodes of Ranvier).

   4. Injury—Peripheral nerve injury leads to death of the distal axons and wallerian degeneration (of myelin). Proximal axonal budding occurs (after a 1-month delay) and leads to regeneration at the rate of about 1 mm/day. Pain is the first modality to return. Nerve injury is characterized as one of three types:

Injury	Pathophysiology	Prognosis
Neurapraxia	Reversible conduction block—local ischemia	Good
Axonotmesis	More severe injury but endoneurium intact	Fair
Neurotmesis	Complete nerve division	Poor

   Nerve stretching also can affect function—8% elongation diminishes microcirculation to the nerve and 15% elongation disrupts axons. Nerve regeneration is influenced by contact guidance (attraction of regenerating nerve to basal lamina of the Schwann cell), neurotrophism (factors enhancing growth), and neurotropism (preferential attraction toward nerves as opposed to other tissues).

   5. Repair—Several methods available.

   a. Direct Muscular Neurotization—Inserts the proximal stump of the nerve into affected muscle belly. Results in less than normal function, but indicated in selected cases.

   b. Epineural Repair—Primary repair of the outer connective tissue layer of the nerve at the site of injury after resecting the proximal neuroma and distal glioma. Care is taken to assure proper rotation and lack of tension on the repair.

   c. Grouped Fascicular Repair—Primary repair is also done after resection of neuroma and glioma, but individual fascicles are reapproximated under microscopic magnification. Used for larger nerves, but no significant improvement in results over epineural repair.

VII. Soft Tissue Repair

A. Four phases of soft tissue repair are described.

1. Hemostasis—Primary platelet plug occurs within 5 minutes. Secondary clotting (via the coagulation cascade) uses fibrin and occurs within the first 10–15 minutes of injury. Fibronectin, a large glycoprotein, binds fibrin and cells and acts as a chemotactic factor. Platelets release factors that activate the next phase of repair.

2. Inflammation—Involves débridement of injured/necrotic tissue utilizing macrophages (facultative anaerobes), and occurs within the first week following injury. It includes three stages: (1) activation (immediate), (2) amplification (48–72 hours), and (3) débridement (using bacteria, phagocytosis, and matrix [biochemical] means). Prostaglandins help to mediate the inflammatory response.

3. Organogenesis—Occurs at 7–21 days and consists of tissue modeling. Mesenchymal precursors differentiate into myofibroblasts. Angiogenesis occurs. Further differentiation leads to the final stage of healing.

4. Remodeling—That of individual tissue lines begins shortly after repair and continues for up to 18 months. Realignment and cross-linking of collagen fibers allows increased tensile strength.

B. Growth factors—Require activation, are redundant, and function with feedback loop mechanisms.

1. Chemotactic Factors—Attract cells. Include prostaglandins (PMNs), prostanoids (PMNs), complement (PMNs and macrophages), platelet derived growth factor (PDGF) (macrophages and fibroblasts), and angiokines (endothelial cells).

2. Competence Factors—Activate dormant (G_o) cells. Includes PDGF and prostaglandins.

3. Progression Factors—Allow cell growth. Induce epidermal growth factor, interleukin-1, and somatomedins.

4. Inductive Factors—Stimulate differentiation. Include angiokines, bone morphogenic protein, and specific tissue growth factors.

5. Transforming Factors—Cause dedifferentiation and proliferation.

6. Permissive Factors—Are enhancing factors; include fibronectin and osteonectin.

VIII. Soft Tissue Implants

A. Introduction—Usually used around the knee (ACL), implants can be allografts, autografts, and synthetics.

B. Allografts—Have no donor site morbidity, but incite an immune response and may transmit infection. The immunogenic response can be reduced with treatment (freeze-drying), but this affects strength. If not harvested sterilely, treatment with ethylene oxide (may have adverse affects), or radiation is required.

C. Synthetic Ligaments—Unlike autografts or allografts, these structures have no initial period of weakness. However, they suffer from wear and are associated with effusions.

Part **3**

Metabolic Bone Disease

I. Normal Bone Metabolism

A. Calcium—Bone serves as a reservoir for over 99% of the body's calcium. Calcium is also important in muscle and nerve function, in the clotting mechanism, and many other areas. Plasma calcium is about equally free and bound (usually to albumin). It is absorbed from the gut (duodenum) via active transport (ATP and calcium binding protein required) that is regulated by 1,25-$(OH)_2$-vitamin D_3, and also absorbed by passive diffusion (jejunum). It is 98% reabsorbed by the kidney (60% in proximal tubule). Dietary requirement of calcium is about 900 mg/day; it increases to about 1500 mg/day for adolescents, in pregnancy, and in postmenopausal females, and to about 2000 mg/day for lactating females. Most people have a positive calcium balance in their first three decades of life and a negative balance after the fourth decade. About 400 mg of calcium is released from bone on a daily basis. Calcium may be excreted in stool. Hypercalcemia can lead to hyperreflexia and convulsions. Hypocalcemia leads to somnolence and areflexia.

B. Phosphate—Besides being a key component of bone mineral, phosphate has an important role in enzyme systems and molecular interactions (metabolite and buffer). Approximately 85% of the body's phosphate stores are in bone. Plasma phosphate is mostly in the unbound form, and is reabsorbed by the kidney (also in the proximal tubule). Dietary intake of phosphate is usually adequate; daily requirement is 1000–1500 mg/day. May excrete in urine.

C. Parathyroid Hormone (PTH)—An 84–amino acid peptide made and secreted from chief cells in the four parathyroid glands, PTH helps regulate plasma calcium. It probably acts via a β_2 receptor in the parathyroid gland. Decreased calcium levels in the extracellular fluid stimulate release of PTH. It acts at three sites:

Site	Action
Bone	Mobilizes calcium and phosphate
	Releases osteocytic perilacunar stores (fast)
	Increases osteocyte number and activity (slow)
Kidney	Increases resorption of calcium (cAMP required)
	Increases excretion of phosphate
	Stimulates 1,25-(OH)$_2$-vitamin D$_3$ (calcitriol) production
Gut	Increases absorption (through vitamin D$_3$)

PTH may also have a role in bone loss in the aged.

D. Vitamin D$_3$—Naturally occurring steroid that is activated by UV irradiation from sunlight or utilized from dietary intake (vitamin D$_2$) (Fig. 2–18). It is hydroxylated to the 25 (OH)-vitamin D$_3$ form in the liver, and is hydroxylated a second time in the kidney. Conversion to the 1,25-(OH)$_2$-vitamin D$_3$ form activates the hormone, whereas conversion to the 24,25-(OH)$_2$-vitamin D$_3$ form inactivates it. The active form works at all three sites:

Site	Action
Bone	Promotion and mobilization of calcium
	Increases osteocyte number and activity
Kidney	Increases phosphate ± calcium resorption
	Encourages production of 24,25-(OH)$_2$-vitamin D$_3$
Gut	Promotes calcium and phosphate absorption
	Acts by inducing calcium binding protein

E. Calcitonin—A 32–amino acid peptide hormone made by clear (C) cells in parafollicles of the thyroid gland, this hormone also has a limited role in calcium regulation. Increased calcium levels in the extracellular milieu cause its secretion. Like PTH, calcitonin secretion is controlled by a β_2 receptor. Its role, still not fully known, is to decrease plasma calcium by working, once again, at three sites:

Site	Action
Bone	Decreases osteoclastic (and osteocytic) resorption
	(Osteoclasts lose ruffled border and clear zone)
Kidney	Decreases resorption of calcium and phosphate
Gut	Increases secretion of electrolytes
	Decreases secretion of acid

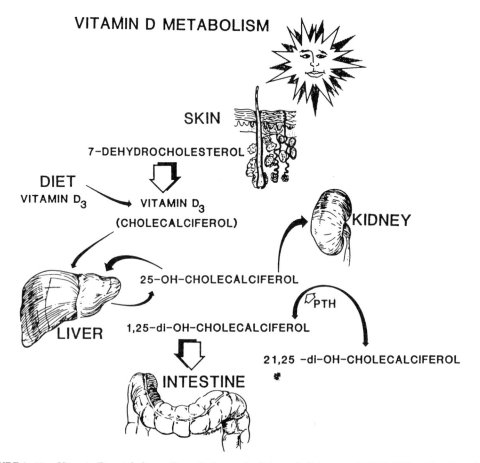

VITAMIN D METABOLISM

SKIN

7-DEHYDROCHOLESTEROL

DIET
VITAMIN D$_3$

VITAMIN D$_3$
(CHOLECALCIFEROL)

KIDNEY

LIVER

25-OH-CHOLECALCIFEROL

PTH

1,25-di-OH-CHOLECALCIFEROL

21,25 -di-OH-CHOLECALCIFEROL

INTESTINE

FIGURE 2–18. Vitamin D metabolism. (From Orthopaedic Science Syllabus, p. 45. Park Ridge, IL., American Academy of Orthopaedic Surgery, 1986; reprinted by permission.)

Calcitonin may also have a physiologic role in fracture healing and treatment of osteoporosis.

F. Other Hormones—The following hormones also have an effect on bone metabolism.
  1. Estrogen—Prevents bone loss by inhibiting resorption (related to calcitonin?). Supplementation is helpful in postmenopausal women but only if it is started within the first 5–10 years after the onset of menopause. The risk of endometrial cancer for patients taking estrogen is reduced when it is combined with cyclic progestin therapy.
  2. Corticosteroids—Increase bone loss (decrease gut absorption by decreasing binding proteins, and decrease bone formation [cancellous bone more affected than cortical bone] through inhibition of collagen synthesis). Adverse effects with therapy may be reduced with alternate-day therapy.
  3. Thyroid Hormones—Affect bone resorption more than bone formation, leading to osteoporosis. Large (thyroid-suppressive) doses of thyroxine can lead to osteoporosis.
  4. Growth Hormone—Causes a positive calcium balance by increasing gut absorption more than its increase in urinary excretion. Insulin and somatomedins participate in this effect.
  5. Growth Factors—TGF, PDGF, and mono/lymphokines have a role in bone and cartilage repair.

G. Interaction—Calcium and phosphate metabolism is affected by an elaborate interplay of hormones and even the levels of the metabolites themselves. Feedback mechanisms play an important role in the regulation of plasma levels of calcium and phosphate. Peak bone mass usually occurs in the third or fourth decade and is greater in men and blacks. After this peak, bone loss occurs at a rate of 0.3–0.5% per year (2–3% per year for untreated females during the sixth through 10th years after menopause).

II. Hypercalcemia
  A. Introduction—Hypercalcemia can present with polyuria, constipation, lethargy, and disorientation. Hyperreflexia, kidney stones, excessive bony resorption ± fibrotic tissue replacement (osteitis fibrosa cystic), weakness, and CNS and GI effects are also common.
  B. Primary Hyperparathyroidism—Caused by overproduction of PTH, usually as a result of a parathyroid adenoma (which usually affects only one gland). Excessive PTH causes a net increase in plasma calcium (from all three sources) and a decrease in plasma phosphate (due to enhanced urinary excretion). This results in increased osteoclastic resorption and failure of repair attempts (poor mineralization from low phosphate). Diagnosis is based on signs and symptoms of hypercalcemia (described above), and characteristic labs (incr. serum calcium, PTH, urinary phosphate; decr. serum phosphate). Bony changes include osteopenia, osteitis fibrosa cystica (fibrous replacement of marrow), "brown tumors" (increased giant cells, extravasation of RBCs, hemosiderin staining and fibrous tissue hemosiderin), and chondrocalcinosis. Radiographs may

demonstrate deformed, osteopenic bones, fractures, "shaggy" trabeculae, and areas of radiolucency. Histologic changes in these tumors include osteoblasts and osteoclasts active on both sides of trabeculae (as seen in Paget's disease), areas of destruction, and wide osteoid seams. Surgical parathyroidectomy is curative.

C. Other Causes of Hypercalcemia
  1. Familial Syndromes—Hypercalcemia can occur from pituitary adenomas associated with multiple endocrine neoplasia (MEN) types I and II, and from familial hypocalciuric hypercalcemia, which is caused by poor renal clearance of calcium.
  2. Other causes of hypercalcemia include malignant disease (most common), hyperthyroidism, Addison's disease, peptic ulcer disease, kidney disease, and sarcoidosis.

III. Hypocalcemia
  A. Introduction—Low plasma calcium can occur from low PTH or vitamin D_3. Hypocalcemia leads to increased neuromuscular irritability (tetany, seizures, Chvostek's sign), cataracts, nail fungal infections, EKG changes (prolonged Q interval), and other signs and symptoms.

  B. Primary Hypoparathyroidism—Decreased PTH causes diminished plasma calcium and increased plasma phosphate (urinary excretion not enhanced due to lack of PTH). Common findings include fungal infections of the nails, hair loss, and blotches of skin with pigment loss (vitiligo). Skull radiographs may show basal ganglion calcification. Iatrogenic hypoparathyroidism can follow thyroidectomy.

  C. Pseudohypoparathyroidism (PHP)—A rare genetic disorder that causes a lack of effect of PTH at the target cells. PTH levels are normal or even high, but its action on the cellular level is blocked by an abnormality at the receptor, the cAMP system, or by a lack of required cofactors (e.g., Mg^{2+}). **Albright** hereditary osteodystrophy, a form of PHP, is associated with **short first, fourth, and fifth MCs and MTs**, brachydactyly, exostoses, obesity, and diminished intelligence.

  D. Renal Osteodystrophy—Chronic renal failure (CRF) leads to inability to excrete phosphate. Often considered a form of osteomalacia, it is commonly associated with long-term hemodialysis. High levels of plasma phosphate lead to a decrease in plasma calcium. This is ordinarily adjusted by PTH, which increases urinary excretion of phosphate. This often leads to hyperplasia of the parathyroid chief cells, resulting in **secondary hyperparathyroidism**. In CRF, however, the phosphate cannot be secreted, and symptoms similar to hypoparathyroidism result. Radiographs may demonstrate a "rugger jersey" spine like that in childhood osteopetrosis, and soft tissue calcification. Labs show abnormal glomerular filtration rate (GFR). Treatment should be directed at relieving urologic obstruction or kidney disease.

  E. Rickets (Adult Osteomalacia)—Failure of mineralization leading to changes in the physis (increased width and disorientation) and bone (cortical thinning, bowing).

1. Vitamin–D Deficiency Rickets—Almost eliminated by addition of vitamin D to milk in the U.S., this disease is still seen in Asian immigrants, patients with dietary peculiarities, premature infants, and with malabsorption (sprue) or chronic parenteral nutrition. Decreased absorption of calcium and phosphate leads to secondary hyperparathyroidism (PTH continues to be produced because of low plasma calcium). Lab studies show low normal calcium (maintained by high PTH), low phosphate (excreted due to effect of PTH), increased PTH, and low levels of vitamin D. Enlargement of the costochondral junction ("rachitic rosary"), bony deformities (bowing of the knees, "codfish" vertebrae), retarded bone growth (defect in hypotrophic zone with **widened osteoid seams** and physeal cupping), muscle hypotonia, dental disease, pathologic fractures (Looser's zones [pseudofracture of compression side of bone], Milkman's fracture [pseudofracture in adults]), and other problems can result. Treatment with vitamin D (5,000 U daily) and calcium (up to 3 g daily) will resolve most deformities.

2. Hereditary Vitamin D–Dependent Rickets—Rare AR disorder that may represent a defect in 1-hydroxylation of vitamin D_3 in the kidney, leading to low levels of and/or defective 1,25-$(OH)_2$-vitamin D_3. The disease features are similar to those of vitamin D–deficient rickets, except that they may be worse and include total baldness. High levels of vitamin D are required to treat this form of rickets—on the order of 20,000–100,000 units per day—followed by maintenance dosage of a vitamin D_3 analogue.

3. Familial Hypophosphatemic Rickets (Vitamin D–Resistant Rickets; a.k.a. "Phosphate Diabetes")—X-linked dominant disorder that is a result of impaired renal tubular reabsorption of phosphate. Affected patients have a normal GFR and an impaired vitamin D_3 response. Phosphate replacement (1–4 g daily) with vitamin D_3 can correct the effects, which are similar to those of the other forms of rickets.

4. Hypophosphatasia—AR disorder caused by low levels of alkaline phosphatase, which is required for the synthesis of inorganic phosphate, important in bone matrix formation. Features are similar to rickets, and treatment may include phosphate therapy. Increased urinary phosphoethanolamine is diagnostic.

IV. Osteopenia

A. Osteoporosis—Age-related decrease in bone mass usually associated with loss of estrogen in postmenopausal women. Osteoporosis is responsible for over 1 million fractures per year (vertebral body most common). It is a quantitative and not a qualitative defect in bone. Sedentary, thin Caucasian women of northern European descent, particularly smokers, heavy drinkers, and patients on phenytoin (impairs vitamin D metabolism), with low-calcium and low–vitamin D diets who breast-fed their infants, are at greatest risk. Cancellous bone is most affected. Clinical features include kyphosis (dowager's hump) and fractures (compression fractures of T11–L1 [ventrally creating a wedge-shaped defect or centrally resulting in "codfish" vertebrae], hip fractures,

TABLE 2–4. METABOLIC

Disease	Etiology	Findings	Radiographs
Hypercalcemia			
Hyperparathyroidism	PTH overproduction—adenoma	Kidney stone, hyperreflexia	Osteopenia, osteitis fibrosa cystica
Familial syndromes	PTH overproduction—MEN/renal	Endocrine/renal abnormalities	Osteopenia
Hypocalcemia			
Hypoparathyroidism	PTH underproduction—idiopathic	Neuromuscular irritability, eye	Calcified basal ganglia
PHP/Albright	PTH receptor abnormality	Short MC/MT, obesity	Brachydactyly, exostosis
Renal osteodystrophy	CRF—decr. phosphate excretion	Renal abnormalities	"Rugger jersey" spine
Rickets (osteomalacia)			
Vit. D–deficient	Decr. vit. D diet; malabsorption	Bone deformities, hypotonia	"Rachitic rosary," wide growth plates, fxs
Vit. D–dependent	Def. 1-hydroxylation in kidney	Total baldness	Poor mineralization
Vit. D–resistent (hypophosphatemic)	Decr. renal tubular phosphate resorption	Bone deformities hypotonia	Poor mineralization
Hypophosphatasia	Decr. alkaline phosphatase	Bone deformities, hypotonia	Poor mineralization
Osteopenia			
Osteoporosis	Decr. estrogen—decr. bone mass	Kyphosis, fractures	Compression vertebral fx, hip fx
Scurvy	Vit. C deficiency—defective collagen	Fatigue, bleeding, effusions	Thin cortices, corner sign
Osteodense			
Paget's disease	Osteoclastic abn—incr. bone turnover	Deformities, pain, CHF, fxs	Coarse trabeculae, "picture frame" vertebrae
Osteopetrosis	Osteoclastic abn—unclear	Hepatosplenomegaly, anemia	Bone w/in bone

a I, increase; D, decrease; N, normal; DD, markedly decreased, NI, normal or increased.

and distal radius fractures are common). Two types of osteoporosis have been characterized:

TYPE	CHARACTERISTICS
Type I (postmenopausal)	Affects trabecular bone primarily; vertebral & distal radius fractures common
Type II (Age-related)	In patients >75 yo (related to poor calcium absorption); affects trabecular and cortical bone; hip/pelvic fractures common

Laboratory studies, including urinary calcium and hydroxyproline and serum alkaline phosphatase, are helpful in evaluation of osteoporosis. Results are usually unremarkable, but hyperthyroidism, hyperparathyroidism, Cushing's syndrome, hematologic disorders, and malignancy should be ruled out. Plain **radiographs** are usually **not helpful unless >30% bone loss** is present. Special studies used in the work-up of osteoporosis include single- (appendicular) and double- (axial) photon absorptiometry, quantitative CT and dual-energy radiographic absorptiometry (DRA). DRA is most accurate with less radiation. Biopsy (after tetracycline labeling) may sometimes be necessary to evaluate the severity of osteoporosis and to identify osteomalacia. Histologic changes in osteoporosis include thinning of trabeculae, decreased size of osteons, and enlargement of haversian and marrow spaces. Physical activity, calcium supplements (more effective in type II, age-related osteoporosis), estrogen-progesterone therapy (in type I, postmenopausal osteoporosis; best when initiated within 6 years of menopause), and fluoride (inhibits bone resorption but bone is more brittle) have a role in therapy. Other drugs, such as intramuscular calcitonin, may also be helpful but are expensive and may cause hypersensitivity reactions. The future of bone augmentation with PTH, growth factors (GF), prostaglandin inhibitors and other modes of therapy remains to be determined.

B. Osteomalacia—Discussed with rickets. Defect in mineralization results in a large amount of unmineralized osteoid (qualitative defect). Osteomalacia is caused by vitamin D–deficient diets, GI disorders, renal osteodystrophy, and certain drugs (aluminum-containing phosphate binding antacids [Al deposition in bone prevents mineralization] and Dilantin). It is commonly associated with Looser's zones (microscopic stress fractures), other fractures, biconcave vertebral bodies, and trefoil pelvis seen on plain radiographs. Biopsy (transiliac) is required for diagnosis (histologically, widened osteoid seams are seen). Femoral neck fractures are common in patients with osteomalacia. Treatment usually includes large doses of vitamin D.

C. Scurvy—Vitamin C (ascorbic acid) deficiency leads to defective collagen growth and repair. Clinical features include fatigue, gum bleeding, ecchymosis, joint effusions, and iron deficiency. Radiographic changes may include thin cortices and trabeculae and metaphyseal clefts (corner sign). Labs are normal. Histologic changes include replacement of primary trabeculae with

BONE DISEASES

	SERUM LAB VALUES[a]				URINARY LAB VALUES[a]		
Ca	PO$_4$	PTH	Other Labs		Ca	PO$_4$	TREATMENT
I	D	I			N	I	Surgical excision
I	D	I			N	I	Treat underlying syndrome
D	I	D			D	D	PTH
D	I	I	Decr. Mg^{2+}		D	D	Ca, vit. D, ± Mg
D	I	I	Incr. BUN/Cr		D	D	Treat kidney disease
N	D	I	Decr. vit. D		D	I	Ca, vit. D
D	D	I	Decr./abnorm. vit. D		D	I	Ca, vit. D incr.
N	DD	N			N	I	Phos, vit. D$_3$
NI	N	N	Decr. AP, Incr. urinary urea		N	N	Phosphate
N	N	N	Special testing		N	N	Ca, estrogen-progesterone, fluoride
N	N	N	Decr. vit. C, Fe		N	N	Vit. C supplementation
N	N	N	Incr. AP, urinary hydroxyproline		N	N	Calcitonin, diphosphonates
N	N	N			N	N	Bone marrow transplant

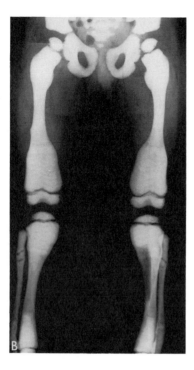

FIGURE 2–19. Typical "marble bone" appearance in osteopetrosis. (From Tachdjian, M.O.: Pediatric Orthopaedics, 2nd ed., p. 795, Philadelphia, W.B. Saunders, 1990; reprinted by permission.)

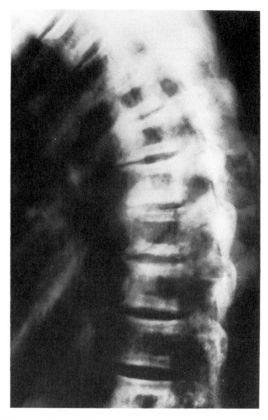

FIGURE 2–20. Typical "rugger jersy" spine in osteopetrosis. (From Tachdjian, M.O.: Pediatric Orthopaedics, 2nd ed., p. 797. Philadelphia, W.B. Saunders, 1990; reprinted by permission.)

granulation tissue, areas of hemorrhage, and widening of the zone of provisional calcification in the physis.

    D. Marrow Packing Disorders—Myeloma, leukemia, and other disorders can cause osteopenia (see Chapter 7, Orthopaedic Pathology).

V. Increased Osteodensity

    A. Paget's Disease—Discussed in Chapter 7, Orthopaedic Pathology.

    B. Osteopetrosis (Marble Bone Disease)—A group of bone disorders that lead to increased sclerosis and obliteration of the medullary canal due to decreased osteoclast function (a failure of bone resorption). Histologically, osteoclasts lack the normal ruffled border and clear zone. The marrow spaces become filled with necrotic calcified cartilage. Empty lacunae and plugging of haversian canals is also seen. The most severe juvenile (AR) "malignant" form leads to a "bone within a bone" appearance on x-rays, hepatosplenomegaly, and aplastic anemia. **Bone marrow transplantation** (of osteoclast precursors) **can be life-saving in childhood.** High doses of calcitriol ± steroids may also be helpful. The AD "tarda" form (Albers-Schönberg disease) demonstrates generalized osteosclerosis (including the typical "rugger jersey" spine, usually without other anomalies (Figs. 2–19 and 2–20). Pathologic fractures through abnormal (brittle) bone are common.

    C. Osteopoikilosis ("Spotted Bone Disease")—Islands of deep cortical bone appear within the medullary cavity and cancellous bone of long bones (especially in the hands and feet). These areas are usually asymptomatic and there is no known incidence of malignant degeneration.

VI. Summary—The characteristic of the various types of metabolic bone disease are summarized in Table 2–4.

Part 4

Arthritides

I. Noninflammatory Arthritides

A. Common Characteristics—This group of arthritides includes osteoarthritis, neuropathic arthropathy, acute rheumatic fever, and other entities discussed elsewhere (acromegaly, osteonecrosis, osteochondromatosis, osteochondritis dissecans). All share similar results on joint fluid analysis, with normal viscosity (high), color (straw), WBCs and differential (200 with 25% PMNs), mucin clot (firm), and glucose and protein (equal to serum).

B. **Osteoarthritis** (degenerative joint disease)—Although it is the most common form of arthritis, very little is known about this disease.

1. Etiology—On a cellular level, osteoarthritis may be a result of a failed attempt of chondrocytes to repair damaged cartilage as well as increased water content (as opposed to a decrease in water content seen with aging); alterations in proteoglycans (shorter chains—decreased chondroitin-to–keratin sulfate ratio); collagen (disrupted by collagenase); and binding of proteoglycans to hyaluronic acid (caused by action of proteolytic enzymes from increased PgE and decreased numbers of link proteins) of affected cartilage. Cartilage degeneration is encouraged by shear stresses and is prevented with normal compressive forces. Excessive stresses and inadequate chondrocyte response lead to degeneration. Interleukin-1 (catabolin) and estradiol lead to degeneration in cartilage; GAGs and polysufuric acid may help prevent it. Genetic predisposition is an important factor.

2. Characteristics—From a larger perspective, osteoarthritis can be primary (from an intrinsic defect—mechanical, immune, vascular, cartilage, etc.), or secondary (from trauma, infection, congenital disorders, etc.). Changes that occur in osteoarthritis begin with deterioration and loss of the bearing surface, followed by development of osteophytes and breakdown of the osteochondral junction; finally, disintegration of the cartilage plus subchondral microfracture exposes the bony surface. Subchondral cysts (from microfractures) and osteophytes, which are part of this process, along with joint space narrowing and eburnation of bone, are demonstrated on radiographs. Microscopic changes include loss of superficial chondrocytes, chondrocyte cloning (>1 chondrocyte per lacunae), replication and breakdown of the tidemark, fissuring, cartilage destruction with eburnation of subchondral "pagetoid" bone and other changes noted elsewhere. Notable features on exam include decreased ROM and crepitus. The knee is the most common joint affected. Treatment begins with supportive measures (activity modification, cane, etc.) and includes NSAIDs and a variety of surgical procedures ranging from arthroscopic débridement to total joint arthroplasties.

C. **Neuropathic Arthropathy** (Charcot Joint)—An extreme form of osteoarthritis caused by a disturbance in the sensory innervation of a joint. Causes include diabetes (foot), tabes dorsalis (lower extremity), **syringomyelia (upper extremity)**, Hansen's disease (#2 cause of neuropathic joints in the upper extremity), myelomeningocele (ankle and foot), congenital indifference to pain (ankle and foot), and other neurologic problems. Typically involves an older patient with an unstable, painless, swollen joint. Can present with hemarthrosis (and is sometimes classified in group IV). It is often confused with infection. Radiographs show advanced destructive changes on both sides of the joint, scattered "chunks" of bone embedded in fibrous tissue, and heterotopic ossification. Treatment is focused on limitation of activity and appropriate bracing. A **Charcot joint is usually a contraindication for a total joint arthroplasty** and other orthopaedic hardware.

D. **Acute Rheumatic Fever** (Sometimes included in the inflammatory group)—Formerly the most common cause of childhood arthritis, acute rheumatic fever is now rarely seen since the advent of antibiotics. Arthritis and arthralgias can follow untreated group A β-hemolytic strep infections, and can present with acute onset of red, tender, and extremely painful joint effusions. Systemic manifestations include carditis, erythema marginatum (painless macules with red margins—usually involving the abdomen and never seen on the face), subcutaneous nodules (extensor surfaces of upper extremities), and chorea. The arthritis is migratory and typically involves multiple larger joints. **Diagnosis is based on Jones criteria** (preceding streptococcal infection with two major criteria [carditis, polyarthritis, chorea, erythema marginatum, subcutaneous nodules] or one major and two minor criteria [fever, arthralgia, prior rheumatic fever, elevated ESR, prolonged PR interval on EKG]). Antistreptolysin O titers are elevated in 80% of affected patients. Treatment includes penicillin and acetylsalicylic acid.

E. Ochronosis—Degenerative arthritis resulting from alkaptonuria, a rare inborn defect of the homogentisic acid oxidase enzyme system (tyrosine and phenylalanine catabolism). Excess homogentisic acid is deposited in joints and then polymerizes (turns black) and leads to early degenerative changes. **Ochronitic spondylitis** which usually occurs in the fourth decade of life, includes progressive degenerative changes and **disc space narrowing** and **calcification**.

II. Inflammatory Arthritides

A. Common Characteristics—Include a wide range of rheumatologic diseases. Rheumatoid arthritis, systemic lupus erythematosus (SLE), juvenile rheumatoid arthritis (JRA), the spondyloarthropathies, and crystalline arthropathies are usually included in this group. Synovial fluid in this group typically demonstrates low viscosity, yellow-green color, 2,000–75,000 WBCs with 50% PMNs, a friable mucin clot, and moderately decreased glucose (25 mg/dl lower than serum glucose). All of these disorders may be associated with an HLA complex region:

Region	Expression	Rheumatologic Disease
Class I	All cells ("self")	Spondyloarthropathies
Class II	Lymphocytes, MOs	RA, SLE
Class III	Complement proteins	SLE

B. **Rheumatoid Arthritis (RA)**—The most common form of inflammatory arthritis, affects 3% of women and 1% of men. Diagnostic criteria, developed by the American Rheumatism Association, require several of the following: morning stiffness, swelling, nodules, positive lab tests, and radiographic findings.

1. Etiology—Unclear, but probably related to cell-mediated immune response (T cell) that incites an inflammatory response initially against soft tissues and later against cartilage (chondrolysis) and bone (periarticular bone resorption). May be associated with infectious etiology or HLA focus (HLA-Dw4). Lymphokines and other inflammatory mediators initiate a destructive cascade that leads to joint destruction. Rheumatoid arthritis cartilage is sensitive to PMN degradation and IL-1 effects (phospholipase A_2, PGE_2, and plasminogen activators).

2. Characteristics—Usually an insidious onset of morning stiffness and polyarthritis. Most commonly the hands (ulnar deviation and subluxation of MCPs) and feet (MTPs—claw toes and hallux valgus) are affected early, but involvement of knees, elbows, shoulders, ankles, and neck is also common. Synovium and soft tissues are first affected, and only later are joints significantly involved. Pannus ingrowth denudes articular cartilage and leads to chondrocyte death. Lab findings include elevated ESR and C-reactive protein, as well as a positive RF (IgM) in most patients. Radiographs demonstrate periarticular erosions and osteopenia. Joint fluid assays can also demonstrate RF, decreased complement levels, and other helpful findings. Systemic manifestations can include pericarditis and pulmonary disease (pleurisy, nodules, and fibrosis). Popliteal cysts in rheumatoids (confirmed by ultrasound) can mimic thrombophlebitis. *Felty's syndrome* is RA with splenomegaly and leukopenia. *Still's disease* is acute-onset RA with fever, rash, and splenomegaly. *Sjögren's syndrome* is an autoimmune exocrinopathy often associated with RA. Symptoms include decreased salivary and lacrimal gland secretion (keratoconjunctivitis sicca complex) and lymphoid proliferation.

3. Treatment—Control of synovitis and pain, maintenance of joint function, and prevention of deformities are the goals of therapy. A multidisciplanary approach involving therapeutic drugs, physical therapy, and sometimes surgery is necessary to achieve these goals. A "pyramid" approach to drug therapy for rheumatoids involves beginning with NSAIDs and slowly progressing to antimalarials, remissive agents (gold and penicillamine), steroids, cytotoxic drugs, and finally experimental drugs. Surgery includes synovectomy (rarely indicated, only if aggressive drug therapy fails), soft tissue realignment procedures (usually not favored because deformity will progress), and various reconstructive procedures. Chemical and radiation synovectomy (dyprosium-165) can be successful if it is done early. Arthroscopic synovectomy, especially in the knee, has proven efficacy. Following all forms of synovectomy, the synovium initially regenerates normally, but with time it will degenerate back into rheumatoid synovial tissue. Evaluation of cervical spine with preoperative radiographs is important.

C. **Systemic Lupus Erythematosus** (SLE)—Chronic inflammatory disease of unknown origin usually affecting women, especially black women. Probably immune complex related. Manifestations include fever, butterfly rash, pancytopenia, pericarditis, nephritis, and polyarthritis. Joint involvement is the most common feature, affecting over 3/4 of SLE patients. Arthritis typically presents as acute, red, tender swelling of PIPs, MCPs, and carpi of the hand as well as the knees and other joints. It is typically not as destructive as RA. Treatment for SLE arthritis usually includes the same medications described for RA. Mortality in SLE is usually related to renal disease. Differential diagnosis includes polymyositis and dermatomyositis, which also present with symmetric weakness ± a characteristic "helotropic" rash of the upper eyelids.

D. **Polymyalgia Rheumatica**—A common disease of the elderly. Aching and stiffness of the shoulder and pelvic girdles, associated with malaise, headaches, and anorexia, are common symptoms. Exam is usually unremarkable. Labs are notable for a markedly increased ESR, anemia, increased alkaline phosphatase, and increased immune complexes. This disorder, which **may be associated with temporal arteritis** (often requiring biopsy for definitive diagnosis), is usually treated symptomatically, with steroid use for refractory cases.

E. **Juvenile Rheumatoid Arthritis** (JRA)

1. Introduction—Discussed also in Chapter 1, Pediatric Orthopaedics. Three major types are recognized based on early involvement (first 6 months). May also be associated with an HLA focus (HLA-DR2, -4, -5, and -8, and HLA-B27 in boys). Treatment includes high-dose aspirin, only occasionally gold or remissive agents (refractory polyarticular), and **frequent ophthalmologic exam** (with slit lamp) for asymptomatic ocular involvement (pauciarticular).

2. Types—Characteristics of the three major types of JRA are given in Table 2–5.

F. **Relapsing Polychondritis**—Rare disorder associated with episodic inflammation, diffuse self-limited arthritis, and progressive cartilage destruction ± systemic vasculitis. The disorder typically involves the ears (thickening of the auricle), inflam-

TABLE 2–5. THREE MAJOR TYPES OF JUVENILE RHEUMATOID ARTHRITIS

TYPE	INCIDENCE	RF/ANA[a]	SEX	NO. JOINTS	OTHER SYMPTOMS
Pauciarticular	30%	−/−	F > M	<4	Iridocyclitis (20%)
Polyarticular	50%	+/+ 20%	F > M	>4	Rash (rule out rheumatic fever)
Systemic	20%	−/−	F = M	Metaphyses, cervical spine	Fever, rash, hepatosplenomegaly

[a] Rheumatoid factor/antinuclear antibodies: −, negative; +, positive.

matory eye disorders, tracheal involvement, hearing disorders, and sometimes cardiac involvement. It may be an autoimmune disorder (type II collagen affected). Treatment is supportive, but dapsone may have a role in the future.

G. Spondyolarthropathies—Enthesopathies (occur at ligament insertion into bone) characterized by positive HLA-B27 (sixth chromosome, "D" focus) and negative RF.

1. **Ankylosing spondylitis** (AS)—Bilateral sacroiliitis ± acute anterior uveitis in a HLA-B27–positive male is diagnostic of this disease. Radiographic changes in the spine include squaring of the vertebra, vertical syndesmophytes, and "whiskering" of the enthesis. Ascending ankylosis of the spine usually begins in the T–L-spine, often causing the entire spine to become rigid. Spinal manifestations include the "chin on chest" deformity, which may require corrective osteotomy of the cervicothoracic junction, difficult cervical **fractures (associated with epidural hemorrhage)**, and severe kyphotic deformities (posterior closing wedge osteotomy). Lower spinal deformities with hip flexion deformities are often helped with bilateral THAs. Acetabular protrusion (medial displacement of the acetabulum beyond the radiographic teardrop) is also associated with AS, and requires special techniques for THA as well as measures to control ectopic ossification. Initial therapy with PT and NSAIDs (phenylbutazone best, but can cause bone marrow depression) can be helpful. Often associated with heart disease and pulmonary fibrosis. Poor prognosis is associated with pulmonary involvement, hip involvement, and younger age at onset.

2. **Reiter's Syndrome**—Classic presentation is a young male with a **triad of urethritis, conjunctivitis, and oligoarticular arthritis**. Painless oral ulcers, penile lesions, and ulcers on the extremities, palms, and soles (keratoderma blennorrhagicum) are also common. The arthritis usually has an abrupt onset of swelling and pain in weight-bearing joints. Recurrence is common and can lead to erosions of MT heads and calcaneal periostitis. About 80% of patients will be HLA-B27 positive, and 60% with chronic disease will have sacroiliitis. Treatment includes NSAIDs, PT, and possibly sulfa drugs in the future.

3. **Psoriatic Arthropathy**—Affects about 7% of patients with psoriasis. Many different HLA loci may be involved, but HLA-B27 is found in 70% of patients with psoriatic arthritis and sacroiliitis. Many forms exist—most patients have the oligoarticular form, which affects the small joints of the hands and feet. Nail pitting, "sau-

sage" digits, and "**pencil in cup**" deformity (of the DIP on x-rays) are well recognized, which may progress to fusion. Treatment is similar to RA.

4. **Enteropathic Arthritis**—About 10–20% of Crohn's disease and ulcerative colitis patients can develop peripheral joint arthritis, and 5% or more may develop axial disease. The arthritis is nondeforming and occurs more commonly in the larger, weight-bearing joints. It usually presents as an acute monarticular synovitis, which may precede any bowel symptoms. Enteropathic arthritis is associated with AS 10–15% of the time.

H. Crystal Deposition Disease

1. **Gout**—A disorder of nucleic acid metabolism causes hyperuricemia, which leads to monosodium urate crystal deposition in joints. Inflammatory mediators (proteases, chemotactic factors, prostaglandins, leukotriene B_4, and free O_2 radicals) are activated by the crystals (inhibited by colchicine). Crystals also activate platelets, phagocytosis (inhibited by phenylbutazone and Indocin), interleukin-1, and the complement system. Local polypeptides may inhibit crystal inflammatory response via glycoprotein "coating." Recurrent attacks of arthritis, especially in males 40–60 yo (usually in the lower extremity—especially the great toe [podagra]), crystal deposition in tophi (ear helix, eyelid olecranon, Achilles; usually seen in chronic form), and renal disease/stones (2% Ca^{2+} vs. normal 0.2%) are characteristic. Gout may be precipitated by chemotherapy for myeloproliferative disorders. Radiographs may show soft tissue changes and "punched out" periarticular erosions with sclerotic overhanging borders. Demonstration of **thin, tapered intracellular crystals that are strongly negative birefringent** (parallel to yellow axis) in joint aspirate is essential for the diagnosis. Initial treatment with Indocin (75 mg tid) is indicated followed by a rheumatology consult. Allopurinol is used to treat chronic gout and prior to chemotherapy for myeloproliferative disorders. Cholchicine can be used for prophylaxis following recurrent attacks.

2. **Chondrocalcinosis**—Caused by several disorders, including calcium pyrophosphate deposition disease (CPPD), ochronosis, hyperparathyroidism, hypothyroidism, and hemochromatosis, which lead to increased calcium ± pyrophosphate crystal deposition. **CPPD, a.k.a. pseudogout**, is a common disorder of pyrophosphate metabolism that occurs in older patients and can occasionally cause acute attacks (again usually in the lower extremities, but

especially the knee). An amplification-loop hypothesis has been proposed. **Short, blunt (rhomboid-shaped) rods that are weakly positive birefringent** are demonstrated with aspiration. Radiographs show fine linear calcification in hyaline cartilage, and more diffuse calcification of menisci and other fibrocartilage. NSAIDs are often helpful in treatment. Intraarticular yttrium-90 injections have also been successful in chronic cases.

3. **Calcium Hydroxyapatite Crystal Deposition Disease**—Also associated with chondrocalcinosis and degenerative joint disease (DJD). It is a destructive arthropathy commonly seen in the shoulder (causing cuff arthropathy—the **"Milwaukee shoulder"**) and in the knee. Treatment is usually supportive.

III. Infectious Arthritides

A. Common Characteristics—Aspirates of acute, red, hot, effusions usually show opaque fluid with >80,000 WBCs (75 + % PMNs), low glucose (>25 mg/dl less than serum values), and positive Gram's stains/cultures. Increased lactate in synovial fluid may also be seen in infectious arthritis.

B. **Pyogenic Arthritis**—Occurs from hematogenous spread or by extension of osteomyelitis. Commonly occurs in children, and is discussed in detail in Chapter 1, Pediatric Orthopaedics. Occurs more commonly in adults who are at risk, including IV drug abusers (esp. SC and sacroiliac joints), sexually active young adults (gonococcal, especially if seen with skin papules), diabetics (feet and lower extremities), rheumatoids, and following trauma (fight bites, open injuries) and surgery (iatrogenic). Histology may demonstrate synovial hyperplasia, numerous PMNs, and cartilage destruction. Destruction of cartilage can be direct (proteolytic enzymes) or indirect (caused by pressure and lack of nutrition). Treatment includes I&D(s) and long-term antibiotics.

C. **Tuberculous Arthritis**—The chronic granulomatous infection caused by *Mycobacterium tuberculosis* usually involves joints by hematogenous spread. Spine and lower extremities are most often involved, typically in Mexicans and Asians. It is 80% monarticular. Radiographically, tuberculous arthritis causes changes on both sides of the joint. Diagnosis is helped with positive PPD, demonstration of acid-fast bacilli and "rice bodies" (fibrin globules) in joint fluid, positive cultures (may take several weeks), and characteristic x-rays (subchondral osteoporosis, cystic changes, notch-like bony destruction at the edge of the joint, and joint space

TABLE 2–6. COMPARISON OF

Arthritis	Age	Sex	Sym?	Joints	Exam
Noninflammatory					
Osteoarthritis	Old	M > F	Asym	Hip, knee, TMC	Dec ROM, crepitus
Neuroapathic	Old	M > F	Asym	Foot, ankle, LE	Effusion, Unstable
ARF	Child	M = F	Asym	Mig; lgr joints	Red tender jnt, rash
Ochronosis	Adult	M = F	Asym	Lg joints/spine	Dec ROM, locking
Inflammatory					
Rheumatoid	Young	F > M	Sym	Hands, feet	Ulnar dev, claw toes
SLE	Young	F > M	Sym	PIP, MCP, knee	Red swollen jnt, rash
JRA	Child	F > M	Sym	Knee, multi	Swollen jnt, nl color
Relapsing polychondritis	Old	M = F	Sym	All joints	Eye, ear involved
Spondyloarthropathies					
AS	Young	M > F	Sym	SI, spine, hip	Rigid spine "chin on chest"
Reiter's synd.	Young	M > F	Asym	Wt-bearing	Urethral D/C, conjunctivitis
Psoriatic	Young	M = F	Asym	DIP, Small jnts	Rash, Sausage digit, pitting
Entereopathic	Young	M > F	Asym	Wt-bearing	Synovitis, GI manifestations
Crystal Deposition Disease					
Gout	Young	M > F	Asym	Gt toe, LE	Tophi, red, swollen
Chondrocalcinosis	Old	M = F	Asym	Knee, LE	Acute swelling
Infectious					
Pyogenic	Any	M = F	Asym	Any joint	Red, hot, swollen
Tuberculous	Old	M > F	Asym	Spine, LE	Indolent, swelling
Lyme disease	Young	M = F	Asym	Any joint	Acute effusion
Fungal	Any	M > F	Asym	Any joint	Indolent
Hemorrhagic					
Hemophilic	Young	M	Asym	Knee, UE (elbow, shoulder)	Decr. ROM, swelling
Sickle cell	Young	M = F	Asym	Hip, any bone	Pain, Decr. ROM
PVNS	Young	M = F	Asym	Knee, LE	Pain, synovitis

narrowing with osteolytic changes on both sides of the joint). Histology may demonstrate characteristic granulomas with Langerhans giant cells. Treatment includes I&D and antibiotics.

D. **Fungal Arthritis**—More common in neonates, AIDS victims, and drug users. Pathogens include *Candida albicans*. KOH prep of synovial fluid is helpful because cultures require prolonged incubation. Arthritis can be treated with 5-flucytosine. Blastomycosis, cocci, and other fungal infections often require treatment with amphotericin (this treatment may sometimes be administered intra-articularly with less side effects).

E. **Lyme Disease**—Acute, self-limited joint effusions (especially in the shoulder and knee) that recur at frequent intervals, caused by the spirochete *Borrelia burgdorferi*, which is transmitted by ticks endemic in 1/2 of the U.S. Sometimes called the "great mimicker"; systemic signs may include a characteristic "bull's-eye" rash **(erythema chronicum migrans)**, and neurologic (Bell's palsy is common) or cardiac symptoms. The disease occurs in three stages (I—rash, II—neurologic symptoms, III—arthritis). Immune complexes and cryoglobulins accumulate in the synovial fluid of affected individuals. Diagnosis is confirmed by ELISA testing, which should be sought in endemic areas after Gram's stain and joint cultures of an infectious aspirate show no organisms. Treatment is with penicillin or tetracycline.

IV. Hemorrhagic Effusions

A. Common Characteristics—Share the same laboratory findings with blood. Can be the result of hemophilia, sickle cell disease, pigmented villonodular synovitis, or other causes discussed elsewhere (neuropathic joint, trauma, tumors).

B. **Hemophilic Arthropathy**—X-linked recessive factor VIII deficiency (hemophilia A—classic or factor IX deficiency; hemophilia B—Christmas disease) associated with repeated hemarthrosis from minor trauma leading to synovitis, cartilage destruction (enzymatic processes), and joint deformity. Severity of disease is related to degree of deficiency (mild, 5–25% levels; moderate, 1–5% levels; severe, 0–1% levels). Repeated episodes of hemarthrosis lead to replacement of the normal joint capsule with dense scar. The knee is most commonly involved, followed by the elbow, ankle, shoulder, and spine. Joint swelling, decreased ROM, and pain are characteristic. A joint aspirate should be obtained in order to rule out a concomitant infection. Radiographs later in the disease process may demonstrate a **"squared off"** patella (Jordan's sign

COMMON ARTHRITIDES

Labs	Radiographs	Systemic	Treatment
Nonspecific	Asymm. narrowing, eburnation, cysts, osteophytes	None	NSAID, Fusion, Osteotomy, TJA
For underlying dis.	Destruction/heterotopic bone	None	Brace, **TJA contraindicated**
ASO titer	Usually normal	Eryth. marg, nodules, carditis	Symptomatic
Urine homogentisic acid	Destruction, disc calcification	Spondylosis	Supportive
ESR, CRP, RF	Symm. narrow, periart. resorp.	Pericard, Pulm. dis.	Pyramid Tx, synovitis, reconstr. surg.
ANA	Less destruction	Card, neph, pancytopenia	Drug therapy like RA
RF/ANA	Juxta-art. rare, osteopenia	Iridocyclitis, rash	ASA; 75% remission
ESR	Normal	Ear, cardiac	Supportive, dapsone?
ESR, alk. phos., CPK, B27	SI arth, bamboo spine	Uveitis	PT, NSAID, osteostomy
ESR, WBC, B27	MT head erosion, periostitis	Urethritis, conjunctivitis, ulcer	PT, NSAID, Sulfa?
ESR, α_2, B27	DIP—pencil in cup	Rash, conjunctivitis	Drug therapy like RA
ESR, B27	Normal	Eryth. nodosum, pyoderma	Tx bowel dis; symptomatic
Uric Acid; −Birefr. cryst.	Soft tissue swell, erosions	Tophi, renal stones	Colchicine, Indocin
+Birefr. rod-shaped cryst.	Art, fibrocart. calcified	Ochronosis, hyperparathyroidism, hypopthyroidism	Sympotomatic, avoid surg
WBC, ESR, bacteria	Joint narrowing (late)	Fever, chills, infect.	I&D, IV antibiotics
PPD, AFB, cultures	Both sides, cysts	Lung, multiorgan	Antibiotics ± I&D
Culture, ELISA	Usually normal	ECM rash, neuro, cardiac	Penicillin, tetracycline
Special studies/cult	Minimal changes	Immunocompromised	5-FU, amphotericin
PTT, factor VIII	Squared-off patell·	Soft tissue bleeding	Support, synovectomy, TJA (unless + inhibitor)
Sickle prep	Osteonecrosis	Infarcts, osteonecrosis	
Aspirate, biopsy	Juxtacortical erosion	None	Surgical excision

[also seen in JRA]), widening of the intercondylar notch, and enlarged femoral condyles that appear to "fall off" the tibia. Ultrasound can be used to diagnose and follow intramuscular bleeding episodes. **Iliacus hematomas can cause femoral nerve palsies**. Management includes balancing of factors, splints, compressive dressings, bracing, and analgesics. Occasionally, steroids are helpful. Surgical management includes synovectomy (for recurrent hemarthroses and synovial hypertrophy refractory to conservative treatment), total joint arthroplasty (end-stage arthropathy), or fusion (especially for the ankle). Synovectomy has been shown to reduce the incidence of recurrent hemarthroses. **The presence of an inhibitor (15% incidence in hemophiliacs) is a relative contraindication to any elective surgical procedure.** Factor levels should be maintained near 100% the first week postop, and 50–75% for the second week. There is an extremely high incidence of HIV positivity in hemophiliacs (up to 90%).

C. **Sickle Cell Disease**—HbSS is found in 1% of North American blacks and leads to local infarction from capillary stasis. Dactylitis with MC/MT periosteal new bone formation, bone infarcts, osteomyelitis (*Salmonella* and staph most common; ESR usually is falsely low), and osteonecrosis (esp. femoral head, which leads to joint destruction and may require THA) are common features of sickle cell patients. Results with total joint arthroplasty are poor due to ongoing negative bone remodeling. *Salmonella* spread can come from gallbladder infection.

D. **Pigmented Villonodular Synovitis** (PVNS)—Synovial disease with exuberant proliferation of villi and nodules. Pain, swelling, synovitis, and a rust-colored effusion are common. The knee is the most frequent site of PVNS, with occasional involvement of the hip and ankle. X-rays show juxtacortical erosions. Treatment is surgical excision of affected synovium.

V. Summary—The characteristics of the various arthritides are summarized in Table 2–6.

Part 5

Osteonecrosis/Osteochondrosis

I. Osteonecrosis

A. Introduction—Osteonecrosis (ON) represents death of bony tissue adjacent to a joint surface from causes other than infection. It is usually caused by loss of blood supply (trauma or other etiology). Osteonecrosis commonly affects the hip joint, leading to eventual collapse. It is more common with steroid and heavy alcohol use and is also associated with blood dyscrasias (e.g., sickle cell disease), dysbarism (Caisson disease), excessive radiation therapy, and Gaucher's disease.

B. Etiology—Theories regarding the etiology of osteonecrosis are varied. It may be related to enlargement of space-occupying marrow fat cells that lead to ischemia of adjacent tissues. Vascular insults and other factors may also be significant. Idiopathic osteonecrosis (Chandler's disease) is diagnosed when no other cause can be identified. Idiopathic/alcohol and dysbaric ON are associated with multiple insults and have been classified by Enneking as described in Table 2–7.

C. Pathologic Changes—Grossly necrotic bone, fibrous tissue, and subchrondral collapse may be seen (Fig. 2–21 and 2–22). Histologically, early changes involve autolysis of osteocytes (14–21 days). This is followed by inflammation invasion of buds of primitive mesenchymal tissue and capillaries. Later, **new woven bone is laid down on top of dead trabecular bone**. This is followed by resorption of the dead trabeculae and remodeling in a process of "creeping substitution." It is during this process that the bone is weakest and collapse and fragmentation can occur.

D. Evaluation—Careful history taking (risk factors) and physical examination (decreased ROM, limp, etc.) should precede additional studies. Evaluation

TABLE 2–7. ENNEKING'S STAGES OF OSTEONECROSIS[a]

Stage	Pain	Radiographs	Pathology	Treatment
I	None	Slight incr. density	Creeping substitution	Observation
II	None	Reactive rim	Rim, reinfarction	Core decompression
III	Occasional	Crescent sign	Fracture	Core decomposition
IV	Limp	Step off flattening	Loose fragments	?
V	Continuous	Collapse	Cartilage flap	Hemiarthroplasty
VI	Severe	Deformed	Advanced arthritis	THA/Girdlestone

[a] Adapted from Emeking, W.F.: Clinical Musculoskeletal Pathology. 3rd Revised ed. Gainsville, University of Florida Press, 1990; pp. 144–155.

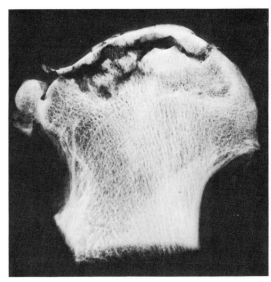

FIGURE 2–21. Fine-grain radiograph demonstrating space between articular surface and subchondral bone: the "crescent sign." (From Steinberg, M.E.: The Hip and Its Disorders, p. 630. Philadelphia, W.B. Saunders, 1991; reprinted by permission.)

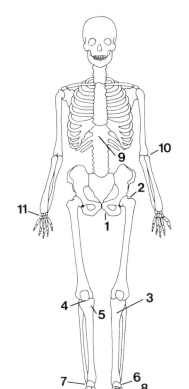

1 Van Neck's
2 Legg-Calve-Perthes
3 Osgood Schlatter
4 Sinding Larson-Johannsen
5 Blount's
6 Sever's
7 Kohler's
8 Freiburg's
9 Scheurmann's
10 Panner's
11 Theimann's

FIGURE 2–23. Locations of common osteocondroses.

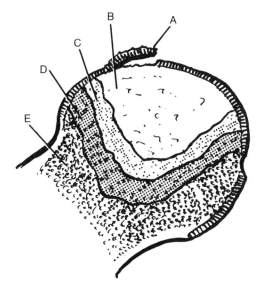

FIGURE 2–22. Pathology of avascular necrosis. *A*, Articular cartilage. *B*, Necrotic bone. *C*, Reactive fibrous tissue. *D*, Hypertrophic bone. *E*, Normal trabeculae. (From Steinberg, M.E.: The Hip and Its Disorders, p. 630. Philadelphia, W.B. Saunders, 1991; reprinted by permission.)

of other joints (especially the contralateral hip) is important in order to identify the disease process early. The process is bilateral in 50% of cases of idiopathic ON and up to 80% of steroid-induced ON. MRI and bone scanning are helpful in the early diagnosis. Femoral head pressure measurement is possible but is invasive. Pressure >30 mm Hg or increased >10 mm Hg with injection of 5cc of saline (stress test) is considered abnormal.

E. Treatment—Replacement arthroplasty of the hip is associated with increased loosening. Nontraumatic ON of the femoral condyle and proximal humerus may improve spontaneously without surgical correction.

TABLE 2–8. FICAT'S STAGES OF OSTEONECROSIS

Stage	Pain	Physical Exam	Radiographs	Bone Scan	MRI	IOP[a]	Treatment
0	None	Normal	Normal	Normal	Normal	Incr.	None
I	Minimal	Decr. int. rot.	Normal	Nondiagnostic	Early changes	Incr.	Core decompression
II	Moderate	Decr. ROM	Porosis/sclerosis	Positive	Positive	Incr.	Strut graft
III	Advanced	Decr. ROM	Flat/crescent sign	Positive	Positive	Incr.	Hemiarthroplasty
IV	Severe	Pain	Acetabular changes	Positive	Positive	Incr.	THA

[a] IOP, intraosseous pressure.

F. Classification—Hip ON has been classified by Ficat, and Table 2–8 highlights important features of the disease process.

II. Osteochondrosis

A. Introduction—Osteochondrosis can occur at traction apophyses in children and may or may not be associated with trauma, inflammation of the joint capsule, or vascular insult/secondary thrombosis. The pathology is similar to that described for osteonecrosis in the adult.

B. Common Osteochondroses—The following are the common osteochondroses. Most are discussed separately in the chapters covering the respective sites of disease (Fig. 2–23).

Disorder	Site	Age
Van neck's disease	Ischiopubic synchrondrosis	4–11
Legg-Calvé-Perthes disease	Femoral head	4–8
Osgood-Schlatter disease	Tibial tuberosity	11–15
Sinding-Larsen-Johansson syndrome	Inferior patella	10–14
Blount's disease (infant)	Proximal tibial epiphysis	1–3
Blount's disease (adolescent)	Proximal tibial epiphysis	8–15
Sever's disease	Calcaneus	9–11
Köhler's disease	Tarsal navicular	3–7
Freiberg's infraction	Metatarsal head	13–18
Scheuermann's disease	Discovertebral junction	13–17
Panner's disease	Capitellum of humerus	5–10
Thiemann's disease	Phalanges of hand	11–19
Kienböck's disease	Carpal lunate	20–40

Part 6

Imaging and Special Studies

I. Nuclear Medicine

A. Bone Scan—Technetium-99m phosphate complexes reflect increased blood flow and metabolism and are absorbed onto the hydroxyapatite crystals of bone in areas of infection, trauma, neoplasia, etc. Whole-body views and more detailed views can be obtained. It is particularly useful in the diagnosis of subtle fractures; avascular necrosis (no focal uptake early, increased uptake in the reparative phase); osteomyelitis (esp. when triple-phase study is done, or in conjunction with gallium or indium scan); and THA and TKA loosening (esp. femoral components; can be used with gallium scan to rule out concurrent infection). Three- or even four-stage studies may be helpful in evaluating diseases such as reflex sympathetic dystrophy and osteomyelitis.

B. Gallium Scan—Gallium-67 citrate localizes in sites of inflammation and neoplasia probably because of exudation of labeled serum proteins. Delayed imaging (usually 24–48+ hours) is required. Frequently used in conjunction with bone scan—a "double tracer" technique. Gallium is less dependent on vascular flow than technetium, and may identify foci that would otherwise be missed. It is difficult to differentiate cellulitis from osteomyelitis.

C. Indium Scan—Indium-111–labeled WBCs accumulate in areas of inflammation and do not collect in areas of neoplasia. Useful in the evaluation of acute osteomyelitis, and possibly TJA infections. Unlike gallium, it is also useful in the presence of pseudarthrosis.

D. Radiolabeled Monoclonal Antibodies—May have a future role in identifying primary malignancies and metastatic disease.

E. Other Studies

1. Bone Mineral Analysis—Single-photon absorptiometry (usually of the distal radius and cortical bone; has limited utility), dual-photon absorptiometry (vertebral bodies and femoral neck), and quantitative CT (larger radiation exposure and can be inaccurate, but can pick up early changes in trabecular bone) can be used to measure bone mineral content for diagnosing osteoporosis and predicting fracture risk.

2. Deep Venous Thrombosis/Pulmonary Embolism (DVT/PE) Scan—Radioactive iodine–labeled fibrinogen accumulates in clot and shows up on scanning. Its limitations include inaccuracy in area of surgical wounds. Radioisotope scanning of lungs may also help in evaluating regional pulmonary blood flow, but it too is limited at present.

3. Single-Photon Emission Computed Tomography (SPECT)— Uses scintigraphy and CT to evaluate overlapping structures. Femoral head ON, patellofemoral syndrome, and healing spondylolytic defects have been evaluated with this technique.

II. Arthrography

A. Shoulder—Can be used with single- or double-contrast technique (better detail). Used for the following studies.

1. Rotator Cuff Tear Diagnosis—Extravasation of contrast through the tear into the subacromial bursa.

2. Adhesive Capsulitis—Diagnosed by demonstrating diminished joint capsule size and loss of the normal axillary fold. May have a role in therapy also by distending the capsule—brisement.

3. Recurrent Dislocations—Arthrography may demonstrate a distended capsule or disruption of the glenoid labrum. Can be used in conjunction with tomograms or CT (computed arthrotomography) to better demonstrate capsular or labial pathology.
4. Other uses include diagnosis of bicipital tendon abnormalities, articular pathology, and impingement syndrome.

B. Elbow—Especially when used with tomography, elbow arthrography can be helpful in the diagnosis of articular cartilage defects/loose bodies and osteochondral fractures.

C. Wrist—Most useful in the evaluation of the post-traumatic wrist to demonstrate ligamentous disruption. Digital subtraction techniques are helpful in this area. Demonstration of communication between compartments is used to determine pathology; however, communication is common in asymptomatic patients in the over-40 age group:

COMMUNICATION	PATHOLOGY
Radius-carpus & midcarpal	S–L or L–T ligament tears
Radius-carpus & distal radius–ulna	TFCC tear

D. Hip—Separate indications in children and adults.
1. Infants and children—useful in diagnosing septic hip (obtain aspirate and assess joint damage), congenital dysplasia of the hip (degree of joint incongruity—interposed limbus), and Legg-Calvé-Perthes (severity of deformity).
2. Adolescent and adult—used to evaluate arthritis (cartilage destruction and loose bodies), osteochondral fractures, chondrolysis, and THA loosening. Digital subtraction arthrography can be useful in patients with suspected loose THAs.

E. Knee—Can be a useful screening tool in patients with equivocal history or findings. Very accurate in diagnosing most meniscal tears (except in posterior horn of lateral meniscus), and demonstrates discoid lateral menisci well. Evaluation of cruciate ligaments is less accurate. Abnormalities of articular cartilage, evaluation of loose bodies (air contrast only recommended), and pathologic synovial tissue (PVNS, popliteal cysts, and plicas) can be demonstrated also.

F. Ankle—Helpful in evaluating torn ligaments acutely, and in assessing chronic osseous and osteocartilaginous abnormalities.

G. Spine—May be useful in conjunction with therapeutic injections (of anesthetics and steroids) into facet joints.

III. Magnetic Resonance Imaging (MRI)

A. Introduction—Excellent study for soft tissue evaluation. Used frequently in the evaluation of osteonecrosis, neoplasm, infection, and trauma. Allows for both axial and sagittal representations. It is contraindicated in patients with pacemakers, cerebral aneurysm clips, or shrapnel in vital locations.

B. Basic Principles—Uses radiofrequency (RF) pulses on tissues in a magnetic field and displays images in any plane desired without the use of ionizing radiation. MRI aligns nuclei with odd numbers of protons/neutrons (with a normally random spin) parallel to a magnetic field. Most magnets used have a strength of about 0.5–1.5 Telsa (1 Telsa is 10,000 Gauss). RF pulses cause deflection of these particles' nuclear magnetic moments, resulting in an image. The use of surface coils decreases the signal-to-noise ratio. Body coils are used for large joints, smaller coils are available for other studies. Sequences have been developed that have either short (T_1) or long (T_2) relaxation times for atoms to return to their normal spin. T_1 images are weighted toward fat, T_2 images are weighted toward water. Typically T_1-weighted images have TR values <1000, T_2 images have TR values >1000. Some tissues appear differently on T_1- and T_2-weighted scans. Water, CSF, acute hemorrhage, and soft tissue tumors appear dark on T_1 studies and light on T_2 studies. Other tissues remain basically the same color on both studies. Cortical bone, rapidly flowing blood, and fibrous tissue are all dark; muscle and hyaline cartilage are gray; and fatty tissue, nerves, slowly flowing (venous) blood, and bone marrow are light. **T_1 images best demonstrate normal anatomy, whereas T_2 images show contrast of abnormal tissues best.**

C. Specific Applications
1. Osteonecrosis—MRI may be the most sensitive method for early detection of ON. It is very specific (98%) and reliable in estimating age and extent of disease. T_1 images demonstrate diseased marrow as dark. MRI allows direct assessment of overlying cartilage.
2. Infection and Trauma—MRI makes use of its excellent sensitivity to increases in free water to demonstrate areas of infection and fresh hemorrhage (dark on T_1 and light on T_2 studies).
3. Neoplasms—MRI has many applications in the study of primary and metastatic bone tumors. Primary tumors, particularly soft tissue components (extraosseous and marrow) are well demonstrated on MRI. Although nuclear medicine studies remain the procedure of choice for seeking metastatic foci in bone, MRI has key a role in evaluating spinal metastases. Benign tumors are typically bright on T_1 images and dark on T_2 images. Malignant bony lesions are often bright on T_2 images. Differential diagnosis, however, is best made based on plain films.
4. Spine—Disc disease is well demonstrated on T_2 images. Degenerated discs lose their water content and become dark on T_2-weighted studies. Herniated discs and their extent are well shown. Recurrent disc herniation can be differentiated from scar based on the following characteristics:

PROBLEM	T_1 IMAGE	T_2 IMAGE
Scar	Decreased	Increased
Free fragment	Increased	Increased
Extruded disc	Decreased	Decreased

Gadolinium-DTPA can also be used to differentiate scar from disc. It enhances edematous structures in T_1 images.

5. Bone Marrow Changes—Best demonstrated by MRI (but nonspecific). Five groups of disorders have been described:

DISORDER	PATHOLOGY	EXAMPLES	MRI CHANGES
Reconversion	Yellow → red	Anemia, metastasis	Decr. T_1 image
Marrow infiltration		Tumor, infection	Decr. T_1 image
Myeloid depletion		Anemia, chemotherapy	Incr. T_1 image
Marrow edema		Trauma, RSD	Decr. T_1, incr. T_2 image
Marrow ischemia		Osteonecrosis	Decr. T_1 image

6. Knee MRI—Arthrography with MRI can be accomplished with installation of saline, creating an iatrogenic effusion. This technique can improve joint definition. Knee derangements are well demonstrated on MRI. ACL rupture can be correctly diagnosed in 95% of cases. Meniscal pathology has been classified into four groups of myxoid changes (Lotysch):

GROUP	CHARACTERISTICS
I	Globular areas of hyperintense signal
II	Linear hyperintense signal
III	Linear hyperintense signal that communicates with the meniscal surface (tears)
IV	Vertical longitudinal tear/truncation

7. Shoulder MRI
   a. Rotator Cuff Tears—Results are improving with use (sensitivity and specificity are about 90%). The following grading system is commonly used:

GRADE	SIGNAL	MORPHOLOGY
0	Normal	Normal
1	Increased	Normal
2	Increased	Abnormal
3	Increased	Discontinuity

   b. Capsular/Labral Tears—MRI is equal to CT arthrography in the presence of an effusion.

8. MRI Spectroscopy—May help with the measurement of metabolic changes (especially ischemic changes) in the future.

IV. Other Imaging Studies

A. Computed Tomography (CT)—Continues to be important in evaluation of many orthopaedic areas. Hounsfield units are used to identify tissue types (-100 = air, -100–0 = fat, 0 = water, 100 = soft tissue, 1000 = bone). Demonstrates bony anatomy better than any other study. Also shows herniated nucleus pulposis better than myelography alone, and may be helpful differentiating recurrent disc herniation vs. scar (like MRI). IV contrast is administered and taken up in scar tissue but not disc material. Used frequently in conjunction with contrast (arthrogram-CT, myelogram-CT, etc.). Sagittal and 3-D reconstruction techniques may expand its indications. Cine-CT (and MRI) may be helpful in evaluation of many joint disorders. CT digital radiography (CT scannogram) can be used for accurate demonstrations of leg length discrepancy with minimal radiation exposure.

B. Ultrasound—has been used successfully in at least three areas in orthopaedics.
   1. Shoulder—May be useful for diagnosing rotator cuff tears.
   2. Hip—Has been shown to be effective in diagnosis and follow-up of developmental hip dysplasia and to identify iliopsoas bursitis in adults.
   3. Knee—Used to assess articular cartilage thickness, identify intra-articular fluid, etc.

TABLE 2–9. NERVE CONDUCTION STUDY RESULTS[a]

	LATENCY	CONDUCTION VELOCITY	EVOKED RESPONSE
Normal study	Normal	Upper extremities: >45 m/s Lower extremities: >40 m/s	Biphasic
Axonal neuropathy	Incr.	Normal or slightly decr.	Prolonged, decr. amplitude
Demyelinating neuropathy	Normal	Decreased (10–50%)	Normal or prolonged, with decr. amplitude
Anterior horn cell disease	Normal	Normal (rarely decr.)	Normal or polyphasic with prolonged duration and decr. amplitude
Myopathy	Normal	Normal	Decr. amplitude, may be normal
Neurapraxia			
Proximal to lesion	Absent	Absent	Absent
Distal to lesion	Normal	Normal	Normal
Axonotmesis			
Proximal to lesion	Absent	Absent	Absent
Distal to lesion	Absent	Absent	Normal
Neurotmesis			
Proximal to lesion	Absent	Absent	Absent
Distal to lesion	Absent	Absent	Absent

[a] Modified from Jahss, MH: Disorders of the Foot. Philadelphia, WB Saunders Company, 1982; reprinted by permission.

TABLE 2–10. ELECTROMYOGRAPHY FINDINGS[a]

	INSERTIONAL ACTIVITY	ACTIVITY AT REST	MINIMAL CONTRACTION	INTERFERENCE
Normal study	Normal	Silent	Biphasic and triphasic potentials	Complete
Axonal neuropathy	Incr.	Fibrillations and positive sharp waves	Biphasic and triphasic potentials	Incomplete
Demyelinating neuropathy	Normal	Silent (occasional activity)	Biphasic and triphasic potentials	Incomplete
Anterior horn cell disease	Incr.	Fibrillations, positive sharp waves, fasciculations	Large polyphasic potentials	Incomplete
Myopathy	Incr.	Silent or incr. spontaneous activity	Small polyphasic potentials	Early
Neurapraxia	Normal	Silent	None	None
Axonotmesis	Incr.	Fibrillations and positive sharp waves	None	None
Neurotmesis	Incr.	Fibrillations and positive sharp waves	None	None

[a] Modified Jahss, M.H.: Disorders of the Foot. Philadelphia, W.B. Saunders Company, 1982; reprinted by permission.

4. Other areas—Helpful in the evaluation of soft tissue masses, hematoma, tendon rupture, abscesses, foreign body location, and intraspinal disorders in infants.

C. Guided Biopsies—Aspiration and core biopsy (using a trephine Craig needle) is helpful in the work-up of musculoskeletal lesions, and is commonly used in conjunction with CT.

D. Myelography—Still useful to evaluate cervical radiculopathy, subarachnoid cysts, and the failed back syndrome. It is the procedure of choice for extramedullary intradural pathology. Can be used in conjunction with other studies (CT).

E. Discography—Although its use is controversial, it is helpful in evaluation of symptomatic disc degeneration. Reproduction of pain with injection and characteristic changes on discograms help identify pathologic discs. It is commonly used in conjunction with CT.

V. Electrodiagnostic Studies

A. Nerve Conduction Studies—Allow evaluation of peripheral nerves and their sensory and motor responses anywhere along their course. Nerve impulses are stimulated and recorded by electronic surface electrodes, allowing calculation of a conduction velocity. Latency (the time between the onset of the stimulus and the response) and the amplitude of the response are measured. Late responses (F and H) allow evaluation of proximal lesions (impulse travels to spinal cord and returns). Somatosensory evoked potentials (SEPs) can be used to study brachial plexus injuries and for spinal cord monitoring.

B. Electromyography—Uses intramuscular needle electrodes to evaluate muscle units. Most studies are done to evaluate denervation, which demonstrates fibrillations (earliest sign—usually at 4 weeks), sharp waves, and an abnormal recruitment pattern.

C. Interpretation—For peripheral nerve entrapment syndromes, distal motor and sensory latencies >3.5 m/s, nerve conduction velocities of <50 m/s, and changes over a distinct interval are considered abnormal (Tables 2–9 and 2–10).

Part **7**

Orthopaedic Infections

I. Introduction—This section serves as an overview of orthopaedic infections. Specific infections unique to particular orthopaedic areas are covered in detail in the appropriate chapters.

II. Soft Tissue Infections

A. Cellulitis—An inflammatory infection of the subcutaneous tissues, usually due to staph or strep (and *Haemophilus* in children). Local erythema, tenderness, and occasionally lymphangitis/lymphadenopathy make up the clinical picture. Ordinarily, mild cases of cellulitis can be treated with an oral penicillinase-resistant penicillin or cephalosporin. Patients with high fever, systemic toxicity, poor host resistance, or underlying skin disease should be admitted for IV antibiotic therapy.

B. Significant Streptococcal Infections—Several serious diseases are related to specific streptococcal infections.

1. Erysipelas—Group A strep causes this progressively enlarging, red, raised, and painful plaque seen predominately in infants, diabetics, elderly, and patients with predisposing skin ulcers. Severe toxicity, fever, leukocytosis, and bacteremia are common. Treatment with high doses of IV penicillin is essential for this life-threatening disease.
2. Necrotizing Fasciitis—Aggressive, life-threatening fascial infection that is often associated with underlying vascular disease (esp. diabetes). Usually follows insignificant trauma (can follow abdominal surgery in diabetics), and rapidly progresses. Can be associated with strep gangrene, and may be polymicrobial with both aerobes and anaerobes. Wide surgical I&D and IV antibiotics are required emergently.

C. Gas Gangrene—Classically caused by *Clostridia* species (G+ rod), but also can develop from G− and sometimes G+ (strep) infections. Clinical presentation usually includes progressive pain; edema (distant from wound); foul smelling, serosanguineous discharge; and feeling of impending doom. May be associated with bowel cancer. Radiographs typically show widespread gas in tissues. Treatment with high-dose penicillin (and aminoglycoside and cephalosporin), hyperbaric oxygen (inhibits toxins), and surgical I&D are required.

D. Tetanus—Potentially lethal neuroparalytic disease caused by an exotoxin of *Clostridium tetani*, a G+ anaerobic rod. Treatment is centered on prophylaxis with proper wound care and tetanus toxoid administration (and TIG for patients with severe wounds and without known previous immunizations). Late management is largely symptomatic.

E. Toxic Shock Syndrome—Severe staph infection that usually develops postoperatively. Fever, hypotension, systemic symptoms, an erythematous macular rash, and a serous exudate (with G+ cocci) are present. Wounds may look benign but require immediate I&D and IV antibiotics.

F. Surgical Wound Infection—There has been a recent increase in the incidence of *Staph. epidermidis* wound infections. *Staph. aureus* is still the most common infection overall, and in trauma patients. Methicillin-resistant staph species infections are also increasing and are best treated with vancomycin.

G. Puncture Wounds of the Foot—Commonly are infected with *Pseudomonas* (from shoewear), and require aggressive débridement and appropriate antibiotics (aminoglycoside and piperacillin) early.

H. Fungal Infections—Multicellular organisms with mycelia (branches) that induce a hypersensitivity reaction in tissues, causing chronic granuloma, abscesses, and necrosis. Surgical treatment and amphotericin-B administration often required. Oral ketoconazole may be effective for some limited infections.

I. Human Immunodeficiency Virus (HIV) Infection—Incidence is increased in the homosexual population but is becoming increasingly common in heterosexual patients. Additionally, well over half of the hemophiliac population is affected. Fetal AIDS is transmitted across the placenta, and affected children typically have a box-like forehead, wide eyes, a small head, and growth failure. The virus primarily affects the lymphocyte and macrophage cell lines and decreases the number of T helper cells (T4 lymphocytes). This disease has increased the importance of blood and body fluid handling precautions in trauma management and surgery. Only advanced stages of HIV infection are classified as acquired immunodeficiency syndrome (AIDS) [class 6 of 6 in the Walter Reed Classification Scheme]. **HIV positivity is not a contraindication to performing required surgical procedures.** There is a 0.3% risk of HIV conversion following parenteral inoculation.

J. Hepatitis—Three types are commonly recognized.
1. Hepatitis A—Common in areas with poor sanitation and public health concerns. Less of a problem in surgical transmission.
2. Hepatitis B—Approximately 200,000 people are infected with the hepatitis B virus each year, and there are over 1 million carriers. Screening and use of a new vaccine has reduced the risk of transmission for health care workers. Immune globulin is administered after exposure in nonvaccinated individuals. Neither vaccine or immune globulin administration has been documented as causing HIV transmission.
3. Non-A, Non-B Hepatitis—The offending virus has recently been identified (hepatitis C virus proposed). It is the most common transfusion-associated hepatitis.

III. Bone and Joint Infections

A. Acute Hematogenous Osteomyelitis—Bone and bone marrow infection caused (most commonly) by blood-borne organisms. Commonly affects children (boys > girls). *Staph. aureus* is the most common offender. Anaerobic infections are also frequently seen, with *Peptococcus magnus* (G+) appearing more frequently than *Bacteroides* (G−). The infection is most common in the metaphyses or epiphyses of long bones (lower extremity > upper extremity). Radiographic changes include soft tissue swelling early, demineralization (10 days to 2 weeks), and sequestra (dead bone with surrounding granulation tissue) and involucrum (periosteal new bone) later. Pain, loss of function, and sometimes a soft tissue abscess are present. Elevated WBC count and ESR and positive blood cultures are usually seen. Bone scan (delayed uptake in bone) ± gallium (in spine infections) or indium (in extremity infections) scans may be helpful in equivocal cases. MRI shows changes usually before plain films (nonspecific low signal intensity in marrow spaces on both T_1 and T_2 images). **Aspiration** is helpful for antibiotic choice. IV antibiotics followed by a course of oral antibiotics after the temperature has normalized (total of 6 weeks or until the ESR returns to normal), immobilization, and for refractory cases surgical drainage (saving bone from further destruction) are usually curative. Recurrence is high for metatarsal lesions (50%), around the knee (25%), and with late diagnosis (25%). Long-term morbidity is >25%.

B. Subacute Osteomyelitis—Usually discovered radiologically in a patient with a painful limp and no systemic (and often no local) signs or symptoms,

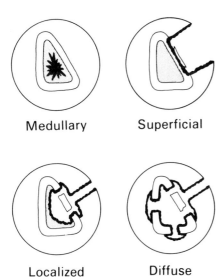

Medullary   Superficial

Localized   Diffuse

FIGURE 2–24. Cierney's anatomic classification of adult chronic osteomyelitis. (From Cierney, G., III: Chronic osteomyelitis: Results of treatment. Instr. Course Lect. 39:495, 1990; reprinted by permission.)

often from partially treated acute osteomyelitis, occasionally developing in a fracture hematoma. Unlike acute osteomyelitis, WBC count and blood cultures are frequently normal. ESR, bone cultures, and radiographs are often useful. Most commonly affects the femur and tibia, and unlike acute osteomyelitis, it can cross the physis even in older children. Radiographic changes include Brodie's abscess, a localized radiolucency usually seen in the metaphyses of long bones. It is sometimes difficult to differentiate from Ewing's sarcoma. When localized to the epiphysis only, other lesions (such as chondroblastoma) must be ruled out. **Epiphyseal osteomyelitis is caused exclusively by Staph. aureus.** Treatment of Brodie's abscess in the metaphysis includes surgical curettage. Epiphyseal osteomyelitis requires surgical drainage only if pus is present (48 hours of IV antibiotics followed by 6 weeks of oral antibiotics is curative otherwise).

C. Chronic Osteomyelitis—Can follow inappropriately treated acute osteomyelitis, trauma, or soft tissue spread, especially in the elderly, immunosuppressed, diabetics, and IV drug abusers (Cierney type C host). *Staph. aureus,* G− rods, and an-

aerobes are frequent offending organisms. Often classified anatomically (Cierney) (Fig. 2–24). Skin and soft tissue are often involved, and fistulous tracts can occasionally develop into epidermoid carcinoma. Periods of quiescence are often followed by acute exacerbations. Nuclear medicine studies are often helpful in determining activity of disease. Combination IV antibiotics (based on deep cultures), surgical débridement, bone grafting (open, vascularized, or bypass [proximal and distal to infected area]), stabilization (avoid IM devices following external fixator use with associated pin tract infections), and soft tissue coverage (flaps) are often required. Amputations are still often necessary.

D. Chronic Sclerosing Osteomyelitis—An unusual infection that involves primarily diaphyseal bones of adolescents. Typified by intense proliferation of the periosteum leading to bony deposition, it may be caused by anaerobic organisms. Insidious onset, dense progressive sclerosis on radiographs, and localized pain and tenderness are common. Malignancy must be ruled out. Surgical and antibiotic therapy are not curative.

E. Chronic Multifocal Osteomyelitis—Caused by an infectious agent appearing in children without systemic symptoms. Normal lab values except for an elevated ESR are common. Radiographs demonstrate multiple metaphyseal lytic lesions, especially in the medial clavicle, distal tibia, and distal femur. Symptomatic treatment only is recommended because this disease usually resolves spontaneously.

F. Osteomyelitis with Unusual Organisms—Several unusual organisms can occur in the appropriate clinical setting (Table 2–11). Radiographs show characteristic features in syphilis (*T. pallidum;* radiolucency in metaphysis from granulation tissue) and tuberculosis (joint destruction on both sides of a joint). Histology can also be helpful (e.g., tuberculosis with granulomas and Langerhan's giant cells).

G. Septic Arthritis—Commonly follows hematogenous spread or extension of osteomyelitis; can also follow diagnostic or therapeutic procedures. Bacteria have a special affinity to exposed collagen matrix. Most cases involve infants (esp. hip), and children (knee). RA (tuberculosis) and drug abuse (*Pseudomonas*) can predispose adults. *Haemophilus influenzae* is the most common organism in children <5 yo (Rx chloramphenicol or a third-generation cephalosporin), staph in children >5 yo (Rx methacillin or oxacillin), and gonococci in adults (pen-

TABLE 2–11. UNUSUAL ORGANISMS FOUND IN OSTEOMYELITIS

Organism	Risk Factor(s)	Sx/Findings	Treatment
Serratia marcescens	IV drug abuse	Axial skeleton	Cotrimoxazole
Pseudomonas aeruginosa	IV drug abuse	Nonspecific	Aminoglycoside
Brucella (G−)	Meat handling	Flat bones	Tetracycline/Septra
Salmonella	Sickle cell disease	Asymptomatic	Ampicillin
Anaerobes	Skin contamination	Tissue culture	Clindamycin/cephalosporin
Fungi	Skin contamination	Special study	Amphotericin B
Treponema pallidum	Sexual contact	Nontender swelling	Penicillin
Mycobacteria	TB/leprosy/fishermen	PPD/granuloma/culture at 30°C	PAS, isoniazid

icillin). Third-generation cephalosporins (ceftraidime, cefsulodin, and aztreonam) are now favored over aminoglycosides (with the possible exception of gentamicin) for the treatment of G− infections. Surgical drainage (often arthroscopically) or daily aspiration is the mainstay of treatment. Open drainage is required for septic hip joints. SI joint sepsis is unusual but is best diagnosed by physical examination (Flexian ABduction Exteral Rotation—FABER most specific) and aspiration. A pannus (much like in inflammatory arthritis) can be seen in tuberculosis infections. Late sequellae of septic arthritis include soft tissue contractures that can sometimes be treated with soft tissue procedures such as quadricepsplasty.

IV. Antibiotics

   A. Indications—Used for prevention of postoperative sepsis, treatment of incipient infection, and in the treatment of established infections. Perioperative use of first-generation cephalosporins is efficacious in cases requiring insertion of hardware.
   B. Specific Antibiotics—Selected antibiotics, their indications, and side effects are listed in Table 2–12.
   C. Other Forms of Antibiotic Delivery
      1. Antibiotic Beads or Spacers—Made of PMMA impregnated with antibiotics (usually an aminoglycoside); useful in eradicating infections with TJA or osteomyelitis with bony defects.

These are inserted only after thorough débridement.
      2. Osmotic Pump—An experimental method for delivery of high concentrations of antibiotics locally. Used mainly for osteomyelitis.
      3. Home IV Therapy—A cost-effective alternative for patients requiring long-term IV antibiotics. This treatment is facilitated with the use of a Hickman or Broviac indwelling catheter.

V. Other Infections

   A. Infected Total Joint Arthroplasty—Covered in Chapter 3, Adult Reconstruction and Sports Medicine, but bears some mention here. Perioperative IV antibiotics are the most effective method of decreasing incidence, but good operative technique, laminar flow (avoiding obstruction between the air source and operative wound), and special "space" suits also have a role. The ESR is the most sensitive indicator of infection, but it is nonspecific. Culture of hip aspirate is very sensitive and specific. C-reactive protein may be helpful also. Acute infections (within 2–3 weeks) can usually be treated with prosthesis salvage, but delayed or chronic infections will require removal. *Staph. epidermidis* and *aureus* are the most common offenders. Polymicrobial organisms may form an overlying glycocalix, making infection control difficult without removal of the prosthesis and vigorous débridement. However, according to Cierny, the host is more im-

TABLE 2–12. ANTIBIOTICS, INDICATIONS, AND SIDE EFFECTS

ANTIBIOTIC	ORGANISMS	COMPLICATIONS/OTHER
Cell Wall Synthesis Inhibitors		
Penicillin	Strep, G+	Hypersensitivity/resistance, hemolytic
Methicillin/oxacillin/naphcillin	Penicillinase resistant	Same as penicillin; nephritis (methicillin); Subcut. Q skin slough (naphcillin)
Carbenicillin/ticarcillin/piperacillin	Better against G−	Bleeding diathesis (carbenicillin)
Cephalosporins		
First generation	Prophylaxis	Cephazolin is the drug of choice
Second generation	Some G+/G−	Cefuroxime/cefotaxime for pediatric septic joint
Third generation	G−, less G+	Hemolytic anemia (bleeding diathesis [moxalactam])
Inhibitors of Cell Membrane Function		
Polymyxin/nystatin	GU	Nephrotoxic
Amphotericin	Fungi	Nephrotoxic
Inhibitors of Protein Synthesis		
Aminoglycosides	G−, Syn, PM	Nephrotoxicitity, ototoxicity (dose related)
Clindamycin	G+, anaerobes	Pseudomembranous enterocolitis
Chloramphenicol	*H. influenzae*, anaerobes	Bone marrow aplasia
Erythromycin	G+ (PCN allergy)	Ototoxic
Tetracycline	G+ (PCN allergy)	Stains teeth/bone (up to age 8)
Fluoroquinolones		
Ciprofloxacin	G−, methicillin resistant *S. aureus*	Cartilage erosion (children); oral therapy increases theophyline levels; antacids reduce absorption
Inhibitors of Nucleic Acid Synthesis		
Vancomycin	Methicillin-resistant *S. aureus, C difficile*	Ototoxic, erythema with rapid IV delivery
Sulfonamides	GU	Hemolytic anemia
Carbapenems		
Imipenam	G+, some G−	Resistance, seizure
Azactam	G−, no anaerobes	

portant than the organism. He defines three types of hosts:

Type	Description	Risk
A	Normal immune response; nonsmoker	Minimal
B	Local or mild systemic deficiency; smoker	Moderate
C	Major nutritional or systemic disorder	High

Use of antibiotic-impregnated cement in revision arthroplasties and antibiotic spacers/beads in infected total joints may be helpful. Reimplantation after thorough débridement and use of PMMA antibiotics has been successful staged at variable intervals. Some advocate frozen sections at the time of reimplantation to assure that local tissues have <5–10 PMNs/high-power field.

B. Allograft infection—May involve up to 20% of allografts; requires aggressive measures to control.

C. Meningococcemia—Can develop in patients with multiple infarcts, such as in electrical burns.

D. Marjolin's Ulcer—Squamous cell carcinoma that develops in patients with chronic drainage from sinus tracts. Seen in untreated chronic osteomyelitis.

E. Nutritional Status and Infection—Nutrition is critical in decreasing the incidence of postoperative infection. Malnutrition is common following multiple trauma.

F. Postsplenectomy Patients—Quite susceptible to streptococci infections and respond poorly to them.

Part 8

Perioperative Problems

I. Pulmonary Complications

A. General Considerations—Pulmonary function tests and air blood gas measurements are often helpful to evaluate baseline status. Thoracic and abdominal surgery can significantly affect these values.

B. Thromboembolism—A common problem in orthopaedic patients, especially with procedures about the hip. Risk is increased with obesity, malignancy, age, CHF, birth control pill use, smoking, **general anesthetics (as opposed to continuous epidural anesthesia)**, and pregnancy. Clinical suspicion is more helpful than physical exam findings (pain, swelling, Homan's sign) for deep venous thrombosis. Useful studies include venography (the "gold standard"), labeled fibrinogen (operative site artifact), plethysmography (poor sensitivity), and ultrasonography (often best for a first study). Prophylaxis is the most important factor in decreasing morbidity and mortality, and the methods commonly used are listed in Table 2–13. The anticoagulation effects of Coumadin can be reversed with vitamin K, or more rapidly with fresh frozen plasma. Once the diagnosis of deep venous thrombosis has been confirmed, initiation of heparin therapy is required (followed by later conversion to long-term coumadin therapy). Treatment is recommended for all thigh DVTs; however, treatment of DVTs occurring below the popliteal fossa is controversial. Pulmonary embolism should be suspected in postoperative patients with acute-onset pleuritic pain, tachypnea, and tachycardia. Initial work-up includes EKG (RBBB, RAD in 25%) chest x-ray (hyperlucency rare), and ABG (normal PaO_2 does not exclude PE). Nuclear medicine ventilation-perfusion (V/Q) scan can be helpful, but pulmonary angiography is required to make the diagnosis if there is any question. Heparin therapy is initiated for patient with a proven PE. More aggressive therapy (thrombolytic agents, vena cava interruption, and other surgical measures) is usually not required.

C. Fat Embolism—Can occur 24–72 hours following trauma (with long bone fractures) and is fatal in 10–15% of cases. Onset may be heralded by tachypnea, tachycardia, mental status changes, and upper extremity petechiae. May be caused by bone marrow fat (mechanical theory) and/or chylomicra changes as a result of stress (chemical theory). Me-

TABLE 2–13. THROMBOEMBOLISM PROPHYLAXIS

Method	Effect	Advantages	Disadvantages
Heparin			
Intravenous	Coagulation cascade—antithrombin III	Reversible, effective	Control, embolization
Subcutaneous	Antithrombin III inhibitor	Reversible	No effect in extremity surgery
Coumadin	Coagulation cascade—vitamin K	Most effective, oral	3–5 days to full effect, control
Aspirin	Inhibits platelet aggregation	Easy, no monitoring	Limited efficacy
Dextran	Dilutional	Effective	Overload, bleeding
Pneumatic compression	Mechanical	Cheap, no bleeding	Bulky

tabolism to free fatty acids, initiation of the clotting cascade, and pulmonary capillary leakage follows. Treatment includes mechanical ventilation with high levels of PEEP. Steroids have a prophylactic role only. Prevention with early fracture stabilization is key.

D. Adult Respiratory Distress Syndrome (ARDS)—Acute respiratory failure secondary to pulmonary edema following trauma, shock, infection, etc. Tachypnea, dyspnea, hypoxemia, and decreased lung compliance are manifestations of ARDS. Normal supportive care is often unsuccessful, and a 50% mortality rate is not uncommon. Fluid overload, aspiration, and microscopic emboli may all contribute to the development of ARDS. Activation of the complement system leads to further progression. Ventilation with PEEP is usually successful, steroids have not been proven to be efficacious.

E. Pneumonia—Aspiration pneumonia can occur in patients with decreased mentation, supine positioning, and decreased GI motility. Simple preventive measures such as raising the head of the bed and the use of antacids and Reglan can help to avoid problems. Appropriate IV antibiotics and pulmonary toilet are required.

F. Pulmonary Complications of Orthopaedic Disorders—Scoliosis can cause pulmonary dysfunction in larger curves. Spontaneous pneumothorax is common in patients with Marfan's syndrome.

II. Other Medical Problems

A. Nutrition—Adequate nutrition should be ensured prior to elective surgery. Malnutrition may be present in 50% of patients on a surgical ward. Several indicators exist (anergy panels, albumin levels, transferrin level, etc.), but **arm muscle circumference measurement is the best indicator of nutritional status.** Wound dehiscence and infection, pneumonia, and sepsis can be a result of poor nutrition. Lack of internal feeding can lead to atrophy of the intestinal mucosae, leading to bacterial translocation. Requirements are significantly elevated as a result of stress. Full enteral or parenteral nutrition (200 mg/kg/day of nitrogen) should be provided for patients who cannot tolerate normal intake. Early elemental feeding through a jejunostomy tube can decrease complications in the multiple trauma patient.

B. Myocardial Infarction—Acute chest pain, radiation, and EKG changes are classic, and warrant monitoring in an appropriate critical care environment where cardiac enzymes and EKGs can be monitored on a continuing basis. Risk is increased with increased age, smoking, elevated cholesterol, hypertension, aortic stenosis, a history of coronary artery disease, and other factors.

C. GI complications—Can range from ileus (treated with nasogastric suction and antacids) to upper GI bleeding. Postoperative ileus is common in diabetics with neuropathy. Upper GI bleeding is more likely in patients with a history of ulcers, NSAID use, and smoking. Treatment includes lavage, antacids, and H_2 blockers. Intra-articular vasopressin (left gastric artery) may be required in more serious cases. Ogilvie's syndrome, which includes cecal distention, can follow total joint surgery. If the cecum is >10 cm on an abdominal flat plate radiograph, then it must be decompressed (usually can be done colonoscopically).

D. Decubitus Ulcers—Associated with advanced age, critical illness, and neurologic impairment. Common sites include the sacrum, heels, and buttocks. Can be a source of infection and increased morbidity. Prevention with constant changing of position, special mattresses, and treatment of systemic illness and malnutrition is essential. Once established, débridement and sometimes flaps are required for treatment.

III. GU Complications

A. Urinary Tract Infection—The most common nosocomial infection (6–8%). Causes increased risk for joint sepsis following TJA (but may not be from direct seeding). Established UTIs should be adequately treated preoperatively. Perioperative catheterization (removed 24 hours postop) may reduce the rate of postoperative urinary tract infection.

B. Prostatic Hypertrophy—Causes postoperative urinary retention. If history, physical (prostate exam), and urine flow studies are suggestive (<17 cc/second peak flow rate), urologic referral should be accomplished preoperatively.

C. Acute Tubular Necrosis—Can cause renal failure in trauma patients. Alkalization of urine is important in the early treatment of this disorder.

D. Renal Injury—NSAIDs can affect the kidney and appropriate screening laboratories are required at regular intervals.

V. Intraoperative Considerations

A. Anesthesia—Regional anesthesia may allow quicker recovery, decreased blood loss, and less postoperative complications, including reduced blood loss and incidence of DVT/PE in THA patients. Controlled hypotension during surgery will help with blood loss, and is a widely accepted technique, especially with THA and spinal fusion. Nitroprusside, nitroglycerine, and isoflurane are all effective. Transient decreases in BP with PMMA insertion are well known. The use of the fiberoptic bronchoscope has benefited surgery on rheumatoids and others with C-spine abnormalities. The use of local anesthetics for arthroscopy is also gaining popularity. **Malignant hyperthermia**, an AD hypermetabolic disorder of skeletal muscle, can be triggered by various anesthetics (especially halothane and succinylcholine) in susceptible patients (e.g., neuromuscular disorders). Patients with Duchenne's muscular dystrophy arthrogryposis and osteogenesis imperfecta are especially at risk. Cell membrane defects affect calcium transport, leading to muscle rigidity and hypermetabolism. Masseter muscle spasm, increased temperature, rigidity, and acidosis are the hallmarks of the disease. Early diagnosis and treatment (with dantrolene, balancing of electrolytes, increasing urinary output, respiratory support, and cooling) are essential.

B. Spinal Cord Monitoring—Usually involves testing the posterior column, but monitoring of other areas is under investigation. Electric monitoring includes the use of somatosensory cortical evoked potentials (SCEPs) to record summed input from stimulation of peripheral areas. Somatosensory spinal evoked potentials (SSEPs) are more invasive, but can be more sensitive. Preoperative recordings are compared to readings (especially latency and amplitude) at critical times during the procedure. The wake-up test is still the standard for monitoring, and relies on lightening of anesthesia and the patient moving selected extremities.

C. Tourniquet—Injuries usually involve the area directly beneath the tourniquet and include nerve and muscle damage. Careful application, wide cuffs, lower pressures (200 mm in upper extremity and 250 mm in lower extremity), and double cuffs help avoid these problems. Equilibrium can be reestablished within 5 minutes following 90 minutes of tourniquet application, but requires 15 minutes following the use of a tourniquet for 3 hours.

V. Other Problems

A. Pain Control—Acutely, pain implies the presence of potential tissue damage, whereas chronic pain (3–6 months) does not. Nociceptors transduce stimuli through substances (P), allowing transmission along peripheral nerves (types A and C fibers) to the dorsal column, spinothalamic tract, and thalamus. Modulation is via brain stem centers and endogenous opiates. Postoperative pain control can be targeted at any step. Local prostaglandin inhibitors (under investigation), and long-acting local anesthetics target transduction of pain. Perispinal opiates affect modulation, and systemic opiates affect perception and modulation of pain.

B. Transfusion—Because of disease transmission, that has become an important issue.

1. Transfusion reactions—Include allergic, febrile, and hemolytic reactions.

a. Allergic reaction—Most common; occurs toward the end of transfusion. Symptoms include chills, pruritus, erythema, and urticaria. It usually spontaneously subsides. Pretreatment with Benadryl and hydrocortisone, if appropriate, in patients with a prior history of allergic reactions.

b. Febrile reaction—Also common; occur after the initial 100–300 cc of packed RBCs have been transfused. Chills and fever are caused by antibodies to foreign WBCs. Treatment is

similar to allergic reaction. Risk is reduced with use of Leukopoor products.

c. Hemolytic Reaction—Less common but most serious. This occurs early in the transfusion, and symptoms include chills, fever, tachycardia, chest tightness, and flank pain. Treatment includes stopping the transfusion, administration of IV fluids, appropriate lab studies, and monitoring in an intensive care setting.

2. Transfusion Risks—include transmission of hepatitis (non-A, non-B [2–3%], B [<1%]), CMV [highest incidence, but not clinically important], HTLV-1, and HIV (<0.04%). Donor deferral for high-risk individuals and more effective screening methods are decreasing these risks.

3. Alternatives to Homologous Blood Transfusion

a. Autologous Deposition—Requires a hemoglobin of 11 and a hematocrit of 33, and long lead times. Iron supplementation during donation is routine. Allows storage of several units prior to elective procedures with large anticipated blood loss.

b. "Cell-Saver"—Intraoperative autotransfusion. Usually requires 400 cc of blood loss to recover 1 unit (250 cc). Can only be used for 4 hours at one time.

c. Autotransfusion—Allows postoperative drain recuperation and use.

d. Acute Preoperative Normovolemic Hemodilution—Allows storage of autologous blood (replace with crystal) immediately preoperatively for use intra/postoperatively.

e. Pharmacologic Intervention—Alternatives including desmopressin (ADH analogue that increases levels of plasma factor VIII), recombinant erythropoietin (stimulates erythrogenesis), and synthetic erythrocyte substitutes are all under research.

f. Judicious Use of Blood Products—Platelet transfusion with massive bleeding/coagulopathies is done based on clinical parameters rather than set platelet thresholds. Fresh frozen plasma is reserved for patients with massive bleeding with significantly abnormal coagulation tests. Cryoprecipitate is used in hemophilia (with less exposure than factor concentrates), and as a source of fibrinogen in consumptive coagulopathies.

SELECTED BIBLIOGRAPHY

AAOS Task Force on AIDS and Orthopaedic Surgery: Recommendations for the Prevention of Human Immunodeficiency Virus (HIV) Transmission in the Practice of Orthopaedic Surgery. Park Ridge, IL, American Academy of Orthopaedic Surgeons, 1989.

Albright, J.A., and Brand, R.A. eds. The Scientific Basis of Orthopaedics, 2nd ed. Norwalk, CT, Appleton & Lange, 1987.

Austin, L.A., and Heath, H., III: Calcitonin: Physiology and pathophysiology. N. Engl. J. Med. 304:269–278, 1981.

Barth, R.W., and Lane, J.M.: Osteoporosis. Orthop. Clin. North Am. 19:845–858, 1988.

Bartlett, P., Reingold, A.L., Graham, D.R., Dan, B.B., Selinger, D.S., Tank, G.W., and Wichterman, K.A.: Toxic shock syndrome associated with surgical wound infections. J.A.M.A. 247:1448–1451, 1982.

Beighton, P., and Horan, F.: Orthopaedic aspects of Ehlers-Danlos syndrome. J. Bone Joint Surg. [Br] 51:444–453, 1969.

Bobyn, J.D., Pilliar, R.M., Cameron, H.U., and Weatherly, G.C.: The optimum pore size for the fixation of porous-surfaced metal implants by the ingrowth of bone. Clin. Orthop. 150:263–270, 1980.

Bonucci, E.: New knowledge on the origin, function and fate of osteoclasts. Clin. Orthop. 158:252–269, 1981.

Booth, F.W.: Physiologic and biochemical effects in immobilization of muscle. Clin. Orthop. 219:15–20, 1987.

Boskey, A.L.: Current concepts of the physiology and biochemistry of calcification. Clin. Orthop. 157:225–257, 1981.

Brighton, C.T.: Structure and function of the growth plate. Clin. Orthop. 136:22–32, 1978.

Bronner, F., and Worreli, R.V.: A Basic Science Primer in Orthopaedics. Baltimore, Wilkins & Wilkins, 1991.

Canalis, E.: Effect of growth factors on bone cell replication and differentiation. Clin. Orthop. 193:246–263, 1985.

Carter, D.R., and Spengler, D.M.: Mechanical properties and composition of cortical bone. Clin. Orthop. 135:192–217, 1978.

Centers for Disease Control: Recommendations for venting transmission of infection with human T-lymphotropic virus type III/lymphadenopathy-associated virus in the workplace. M.M.W.R. 34 (45):682–695, 1985.

Chesney, R.W.: Current clinical applications of vitamin D metabolite research. Clin. Orthop. 161:285–314, 1981.

Cierney, G., III: Chronic osteomyelitis: Results of treatment. Instr. Course Lect. 39:495–508, 1990.

Claes, L.: Biomechanical properties of human ligaments. Aktuel Probl. Chir. Orthop. 26:10–17, 1983.

Culp, R.W., Eichenfield, A.H., Davidson, R.S., et al.: Lyme arthritis in children: An orthopaedic perspective. J. Bone Joint Surg. [Am.] 69:96–99, 1987.

Dee, R., Mango, E., and Hurst, L.C.: Principles of Orthopaedic Practice. New York, McGraw Hill Book Co., 1989.

DeLee, J.C., and Rockwood, C.A., Jr.: Current concepts review. The use of aspirin in thromboembolic disease. J. Bone Joint Surg. [Am.] 62:149–152, 1980.

Ficat, R.P., and Arlet, J.: Ischemia and Necroses of Bone. Baltimore, Williams & Wilkins, 1980.

Fitzgerald, R.H., Jr.: Orthopaedic sepsis in osteomyelitis: Antimicrobial therapy for the musculoskeletal system. Instr. Course Lect. 31:1–9, 1982.

Fitzgerald, R.H., Jr., Ruttle, P.E., Arnold, P.G., Kelly, P.J., and Irons, G.B.: Local muscle flaps in the treatment of chronic osteomyelitis. J. Bone Joint Surg. [Am.] 67:175–185, 1985.

Frankel, V.H., and Burnstein, A.H.: Orthopaedic Biomechanics. Philadelphia, Lea & Febiger, 1970.

Friedlaender, G.E.: Bone grafts: The basic science rationale for clinical applications. J. Bone Joint Surg. [Am.] 69:786–790, 1987.

Friedlaender, G.E., Mankin, H.J., and Sell, K.W., eds.: Osteochondral Allografts: Biology, Banking, and Clinical Applications. Boston, Little, Brown and Company, 1983.

Friedlaender, G.E. ed.: Bone grafting. Orthop. Clin. North Am., (2), 1987.

Garrett, W.E., Jr., Seaber, A.V., Boswick, J., Urbaniak, J.R., and Goldner, J.L.: Recovery of skeletal muscle after laceration and repair. J. Hand Surg. [Am.] 9:683–692, 1984.

Ger, R.: Muscle transposition for treatment and prevention of chronic posttraumatic osteomyelitis of the tibia. J. Bone Joint Surg. [Am.] 59:784–791, 1977.

Glimcher, M.J., and Kenzora, J.E.: The biology of osteonecrosis of the human femoral head and its clinical implications: I. Tissue biology. II. The pathological changes in the femoral head as an organ and in the hip joint. III. Discussion of the etiology and genesis of the pathological sequelae; Comments on treatment. Clin. Orthop. 138:284–309; 139:283–312; 140:273–312, 1979.

Goldberg, V.M., and Stevenson, S.: Natural history of autografts and allografts. Clin. Orthop. 225:7–16, 1987.

Greech, P., Martin, T.J., Barrington, N.A. and Ell, P.J.: Diagnosis of Metabolic Bone Disease. Philadelphia, W.B. Saunders, 1985.

Gustilo, R.B., Gruninger R.P. and Tsukayama, D.T.: Orthopaedic Infection: Diagnosis and Treatment. Philadelphia, W.B. Saunders, 1989.

Harcke, H.T., Grissom, L.E., and Finkelstein, M.S.: Evaluation of the musculoskeletal system with sonography. AJR 150:1253–1261, 1988.

Hauzeur, J.P., Pasteels, J.L., Schoutens, A., et al.: The diagnostic value of magnetic resonance imaging in non-traumatic osteonecrosis of the femoral head. J. Bone Joint Surg. [Am.] 71:641, 1989.

Hill, C., Mazas, F., Flamant, R., and Evrard, J.: Prophylactic cefazolin versus placebo in total hip replacement. Lancet 1:795–797, 1981.

Hungerford, D.S., ed.: Avascular necrosis of the femoral head. Hip 11:247–330, 1983.

Jahss, M.H.: Disorders of the Foot. Philadelphia, W.B. Saunders, 1982.

Jardon, O.M., Wingard, D.W., Barak, A.J., and Connolly, J.F.: Malignant hyperthermia. A potentially fatal syndrome in orthopaedic patients. J. Bone Joint Surg. [Am.] 61:1064–1070, 1979.

Kanis, J.A.: Vitamin D metabolism and its clinical application. J. Bone Joint Surg. [Br.] 64:542–560, 1982.

Kelly, W.N., Harris, E.D., Ruddy, S., and Sledge, C.B.: Textbook of Rheumatology. Philadelphia, W.B. Saunders, 1981.

Kleerekoper, M.B., Tolia, K., and Parfitt, A.M.: Nutritional endocrine, and demographic aspects of osteoporosis. Orthop. Clin. North Am. 12:547–558, 1981.

Kneeland, J.B., Middleton, W.D., Carrera, G.F., et al: MR imaging of the shoulder: Diagnosis of rotator cuff tears. AJR 149:333–337, 1987.

Lane, J.M., Healey, J.H., Schwartz, E., Vigorita, V.J., Schneider, R., Einhorn, T.A., Suda, M., and Robbins, W.C.: Treatment of osteoporosis with sodium fluoride and calcium: Effects on vertebral fracture incidence and bone histomorphometry. Orthop. Clin. North Am. 15:729–745, 1984.

Lane, J.M., and Vigorita, V.J.: Osteoporosis. J. Bone Joint Surg. [Am.] 65:274–278, 1983.

Mallouh, A., and Talab, Y.: Bone and joint infection in patients with sickle cell disease. J. Pediatr. Orthop. 5:158–162, 1985.

McCollough, N.C., III; Enis, J.E., Lovitt, J., Lian, E.C., Niemann, K.N.W., and Loughlin, E.C., Jr.: Synovectomy or total replacement of the knee in hemophilia. J. Bone Joint Surg. [Am.] 61:69–75, 1979.

McKibbin, B.: The biology of fracture healing in long bones. J. Bone Joint Surg. [Br.] 60:150–162, 1978.

McKusick, V.A.: Heritable Disorders of Connective Tissue. 4th ed. St. Louis, C.V. Mosby, 1972.

Mitchell, M.D., Kundel, H.L., Steinberg, M.E., et al.: Avascular necrosis of the hip: Comparison of MR, CT, and scintigraphy. AJR 147:67–71, 1986.

Moskowitz, R.W., Howell, D.S., Goldberg, V.M., and Mankin, H.H.: Osteoarthritis: Diagnosis and Management. Philadelphia, W.B. Saunders Company, 1984.

Murphy, E.F., and Burstein, A.H.: Physical properties of materials including solid mechanics. In AAOS Atlas of Orthotics: Biomechanical Principles and Application. St. Louis, C.V. Mosby, 1975.

Nordin, B.E.C., Horsman, A., Marshall, D.H., Simpson, M., and Waterhouse, G.M.: Calcium requirement and calcium therapy. Clin. Orthop. 140:216–239, 1979.

Orthopaedic Knowledge Update Home Study Syllabus I, II, and III. Chicago, American Academy of Orthopaedic Surgeons, 1984, 1987, 1990.

Orthopaedic Science Syllabus. Chicago, American Academy of Orthopaedic Surgery, 1986.

O'Sullivan, M.E., Chao, E.Y.S., and Kelly, P.J.: Current concepts review. The effects of fixation on fracture-healing. J. Bone Joint Surg. [Am.] 71:306, 1989.

Owen, R., Goodfellow, J., and Bullough, P.: Scientific Foundations of Orthopaedics and Traumatology. Philadelphia, W.B. Saunders, 1982.

Palmer, A.K., Werner, F.W., Murphy, D., and Glisson, R.: Functional wrist motion: A biomechanical study. J. Hand Surg. [Am.] 10:39–46, 1985.

Perry, J.: Anatomy and biomechanics of the hindfoot. Clin. Orthop. 177:9–15, 1983.

Person, D.A., and Sharp, J.T.: The etiology of rheumatoid arthritis. Bull. Rheumat. Dis. 27:888–893, 1977.

Petty, W.: The effect of methylmethacrylate on bacterial phagocytosis and killing by human polymorphonuclear leukocytes. J. Bone Joint Surg. [Am.] 60:752–757, 1978.

Prevention and treatment of postmenopausal osteoporosis. Med Lett 29:75–77, 1987.

Pyeritz, R.E.: The Marfan Phenotype: Pleiotrophy and Variability as Clues to Genetic Heterogeneity. St. Louis, C.V. Mosby, 1982.

Pykett, I.L., Newhouse, J.H., Buonanno, F.S., Brady, T.J., Goldman, M.R., Kistler, J.P., and Pohost, G.M.: Principles of nuclear magnetic resonance imaging. Radiology 143:157–168, 1982.

Raisz, L.G., and Kream, B.E.: Regulation of bone formation. N. Engl. J. Med. 309:29–35, 1983.

Robinson, H.J., Jr., Hartleben, P.D., Lund, G., et al: Evaluation of magnetic resonance imaging in the diagnosis of osteonecrosis of the femoral head. Accuracy compared with radiographs, core biopsy, and intra-osseous pressure measurements. J. Bone Joint Surg. [Am.] 71:650, 1989.

Rosner, I.A., Goldberg, V.M., and Moskowitz, R.W.: Estrogens and osteoarthritis. Clin. Orthop. 213:77–83, 1986.

Salter, R.B., Minster, R.R., Clements, N.: Bell, R.S., and Bogoch, E.R.: Continuous passive motion and the repair of full thickness articular cartilage defects: A one-year follow-up. Orthop. Trans. 6:266–267, 1982.

Schenkar, D.L., Roeckel, I.E., Bailey, H.L., and Brower, T.D.: Thrombocytopenia and its management in the surgical patient needing multiple reconstructive procedures. Am. J. Surg. 13:572–574, 1977.

Smith, R.L., Schurman, D.J., Kajiyama, G., et al: The effect of antibiotics on the destruction of cartilage in experimental infectious arthritis. J. Bone Joint Surg. [Am.] 69:1063–1068, 1987.

Steinberg, M.E., The Hip and its Disorders. Philadelphia, W.B. Saunders, 1991.

Vaes, G.: Cellular biology and biochemical mechanism of bone resorption: A review of recent developments on the formation, activation, and mode of action in osteoclasts. Clin. Orthop. 231:239–271, 1988.

Wahner, H.W., Dunn, W.L., and Riggs, B.L.: Assessment of bone mineral. Part 1 and Part 2. J. Nucl. Med. 25:1134–1141; 1241–1253, 1985.

Wallach, S.: Hormonal factors in osteoporosis. Clin. Orthop. 144:284–292, 1979.

Watanabe, A.T., Carter, B.C., Teitelbaum, G.P., et al: Common pitfalls in magnetic resonance imaging of the knee. J. Bone Joint Surg. [Am.] 71:857, 1989.

Woo, S.L-Y., and Buckwalter, J.A., eds.: Injury and Repair of the Musculoskeletal Soft Tissues. Park Ridge, IL, American Academy of Orthopaedic Surgeons, 1988.

CHAPTER 3

Adult Reconstruction and Sports Medicine

I. Hip Reconstruction
   A. Introduction—The following sections concentrate on specific procedures. Individual disease processes affecting the hip are covered elsewhere.
   B. Arthrodesis—Favored in **young** patients with **unilateral** hip disease (usually posttraumatic) with a **good back and ipsilateral knee**. Return to normal activity, including manual labor, can be expected with excellent pain relief. Indications include arthritis, failed osteotomies, and failed cup arthroplasty in young patients. Preoperative immobilization (hip spica) is commonly used to acquaint the patient with postoperative expectations. Later conversion to THA is possible if hip abductors are preserved. Fusion in neutral abduction and rotation with **30 degrees of flexion** is recommended; **avoid abduction** and internal rotation. Fixation is with Barr bolts or AO Cobra plate (more stable but disrupts abductors). Complications include nonunion, malposition (most common), degenerative joint disease (DJD), or instability of ipsilateral knee, back, and contralateral hip. Should not be done bilaterally but can be done with contralateral THA.
   C. Resection Arthroplasty—indicated for incurable infection (esp. after failed THA), postradiation osteonecrosis, or in patients with minimal or no ambulation potential and poor mental status/medical risk. Shortening of 2–5 cm and severe Trendelenburg gait can be expected, and most patients will require support to ambulate. Can be done bilaterally.
   D. Femoral Osteotomy—Although used commonly in Europe for advanced DJD, its use in the U.S. is usually restricted to localized structural defects that can be redirected to a non–weight-bearing area. Intertrochanteric osteotomies are commonly done after x-rays in abduction, adduction, internal rotation, and external rotation are studied to plan for the best correction. Congruence achieved in adduction is a major criterion for selecting a valgus osteotomy. An increased neck-to-shaft angle, superolateral joint space narrowing, sphericity of the femoral head, and congruence achieved in abduction are all criteria for selecting a varus osteotomy.

A varus extension osteotomy is most commonly required. Best results are in younger, nonobese patients with good ROM and radiographs with focal defects.
   E. Pelvic Osteotomies (see Chapter 1, Pediatric Orthopaedics)—Can allow redirection of acetabular cartilage (Steel, Sutherland, Salter, Dome/Dial) or augment the acetabulum with extra-articular bone (Chiari, shelf). Redirection osteotomies require a congruent joint space (relatively early arthritis with >50% joint space and >60% ROM remaining); the Chiari and shelf procedures are salvage procedures (articular cartilage reduced by >1/2). Table 3–1 summarizes the salient features of each.
   F. Resurfacing Arthroplasty—Femoral resurfacing implants (e.g., Wagner) became popular in the late 1970s; however, because of poor design and frequent failure (20–50% at 5 years), they are not currently indicated. Failure was frequently at the femoral neck due to disruption of the vascular supply and thinning of the acetabulum. Revision is difficult due to large acetabular bone loss.
   G. Hemiarthroplasty—Requires a normal acetabulum and therefore is rarely used for arthritis. May be indicated with osteonecrosis or hip fracture. Can be converted later to THA.
   H. Total Hip Arthroplasty (THA)
      1. Indications—Expanded from the original primary indication of incapacitating pain in >65-year-old patients refractory to all medical and surgical therapy (short of resection arthroplasty); now includes rheumatoid arthritis (RA), osteonecrosis, DDH, fractures, failed reconstruction, tumors, etc. It should also be considered in younger patients with significant back or ipsilateral knee DJD (who are not candidates for fusion). Conservative therapy, including weight loss, various NSAIDs, limitation of activity, and use of a cane (in contralateral hand) should be exhausted prior to considering THA. Persistent symptoms of pain with limited ambulation, night pain, and severe quality-of-life impact despite conserva-

TABLE 3–1. FEATURES OF VARIOUS PELVIC OSTEOTOMIES

Procedure	Osteotomies	Indication	Other
Salter	Innominate/open wedge	Youth/anterior deficiency	Poor lateral coverage/length
Steel	Both rami, innominate	Incr. redirection rad.	Incr. instability, complex
Sutherland	Pubis, innominate	Can medialy displace	Less rotation
Dome/Dial	Acetabulum subchondral	Good cartilage	Osteonecrosis and penetration
Chiari	Innominate/displaces roof	Salvage	Loses cartilage-cartilage continuity

tive therapy are now recognized as the principle indications for THA. Contraindications include pre-existing medical problems that have not been optimized (cardiac, pulmonary, GI, etc.), physiologic age >80, nonambulators, and the skeletally immature. Specific contraindications include active infection, rapid destruction of bone, neurotrophic joint, abductor mass loss, and progressive neurologic disease.

2. Preoperative Work-Up—careful preoperative evaluation to include medical evaluation, laboratory studies, dental evaluation and careful surgical planning (approach, templating, etc.) is necessary. Pre- and postoperative antibiotics have been recommended, and careful preparation of the patient and the room is indicated to decrease the incidence of infection. The use of laminar flow, special surgical exhaust systems, and special drapes may reduce rates of infection. Deep venous thrombosis (DVT) prophylaxis usually includes the use of coumadin (Warfarin) perioperatively.

3. Surgical Approach—Many favor the anterolateral approach (with or without a greater trochanteric osteotomy); however, the posterior approach is also commonly used (may be increased incidence of posterior dislocation but component positioning is the most critical factor).

4. Components
   a. Femoral Component—designed either for cemented or noncemented (press fit and/or porus ingrowth) use. Other differences are based on metal type and design properties. Stainless steel or "supermetal" alloys (Co-Cr-Mo) have been used most frequently, but newer implants using titanium may allow increased implant load transmission to the cement and bone in the calcar region. Poor wear characteristics of titanium have lead to component use of Co-Cr heads on titanium stems. Macrophages and foreign body giant cells at the bone-cement interface may contribute to fibrous membrane and loosening (cement disease histiocytosis). Macrophages affected by cement particles may be able to generate PGE_2 and collagenase, leading to resorption of bone at the bone-cement interface. However, mechanical loosening is also a problem (loosening in torsion most common). Press-fit prostheses rely on bone formation about the stem to allow a tight fit. Porous-coated implants have surface openings of 50–400 μ to allow bone ingrowth. Initial stability is best achieved by maximum interference fit (minimizes micromotion and maximizes surface contact). Stems are often

not treated distally to allow later removal for revision. Complications are still not fully understood but may include metal ion disease and loosening. Additionally, **postoperative thigh pain** is common and may last up to a year or more. Newer component materials, coatings, and designs may allow better results in the future. Hydroxyapatite coatings and fibermesh (as opposed to beaded design) allow better ingrowth in animal models. Cemented stems are best for older patients (>65 years physiologic age) with poor bone quality (e.g., type "C" bone with thin cortices and no fluting). Uncemented stems are best for younger patients and in revision surgery. Collared designs appear to have decreased subsidence rates and have higher load-to-failure ratios.

   b. Femoral Head—Available in different diameters. The smaller diameter heads (22 mm) allow less stress/torque but may result in increased central acetabular wear and dislocation. Larger head sizes (up to 32 mm) allow increased ROM and reduced dislocation, but have less net wall thickness for long-term wear. Heads of 26–28 mm appear to be the ideal compromise and are most commonly used.

   c. Acetabular Component—Like the femoral component, is designed either for cemented or noncemented use. Noncemented prostheses rely on a macro-lock screw in design; increased incidence of loosening has been experienced with these. Porous coated designs usually rely on temporary fixation with screws. Placement of these screws anteriorly has been demonstrated to be dangerous **(iliac vein at risk with anterosuperior screws; obturator artery at risk with anteroinferior screws)**.

   d. Acetabular Cup—Typically ultrahigh-molecular-weight polyethylene (UHMWPE). Thickness is based on femoral head size and can include a lip of 10–20 degrees ("dial-a-prayer") that may reduce incidence of postoperative dislocation.

5. Component Position—The femoral component should be placed in slight valgus with the neck in 5–10 degrees of anteversion. The acetabulum should be placed in 10–15 degrees of anteversion and 45 degrees of vertical inclination.

6. Complications
   a. Loosening—The most common long-term complication. Can be based on radiologic or clinical grounds. Radiologic loosening is based on change in position of a prosthesis, 2 mm or more of circumferential lucency, ce-

TABLE 3–2. MODES OF FEMORAL STEM LOOSENING

MODE	MECHANISM	CAUSE	FINDINGS/RESULTS
I	Pistoning	Subsidence	Stem in cement or cement mantle
II	Medial stem pivot	Medial migration	Proximal medial, distal lateral shift
III	Calcar pivot	Distal toggle	Windshield wiper effect
IV	Cantilever bending[a]	Proximal resorption	Medial migration, defect, or *fracture of proximial stem*

[a] Most common.

ment fracture, and especially progressive enlargement of a radiolucent line on serial radiographs. There is a 10–40% incidence of radiographic loosening at 10 years. Early loosening (the first 5 years) is usually from the femoral component at the prosthesis-cement interface; late loosening is usually from the acetabular component. Loosening is more frequent with younger patients, rheumatoids, heavy patients, and prior hip surgery. Diagnosis and treatment of loosening is largely based on patient's symptoms. Bone scans may be helpful but are not specific. Arthograms are not usually helpful but can sometimes be reliable, particularly if patient is allowed to ambulate after injection. Aspiration and culture is an important part of this procedure, or is done separately to rule out septic loosening. Injection of anesthetic into the joint is also helpful in establishing the diagnosis of symptomatic loosening. The ultimate treatment for patients with increased symptoms, progressive radiographic loosening (subsidence), and failure to respond to conservative therapy may be surgical intervention and replacement if

necessary. Specific points regarding stem and cup loosening follow.

(1) Stem Loosening—Four modes of femoral stem loosening have been described (Gruen) (Table 3–2; Fig. 3–1). **Cracks most commonly begin on the anterolateral surface** of the femoral prosthesis. These are much less common now with stronger metal alloys. Cement loosening of the femoral stem has also been characterized by Gruen (Fig. 3–2).

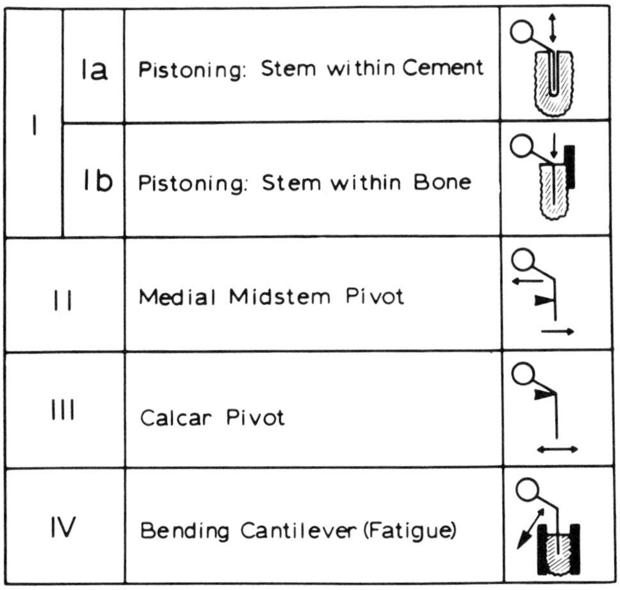

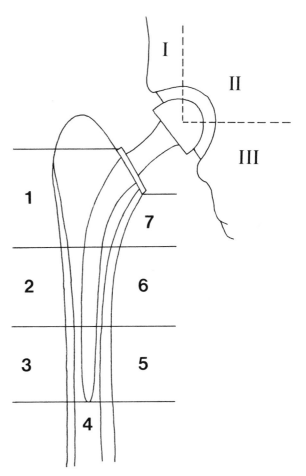

I	Ia	Pistoning: Stem within Cement	
	Ib	Pistoning: Stem within Bone	
II		Medial Midstem Pivot	
III		Calcar Pivot	
IV		Bending Cantilever (Fatigue)	

FIGURE 3–1. Modes of femoral stem failure. (From Gruen, T.A., McNeice, G.M., and Amstutz, H.C.: Modes of failure of cemented stem-type femoral components. Clin. Orthop. Rel. Res. 141:19, 1979; reprinted by permission.)

FIGURE 3–2. Composite diagram demonstrating zones of loosening in THA. (Modified from Gruen, T.A., McNeice, G.M., and Amstutz, H.C.: Modes of failure of cemented stem-type femoral components. Clin. Orthop. Rel. Res. 141:17–27, 1979; and DeLee, J.C., and Charnley, J.: Radiologic demarcation of cemented sockets in total hip replacement. Clin. Orthop. Rel. Res. 121:20–32, 1976).

(2) Cup Loosening—Described based on three zones (DeLee): I = superior, II = middle 90 degrees, 3 = inferior (Fig. 3–2). The acetabular cup is considered loose if there is a radiolucency ≥2 mm in all three zones, **progressive loosening** in one or two zones, or change in position of cup. Loosening between the cement and cup is unusual (vs. femoral stem). The popular use of press-fit components in the acetabulum, even with cemented stems (hybrid design), has reduced cup loosening problems.

b. Implant Failure
(1) Stem Failure—Increased incidence with heavy, active patients; varus position of stem; stems with decreased cross-sectional area and long necks; stainless steel components; and poor support in the proximal 1/3 (bending cantilever fatigue). Fracture usually begins in the middle 1/3 of the anterolateral aspect of stem and progresses medially.
(2) Acetabular Wear—Although initially a big concern, wear rates of less than 0.1 mm/year can be expected, partly due to UHMWPE. Wear rates can be increased with loose prostheses or acrylic debris. Metal backing of prosthesis has reduced stresses in cement and trabecular bone and decreased polyethylene wear. Proximal femoral osteolysis is associated with polyethylene wear and can lead to further loosening of the stem.

c. Dislocation—Occurs in 1–4% of primary THAs. Most commonly caused by looseness of the hip (improper neck length), and component malposition (combined retroversion → posterior dislocation; combined anteroversion → anterior dislocation). Dislocations are much more common in revision THA. Careful testing with trial components with correction of neck length, impingement, and repair of the trochanter may avoid this complication. Late dislocation may be related to gradual stretching of the pseudocapsule. Patient education is also a critical factor. After reduction, treatment with 3–6 weeks of immobilization in abduction with a brace or hip spica may be indicated. Recurrent dislocation should be treated with aspiration (to rule out sepsis), and revision if indicated. Posterior dislocations are more common than anterior dislocations. Dislocation may be more common in radiation therapy (XRT) osteonecrosis—acetabular components should be placed more horizontally in these patients.

d. Heterotopic Bone—Increased incidence in males, ankylosing spondylitis, DISH, post-traumatic arthritis, heterotopic osteoarthritis, and patients who previously formed heterotopic bone. Treatment with low-dose XRT (1000 centi Gy [rads]) immediately postoperatively has been most effective in prophylactically treating patients at risk. Indomethacin (1 month preop, 3 months postop) has also been shown to be a useful prophy-

laxis. These agents may affect porus ingrowth and therefore are usually indicated only for cemented components.

e. Thromboembolic Disease—most common serious complication of THA, and a significant cause of postop mortality. Increased incidence can be expected with older patients, osteoarthritis (vs. RA), prior history, obesity, and long operations with large blood loss. Other factors include CHF, malignancy, and prolonged immobility. Adjusted-dose coumadin appears to be the best prophylaxis. Other schemes include minidose heparin, enteric-coated aspirin, dextran, and pneumatic devices. B-mode ultrasound can be helpful to diagnose DVTs, but venography is still best. Ventilation-perfusion (V/Q) scan and pulmonary angiography may be required to establish the diagnosis of pulmonary embolism (PE) prior to starting a heparin drip, which is followed by 3–6 months of coumadin therapy. Venous traps are reserved for high-risk patients.

f. Intraoperative Complications—Can include fracture (esp. medial calcar), which is treated with cerclage wiring and in some cases longer femoral stems; neurovascular injury (common peroneal branch of sciatic is more common and will result in footdrop; significant vascular injury can result from acetabular screws placed anteriorly [superiorly and inferiorly]), shaft penetrations (esp. laterally with revision when medial cement is not removed early); and various other catastrophes. Hypotension during cement insertion may be associated with complement activation and is usually transient.

g. Greater Trochanteric Problems—Nonunions of the trochanter after osteotomy may do well after wire removal or may require reapproximation. Fortunately, this is being used less commonly now. Newer cable fixation devices may create a resurgence of its use. Greater trochanter bursitis is common but usually responds to hip abductor strenthening and steroid injection.

h. Infection—Perhaps the most devastating and dreaded complication. It often results in removal of components, increased morbidity, and often mortality. Incidence is increased with obesity, diabetes, sickle cell disease, osteonecrosis, alcoholism, RA, postop urinary instrumentation, and patients on immunosuppressive drugs and steroids. Also increased with longer procedures, revisions, and improper operating technique. Use of IV antibiotics, Ultraclean Air, UV lights, decreased traffic and conversation, and containment devices all help decrease rates. Most common organisms include *Staph. aureus* (penicillin, cefazolin), streptococcus (penicillin), *E. coli* (amphotericin ± gentamycin), and *Pseudomonas* (gentamycin, ticarcillin). Presentation usually involves pain (especially at rest), and laboratory studies are often not helpful (however, ESR and C-reactive protein levels are elevated). Bone scan/indium scan and aspiration are most helpful. Tissue biopsies at the time of débridement (with frozen section confirmation of >5 PMNs/high-power field) are also useful to diagnose infection. Acute infections (within the first 12 weeks) are managed with I&D (superficial only if not deep with aspiration of hip joint; posterolateral incision if in joint to allow better drainage), preservation of hardware if it is not loose, and IV antibiotics for 4–6 weeks followed by oral antibiotics for at least an additional 6 weeks. Close follow-up and guarded prognosis are necessary. Deep delayed infections (3–24 months postop) require removal of prosthesis and all cement as well as long-term antibiotics. Exchange arthroplasty for less virulent organisms should follow at least a several-week delay. Late hematogenous infections occur 24+ months after surgery and can follow an infection elsewhere. Removal of components and all cement is required, and an extended delay should precede a decision to insert a replacement prosthesis. Recurrence following replantation may be as high as 13%, and is greater with retained cement and in replantations within 1 year following component removal. For virulent organisms such as *Pseudomonas*, a resection arthroplasty should be done.

    i. Other Problems—include nerve injury (sciatic > femoral > obturator—rare with good technique), and urinary retention (lower with preop and 24-hour postop indwelling catheters). Sciatic nerve injury is often transient and the result of traction from excessive lengthening. Femoral nerve injury is usually secondary to excessive retraction of the psoas muscle.

  7. Revision THA—Associated with less satisfactory results, increased operative time, blood loss, infection, and other complications. Additionally, revisions are less durable. Painful loosening is the major indication for revision, although impending fracture, component

malposition with recurrent dislocation, or other problems that would make a revision more difficult can be an indication. Removal of hardware and all previous cement is often followed by placement of a porous ingrowth prosthesis. Revision femoral stem length should be 1–3 cm longer than original stem. **If there is femoral cortical disruption, the revision stem should extend two to three shaft diameters distal** to the defect. The use of cement in revision surgery should only be considered in patients who are terminally ill or have very poor bone, who are not candidates for allograft. Bone grafting is often required, sometimes using allografts when host bone is severely deficient. The use of large bulk allografts is controversial due to migration and loosening.

  8. Special Problems
    a. Acetabular Bony Defects—Classified by the AAOS into five types (Fig. 3–3):

Type	Description	Example	Bone Graft
I	Segmental	Wall defect	Cortical-cancellous
II	Cavitary	Cyst	Cancellous
III	Combined	DJD	Both
IV	Pelvic discontinuity	Fx/DDH	Bone graft first
V	Arthrodesis	Fusion	Attention to landmarks

Principles of bone grafting involve restoration of the center of rotation, acetabular continuity/integrity, containment of prosthesis and graft, and rigid fixation of bone graft. Infection and graft resorption continue to be problems.

    b. Otto Pelvis (Arthrokatadysis)—Primary protrusio acetabuli characterized by progressive protrusio in middle-aged women. Can be bilateral in 1/3 of patients and causally related to osteomalacia. Large cortical-cancellous bone grafting may be required using the patient's femoral head in a primary arthroplasty as well as a large acetabular component.

  9. Additional Points—Childhood hip subluxation is the most common cause of hip DJD in patients younger than 40 yo. Surgery in hips with developmental dysplasia (DDH) has been based on anatomic reconstruction; however, recent studies suggest that proximal placement of acetabular components without lateralization may be superior to use of large grafts. Smaller pelvis size may make surgery difficult. Superolateral bone grafting may be required in severe cases. Other forms of childhood hip disease that often result in THA include Perthes disease, and slipped capital femoral epiphysis (SCFE). (Fig. 3–4). Postoperative range of motion is most dependent upon preoperative motion in the hip.

II. Knee Reconstruction

  A. Osteotomy—Indicated in selected cases of unicompartmental degenerative arthritis of the knee to transfer weight-bearing load to an uninvolved tibiofemoral joint surface. Most commonly per-

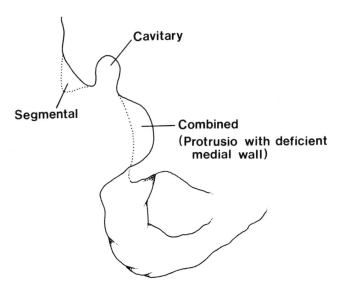

FIGURE 3–3. Acetabular defects (AAOS classification scheme). Pelvic discontinuity and hip arthrodesis not shown.

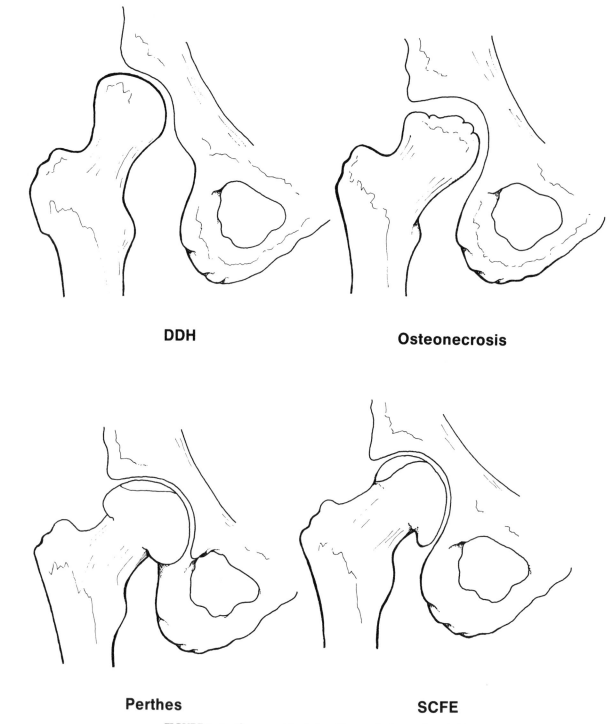

DDH

Osteonecrosis

Perthes

SCFE

FIGURE 3–4. Common hip deformities producing early arthritis.

formed for medial compartment disease, can also be done for lateral compartment disease.

1. Medial Compartment Disease—Valgus osteotomy of the proximal tibia is indicated with medial tenderness only, less than 15 degrees of fixed varus deformity, and radiographically intact lateral and patellofemoral compartments. **Contraindications** also include **lateral subluxation** of the tibia on the femur **>1 cm** (which indicates articular incongruity), tibial plate bone loss, **flexion contracture >15 degrees**, limitation

of flexion beyond 90 degrees, peripheral vascular disease, and instability. Full-length radiographs are necessary preoperatively to correct the mechanical axis of the limb. A lateral closing wedge osteotomy held with staples (stepped Coventry or standard) and fibular (or tibiofibular articulation) shortening is the standard method. Overcorrection of the mechanical axis 2–3 degrees beyond neutral provides the best results. Best results are in young, heavy patients with good bone stock. Complications include **undercorrection (most common),** overcorrection, penetration of the articular surface, avascular necrosis (AVN) of the plateau fragment, patella Baja, peroneal nerve injuries, and anterior compartment syndrome. The most important factor influencing the long-term results of proximal tibial osteotomies is adequacy of correction of the angular deformity. Usually considered as a temporizing procedure that will last 7–10 years prior to consideration for a total knee arthroplasty. TKA may be more difficult after upper tibial osteotomy but it is possible. Therefore, it is rarely indicated in a patient over 60 years old.

2. Lateral Compartment Disease—Varus osteotomy; usually involves a medial closing wedge osteotomy of the distal femur (supracondylar region) fixed with a plate. The femoral osteotomy is sometimes reserved for valgus deformities of >12 degrees and >10 degrees deviation of the knee joint from the horizontal. Preoperative range of motion of at least 90 degrees, <15-degree flexion contracture, and no associated instability are required. Medial displacement of the distal fragment will help maintain the mechanical axis of the limb in the center of the knee joint by restoring the axis of the femoral shaft to its preoperative position. Plate fixation of the distal femur is usually indicated.

B. Arthrodesis—Indicated in a patient with uncontrollable septic arthritis and complete joint destruction, young patients with severe ligamentous and articular damage, neuropathic joint disease, and patients with failed total knee replacements. Successful arthrodesis is possible in about 80% of failed condylar components but only 55% of hinged prostheses (may be less with the use of intramedullary fixation). Fusion in 10–15 degrees of flexion and 0–7 degrees of valgus is preferred. Complications include delayed/non/malunion.

C. Débridement—Débridement and drilling of subchondral bone may allow for formation of granulation tissue with metaplasia into fibrocartilage, and has had some temporary success. This procedure, to include abrasion chondroplasty, is typically done arthroscopically.

D. Arthroplasty—Includes unicompartmental and total knee arthroplasty, both with separate indications.

1. Unicompartmental Arthroplasty—Reserved for patients with single-compartment disease (DJD or osteonecrosis) who are not candidates for HTO (usually because of age). Achieves better ROM, preserves the cruciate ligaments, and preserves bone stock (vs. TKA). Usually reserved for older, sedentary patients who are not obese; contraindicated with significant fixed deformities, in inflammatory arthritis, in young patients, active obese patients, or those with dynamic instability or severely decreased ROM. Technique is important as the tibial implant must be placed at right angles to the mechanical axis of the tibia, and overcorrection should be avoided. Complications include loosening most commonly.

2. Total Knee Arthroplasty
   a. Indications—Disabling knee pain and decreased function from arthritis/arthropathy that involves at least two compartments in a patient who has failed all nonoperative treatment. **Contraindicated with nonfunctioning extensors,** severe neuromuscular dysfunction, **active sepsis, prior surgical fusion,** and in a **neuropathic joint.**

   b. Implant Design—Most commonly are "conforming" implants. Other types of implants include "linked" prostheses, which are fully constrained (tibial loosening, increased wear, and high infection rates have limited their use to patients with markedly unstable knees, especially after failure of prior TKAs); and "resurfacing implants," which retain both cruciate ligaments (also rarely used due to exacting surgical technique and soft tissue balancing required). Conforming implants have condylar metallic femoral components and metal-backed polyethylene tibial components. All such implants sacrifice the anterior cruciate ligament (ACL) and some ("posterior stabilized") designs also sacrifice the posterior cruciate ligament (PCL). Although posterior stabilized designs are used routinely by some surgeons, they are often indicated for large fixed contractures requiring removal of the PCL, and in postpatellectomy knees. **PCL sacrifice may cause difficulty with climbing stairs** in some patients and may cause increased shear stresses on the prosthesis.

   <u>Goals in TKA</u>

   1. Horizontal joint in stance phase of gait
   2. Restoration of the anatomic and mechanical axes
   3. Flexion gap equal to the extension gap
   4. Proper soft tissue balance
   5. Good patellar placement/alignment

   c. Surgical Technique—Correction of the following deformities may be required:

DEFORMITY	CORRECTION
Fixed varus	Elevate medial capsular sleeve, resect medial osteophytes
Lateral subluxation	Release popliteus tendon
Fixed valgus	Lateral approach, release IT band, LCL, Posterolateral capsule
Fixed flexion	Remove anterior osteophytes, elevate capsule & PCL, resect gastrocnemius, ± posterior capsulotomy
Limited flexion	Quadricepsplasty (V–Y) or patella tendon Z-plasty

Close attention to technique is also essential, and special emphasis should be placed on resecting the tibial surface at 90 degrees, avoiding notching of the anterior femoral surface, making proper cuts, and allowing proper tracking of the patella. Maximum coverage of the tibial plateau is essential. Correct alignment is best assured with the use of both extra- and intramedullary guides to achieve a normal mechanical axis (Fig. 3–5). Lateral parapetallar incisions are best for severe valgus knees (>15 degrees). Addi-

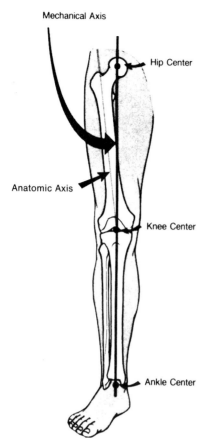

FIGURE 3–5. Knee axes. (From Rohr, W.L.: Primary total knee arthroplasty. In Chapman's Operative Orthopaedics, p. 718. Philadelphia, J.B. Lippincott, 1988; reprinted by permission.)

tionally, appropriate trials should be inserted prior to the final prosthesis to check for flexion and extension gaps (Fig. 3–6). An increased **flexion gap** (loose in flexion and tight in extension) is more common and can be corrected by resecting more of the distal femur. An increased **extension gap** (loose in extension and tight in flexion) is usually the result of a technical error and can be corrected by resecting the posterior femoral condyles or converting the flat tibial surface to a posteriorly sloping surface. When the knee is tight in both flexion and extension, more proximal tibia should be resected. The patella height can also result in tight flexion and may require additional patellar resection. Close attention to patella tracking is important, and the superolateral geniculate artery should be preserved. Bone grafting is indicated for defects involving >50% of the tibial plateau or if >5 mm of cement is needed to fill a defect. In general, bone stock should be preserved whenever possible, and large defects should be replaced with allograft bone.

d. Design—Hybrid TKAs with uncemented femoral components and cemented tibial and patellar components are often successful. Controversy regarding patella resurfacing has swung toward resurfacing in most cases (and all rheumatoids). The original patella height should be restored. Resurfacing leads to less patellofemoral pain and better stair climbing ability. Patellar alignment is enhanced with placing the femoral component in slight external rotation. Less than 20

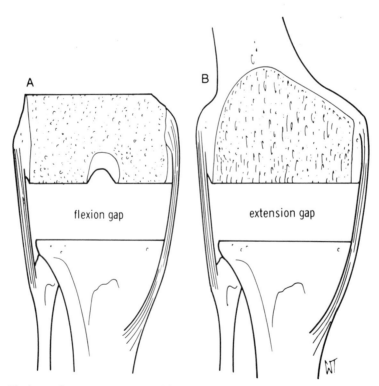

FIGURE 3–6. Flexion and extension gap in total knee arthroplasty. (From Scuderi, G.R., and Insall, J.N.: The posterior stabilized knee prosthesis. Orthop. Clin. North Am. 20(1):73, 1989; reprinted by permission.)

TABLE 3–3. TKA COMPLICATIONS

COMPLICATION	RISK FACTOR(S)	RECOMMENDATION/TREATMENT
Patella fracture	Sacrifice of lateral Geniculate Artery Thin/small patella	Preserve artery Minimally displaced fracture: Immobilize in extension Displaced fracture: Removal of component and patellectomy
Patella dislocation	Int rotated femoral component	Place femoral component in external rotation
Component loosening	Poor alignment Infection	Careful preparation, Aseptic technique Exchange arthroplasty
Tibial tray wear	Thin (<8 mm) components	Thicker trays/exchange
Peroneal nerve palsy	Flexion/valgus knee	Flex knee post-op
Supracondylar fracture	Anterior femoral notching	Avoid notching; ORIF
Skin slough	Prior incisions	Plan incisions accordingly
Decreased ROM	Poor rehabilitation	Manipulation under anesthesia (long term results unchanged)

mm of patella thickness is a relative contra-indication for patellar resurfacing. Metal-backed patella components have been uniformly unsuccessful, leading to wear fracture and metal debris in joints. Cementless implants may allow better wear, may cause less toxicity to surrounding tissues, and make revision easier. However, exacting technique is required. Loosening rates are higher, tibial components have poor ingrowth and subsidence (micromotion), metal-backed patellas wear easily, and these are contraindicated in patients with severe osteoporosis. Additionally, 3–6 months are usually required to achieve maximum pain relief.

 e. Complications—Outlined in Table 3–3:

 f. Revision TKA—The key to successful revision surgery is restoration of the original joint line. Radiographs taken prior to the index procedure and of the opposite knee are helpful. The adductor tubercle and the tip of the fibula as well as other landmarks are used to determine component position preoperatively. **The MCL must be intact in order to use a nonconstrained prosthesis.** The following instability patterns usually result from component malposition:

EXTENSION	FLEXION	PROBLEM
Loose varus or valgus	Loose varus or valgus	Tibial malposition
Tight	Loose varus or valgus	Femoral malrotation
Tight	Loose varus and valgus	Joint line malposition

III. Knee Disorders

 A. History—Several key historical points should be sought:

HISTORY	SIGNIFICANCE
Pain after sitting/stair climbing	Patellofemoral etiology
Dashboard injury	PCL tear/dislocation
Locking/pain with squatting	Meniscal tear
Noncontact injury with "pop"	ACL tear
Contact injury with "pop"	Colateral ligament, meniscus, patella dislocation

HISTORY	SIGNIFICANCE
Acute swelling	ACL, peripheral meniscus tear, osteochondral fx, ± capsule tear
Knee "gives way"	Ligamentous laxity, patella subluxation/dislocation, meniscal tear, chondromalasia of patella

 B. Physical Exam—The following are key exam points, and often are best elicited under anesthesia:

EXAM	METHOD	SIGNIFICANCE
Standing/gait	Observe gait	Based on pathology
Deformity	Observe patient standing	Based on pathology
Effusion	Patella: ballot/milk	Ligament/meniscus injury (acute), arthritis (chronic)
PMT	Palpate for tenderness	Based on location (joint line tenderness = meniscus)
ROM	Active and passive	Block = meniscus injury (bucket handle), Loose body, ACL tear impinging
Patella crepitus	With passive ROM	Patellofemoral pathology
Patella grind	Push patella with quadriceps contraction	Patellofemoral pathology
Patella apprehension	Push patella lat. at 20–30° flexion	Patella subluxation/dislocation
Q angle	ASIS-patella-tibial tubercle	Incr. with patella malalignment
Patella tilt	Tilt up laterally	>15° = Lax <0° = tight lateral constraint
Patella glide	Like apprehension	>50° = incr. medial const laxity
Active glide	Lat. excursion with quad. contraction	Lat. > prox. excursion = incr. functional Q angle quadriceps
Quadriceps circumference	10 cm (VMO), 15 cm (quad.)	Atrophy from inactivity
Symmetric extension	Heel from ground	Contracture, displaced meniscal tear, or other mechanical block

EXAM	METHOD	SIGNIFICANCE
McMurray	Ext./int. rotation varus/valgus stress-extension	Meniscal pathology or chondromalacia of articular surface
Varus/valgus stress	30°	MCL/LCL laxity (grade I–IV)
Varus/valgus stress	0°	MCL/LCL and PCL/post. capsule
Apley's	Prone-flexion compression	DJD, meniscal path
Lachman	Tibia forward at 30° flexion	ACL (most sensitive)
Finacetto	Lachman with Tibia subluxing beyond post horns of menisci	ACL (severe)
Ant. drawer	Tibia forward at 90° flexion	ACL
Int. rotation drawer	Foot int. rotated with drawer	Tighter = (normal), looser = ALRI
Ext. rotation drawer	Foot ext. rotation with drawer	Loose (normal), looser = AMRI
Pivot shift	Flexion with int. rotation and valgus	ALRI
Flexion-rotation drawer	Shift with axial load, less valgus	ALRI
Slocum	On back/side flexion and pivot	ALRI
Pivot jerk	Extension with int. rotation and valgus	ALRI
Post. drawer	Tibia backward at 90° flexion	PCL
Tibia sag	Flex 90°, observe	PCL
90° quad. act	Extend flexed knee	PCL
Ext. rotation recurvatum	Pick up great toes	PLRI
Reverse pivot	Extension with ext. rotation and valgus	PLRI
Ext. rotation at 30 + 90° flexion	Incr. and ext. rotation associated with PLRI	PLRI
Posterolateral drawer	Post. drawer, lat. > med.	PLRI

C. Radiographs—In addition to standard views, special views or certain findings can be helpful:

VIEW/SIGN	FINDING	SIGNIFICANCE
Lateral—hip & knee flexed	Sag	PCL disruption
Varus/valgus stress view	Opening	Collateral ligament injury; Salter-Harris fracture
Lateral capsule (Segund) sign	Small tibial avulsion	ACL tear
Pellegrini-Stieda lesion	Med. femoral condyle avulsion	Chronic MCL injury
Lateral-high patella	Patella alta	Patellofemoral path
Congruence angle	$\mu = -6°$ $SD = 11°$	Patellofemoral path
Tooth sign	Irregular ant. patella	Patellofemoral chondrosis
Arthrogram	Dye outline	Meniscal tear
MRI	Intra-articular path	Specific for lesion
Square lateral condyle	Thick joint space	Discoid meniscus
Fairbank's changes	Square condyle, peak eminences, ridging, narrowing	Early DJD (post. menisectomy)

D. Specific Injuries/Treatment

1. ACL Injury—Usually injured in noncontact maneuvers such as rapid deceleration and direction change or cutting while running, hyperextension or hyperflexion, and landing after jumping. Typically presents with an acute hemarthrosis (>70% of patients with an acute hemarthrosis will have an ACL tear!), and commonly (>50%) associated with a meniscal tear. Initial symptoms may be of posterolateral knee pain. The Lachman test (30° flexion) is the most sensitive test acutely on exam. Later, patients will complain of instability without swelling. If patients have persistent effusions, then a missed meniscal tear is more likely and arthroscopy should be considered. If untreated, ACL-injured patients will either do well (including with sports), require modification of sport activities, or do poorly in equal numbers. Functional bracing is probably effective for low-grade laxity under low-load conditions but is not effective for higher levels of activity. Bracing probably works by preventing full extension. Activity level and anticipated demands become the key factors in deciding among treatment options. Surgical options are best used for active, athletic individuals with knee laxity or individuals who have failed conservative management with functional instability that affects their daily living. All candidates must be motivated for an extensive postoperative rehab program. Most extra-articular procedures include rerouting or tenodesis of portions of the IT band to the lateral femoral condyle (Krakow's point) and can be successful by themselves or combined with an intra-articular procedure. Primary repair (done only rarely, usually in children) is usually supplemented with intra-articular augmentation. ACL reconstruction preserves meniscal repairs, and can be done acutely or late. Typically, mid-third patella tendon autograft is selected for its strength and reproducibility. Failing this, allografts have been successful. Cryopreservation decreases their antigenicity. Bovine and synthetic grafts have not had good results in general. All associated intra-articular pathology should be treated prior to ACL reconstruction. Meniscal pathology is common in ACL-deficient knees (>50%) and must be addressed prior to ACL reconstruction. Meniscal tears may recur in ACL-deficient knees (40%), and may influence the decision to proceed with ACL reconstruction. Postoperative rehab includes isometrics, straight leg raising, and progressive weight bearing and isokinetics. Avoidance of active terminal extension (past 45 degrees flexion) is recommended for the initial postop period due to increased strain on the graft. Active quadriceps exercises are not allowed at >45 degree of flexion, and return to normal activities is usually delayed 9–12 months. The ACL graft should be placed isometrically, restoring the anatomy and biomechanics of the knee. Interface screws for bony fixation and spiked washers for soft tissue fixation seems to be the most successful. The points of fixation are the weakest portion of the repair initially. Later, revas-

cularizing graft tissue is weakest. Complications from ACL reconstruction include patella tendon rupture, infection, venous thrombosis, saphenous neuroma, and infrapatellar contraction syndrome (patella infera—entrapment of the patella due to fibrosis of the infrapatellar fat pad and retinaculum).

2. PCL Injury—Strength (twice as strong as the ACL), and location (near the central axis of the joint) may account for less injuries to this structure. Injury is from violent posterior tibial displacement (dashboard injury), or sudden hyperextension of the knee. Commonly associated with medial collateral ligament (MCL), posteromedial joint capsule, and ACL tears. Exam findings include posterior drawer and, when associated with collateral ligament tears, varus or valgus instability at 0 degrees. Patients seem to do well with nonoperative treatment unless they have rotational instability, although many develop patellofemoral pain. Acute tears that are diagnosed early are sometimes repaired primarily ± augmentation. Hamstring exercises are avoided in the early postop period. PCL bony avulsion is repaired acutely; nonoperative treatment is recommended initially otherwise. Late development of patellofemoral and medial compartment DJD is common. Surgical repair is reserved for patients with disability (swelling, activity-related pain) and has moderate success (isometric point important).

3. MCL Injury—One of the most commonly injured knee ligaments. Injury typically is from valgus stress. Associated injuries occur commonly with more severe strains and include medial meniscal tears and vastus medialis obliques rupture. Tears of the MCL, ACL, and peripheral medial meniscus (O'Donoghue's triad) does best with surgical repair. The most common triad however, is MCL, ACL, and lateral meniscal tears. Severity of isolated MCL injuries is based on a standard system:

Grade	Opening	Tears	Instability
I	0–5 mm	Minimal	None
II	5–10 mm	Partial	Some
III	10–15 mm	Significant	Moderate
IV	>15 mm	Complete	Gross

Exam is notable for tenderness at the femoral or tibial attachment, and pain/instability with valgus testing at 30 degrees of flexion. Treatment of grade I lesions is symptomatic. Grade II injuries are usually treated in a hinged knee brace for 6 weeks. During the first 3 weeks of therapy, ROM in the brace is limited to about 30–60 degrees; then ROM is left unrestricted. Grade III injuries were fixed operatively in the past, however, casting in 45 degrees of flexion for 2–3 weeks, followed by bracing in restricted ROM, may be as effective for isolated injuries. Chronic instability may require reconstruction using semimembranosus tendon (Slocum), or advancing the tibial MCL (Mauck).

4. Lateral Collateral Ligament (LCL) Injury—Usually a result of varus stress on the knee, and often associated with tears of the arcuate complex, ACL tears, biceps avulsion, and lateral meniscus tear. Varus laxity on exam is graded I–IV as described above. Treatment is similar to MCL injuries, but slower healing of the LCL requires longer periods of protection. Complete tears are frequently managed operatively with direct repair ± augmentation with biceps tendon.

5. Combined Injuries—Lead to instability (Fig. 3–7), most commonly anterolateral rotatory instability (ALRI) and posterolateral rotatory instability (PLRI).
   a. ALRI—From tear of the ACL, lateral capsule, and arcuate complex. Exam shows anterior instability (Lachman, drawer), lateral instability (varus stress at 30 degrees of flexion), and a combination of the two (pivot shift/jerk). ACL reconstruction with capsular repair will usually correct this instability.
   b. PLRI—Results from a tear of the posterolateral capsule and arcuate complex (± PCL). Exam demonstrates positive external rotation recurvatum, and reverse pivot shift, increased external rotation at 30 degrees and 90 degrees, and posterolateral drawer. Treatment may include arcuate complex advancement (Hughston), or Clancy repair with tenodesis of biceps tendon. Biceps reinforcement may be needed in some cases.
   c. Anteromedial Rotatory Instability (AMRI)—Involves injury to the medial structures (especially the posterior oblique ligament) ± ACL. It is best diagnosed with anterior drawer testing in external rotation and the presence of valgus laxity at 30 degrees of flexion. Treatment includes repair/plication.

6. Meniscal injuries
   a. Meniscal tears—Commonly occur as a result of valgus–external rotation (ER) or varus–internal rotation (IR) stress and more com-

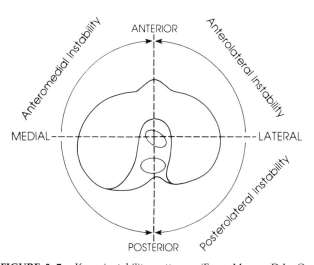

FIGURE 3–7. Knee instability patterns. (From Magee, D.J.: Orthopedic Physical Assessment, p. 285. Philadelphia, W.B. Saunders, 1987; reprinted by permission.)

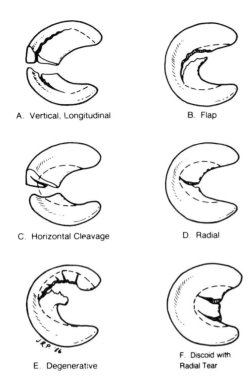

A. Vertical, Longitudinal

B. Flap

C. Horizontal Cleavage

D. Radial

E. Degenerative

F. Discoid with Radial Tear

FIGURE 3–8. Common knee meniscal tears with suggested lines of meniscal resection. (From Rosenberg, T.D., Paulos, L.E., Parker, R.D., and Abbott, P.J.: Arthroscopic surgery of the knee. In Chapman's Operative Orthopaedics, p. 1590. Philadelphia, J.B. Lippincott, 1988; reprinted by permission.)

monly involve the medial meniscus (3:1). Common tears (Fig. 3–8) include "bucket handle" tears (vertical longitudinal tear with displacement of the inner margin), and "parrot beak" tears (oblique vertical tear). Tears of the posterior horn of the menisci are more common. Degenerative tears (in patients >30 yo) are often more chronic and less symptomatic. Joint line tenderness and blocked motion combined with a history of intermittent swelling, locking, and popping are characteristic. Arthroscopy has become the standard of care in the management of meniscal pathology. Partial meniscectomy is usually done when tears involve the inner (avascular) 2/3 of the meniscus. Peripheral 1/3 lesions do well with meniscal repair with suture to the capsule (**meniscoresis**), especially vertical tears at or near the periphery over 10 mm in length. Care to **protect saphenous (medial) and peroneal (lateral) nerves is** important. Meniscal injuries in children are rare, but they do occur. A discoid meniscus (round rather than crescent shaped) usually occurs on the lateral side (90%), and can cause symptoms of popping, clicking, swelling, and locking. In patients who do not respond to conservative care, arthroscopic partial meniscectomy if the inner segment is unstable or torn (saucerization) is favored.

b. Meniscal Cysts—Abnormal multiloculated collections of mucinous material that prob- ably represent degeneration of horizontal cleavage tears. Cysts are more common in the lateral meniscus. Partial meniscectomy (± percutaneous drainage of the cyst) is usually curative.

c. Popliteal (Baker's) Cyst—Often associated with posterior lesions of the medial meniscus. **Located between the semimembranosus tendon and the medial head of the gastrocnemius tendon.** Partial meniscectomy for meniscal tears will usually lead to resolution of the cyst. In the absence of meniscal pathology, removal of the cyst, closure of the communication with the joint, and suture of the medial head of the gastrocnemius to the posterior capsule can be performed in symptomatic individuals. In children, popliteal cysts are not usually associated with intra-articular pathology and may respond to aspiration and steroid injection.

7. Loose Bodies—Loose body formation can be from synovial osteochondromatosis, osteochondral fractures, or joint surface degeneration. Loose bodies within the synovium remain active and can grow. The central nidus does not receive nutrition, however, and undergoes necrosis and calcification. Loose bodies can cause mechanical symptoms, and may be removed arthroscopically. Loose bodies are commonly located in the lateral gutter.

8. Synovectomy—Indicated in refractory rheumatoid arthritis, pigmented villonodular synovitis, synovial chondromatosis, and hemophilic synovitis. Chemical agents are rarely used because of associated cartilage damage. Radiation synovectomy is effective but can be associated with complications. Arthroscopic synovectomy is often successful, especially with the use of posterior portals.

9. Chondromalacia—Chondromalacia of the posterolateral femoral condyle is common in wrestlers. Patella chondromalacia is discussed below.

10. Osteochondritis Dissecans—Discussed in Chapter 1, Pediatric Orthopaedics. Suprapatellar plica is discussed below.

E. **Patellofemoral Disorders**—Commonly present with aching anterior knee pain, worsened with prolonged sitting and climbing stairs, swelling, buckling, or even frank dislocation. PE should include evaluation of alignment, tracking, tenderness/crepitus, and stability. The patella tilt, and active and passive patella glide tests should be accomplished. One should check for the "J" sign (lateral deviation of the patella in terminal extension). Radiographs including Merchant view (to include evaluation of the congruence angle) should be reviewed. Also, evaluation of patella alta and baja should be based on a lateral view with the knee flexed 20–70 degrees. Patella alta = patella tendon >1.2 times the length of the patella (Insall).

1. Patellofemoral Chondrosis (Chondromalacia Patellae)—One of the more common causes of knee pain, it is commonly divided into four

grades, based on appearance of the cartilage (Outerbridge, modified by Insall):

GRADE	APPEARANCE
I	Swelling and softening (closed chondromalacia)
II	Fissuring within the softened areas
III	Breakdown of cartilage surface (fasciculation)
IV	Erosion changes and exposure of subchondral bone (also involves "mirror surface" of femur).

Treatment includes activity modification, NSAIDs, rest, ice, and quadriceps strengthening (not active extension vs. resistance). Surgical treatment is rarely indicated but includes débridement, realignment procedures (with objective evidence of malalignment, increased Q angle, abnormal tracking, incongruence, etc.), and patellectomy (last resort). Patellectomy is often curative, but reduces extension power 30–45% and should be considered a salvage procedure. Other procedures for advanced patellofemoral arthrosis include anterior tibial tubercle elevation (Maquet) [associated with a high complication rate], tibial tubercle transfer (distal medial—Hauser [may develop late DJD]; medial with distal still attached—Elmslie-Trillat), anteromedialization (Fulkerson), and patellar resurfacing [resurfacing with tissue has been unsuccessful; prosthetic replacement is under investigation]. Heel inversion, varus—if associated may be improved with foot orthosis.

2. Patellar Tracking Disorders/Instability—Can be caused by extensor mechanism malalignment (increased Q angle [>15 degrees]), patellar hypermobility (± dislocation check at 45 degrees flexion) and other problems. Often associated with generalized ligamentous laxity. Management includes extensive quadriceps rehabilitation (quadriceps strenghtening, avoiding excessive flexion) and patellar support brace. Surgical management includes lateral release for patients with tight lateral restraints (combined with medial reefing), with laxity medial restraints [>75 degree passive lateral glide]) and realignment procedures. Patella subluxation can cause painful "giving way" with twisting (increased excursion with high Q angle).

3. Lateral Patellar Compression Syndrome—Anterior knee pain with a tight, tender lateral retinaculum. Patients also demonstrate decreased passive medial patellar excursion (normal = 15 mm) and may be associated with a bipartite patela. If conservative therapy fails, a lateral release will often be successful.

4. Patella Alta/Baja—Patella alta (high-riding patella) may be associated with patellar instability, which can be treated with a realignment procedure. Patella baja (low-riding patella) can be a result of a neuromuscular disorder (e.g., polio) or a complication of intra-articular procedures. This is a difficult problem without a good solution.

5. Patellar Tendinitis (Jumper's Knee)—Inflammation of the patellar tendon of athletes involved in jumping sports (e.g., basketball). Tenderness over the patellar tendon, especially with resisted extension, is common. Excessive foot pronation and running hills can exacerbate these symptoms. Most cases are treated conservatively; however, a nidus of necrotic debris and pseudocysts can be treated with surgical excision. Steroid injections are contraindicated (increased risk of patellar tendon rupture). In adolescents, x-ray changes (sclerosis, decalcification, and fragmentation) are sometimes seen in the distal patella. This condition is sometimes referred to as Sinding-Larsen-Johansson syndrome.

6. Suprapatellar Plica (Shelf Syndrome)—Often difficult to differentiate from patella disorders. Symptoms of pain and tightness are aggravated by sitting and activity. Patients complain of popping, catching, and sometimes giving way. Thick synovial fold running medially under the patella over the medial femoral condyle can often be palpated and is tender. Hamstring tightness can exacerbate symptoms and stretching is often helpful. About 95% will improve with rehabilitation. Repetitive use and multiple procedures can lead to thickening and fibrosis of the plica. In later stages chondromatasia of the medial femoral cordyle may be present. Often will result in problems requiring athroscopic débridement.

IV. Shoulder Injury/Reconstruction

A. Subacromial Impingement Syndrome—A common disorder of middle-aged patients, impingement of the humerus (and interposed rotator cuff) occurs under an anterior acromial traction spur and coracoacromial ligament. This frequently leads to rotator cuff disease from mechanical wear (especially with large "hooked" acromions), and has been classified in three stages (Neer) (Table 3–4). Diagnosis is based on typical symptoms of pain, tenderness, including pain with passive flexion of the shoulder past 90 degrees (impingement sign), and pain with internal rotation of the flexed shoulder (impingement reinforcement sign [Hawkins]), both of which are not painful after injection of local anesthetic in the subacromial area (impingement test). Decreased strength with abduction (drop arm sign) and external rotation are consistent with rotator cuff pathology. Tenderness in the bicipital sulcus, positive forearm supination test (Yergason), and positive straight arm raising (Speed) are consistent with involvement of the long head of the biceps tendon. Radiographs should include normal views (decreased acromial-humeral interval on AP view with large cuff tears) as well as supraspinatus outlet view (transcapular "Y" view with 10 degrees of caudal tilt [Bigliani and Morrison] showing acromion types I [flat], II [curved], and III [(hooked)], and 30 degrees' caudal tilt AP view (to demonstrate subacromial spurs.) Arthrography can be useful in equivocal cases, but generally is not required to make the diagnosis. It is often the most reliable diagnostic sign/test for confirming chronic rotator cuff tears. Ultrasonography and MRI are also becoming increasingly useful. Treatment initially includes therapy, rest, and other conservative measures. Acromioplasty en-

TABLE 3–4. STAGES OF SUBACROMIAL IMPINGEMENT SYNDROME

STAGE	AGE	PATHOLOGY	CLINICAL COURSE	TREATMENT
I	<25	Edema and hemorrhage	Reversible	Conservative
II	25–40	Fibrosis and tendinitis	Activity-related pain	Therapy/operative
III	>40	AC spur and cuff tear	Progressive disability	Acromioplasty/repair

larges the space for the rotator cuff tendons and is often successful. Acromioplasty can be done arthroscopically (results controversial) or open. Rotator cuff repair of smaller tears can be accomplished directly (tendon-tendon or tendon-bone). Larger tears require tendon mobilization and insertion into a bony trough [McLaughlin]. In younger patients with glenohumeral instability (with secondary impingement), acromioplasty has a high failure rate. Failure is also more common with incomplete decompression, other pathology (cervical spondylosis), and with workers' comp injuries. Associated suprascapular neuropathy may benefit from early cuff repair.

B. Cuff Tear Arthropathy—May actually be considered a fourth stage of the impingement syndrome, and includes glenohumeral joint degeneration secondary to a long-standing cuff tear. Shoulder arthroplasty will offer pain relief and, if the anterior deltoid is preserved, reasonable function.

C. Shoulder Instability—The shoulder is the most commonly dislocated joint in the body, and instability (anterior >> posterior) is very common in males > females. Instability from traumatic shoulder dislocation/subluxation must be carefully differentiated from multidirectional instability prior to proceeding with surgical options. Reduction is best accomplished in the "zero position" (Saha): 165 degrees of flexion, 45 degrees of IR. Redislocation is common, especially in younger patients. Diagnosis of instability is largely based on history (trauma) and clinical exam (apprehension test—90 degrees of flexion, adduction, and internal rotation; compression/relocation test [humeral head depression with abduction and external rotation and humerus relieves pain until depression is released]), and radiographs (Hill-Sachs or Bankart lesion) are also important. Classification is based on frequency, cause, direction, and degree. Most surgical candidates have recurrent traumatic anterior dislocation (**TUBS**—Traumatic Unilateral Bankart lesion in which Surgery is often indicated). Anterior subluxation without frank dislocation is associated with pain and weakness—the "dead arm syndrome." This is often seen in baseball players with excessive throwing and with forceful external rotation in abduction. Nonoperative treatment includes several months of deltoid and rotator cuff strengthening exercises (Rockwood 5 + 2). Failing this, there are several operative procedures available:

PROCEDURE	ESSENTIAL FEATURES	COMPLICATIONS
Bankhart	Ant. capsule reattachment to glenoid	Standard

PROCEDURE	ESSENTIAL FEATURES	COMPLICATIONS
Staple capsulorraphy	Capsule reattachment and tightening	Staple migration
Putti-Platt	Subscapularis advance/capsule coverage	Decr. ER
Mag-Stack	Subscapularis moved from lesser tuberosity to the greater tuberosity	Decr. ER
Boyd-Sisk	Biceps LH moved lat./post.	
Bristow	Coracoid transfer to glenohumeral neck	Nonunion, migration
Bone block	Ant. bone block	Nonunion, migration
Osteotomy	Wedge of bone blocks dislocation	
Capsular shift	Inf. capsule → superior, superior capsule → inf.	"Relatively few

a preferred method, especially with MDI.

Inexact hardware placement (if used) can sometimes result in nerve injuries (supracapsular nerve) and migration. Repair of Bankart/Perthes' lesions is an integral part of repair. Postop redislocation is rare. Recurrent symptoms can occur and can be diagnosed with apprehension test. A traumatic shoulder instability is often related to underlying multidirectional instability (MDI) and usually with respond to nonoperative treatment. Surgery, done as a last resort, should be an inferior capsular shift. (**AMBRI**)—Atraumatic, Multidirectional, Bilateral, Rehabilitation and rarely Inferior capsular shift).

D. Shoulder Inflammatory Disorders
1. Milwaukee Shoulder—May actually be classified as a form of rotator cuff arthropathy. Large rotator cuff defects, glenohumeral DJD, and joint effusions with calcium phosphate crystals characterize the disorder. Like rotator cuff arthropathy, TSA and rotator cuff repair may be required for advanced cases, but may be associated with poor results.
2. Frozen Shoulder (Adhesive Capsulitis)—Decreased shoulder ROM, often following trauma, leads to this disorder, which often requires several years to resolve. Risk factors for development of adhesive capsulitis include female sex, age (50–60), diabetes, hypothyroid disease, postop status (neurosurgery), and injury. Diagnosis is clinical, and arthrography demonstrates decreased capsular space (not necessary for diagnosis). Treatment includes moist heat and gradually progressing ROM exercises. More aggressive treatment modalities, including brisement, manipulation, and surgical débridement, are usually not necessary. Brise-

ment (distention of the shoulder capsule) may lead to rupture of the capsule and not affect the pathologic axillary fold.

3. Calcific Tendonitis—Calcific deposits are common about the rotator cuff (esp. the supraspinatus tendon) and subacromial bursa. Probably related to avascular changes, it frequently affects late middle-age patients. The calcium deposit can be a semiliquid (acute) or chalky (chronic). Acutely, severe pain and tenderness are common. Chronically, symptoms are less intense and gradual onset ± mechanical symptoms is elicited. Needling, steroid injection(s), NSAIDs, physical therapy, and eventually surgical excision may be required for treatment.

E. Shoulder Arthritis

1. Glenohumeral—Although less common than the hip, spine, and knee, primary osteoarthritis of the shoulder is more common than that in the elbow and ankle. It typically presents in male laborers in the sixth and seventh decades. Radiographs demonstrate progressive joint space narrowing and bony deformity (anterior/inferior osteophytes). Flattening of the head, sclerosis, and subchondral cysts are also seen. Clinically, progressive pain and stiffness, difficulty with sleeping on the affected side, and decreased ROM are common. Shoulder arthroplasty has been very successful in patients who fail a nonoperative regimen. It is most successful with osteoarthritis and less effective (decreased ROM) in rheumatoid and post-traumatic arthritis. Use of the glenoid component depends on the condition of the glenoid (best judged on an axillary lateral radiograph, and at the time of operation), and other factors (not indicated with massive rotator cuff atrophy/tears with high-riding humeral head [hemiarthroplasty with a large head component favored]). Glenoid degeneration is usually posterior in DJD and central in RA. The most common late complication of nonconstrained TSA is glenoid component loosening. Internal rotation contractures may require subscapularis lengthening with surgery. The **humeral component should** be placed in **30–40 degrees of retroversion**. Less retroversion (20 degrees) is recommended in patients with four-part fractures, and **neutral rotation is the favored position** for TSA in patients **with unreduced posterior fracture-dislocations**. Radiographic glenoid loosening is common but does not correlate with clinical loosening. Glenohumeral arthrodesis is an infrequent procedure and is only indicated with infection and unsalvageable loss of rotator cuff and deltoid muscles. The favored position is 20–30 degrees of flexion, 40 degrees abduction, and 25–45 degrees of IR. Excessive external rotation should be avoided.

2. Acromioclavicular (AC) Joint—Arthritis of the AC joint is best diagnosed radiographically (10-degree cephalic tilt view), and clinically (local tenderness and pain with adduction of the affected side arm across the chest) and diagnostic injection. Surgical treatment (open or arthroscopic) includes distal clavicle resection (up to the coracoclavicular ligaments). Osteolysis of

the distal clavicles is more common in young weight lifters, and usually responds to nonoperative treatment but occasionally requires surgical resection of the distal end of the clavicle.

F. Biceps Tendon (Rupture)

1. Bicipital tendonitis is rarely a primary condition and is usually secondary to rotator cuff pathology. Tendonodesis yields unsatisfactory results over time.

2. Proximal—Associated with subacromial impingement and is often attritional, usually involving the musculotendinous junction of the long head. Typically occurs in middle-aged patients while lifting and causes a bulging contour of the arm (Popeye muscle). Surgical treatment is usually not necessary but may include tenodesis of the long head into the bicipital groove of the humerus.

3. Distal—Usually represents an avulsion injury to the distal tendon at its insertion (radial tuberosity). This injury occurs more frequently in young patients with sudden or unexpected lifting of heavy loads. **Surgery** is usually indicated and is best accomplished through **two separate approaches** (Boyd and Anderson).

G. Nerve Disorders

1. Suprascapular Neuropathy—Compression of the suprascapular nerve. Can follow a fall and may present with weakness in abduction and external rotation. EMG studies should be used to confirm the diagnosis.

2. Serratus Anterior Palsy—Can occur by compression of the long thoracic nerve or overuse (tennis, gymnastics). Weakness with adduction and forward flexion, winging of the scapula, and pain with tilting of the head to the contralateral side are characteristic. EMG may demonstrate fibrillation potentials within the serratus anterior muscle. Initial treatment is rest and avoiding traction on the long thoracic nerve.

3. Axillary Nerve Palsy—May occur with anterior subluxation. It is characterized by painless motion and deltoid atrophy.

V. Common Sports Medicine Problems

A. Introduction—Several injuries and disorders unique to sports medicine do not fit easily into other categories, but are important considerations. For this reason, they will be discussed in this section.

B. Physiologic/Psychological Problems

1. Menstrual Cycle Irregularities—Common in female athletes, especially runners, and related to changes in sex hormone production. Also associated with decreased bone mineral content and increased stress fractures; may be related to eating disorders. Also are more frequent in women <115 pounds and those with weight loss >10 pounds. Complete work-up to rule out other causes is necessary prior to initiating therapy with sequential hormone replacement.

2. Eating Disorders

   a. Anorexia Nervosa—Fear of becoming obese leads to this obsession of inadequate caloric intake with excessive exercise that can lead to death in 15–20% of patients, usually secondary to cardiac arrhythmias.

   b. Bulimia—Association with binge eating, weight fluctuations, abdominal pain, and sleep abnormalities.

C. Stress Fractures—Common in athletes, especially in white women, with advancing age, and with underlying metabolic bone disease. Focal structural and muscle weakness and repetitive muscle pull are common. Check for pronated feet and increased external tibial torsion. Metatarsal (**and metatarsal neck** in **distance runners**, **and metatarsal base** in **ballet dancers**), calcaneus, and tibia are common sites. Tibial stress fractures are common in runners and can be diagnosed with bone scanning. Stress fractures of the tarsal navicular should be considered in all athletes with persistent midfoot pain. Bone scans and tomography are helpful. Treatment for stress fractures includes altering activity levels, including avoiding running and jumping for 6–12 weeks. Chondral stress fractures may occur in the medial femoral condyle. Bone scan is often helpful in diagnosis. Arthroscopic débridement and drilling are helpful.

D. Running Injuries—Includes jumper's knee, stress fractures (discussed above), and the following:

   1. Iliotibial Band Friction Syndrome (Runner's Knee)—Pain in the lateral femoral epicondyle from excessive downhill running may be caused by popliteus tendinitis. Activity modification, IT band stretching, and NSAIDs may resolve symptoms.

   2. Pes Anserinus Bursitis—Pain 6 cm below the joint line in the medial tibia, with swelling and tenderness, is characteristic. Treatment is similar to that for runner's knee (NSAIDS, rest, ice, stretching, strengthening). Sometimes a bone scan is necessary to rule out stress factors in equivocal cases. Check for lower extremity malalignment.

   3. Medial-Tibial Stress Syndrome (Shin Splints)—Exercise-related pain in the posterior mid to distal 1/3 of the tibia can be related to periostitis at the origin of the posterior tibialis. Exam is notable for local tenderness with pain on resisted plantar flexion and inversion. Radiographs may demonstrate periosteal change several weeks after onset of symptoms. Conservative treatment is usually successful; however, in chronic cases, posteromedial fascial release may be indicated.

   4. Exertional Compartment Syndrome—Can be exercise induced, usually involves the anterior or deep posterior leg compartment, and leads to pain shortly after exercise is started. Other diagnoses, such as periostitis, stress fractures, nerve compression, and muscle herniation, must be ruled out. Bone scan is helpful (periostitis causes linear streaking, stress fractures show localized uptake). Compartment pressure measurements before and after exercise are also helpful (intracompartment pressures increase to >40 mm Hg during exercise and fail to return to <15 mm Hg after 30 minutes of rest). Fasciotomies may be required for chronic cases not responsive to other treatments (stretching, rest, strengthening).

   5. Herniation of Muscle through Fascia—Sural nerve often affected in lower extremities with activities; diagnosis by lidocaine block.

   6. Postexercise Muscle Pain—Caused by eccentric muscle contraction resulting in acute injury to type II muscle fibers at the myotendinous junction. Treatment is supportive.

   7. Partial Rupture of the Medial Gastrocnemius—Occurs in middle-aged recreational athletes during explosive push-off activities. Thompson test is negative, and diffuse posterior ecchymosis and pain with forced ankle dorsiflexion are common. Treatment includes ice, rest, calf support, and NSAIDS. There is usually a permanent loss of gastrocnemius strength.

E. Other Factors

   1. Sex Differences—Men typically are taller, heavier, and have less body fat than women. Additionally they have a greater MVO_2, larger cardiac output, higher hemoglobin, and more muscular strength.

   2. Warm-Up Activities—Increase muscle tone, blood flow, flexibility, and nerve conduction velocity. They also have a positive influence on muscle mechanics and ROM.

   3. Rehabilitation after Injury—Early ROM → isometric and flexibility exercises → progressive resistance and dynamic exercises → mainstreaming (sports-specific activities), ±cross-training in another sport if required. Normal quadriceps and hamstring strength is required prior to return to full activity—NSAID's have a role acutely. Continuous passive motion (6–8 hours/day) can help with joint surface regeneration and decrease contractures.

   4. Drug Abuse—Can lead to increased risk of sudden death. Stimulants (increased alertness, increased hostility), narcotics (increased pain threshold), steroids (increased lean tissue mass and muscle hypertrophy but increased risk of musculotendinous rupture), β blockers (improve fine motor control), and diuretics (abused in sports with weight classifications) are all problems.

   5. Sudden Death—Cardiac (congenital abnormalities in patients <35 yo, ASCVD in >35-yo patients), thermoregulatory (hyperthermia in patients >50, hypothermia with water sports), and dietary deficiencies usually involved.

   6. Exercise—Regularly, can decrease heart rate and blood pressure, decrease insulin requirements in diabetics, decrease cardiovascular risk, and increase lean body mass. Training can also induce a higher rate of lipid utilization and decrease psychological stress. Aerobic threshold (anaerobic metabolism beginning point) can be measured with the ventilation/O_2 consumption and predicts endurance performance (and onset of lactic acidosis). It is a useful tool in evaluation of training of endurance athletes.

F. Upper Extremity Training Injuries—Common.

   1. Shoulder—Athletes who participate in overhead sports can have both impingement and instability. Impingement pain is nonspecific and occurs with repetitive overhead throwing. This type of impingement, commonly referred to as secondary impingement, usually responds to

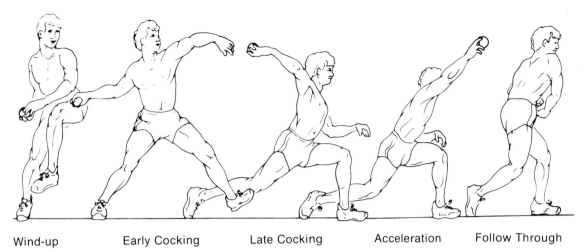

Wind-up   Early Cocking   Late Cocking   Acceleration   Follow Through

FIGURE 3–9. Throwing phases. (From Jobe, F.W., and Glousman, R.E.: Throwing injuries in the athlete. In Orthopaedic Knowledge Update Home Study Syllabus III, p. 294. Chicago, American Academy of Orthopaedic Surgery, 1990; reprinted by permission.)

aggressive rehabilitation of the rotator cuff muscles. The five phases of throwing (Fig. 3–9) are: (1) wind-up, (2) early cocking (deltoid, cuff), (3) late cocking (cuff, deltoid), (4) acceleration (minimum activity), and (5) follow through (most activity-deliberate; stresses the posterior capsule). Posterior glenohumeral pain with subluxation occurs during late cocking and acceleration phases. "Little League" shoulder is caused by proximal physeal stress fracture resulting from repetitive strain from throwing. Patients may develop external rotation contractures and may not be able to internally rotate their arms. Widening of the physis and periosteal reaction may be seen on radiographs. Treatment is sports/activity limitation or modification.
2. Elbow—Elbow problems in training athletes include medial epicondyle stress fractures (Little Leaguer's elbow and its adult counterpart), ulnar neuritis, and ulnar collateral ligament (UCL) rupture. Most respond to conservative treatment but occasionally surgical reconstruction (débridement, transposition of ulnar nerve, ligament reconstruction with peroneus longus graft) is indicated. Osteochondrosis/osteonecrosis dessicans of the capitellum (Panner's disease) and other injuries are common in adolescent athletes. UCL injuries occur most commonly during the acceleration phase of throwing.
G. Cervical Spine Injury—Covered in Chapter 6, Spine. "Stingers" or temporary neurapraxia usually, from a compression-type injury is not associated with any structural abnormalities, and treatment is supportive.

VI. Arthroscopy

A. Shoulder Arthroscopy
1. Indications—Increasingly popular for evaluation and treatment of impingement and instability that has failed nonoperative treatment. Many feel it is indicated prior to any open shoulder procedure.
2. Set Up—Commonly done in lateral decubitus position with arm suspended with a pulley. The arm is abducted 50–70 degrees and flexed about 20 degrees. The beach chair position can be used (without a pulley) and allows easier transition to open procedures.
3. Portals
   a. Posterior—Created first, 2 cm distal to posterolateral corner of acromion with entry parallel to glenoid. Suprascapular artery and nerve are superomedial, axillary nerve and PCH artery are inferior to this portal.
   b. Anterior—Created from inside out using Wissinger rod introduced through posterior portal. Rod is aimed 1 cm medial and inferior to anterolateral corner of acromion. A canula is introduced retrograde over the rod. Cephalic vein is lateral, brachial plexus and axillary artery are medial, and axillary nerve is inferior to this portal.
   c. Superior (Nevaiser) Portal—Rarely used; 1 cm medial to medial edge of acromion and angled 45 degrees. Major risk to spinal accessory nerve branches (medially), suprascapular artery and nerve (anteromedial), and supraspinatus tendon (with abduction >45 degrees).
   d. Lateral—Used for bursoscopy; 2 cm lateral to acromion, angled anteriorly and in line with possible deltoid splitting incision for open cuff repair.
4. Technique—Systematic exam of joint should include evaluation of biceps, glenohumeral ligaments, labrum, articular surfaces, rotator cuff, and capsule.
   a. Instability—Can place fixation for glenoid labral pathology (Bankhart lesion), and some do a modified capsular shift arthroscopically. Fixation of labial tears with staples, screws, sutures, and absorbable devices (future) has been advocated.
   b. Labial Lesions—Anteroinferior (Bankhart) lesions are associated with glenohumeral instability and repair will stabilize joint (resection is contraindicated). Superior lateral an-

terior to posterior (SLAP) lesions should also be repaired if the biceps anchor is disrupted (types I and III); otherwise they can be débrided.

    c. Impingement—Arthroscopic subacromial decompression using bursoscopy is becoming increasingly popular. Less abduction (15–20 degrees of the arm is used) and lateral portals are employed. Coracoacromial ligament is cut with electrocautery, then bursoscopy is used to resect/flatten the acromion.

B. Elbow Arthroscopy
  1. Indications—Somewhat limited; includes loose body removal, osteochondritis dissecans, lysis of adhesions, débridement, synovectomy, and evaluation/treatment of intra-articular fractures.
  2. Set Up—Usually done supine with armboard and elbow flexed 90 degrees and 10–15 pounds Buck's traction. May be done prone with forearm off table. The 2.7-mm scope is useful, especially in posterior compartment.
  3. Portals
    a. Anterolateral—3 cm distal and 1 cm anterior to lateral epicondyle (through extensor carpi radialis brevis); **radial nerve**, PABC nerve, and LABC nerve **at risk**.
    b. Anteromedial—2 cm distal and 2 cm anterior to medial epicondyle (through pronator teres, flexor carpi radialis); brachial artery, median nerve, and medial antebrachial cutaneous nerve at risk.
    c. Posterolateral—3 cm proximal to olecranon and lateral (through triceps); ulnar nerve, posterior antebrachial cutaneous nerve and medial brachial cutaneous nerve at risk.
    d. Posteromedial—Too risky (brachial artery, median nerve)
  4. Technique—Based on systematic exam of joint; specific technique based on indication.

C. Wrist Arthroscopy
  1. Indications—Again, limited in most cases, but includes soft tissue injuries (TFCC), intra-articular fractures, and for diagnostic purposes.
  2. Set Up—Usually done on an arm board with 8–10 pounds of traction.
  3. Portals—Based on dorsal compartments and area of interest.
    a. Radiocarpal—3–4 portal for scope, 6U portal for inflow, 4–5 portal for instruments
    b. Midcarpal—RMC portal for scope, UMC portal for instruments
  4. Technique—Procedure specific; usually diagnostic or TFCC débridement.

D. Hip Arthroscopy
  1. Indications—Extremely limited at present, mostly used for loose body removal, I&D, and diagnosis.
  2. Set up—Requires significant distraction of the hip (50 pounds) long instruments and scope, and image intensifier. Patient is placed in lateral decubitus position with well-padded peroneal post.
  3. Portals
    a. Greater Trochanter—Two portals are usually required—one anterior and another posterior (anterior is near femoral cutaneous nerve).
    b. Anterior—At ASIS (near lateral femoral cutaneous nerve); used for inflow.
  4. Technique—Again limited by indications.

E. Knee Arthroscopy
  1. Indications—Most commonly done arthroscopy, has a number of proven applications, including correcting meniscal pathology, intra-articular ACL reconstruction, correction of patellar tracking abnormalities, abrasion arthroplasty, loose body removal, and synovectomy.
  2. Set Up—Usually done with patient supine with leg flexed in a knee holder and opposite leg suspended.
  3. Portals
    a. Superomedial/Lateral—For inflow canal; directed into superior patellar pouch.
    b. Inferolateral/Medial—Usually placed 1 cm superior to joint and 1 cm lateral to the patellar tendon.
    c. Posteromedial—Located 1 cm above the joint line and 1 cm posterior to the femoral condyle. Occasionally for PCL or posterior horn meniscal tears.
  4. Techniques
    a. Meniscal Tears (Partial Meniscectomy)—Probing of the meniscus helps identify the pattern of the tear. Relocation of displaced tears is best. Excision with baskets and removal with forceps is followed by trimming the meniscal rim.
    b. Repair of Meniscal Tears—Usually reserved for acute tears >1 cm in the peripheral 1/3 of the meniscus. Repair is usually via contralateral portal. Dissection to capsule and visualization of needles is essential to avoid the peroneal nerve (lateral) and saphenous nerve and vein (medial).
    c. ACL Repair—Limited to avulsions or tears of the proximal 25% of the ligament and usually requires supplementation. Techniques are similar to the femoral side of ACL reconstruction.
    d. ACL Reconstruction—Uses central 1/3 patella tendon grafts, medial hamstring tendon grafts, allografts, or (rarely) synthetic grafts to recreate the ACL. Special guides help with femoral tunnel placement (10 o'clock position, 7 mm from posterior cortex [best determined with tensiometer]) and tibial tunnel placement (located at anteromedial portion of ACL origin and drilled at least 3–4 cm distal to the joint). Retention of the ACL stump may improve healing/strength. Fixation is with Kurosaka screws (bone-patella-bone graft) or staples (soft tissue). Pretensioning of grafts may also be important.
    e. PCL Repair—Indications unclear and technically difficult.
    f. Patellofemoral Instability—Lateral release is done only for lateral retinacular tightness. Electrocautery is used for arthroscopic lateral release. Dynamic patellar realignment (with sensory but not motor block) may be helpful in determining appropriate procedures.
    g. DJD abrasion arthroscopy of exposed bone,

combined with débridement, can have limited success and delay the need for TKA.

h. Osteochondritis Dissecans Repair—Has been successful with cannulated compression screw fixation. Débridement of interposed fibrous tissue ± bone grafting is useful prior to fixation.

F. Ankle Arthroscopy
1. Indications—Diagnostic for patients with chronic pain/swelling; therapeutic for loose bodies, impingement, intra-articular fractures, etc.
2. Set Up—Patient is usually supine with thigh and ankle holder. Distraction is often necessary (external device). A 4.0- or 2.7-mm scope can be used.
3. Portals
a. Anteromedial—Just medial to anterior tibial tendon at joint line (avoid saphenous vein and nerve).
b. Anterolateral—Just lateral to peroneus tertius at joint line (avoid superior peroneal nerve branches).
c. Posterolateral—Inflow; lateral to Achilles 2 cm proximal to tip of fibula.
d. Posteromedial—Usually not recommended because of concomitant neurovascular risk.
4. Techniques—Systematic exam important; removal of loose bodies and excision of synovial impingement lesions effective.

Selected Bibliography

Altchek, D.W., Warren, R.F., Wickiewicz, T.L., et al.: Arthroscopic acromioplasty. Technique and results. J. Bone Joint Surg. [Am.] 72:1198, 1990.

American Academy of Orthopaedic Surgeons: Athletic Training and Sports Medicine. Chicago, American Academy of Orthopaedic Surgeons, 1984.

Amstutz, H.C., Friscia, D.A., Dorey, F., and Carney, B.T.: Warfarin prophylaxis to prevent mortality from pulmonary embolism after total hip replacement. J. Bone Joint Surg. [Am.] 71:321, 1989.

Andersson, C., Odensten, M., Good, L., and Gillquist, J.: Surgical or non-surgical treatment of acute rupture of the anterior cruciate ligament. A randomized study with long-term follow-up. J. Bone Joint Surg. [Am.] 71:965, 1989.

Andrews, J.R.: Bony injuries about the elbow in the throwing athlete. Instr. Course Lect. 34:323–331, 1985.

Andrews, J.R., St. Pierre, R.K., and Carson, W.G., Jr.: Arthroscopy of the elbow. Clin. Sports Med. 5:653–662, 1986.

Andriacchi, T.P., Galante, J.O., and Fermier, R.W.: The influence of total knee-replacement design on walking and stair-climbing. J. Bone Joint Surg. [Am.] 64:1328–1335, 1982.

Arnoczky, S.P., and Warren, R.F.: Microvasculature of the human meniscus. Am. J. Sports Med. 10:90–95, 1982.

Baker, C.L., Jr., Norwood, L.A., and Hughston, J.C.: Acute combined posterior cruciate and posterolateral instability of the knee. Am. J. Sports Med. 12:204–208, 1984.

Barrett, W.P., Franklin, J.L., Jackins, S.E., et al.: Total shoulder arthroplasty. J. Bone Joint Surg. [Am.] 69:865–872, 1987.

Barrow, G.W., and Saha, S.: Menstrual irregularity and stress fractures in collegiate female distance runners. Am. J. Sports Med. 16:209–216, 1988.

Bayley, J.C., Scott, R.D., Ewald, F.C., and Holmes, G.B., Jr.: Failure of the metal-backed patellar component after total knee replacement. J. Bone Joint Surg. [Am.] 70:668, 1988.

Becker, D.A., and Cofield, R.H.: Tenodesis of the long head of the biceps brachi for chronic bicipital tendinitis. Long-term results. J. Bone Joint Surg. [Am.] 71:376, 1989.

Briggs, C.A., and Elliott, B.G.: Lateral epicondylitis: A review of structures associated with tennis elbow. Anat. Clin. 7:149–153, 1985.

Buchholz, H.W., Elson, R.A., Engelbrecht, E., Lodenkamper, H., Rottger, J., and Siegal, A.: Management of deep infection of total hip replacement. J. Bone Joint Surg. [Br.] 63:342–353, 1981.

Bullough, P.G., DiCarlo, E.F., Hansraj, K.K., et al.: Pathologic studies of total joint replacement. Orthop. Clin. North Am. 19:611–625, 1988.

Callaghan, J.J., Dysart, S.H., and Savory, C.G.: The uncemented porous-coated anatomic total hip prosthesis. Two-year results of a prospective consecutive series. J. Bone Joint Surg. [Am.] 70:337, 1988.

Canner, G.C., Steinberg, M.E., Heppenstall, R.B., and Balderston, R.: The infected hip after total hip arthroplasty. J. Bone Joint Surg. [Am.] 66:1393–1399, 1984.

Cash, J.D., and Hughston, J.C.: Treatment of acute patellar dislocation. Am. J. Sports Med. 16:244–249, 1988.

Caspari, R.B.: Shoulder arthroscopy: A review of the present state of the art. Contemp. Orthop. 4:523–531, 1982.

Cass, J.R., Morrey, B.F., Katoh, Y., et al.: Ankle instability: Comparison of primary repair and delayed reconstruction after long-term follow-up study. Clin. Orthop. 198:110–117, 1985.

Chandler, H.P., Reineck, F.T., Wixson, R.L., and McCarthy, J.C.: Total hip replacement in patients younger than 30 years old: A five-year follow-up. J. Bone Joint Surg. [Am.] 63:1426–1434, 1981.

Chapman, Michael W., ed.: Operative Orthopaedics. Philadelphia, J.B. Lippincott, 1988.

Charnley, J., and Cupic, Z.: The nine and ten year results of the low friction arthroplasty of the hip. Clin. Orthop. 95:9–25, 1973.

Chick, R.R., and Jackson, D.W.: Tears of the anterior cruciate ligament in young athletes. J. Bone Joint Surg. [Am.] 60:970–973, 1978.

Claes, L., Burri, C., Neugebauer, R., Piehler, J., and Mohr, W.: Animal experiments for comparison of various alloplastic materials in ligament replacements. Aktuel Probl. Chir. Orthop. 26:101–107, 1983.

Clancy, W.G., Jr., Ray, J.M., and Zoltan, D.J.: Acute tears of the anterior cruciate ligament, surgical versus conservative treatment. J. Bone Joint Surg. [Am.] 70:1483, 1988.

Cofield, R.H.: Arthroscopy of the shoulder. Mayo Clin. Proc. 58:501–508, 1983.

Cofield, R.H.: Total shoulder arthroplasty with the Neer prosthesis. J. Bone Joint Surg. [Am.] 66:899–906, 1984.

Cofield, R.H., and Briggs, B.T.: Glenohumeral arthrodesis: Operative and long-term functional results. J. Bone Joint Surg. [Am.] 61:668–677, 1979.

Copeland, S.A., and Taylor, J.G.: Synovectomy of the elbow in rheumatoid arthritis: The place of excision of the head of the radius. J. Bone Joint Surg. [Br.] 61:69–73, 1979.

Coventry, M.B.: Proximal tibial varus osteotomy for osteoarthritis of the lateral compartment of the knee. J. Bone Joint Surg. [Am.] 69:32–38, 1987.

Coventry, M.B.: Upper tibial osteotomy. Clin. Orthop. 182:46–52, 1984.

Coventry, M.B.: Upper tibial osteotomy for gonarthrosis. Orthop. Clin. North Am. 10:191–210, 1979.

Coventry, M.B.: Upper tibial osteotomy for osteoarthritis. J. Bone Joint Surg. [Am.] 67:1136–1140, 1985.

Cox, J.S.: Patellofemoral problems in runners. Clin. Sports. Med. 4:699–715, 1985.

Crenshaw, A.H., ed., Campbell's Operative Orthopaedics, 7th ed., St. Louis, C.V. Mosby Co., 1987.

Daniel, D.M., Stone, M.L., Barnett, P., et al.: Use of the quadriceps active test to diagnose posterior cruciate-ligament disruption and measure posterior laxity of the knee. J. Bone Joint Surg. [Am.] 70:386–391, 1988.

Davey, J.R., Rorabeck, C.H., and Fowler, P.J.: The tibialis posterior muscle compartment. An unrecognized cause of exertional compartment syndrome. Am. J. Sports Med. 12:391–397, 1984.

Dee, R., Mango, E., and Hurst, L.C.: Principles of Orthopaedic Practice. New York, McGraw Hill Book Co., 1989.

DeHaven, K.E.: Diagnosis of acute knee injuries with hemarthrosis. Am. J. Sports Med. 8:9–14, 1980.

DeLee, J.C., Riley, M.B., and Rockwood, C.A., Jr.: Acute straight lateral instability of the knee. Am. J. Sports Med. 11:404–411, 1983.

Dorr, L.D., and Boiardo, R.A.: Technical considerations in total knee arthroplasty. Clin. Orthop. 205:5–11, 1986.

Dorr, L.D., Sakimura, I., and Mohler, J.G.: Pulmonary emboli followed total hip arthroplasty: Incidence study. J. Bone Joint Surg. [Am.] 61:1083–1087, 1979.

Engh, C.A.: Hip arthroplasty with a Moore prosthesis with porous coating: A five-year study. Clin. Orthop. 176:52–66, 1983.

Epps, C.H., ed.: Complications in Orthopaedic Surgery, 2nd ed. Philadelphia, J.B. Lippincott Company, 1986.

Feagin, J.A., Jr.: The Crucial Ligaments. New York, Churchill Livingstone, 1988.

Ferguson, A.B., Jr.: Elevation of the insertion of the patellar ligament for patellofemoral pain. J. Bone Joint Surg. [Am.] 64:766–771, 1982.

Fox, E.L.: Sports Physiology. Philadelphia, W.B. Saunders, 1979.

Friedman, M.J, and Fox, J.M., Course Directors: Arthroscopy of the Upper and Lower Extremity. Syllabus American Academy of Orthopaedic Surgeons Review Course, North Hollywood, CA, November 29–December 1, 1990.

Frisch, R.E., Gotz-Welbergen, A.V., McArthur, J.W., Albright, T., Witschi, J., Bullen, B., Birnholz, J., Reed, R.B., and Hermann, H.: Delayed menarche and amenorrhea of college athletes in relation to age of onset of training. J.A.M.A. 246:1559–1563, 1981.

Fulkerson, J.P., and Shea, K.P.: Current concepts review. Disorders of patellofemoral alignment. J. Bone Joint Surg. [Am.] 72:1424, 1990.

Galante, J.O.: Current concepts review. Causes of fractures of the femoral component in total hip replacement. J. Bone Joint Surg. [Am.] 62:670–673, 1980.

Garvin, K.L., Pellicci, P.M., Windsor, R.E., et al.: Contralateral total hip arthroplasty or ipsilateral total knee arthoplasty in patients who have a long-standing fusion of the hip. J. Bone Joint Surg. [Am.] 71:1355, 1989.

Goldberg, V.M., Figgie, M.P., Figgie, H.E., III, Heiple, K.G., and Sobel, M.: Use of a total condylar knee prosthesis for treatment of osteoarthritis and rheumatoid arthritis. Long term results. J. Bone Joint Surg. [Am.] 70:802, 1988.

Grood, E.S., Stowers, S.F., and Noyes, F.R.: Limits of movement in the human knee: Effect of sectioning the posterior cruciate ligament and posterolateral structures. J. Bone Joint Surg. [Am.] 70:88–97, 1988.

Gruen, T.A., McNeice, G.M., and Amstutz, H.C.: Modes of failure of cemented stem-type femoral components. Clin. Orthop. 141:17–27, 1979.

Guhl, J.F.: Arthroscopy and arthroscopic surgery of the elbow. Orthopedics 8:1290–1296, 1985.

Haddad, R.J., Jr., Cook, S.D., and Thomas, K.A.: Biological fixation of porous-coated implants. J. Bone Joint Surg. [Am.] 69:1459–1466, 1987.

Halverson, P.B., McCarty, D.J., Cheung, H.S., and Ryan, L.M.: Milwaukee shoulder syndrome: Eleven additional cases with involvement of the knee in seven (basic calcium phosphate crystal deposition disease). Semin. Arthritis Rheum. 14:36–44, 1984.

Harris, W.H.: Advances in total hip arthroplasty: The metal-backed acetabular component. Clin. Orthop. 183: 3–11, 1984.

Harris, W.H., and White, R.E., Jr.: Advantages of metal-backed acetabular components for total hip replacement: A clinical assessment with a minimum 5-year follow-up. Hip 11:240–246, 1983.

Hastings, D.E.: The non-operative management of collateral ligament injuries of the knee joint. Clin. Orthop. 147:22–28, 1980.

Haupt, H.A., and Rovere, G.D.: Anabolic steroids: A review of the literature. Am J. Sports Med. 12:469–484, 1984.

Hawkins, R.J., Brock, R.M., Abrams, J.S., et al.: Acromioplasty for impingement with an intact rotator cuff. J. Bone Joint Surg. [Br.] 70:795–797, 1988.

Hawkins, R.J., Koppert, G., and Johnston, G.: Recurrent posterior instability (subluxation) of the shoulder. J. Bone Joint Surg. [Am.] 66:169–174, 1984.

Hawkins, R.J., Misamore, G.W., and Hobeika, P.E.: Surgery for full-thickness rotator-cuff tears. J. Bone Joint Surg. [Am.] 67:1349–1355, 1985.

Hawkins, R.J., and Neer, C.S., II: A functional analysis of shoulder fusions. Clin. Orthop. 223:65–76, 1987.

Hernborg, J.S., and Nilsson, B.E.: The natural course of untreated osteoarthritis of the knee. Clin. Orthop. 123:130–137, 1977.

Holden, D.L., James, S.L., Larson, R.L., and Slocum, D.B.: Proximal tibial osteotomy in patients who are fifty years old or less. A long-term follow-up study. J. Bone Joint Surg. [Am.] 70:977, 1988.

Hughston, J.C., Bowden, J.A., Andrews, J.R., and Norwood, L.A.: Acute tears of the posterior cruciate ligament: Results of operative treatment. J. Bone Joint Surg. [Am.] 62:438–450, 1980.

Hungerford, D.S., and Lennox, D.W.: Rehabilitation of the knee in disorders of the patellofemoral joint: Relevant biomechanics. Orthop. Clin. North Am. 14:397–402, 1983.

Insall, J.N., Hood, R.W., Flawn, L.B., and Sullivan, D.J.: The total condylar knee prosthesis in gonarthrosis: A five to nine-year follow-up of the first one hundred consecutive replacements. J. Bone Joint Surg. [Am.] 65:619–628, 1983.

Insall, J.N., and Kelly, M.: The total condylar prosthesis. Clin. Orthop. 205:43–48, 1986.

Jackson, R.W., and Rouse, D.W.: The results of partial arthroscopic meniscectomy in patients over 40 years of age. J. Bone Joint Surg. [Br.] 64:481–485, 1982.

Jobe, F.W., Tibone, J.E., Perry, J., and Moynes, D: An EMG analysis of the shoulder in throwing and pitching: A preliminary report. Am. J. Sports Med. 11:3–5, 1983.

Johnson, L.L.: Arthroscopy of the shoulder. Orthop. Clin. North Am. 11:197–204, 1980.

Kavanagh, B.F., Dewitz, M.A., Ilstrup, D.M., et al.: Charnley total hip arthroplasty with cement, fifteen-year results. J. Bone Joint Surg. [Am.] 71:1496, 1989.

Keating, E.M., Ritter, M.A., and Faris, P.M.: Structures at risk from medially placed acetabular screws. J. Bone Joint Surg. [Am.] 72:509, 1990.

Kellett, J.: Acute soft tissue injuries: A review of the literature. Med. Sci. Sports Exerc. 18:489–500, 1986.

Kennedy, J.C.: Application of prosthetics to anterior cruciate ligament reconstruction and repair. Clin. Orthop. 172:125–128, 1983.

Kilgus, D.J., Amstutz, H.C., Wolgin, M.A., et al.: Joint replacement for ankylosed hips. J. Bone Joint Surg. [Am.] 72:45, 1990.

Krackow, K.A., and Brooks, R.L.: Optimization of knee ligament position for lateral extraarticular reconstruction. Am. J. Sports Med. 11:293–302, 1983.

Landy, M.M., and Walker, P.S.: Wear of ultra-high-molecular-weight polyethylene components of 90 retrieved knee prostheses. J. Arthop. suppl., pp. S73–S85, 1988.

Liechti, R.: Hip Arthrodesis and Associated Problems. Berlin, Springer-Verlag, 1978.

Ling, R.S.M.: Complications of Total Hip Replacement. Edinburgh, Churchill Livingstone, 1984.

Lynch, A.F., Bourne, R.B., Rorabeck, C.H., et al.: Deep-vein thrombosis and continuous passive motion after total knee arthoplasty. J. Bone Joint Surg. [Am.] 70:11–14, 1988.

Lyons, W.W., Berquist, T.H., Lyons, J.C., Rand, J.A., and Brown, M.L.: Evaluation of radiographic findings in painful hip arthroplasties. Clin. Orthop. 195:239–251, 1985.

Maloney, W.J., and Harris, W.H.: Comparison of a hybrid with an uncemented total hip replacement. A retrospective matched-pair study. J. Bone Joint Surg. [Am.] 72:1349, 1990.

Maquet, P.: Mechanics and osteoarthritis of the patellofemoral joint. Clin. Orthop. 144:70–73, 1979.

McDaniel, W.J., Jr., and Dameron, T.B., Jr.: The untreated anterior cruciate ligament rupture. Clin. Orthop. 172:158–163, 1983.

McDonald, D.J., Fitzgerald, R.H., Jr., and Ilstrup, D.M.: Two-stage reconstruction of a total hip arthroplasty because of infection. J. Bone Joint Surg. [Am.] 71:828, 1989.

Medlar, R.C., and Lyne, E.D.: Sinding-Larsen-Johansson disease: Its etiology and natural history. J. Bone Joint Surg. [Am.] 60:1113–1116, 1978.

Miller, M.D., Wirth, M.A., and Rockwood, C.A., Jr.: Thawing the frozen shoulder: The patient patient. Orthop. Trans., In press.

Mink, J.H., Levy, T., and Crues, J.V., III: Tears of the anterior cruciate ligament and menisci of the knee: MR imaging evaluation. Radiology 167:769–774, 1988.

Morrey, B.F., Askew, L.J., An, K.N., and Chao, E.Y.: A biomechanical study of normal functional elbow motion. J. Bone Joint Surg. [Am.] 63:872–877, 1981.

Morrey, B.F., Bryan, R.S., Dobyns, J.H., and Linscheid, R.L.: Total elbow arthroplasty: A five-year experience at the Mayo Clinic. J. Bone Joint Surg. [Am.] 63:1050–1063, 1981.

Muburak, S., and Hargens, A.: Exertional Compartment Syndrome. St. Louis, C.V. Mosby, 1982.

Neer, C.S., II: Impingement lesions. Clin. Orthop. 173:70–77, 1983.

Neer, C.S., II, and Foster, C.R.: Inferior capsular shift for involuntary inferior and multidirectional instability of the shoulder: A preliminary report. J. Bone Joint Surg. [Am.] 62:897–908, 1980.

Neviaser, R.J.: Symposium on disorders of the shoulder. Orthop. Clin. North Am. 11:185–373, 1980.

Norris, T.R., and Bigliani, L.U.: Analysis of Failed Repair for Shoulder Instability—A Preliminary Report. Philadelphia, Decker, 1984.

Noyes, F.R., Bassett, R.W., Grood, E.S., and Butler, D.L.: Arthroscopy in acute traumatic hemarthrosis of the knee. Incidence of anterior cruciate tears and other injuries. J. Bone Joint Surg. [Am.] 62:687–695, 1980.

Noyes, R.F., Grood, E.S., Torzilli, P.A.: Current concepts review: The definitions of terms for motion and position of the knee and injuries of the ligaments. J. Bone Joint Surg. [Am.] 71:465–472, 1989.

Orthopaedic Knowledge Update Home Study Syllabus I, II, and III, Chicago: American Academy of Orthopaedic Surgeons, 1984, 1987, 1990.

Pappas, A.M., Zawacki, R.M., and McCarthy, C.F.: Rehabilitation of the pitching shoulder. Am. J. Sports Med. 13:223–235, 1985.

Paulos, L., Noyes, F.R., Grood, E.S., and Butler, D.L.: Knee rehabilitation after anterior cruciate ligament reconstruction and repair. Am. J. Sports Med. 8:140–149, 1981.

Pellicci, P.M., Wilson, P.D., Jr., Sledge, C.B., Salvate, E.A., Ranawat, C.S., and Poss, R.: Revision total hip arthroplasty. Clin. Orthop. 170:34–41, 1982.

Perrin, T., Dorr, L.D., Perry, J., Gronley, J., and Hull, D.B.: Functional evaluation of total hip arthroplasty with five- to ten-year follow-up evaluation. Clin. Orthop. 195:252–260, 1985.

Picetti, G.D., III, McGann, W.A., and Welch, R.B.: The patellofemoral joint after total knee arthroplasty without patellar resurfacing. J. Bone Joint Surg. [Am.] 72:1379, 1990.

Post, M., Silver, R., and Singh, M.: Rotator cuff tear: Diagnosis and treatment. Clin. Orthop. 173:78–91, 1983.

Rand, J.A., and Bryan, R.S.: Results of revision total knee arthroplasties using condylar prosthesis. A review of fifty knees. J. Bone Joint Surg. [Am.] 70:738, 1988.

Rand, J.A., Peterson, L.F.A., Bryan, R.S., et al.: Revision total knee arthroplasty. Instr. Course Lect. 35:305–318, 1986.

Rockwood, C.A., Jr., and Matsen, F.A., eds. The Shoulder. Philadelphia, W.B. Saunders Co., 1990.

Rose, R.M., Crugnola, A., Ries, M., Cimino, W.R., Paul, I., and Radin, E.L.: On the origins of high in vivo wear rates in polyethylene components of total joint prostheses. Clin. Orthop. 145:277–286, 1979.

Rosenberg, T.D., Paulos, L.E., Parker, R.D., Coward, D.B., and Scott, S.M.: The forty-five degree posteroanterior flexion weight-bearing radiograph of the knee. J. Bone Joint Surg. [Am.] 70:1479, 1988.

Salvati, E.A., Wilson, P.D., Jr., Jolley, M.N., Vakili, F., Aglietti, P., and Brown, G.C.: A ten-year follow-up study of our first 100 consecutive Charnley total hip replacements. J. Bone Joint Surg. [Am.] 63:753–767, 1981.

Sarmiento, A., Ebramzadel, E., Gogan, W.J., et al.: Total hip arthroplasty with cement. A long-term radiographic analysis in patients who are older than fifty and younger than fifty years. J. Bone Joint Surg. [Am.] 72:1470, 1990.

Schneider, R., Abenavoli, A.M., Soudry, M., and Insall, J.: Failure of total condylar knee replacements: Correlation of radiographic, clinical, and surgical findings. Radiology 152:309–315, 1984.

Schoifet, S.D., and Morrey, B.F.: Treatment of infection after total knee arthroplasty by debridement with retention of the components. J. Bone Joint Surg. [Am.] 72:1383, 1990.

Schutzer, S.F., and Harris, W.H.: Deep-wound infection after total hip replacement under contemporary aseptic conditions. J. Bone Joint Surg. [Am.] 70:724–727, 1988.

Scott, W.N.: Symposium on total knee arthroplasty (foreword). Orthop. Clin. North Am. 13:1–249, 1981.

Scuderi, G.R., and Insall, J.N.: The posterior stabilized knee prosthesis. Orthop. Clin. North Am., 20:71–78, 1989.

Sculco, T.P., and Ranawat, C.: The use of spinal anesthesia for total hip-replacement arthoplasty. J. Bone Joint Surg. [Am.] 57:173–177, 1975.

Shoji, H., Yoshino, S., and Kajino, A.: Patellar replacement in bilateral total knee arthroplasty. A study of patients who had rheumatoid arthritis and no gross deformity of the patella. J. Bone Joint Surg. [Am.] 71:853, 1989.

Silva, I., Jr., and Silva, D.M.: Tears of the meniscus as revealed by magnetic resonance imaging. J. Bone Joint Surg. [Am.] 70:199, 1988.

Stoller, D.W., Martin, C., Crues, J.V., III, et al.: Meniscal tears: Pathologic correlation with MR imaging. Radiology 163:731–735, 1987.

Stulberg, B.N., Insall, J.N., Williams, G.W., and Ghelman, B.: Deep-vein thrombosis following total knee replacement: An analysis of six hundred and thirty-eight arthroplasties. J. Bone Joint Surg. [Am.] 66:194–201, 1984.

Tibone, J.E., Elrod, B., Jobe, F.W., et al.: Surgical treatment of tears of the rotator cuff in athletes. J. Bone Joint Surg. [Am.] 68:887–891, 1986.

Total hip joint replacement in the United States. J.A.M.A. 248(15):1817–1821, 1982.

Walker, P.S.: Human Joints and Their Artificial Replacements. Springfield, IL, Charles C Thomas, 1977.

Warren, R.F.: Instability of shoulder in throwing sports. Instr. Course Lect. 34:337–348, 1985.

Windsor, R.E., Insall, J.N., and Vince, K.G.: Technical considerations of total knee arthroplasty after proximal tibial osteotomy. J. Bone Joint Surg. [Am.] 70:547, 1988.

CHAPTER 4

Foot and Ankle Disorders

I. Introduction

A. Overview—This chapter provides an overview of common foot disorders in adolescents and adults. (Childhood foot disorders are covered in Chapter 1, Pediatric Orthopaedics. Anatomy of the foot and ankle is covered in Chapter 10, Anatomy.) Foot and ankle problems have recently been given renewed emphasis in orthopaedics. The foot is responsible for support, balance, locomotion, and sensation for the lower extremity, and failure to consider all aspects of the foot in providing care can result in serious complications.

B. History and Physical Examination—A careful history should detail all foot complaints, including nature, onset, and relationships of problems, and be able to identify foot disorders that can affect the entire lower extremity. The physical exam should progress through an orderly series of steps, comparing both feet, and must include the following:

EXAM	FEATURES
Inspection	Check shoewear, feet standing and sitting
Gait	Evaluate limp, arm swing, toe-in/out, heels
Palpation	Anatomic approach
ROM	Ankle (DF 20°, PF 50°)
	Subtalar (eversion 5°, inversion 15°)
	Forefoot (adduction 20°, abduction 10°)
	1st MTP joint (flexion 45°, extension 80°)
	Digits (similar to hand)
Neurologic exam	Muscle, sensory, reflex (Achilles-S1)
Special tests	For individual disorders

Radiographs should usually include AP and lateral taken with weight bearing (to evaluate foot biomechanics) ± non–weight bearing (for completeness). Obliques are also helpful and should be taken routinely. Special views include sesamoid views, calcaneal axial views, and oblique medial views (for the talocalcaneal joint). CT scans, MRIs and Bone scans are often helpful for particular problems.

II. The Great Toe

A. Hallux Valgus (Bunion)

1. Introduction—Lateral deviation of the great toe secondary to altered foot mechanics and aggra-vated by improper shoewear. There is also a familial tendency. As the deformity progresses, soft tissues become stretched and bone deformities increase. When the valgus angle of the first MTP joint exceeds 30–35 degrees, pronation of the great toe results and other structures are also affected (plantar shift of abductor hallucis and lateral shift of sesamoid and intrinsics, and often hammering of second toe). The primary etiology of hallux valgus is unclear, but both lateral deviation of the great toe and metatarsus primus varus have been implicated. The term "bunion" applies to the "turnip" shape of the prominent medial eminence that results in hallux valgus, but it is frequently inadequate to address only this prominence and not consider other structures. Well over 100 procedures have been described to correct hallux valgus, indicating that no one "cure-all" exists.

2. Evaluation—History should elicit typical symptoms (pain, cosmetic deformity, pain in adjacent toe, etc.). Physical exam should include standing evaluation (accentuates deformity), ROM check, and evaluation of first metatarsal–cuneiform joint for hypermobility. Radiographic evaluation includes checking the hallux valgus angle (HVA; normal <15 degrees), intermetatarsal angle (IMA; normal <9 degrees), and distal metatarsal articular angle (DMAA; normal <10 degrees of lateral deviation) (Fig. 4–1), as well as checking for arthritis, size of the medial eminence, joint incongruity, and hallux valgus interphalangeus (deviation of the distal interphalangeal joint). Evaluation for hypermobile joints is also important because osteotomies may be indicated in these patients.

3. Treatment—Initial treatment is conservative with change in shoewear (wide toe box, soft leather), orthotics to attempt to correct the deformity, and eventually surgery. Several surgical procedures are described based on the deformity (Fig. 4–2).

a. **Prominent Medial Eminence**—In younger patients with a prominent "bunion" who do not have a significant IMA or HVA, **simple exostectomy (Silver)** can be performed. Complications of this procedure are usually

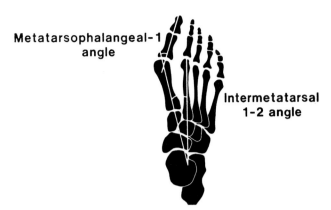

FIGURE 4–1. Hallux valgus: First MTP angle (MPA) >15 degrees, first and second intermetatarsal angle (IMA) >9 degrees. (From Johnson, K. A.: Surgery of the Foot and Ankle, p. 7. New York, Raven Press, 1989; reprinted by permission.)

a result of improper indications and includes recurrence and stiffness.

  b. **Hallux Valgus Interphalangeus**—When the deformity is located at the interphalangeal joint, an **Aiken procedure** may be appropriate. This consists of a closing wedge osteotomy of the proximal phalanx (for hallux valgus interphalangeus) combined with excision of the medial eminence. This is usually reserved for patients with congruent MTP joints or can be combined with other procedures proximally. Complications of this procedure include inadequate correction and malunion, nonunion is less of a problem.

  c. **Mild to Moderate Hallux Valgus**—Distal soft tissue procedures are often adequate.

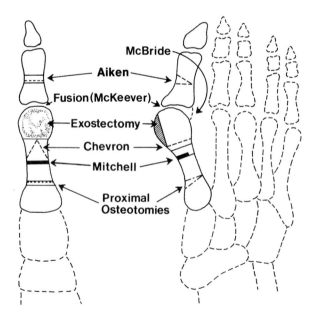

(Lateral View)   **(AP View)**
FIGURE 4–2. Bunion surgery composite.

This usually includes release of adductor hallucis, transverse metatarsal ligament, and lateral capsule combined with excision of the medial eminence and plication of the capsule medially (**modified McBride**). This is usually reserved for mild hallux valgus, or can be combined with a proximal procedure (usually a crescentic metatarsal (MT) osteotomy). Contraindications include impaired vascular status or advanced MTP degenerative joint disease (DJD). Complications of soft tissue procedures include recurrence; hallux varus (static from overcorrection [correct with Keller or fusion], dynamic from intrinsic imbalance [correct with tendon graft or plantar release]); claw toe (loss of intrinsic control—treat with IP fusion); and loss of MTP motion.

  d. **Significant Metatarsus Primus Varus**—As a general rule, when the intermetatarsal angle exceeds 15 degrees or the tibial sesamoid is lateral to a line drawn midway through the axis of the first metatarsal, **proximal MT osteotomies** are indicated. These procedures are often done in conjunction with distal soft tissue procedures. Metatarsal length should be the prime consideration when choosing the type of osteotomy in order to avoid transfer metatarsalgia.

  (1) **Crescentic**—Allows redirection of the MT without loss of bone. Complications include malunion, delayed union, nonunion, and transfer metatarsalgia (not from shortening but if the first MT is dorsiflexed).

  (2) **Opening Wedge**—Lengthens the MT, requires bone grafting and can cause excessive tightness of soft tissues, instability, and dorsiflexion of the first metatarsal.

  (3) **Closing Wedge**—Shortens the MT, can sometimes lead to a dorsiflexion deformity and a transfer lesion (to second MT).

  e. **Moderate Hallux Valgus in Younger Patients**—In general, patients <50 yo with moderate hallux valgus (HVA <30 degrees) and without significant metatarsus primus varus (IMA <13–15 degrees) may be candidates for **distal MT osteotomies**.

  (1) **Chevron**—Corrects mild to moderate deformities and should be done only if bunion deformity is passively correctable. Relies on redirecting the first MT head to correct abnormal shape from long-standing valgus drift. The "chevron" cut is made in the lateral plane. Complications include avascular necrosis (AVN) (increased with lateral release), malunion, excessive shortening (from bone resorption), MTP stiffness, and metatarsalgia (from excessive dorsiflexion at the osteotomy site).

  (2) **Mitchell**—A double step-cut osteotomy that is done more proximally (but still is distal); good for moderate deformities. Can cause transfer lesion, and can result in AVN or malunion.

f. **Hypermobile Metatarsocuneiform Joint**—Although somewhat unusual, this problem is best treated with **metatarsal-cuneiform arthrodesis,** which is usually combined with a distal soft tissue procedure.

g. **Moderate to Significant Hallux Valgus in Older Patients (Salvage)**—Options include arthroplasty and MTP fusion. The decision is based on the activity demands of the patient and where there is associated disease (such as rheumatoid arthritis [RA]). **Keller resection arthroplasty,** although very popular in the past, is now considered to have very few indications, except in people with very limited demands on their feet. It is contraindicated in younger patients and in patients with short first metatarsals. The procedure combines soft tissue release and removal of the medial eminence with resection of the proximal end of the proximal phalanx. Complications include transfer metatarsalgia (helped with MT bar), recurrence (reduced with medullary pin and night splinting), hallux varus, and hallux extensus (also minimized with use of medullary pin). **Silicone arthroplasty** is likewise unpopular due to associated synovitis and lymphadenopathy. It may have limited application in older patients with very limited activities and generalized foot disorders or significant first MTP DJD. **Metatarsal phalangeal arthrodesis** is the procedure of choice for hallux valgus associated with advanced DJD, rheumatoid hallux valgus, advanced hallux valgus (IMA >20 degrees, HVA >40 degrees), severely subluxated or dislocated MTP joints, or hallux valgus that has failed previous procedures. The joint should be fused in 10–15 degrees valgus and 25–30 degrees dorsiflexion. Complications include malunion, nonunion, and IP DJD.

h. **Summary**—Surgical procedures for treatment of hallux valgus are summarized in Table 4–1.

B. Hallux Rigidus (Hallux Limitus)—Limitation of motion and pain at the MTP joint of the great toe secondary to repetitive microtrauma and degenerative arthritis. It is more common in blacks and usually begins with an atraumatic event, possibly osteochondritis dissecans, and progresses to advanced degenerative changes at the first MTP joint. Affected feet are often long, narrow, and pronated with unstable arches, frequently with a hypermobile or elevated (and long) first MT. On exam, decreased ROM, especially dorsiflexion (DF), is common. Radiographs characteristically demonstrate degeneration and bony proliferation dorsally. Nonsurgical treatment includes use of molded firm inserts with rigid bar or a rocker-bottom shoe. Limited steroid injections are also occasionally beneficial. Surgical options include those listed in Table 4–2.

C. Hallux Varus—Usually a result of failed bunion surgery (excessive exostosis removal, medial overplication, or **lateral sesamoid excision**), but can be congenital. Surgery should address the offending cause and can include medial capsular release (for overplication of the capsule or excessive lateral release) ± split extensor hallucis longus (EHL) transfer (for excessive medial eminence resection). Severe cases may require first MTP fusion.

D. Hallux Flexus (Dorsal Bunion)—Caused by plantar flexion of the great toe at the MTP and elevation of the first MT. It is the result of muscle imbalance, hallux rigidus, or bunion surgery (malunion of a MT osteotomy). Transfer of the short flexors and hallux abductor and adductor (McKay) may be indicated in severe deformities. Corrective osteotomy may be required if the deformity was caused by malunion of a previous osteotomy. Arthrodesis may be necessary in some cases.

E. Hallux Extensus—Loss of flexor function leads to an imbalance and a "cock-up" toe. Can be iatrogenic (e.g., after excision of both sesamoids) or developmental. Treatment includes flexor repair (if recognized early), EHL transposition to the first MT neck (Jones procedure—with functional flexor hallucis brevis [FHB] and nonfunctional flexor hallucis longus [FHL]), and IP arthrodesis (for functional FHL and nonfunctional FHB). MTP arthrodesis is often required if there is associated MTP dislocation or significant subluxation.

TABLE 4–1. SURGICAL TREATMENT OF HALLUX VALGUS

PROCEDURE	INDICATION	ESSENTIAL FEATURES	COMPLICATIONS
Exostectomy	Large medial eminence	Excise prominent bunion	Recurrence
Aiken	Hallux valgus interphalangeus	Prox. phalanx osteotomy ± med. eminence resection	Recurrence, malunion
Distal soft tissue	Mild hallux valgus	Lat. release, med. eminence resection	Recurrence, hallux varus
Crescentic	Incr. IMA	Proximal dome	Mal/nonunion
Open wedge	Short MT	Proximal	Instability, mal/nonunion
Closed wedge	Long MT	Proximal	Transfer metatarsalgia, mal/nonunion
Chevron	Mild deformity	Distal cut from side	AVN, stiff joint
Mitchell	Moderate deformity	Distal, double step-cut	AVN, malunion, transfer metatarsalgia
MTC fusion	Hypermobile MTC joint	MTC fusion and soft tissue procedure	Mal/nonunion
Keller arthroplasty	DJD, older patients	Soft tissue + prox. phalanx resection	Recurrence, transfer metatarsalgia, hallux varus/extensus
Silicone arthroplasty	Limited activity	Resection interposition	Synovitis
MTP fusion	Severe DJD, rheumatoid arthritis	MTP fusion	Interphalangeal DJD, nonunion

TABLE 4–2. SURGICAL TREATMENT OF HALLUX RIGIDUS

PROCEDURE	INDICATION	ESSENTIAL FEATURES	COMPLICATIONS
Cheilectomy	Young, active patient	Remove osteophytes	Undercorrection, recurrence
Keller arthroplasty	Moderate DJD, older patient	Prox. phalanx base resection	Recurrence, transfer metatarsalgia, hallux varus/extensus
MTP fusion	Advanced DJD, active patient	25–30° dorsiflexion, 15° valgus	Nonunion, interphalangeal DJD
Silicone arthroplasty	Limited activity	Silicone stem(s)	Silicone synovitis

F. Sesamoid Disorders—Can be difficult to diagnose. Careful history and physical exam and special radiographs (axial projections) can be helpful. **Surgical excision of a sesamoid is contraindicated in patients who have had the adjacent sesamoid removed previously** (because of significant risk of a cock-up deformity of the great toe). The following sesamoid problems should be considered:
1. Sesamoiditis—Inflammation and swelling around the sesamoid (tibial > fibular) and the tendon of the FHB can be a localized event, or can be secondary to trauma, infection, AVN, stress fractures, or a systemic disorder. Symptoms include pain on weight bearing and with dorsiflexion of the great toe and pain with direct palpation. Treatment includes activity limitation, padding, and taping the great toe in a plantar-flexed position. Rarely, sesamoid excision is necessary in refractory cases.
2. Fractures—Sesamoid fractures are uncommon but can occur, usually in the tibial sesamoid. Symptoms include pain and swelling following a traumatic episode. Differential includes bipartite sesamoid (25–30% incidence, 85% of these are bilateral). Treatment includes immobilization for 6 weeks, although sesamoid removal is often required (especially if initial treatment is delayed).
3. Sesamoid Prominence/Arthritis—x-rays including sesamoid views can help to diagnose prominence, which can be corrected with an insert or shaving of the bone, and arthritis (treated with NSAIDs, shoewear, and occasionally sesamoidectomy).
4. "Turf Toe"—Sesamoid injuries (especially the tibial sesamoid) are often the result of this sports injury. Work-up should include radiographs of the sesamoid and a bone scan. Conservative treatment is usually successful. Occasionally, partial or complete sesamoid excision is required.

III. Lesser Toes

A. Lesser Toe Deformities—Includes mallet toe, hammer toe, and claw toe. The incidence of these deformities is increased in shoe-wearing societies (related to small toe box), and in the older population. Mallet toe involves only the DIP (flexion), whereas hammer toe and claw toe can involve all three joints of the toe. The distinction between hammer toe and claw toe is somewhat convoluted, but is based on flexion/extension of the joints (Fig. 4–3):

DEFORMITY	MTP JOINT	PIP JOINT	DIP JOINT
Mallet toe	Neutral	Neutral	Flexion
Hammer toe	Neutral or extension	Flexion	Any position (ext. > flex.)
Claw toe	Hyperextension	Flexion	Flexion

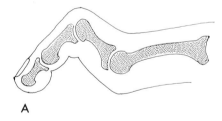

A

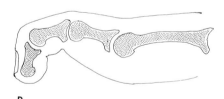

B

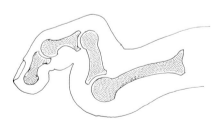

C

FIGURE 4–3. Lesser toe deformities. *A,* Hammer toe. *B,* Mallet toe. *C,* Claw toe. (From Tachdjian, M. D.: Congenital deformities. In Disorders of the Foot, Jahss, M. H., ed., p. 212. Philadelphia, W. B. Saunders Company, 1982; reprinted by permission.)

Additionally, claw toes usually involve all of the lesser toes and are often associated with neuromuscular disorders and midfoot and hindfoot deformities. Hammer toes, in contrast, may involve only one toe (usually the second), present in an older population, and are not associated with other disorders. For all of the lesser toe deformities, it is critical to determine if the deformity is flexible (passively correctable) or rigid, because treatment differs. Left untreated, all of these disorders can develop painful callosities (hard corns) over the affected joints and on the end of the distal phalanx (end corn), and intractable plantar keratosis under the metatarsal heads.

1. Mallet Toe—flexion of DIP of lesser toes, esp. second toe. Treatment includes shoewear modification (toe crest pad, wide toe box) or, failing this, surgery. Flexible deformities, which are uncommon, should be treated with flexor tenotomy. Fixed deformities (more common) are best treated with resection of the head and neck of the middle phalanx and flexor tenotomy or fusion of the DIP joint.

2. Hammer Toe—As noted above, can involve all three joints late because long-standing contractures often lead to extension at the MTP joint. Development of hammer toe is usually related to shoewear and is also associated with flexor digitorum longus (FDL) tightness, insensate feet, and trauma (mild compartment syndrome). The intrinsics (which flex the MTP and extend the IP joints) are overcome by the extrinsic mechanism and result in the characteristic deformities. Physical examination should determine if the affected toe(s) are flexible or rigid and if MTP extension (if present) corrects with weight bearing. Flexible hammer toe should be treated nonoperatively, initially with shoewear modifications (high/wide toe box, toe crest pad) and orthotics (MT bar, Plastozote inserts, etc.). Failing this, a **Girdlestone Taylor** procedure (split FDL transfer to the extensor apparatus) should be considered. Fixed hammer toe usually requires operative intervention. **DuVries arthroplasty** (resection of the head and neck of the proximal phalanx) is usually successful for the second through fourth toes, and should be combined with extensor tenotomy and dorsal capsulotomy with MTP joint extension (with weight bearing) or fusion of the PIP joint.

3. Claw Toe—Often associated with neuromuscular disease, and neurology consultation may be appropriate. Etiology of claw toe also includes severe arthritis, advanced age (decreased muscle tone and reliance of toe gripping for balance), and metabolic disease, and often it is idiopathic. Claw toe results from simultaneous contraction of the extensors and flexors. Treatment of claw toe should follow correction of other foot abnormalities (e.g., pes cavus) if they are present. If the deformity is flexible, then the **Girdlestone Taylor** procedure and extensor tenotomy and dorsal capsulotomy (± collateral ligament resection) will usually correct it. If it is fixed, **DuVries arthroplasty** should be combined with MTP joint soft tissue release (including both flexors in severe deformities) and

K-wire fixation. The **Hibbs** procedure (transfer of the common extensor to the third cuneiform) may be indicated for neuromuscular clawtoe.

B. Subluxation/Dislocations of the second MTP Joint.

1. Introduction—Can develop into hammer toe and can follow trauma, synovitis, chronic changes from footwear, hallux valgus (or can cause it), etc. If the disorder is secondary to hallux valgus, then an appropriate bunion procedure must be accomplished first or subluxation/dislocation of the second MTP joint will recur. The second ray is affected because it is the longest in the foot and is subjected to more pressure than lesser rays. Symptoms include pain (different from neuroma because there is no pain with compression of the transverse MT arch and it is not radicular), swelling, malalignment, and dysfunction. Capsular instability, which is a large part of the disease, can be diagnosed by performing a drawer-like maneuver of the MTP joint (Thompson-Hamilton sign). Radiographs may show subluxation of the MTP joint.

2. Treatment—Conservative treatment consists of shoewear modification (wide toe box and small heel and toe cradle with addition of a deeper box if more advanced), taping of the toe, MT pads, NSAIDs, and judicious use of steroid injections. Surgery, if this fails, attempts to restore the balance of forces across the joint. This includes FDL release or transfer for flexible deformities, and shortening metatarsal osteotomy (for long second MT), or resection arthroplasty (± syndactylization) for rigid deformities. Complications include recurrence, vascular compromise, and transient swelling and pain.

C. First Ray Insufficiency Syndrome (Morton's Foot)—Deficient development of the first metatarsal can make the lesser metatarsals relatively longer than normal and lead to increased stresses, especially over the second MT head. Treatment includes shoe inserts and strengthening exercises. Surgical correction may include osteotomies of the lesser metatarsals.

D. Freiberg's Infraction (See also Chapter 2, Basic Sciences)—Osteonecrosis of the second > third metatarsal head with dorsal proximal subluxation. Symptoms include MTP pain with weight bearing and limited ROM. Radiographs show sclerosis and flattening of the affected MT head. Nonoperative treatment includes orthotics and casting. Surgery in refractory cases includes synovectomy and dorsal cheilectomy (if less advanced) or condylectomy (if advanced).

E. Fifth Toe Deformities—The fifth toe is unique because of its border location and lack of support by the other toes. Two deformities are common: the cock-up deformity and an overlapping deformity.

1. Cock-Up Deformity of the Fifth Toe—This deformity, which probably is related to shoewear, results in a proximal phalanx that may be almost perpendicular to the fifth MT shaft. Treatment usually requires operative intervention. The **Ruiz-Mora** procedure (removal of the proximal phalanx through an elliptical plantar incision) or DuVries arthroplasty with syndactylization of the fourth and fifth toes is recommended.

2. Overlapping Deformity of the Fifth Toe—This is a congenital deformity where the fifth toe is externally rotated and compressed with a contracture of the dorsal MTP joint capsule and extensor tendon. Symptoms develop from shoewear, but patients (or their parents) are often more concerned about cosmesis. Several procedures have been described to correct this problem, including the following:

PROCEDURE	FEATURES
DuVries	Excision of contractures (EDL and capsule) ± syndactylization
Wilson	V–Y-plasty with EDL and capsule sectioning
Lapidus	EDL sectioned and rerouted through prox. phalanx (tibial → fibular) and sutured to abductor digiti minimi

IV. Hyperkeratotic Disorders

A. Introduction—Hyperkeratotic disorders include corns and calluses, which are localized keratoses caused by abnormal pressure. This pressure can be intrinsic (usually bony prominences) or extrinsic (shoewear) and leads to proliferation of horny layers of the epidermis. These disorders are often self-treated by patients with salicylic acid preparations.

B. Hard Corn (Heloma Durum)—Occurs on exposed surfaces of the toes (especially on the fibular side of the fifth toe). (Fig. 4–4). Also occurs in conjunction with the lesser toe deformities discussed above. Nonoperative treatment consists of reducing the horny accumulation (with a pumice stone or Dremel tool), modifying shoewear (large toe box, adding padding), and orthotics. Operative treatment may include **DuVries condylectomy** for deformities located on the fifth toe, and hammer/claw toe correction as appropriate.

C. Soft Corn (Heloma Molle or Clavus)—Forms over a phalangeal condyle between the toes, most commonly between the fourth and fifth toes where the head of the fifth proximal phalanx abuts the base of the fourth proximal phalanx (Fig. 4–5). The keratosis that develops is similar to a hard corn but the overlying tissue becomes macerated because of its location. Nonoperative treatment includes the use of lamb's wool or gauze or Carfussin between the toes. Operative options include excision of offending condyles (fifth toe) or excision of offending exostoses (other toes). DuVries arthroplasty is often helpful for a fourth interspace corn, and is often combined with fusion for corns associated with the other lesser toes.

D. Callosities (Tyloma)—Form over bony prominences, especially on the plantar surface and heel. They can be normal in athletic patients with generalized callosities, especially in the forefoot. **Intractable plantar keratosis** refers to symptomatic, well-localized plantar callosities that typically have a small centralized core. These callosities are commonly located beneath the tibial sesamoid or under the fibular condyle of the first MT head, or diffusely under any metatarsal head. Etiology includes offending footwear, osseous abnormalities (longer plantar-flexed MT, sharp condylar processes [fibular side]), and varus or valgus position of the forefoot. Treatment includes trimming, change in shoewear (wide toe box, soft sole, low heels), orthotics (soft MT support), and other supportive measures. Operative options are directed

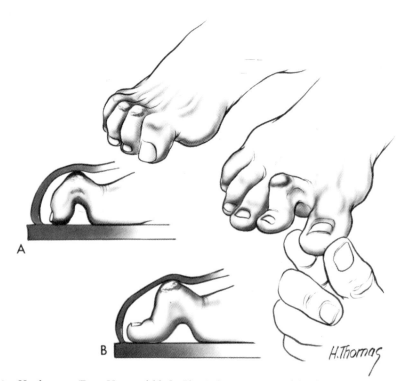

FIGURE 4–4. Hard corns. (From Hoppenfeld, S.: Physical examination of the foot by complaint. In Disorders of the Foot, Jahss, M. H., ed., p. 113. Philadelphia, W. B. Saunders Company, 1982; reprinted by permission.)

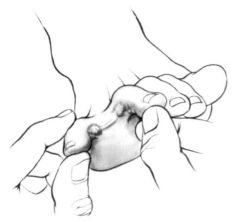

FIGURE 4–5. Soft corns. (From Hoppenfeld, S.: Physical examination of the foot by complaint. In Disorders of the Foot, Jahss, M. H., ed., p. 114. Philadelphia, W. B. Saunders Company, 1982; reprinted by permission.)

at the underlying problem. Sesamoid prominences are best treated with shaving of the plantar half of the sesamoid (favored over excision). Metatarsal condylar prominences may be treated with a **Fowler arthroplasty** (proximal phalengectomy and plantar metatarsal condylectomy). Larger, diffuse lesions that may be caused by elongated or plantar-flexed metatarsals may be corrected with a **Giannestras (oblique) metatarsal osteotomy**.

E. Tailor's Bunion (Bunionette)—Enlargement of the fibular side of the fifth MTP often leads to corns and callosities in this area. Soft tissue hypertrophy, wide fifth MTP head, or lateral deviation of the fifth MT shaft leads to thickening of the bursa overlying this area. Extrinsic pressure (shoewear) can lead to associated keratoses. Treatment includes modification of shoewear (broad-toed shoes, padding) and other supportive measures. Surgery for a wide MT head involves fifth MT lateral ± plantar condylectomy. For deformities with lateral deviation of the fifth MT, a **Sponsel oblique neck osteotomy** (angulated 40–45 degrees proximally) is often successful.

F. High Dorsum of Base of First Metatarsal–Cuneiform Joint—Similar to carpal boss in the hand, this is a congenital disorder that can lead to symptoms from irritation and early DJD. Shoewear modifications are usually helpful. Occasionally, cheilectomy or fusion is required, but surgery should be avoided in most cases.

V. Nerve Disorders

A. Morton's Neuroma—Interdigital plantar neuroma associated with perineural fibrosis and myxoid degeneration of the intermetatarsal plantar digital nerves. Usually occurs at the 3–4 interspace, less commonly the 2–3 interspace. The 3–4 interspace is innervated by branches of both the medial and lateral plantar nerves, and this has been suggested to contribute to the etiology of the disorder. Other causes suggested include increased mobility of the third and fourth digits and both intrinsic and extrinsic compression of affected nerves. The typical presentation is a 55-yo woman with unilateral burning foot pain. Morton's neuroma is bilateral 15% of the time but rarely involves more than one interspace in the same foot simultaneously. The pain can be localized between the MT heads and is aggravated by activities and direct palpation. Approximately $\frac{1}{3}$ of the time a discrete painful mass can be identified by palpation. Initial treatment includes use of a broad, soft-soled shoe with a low heel, soft MT supports, and injection (which can be diagnostic and therapeutic). Surgical excision of the neuroma is usually successful. The dorsal incision is usually favored due to the possibility of scarring with a plantar incision. The **plantar approach is indicated for recurrent Morton's neuroma**.

B. Tarsal Tunnel Syndrome—Entrapment of the tibial nerve or its branches beneath the flexor retinaculum (laciniate ligament, which extends from the medial malleolus to the medial tubercle of the calcaneus). Etiology includes posttraumatic changes, local soft tissue compression (ganglion, lipomas, etc.), and foot deformities (coalition, pronation deformities, etc.). Symptoms are similar to carpal tunnel (burning pain [which may radiate proximally to midcalf], sensory disturbance over the toes and plantar foot, impaired push off [intrinsic weakness]), and EMG/NCS is helpful. Accurate diagnosis depends on the presence of characteristic symptoms, a positive Tinel's sign over the compression, *and* positive EMG/NCS studies (abductor hallucis and abductor digiti quinti affected). Conservative treatment includes NSAIDs, casting, orthotics (especially with pronated feet to relieve pressure on the neuroma), and injections. Failing this, surgical release of the flexor retinaculum behind the medial malleolus with distal exploration of the medial and lateral plantar nerves can be effective if all three diagnostic criteria are met.

C. Entrapment of the First Branch of the Lateral Plantar Nerve (to Abductor Digiti Quinti)—This nerve may be compressed in the deep tissues on the lateral side of the calcaneus (abductor hallucis, proximal plantar fascia), and may be the cause of heel pain in some patients. The pain is worse with compression of the nerve and may respond to rest, heel pads, arch supports, NSAIDs, contrast baths, and occasional steroid injections. Surgical release of the nerve where it is compressed between the deep fascia of the abductor hallucis and the medial margin of the quadratus plantae muscle is usually successful.

D. Other nerve entrapments include the following:

Nerve	Cause	Symptoms/Findings	Treatment
Superficial peroneal	Fascia/muscle	Dorsal foot pain and EMG/NCS	Lateral heel wedge injections, release
Deep peroneal	Inf. extensor retinaculum	Pain/paresthesias	Lower heels, NSAIDs occasionally release
Sural	Fracture, sprains	Pain/paresthesias	NSAIDs, injection occasionally release

E. Incisional Neuromas—Can occur usually following other procedures about the foot. Diagnosis is established by a positive Tinel's sign, local tenderness, and relief with trigger point injection. Three types of neuromas are common in the foot:

NEUROMA	COMMON LOCATIONS	COMMENTS
Stump end	Sural, sup. peroneal, dorsomedial	Nerve severed, can be severe
Scar entrapment	Dorsomedial, deep peroneal	Normal nerve trapped
Forme fruste	Anywhere, superficial	May resolve by 12 months

Treatment should include prevention, massage, local therapy, and surgery as a last resort to release scar, and transplantation of nerve endings if necessary.

VI. Tendon Injuries and Disorders

  A. Introduction—**Tenosynovitis** (tendon sheath inflammation), and **peritendinitis** (inflammation around a tendon that has no sheath) are common afflictions in the foot. These disorders present with localized warmth, erythema, and pain with motion. Treatment includes rest, ice, and elevation early, and immobilization and limited injection late. **Tendonitis** (inflammation and degeneration within the tendon itself) is often more chronic in nature and can lead to tendon rupture.

  B. Tendons Affected by Shoe Irritation—Commonly involves two areas in the feet.

    1. EHL Impingement—Can be caused by the shoe vamp (that portion of the shoe covering the instep) and may lead to formation of a protective fibroma at the first MT head. Excision of the fibroma and EHL repair is sometimes required in chronic cases refractory to changes in shoewear.

    2. Achilles Tendon Irritation (Pump Bump)—Retrocalcaneal bursitis that occurs in women who wear shoes with closely contoured heel counters. Chronic cases can lead to a reactive exostosis of the posterosuperior tuberosity of the calcaneus (**Haglund's deformity**) and inflammation at the Achilles tendon insertion. Treatment includes shoewear modifications and occasionally osteotomy of the calcaneus or removal of the prominence by simple exostectomy.

  C. Chronic Tenosynovitis/Tendonitis—Typically involves the tibialis posterior and flexor hallucis longus tendons, but can also involve the peroneal and tibialis anterior tendons. Chronic degeneration can lead to attritional tears and tendon rupture.

    1. Tibialis Posterior Tendonitis/Rupture—May present with intermittent pain, tenderness, swelling, and crepitus behind the medial malleolus. Patients with subsequent tendon rupture will develop a progressive flatfoot deformity and medial foot and ankle pain. On exam, these patients will have a flattened arch, a valgus heel, talonavicular sagging (seen also on weight-bearing radiographs), and limited heel inversion with toe standing ("too many toes" sign [Johnson]) and motor exam. The single

heel rise test may also be helpful (patient is unable to rise off toes of affected foot with opposite foot elevated). Diagnostic ultrasound and MRI are sometimes helpful if the exam is equivocal. Treatment of tibialis posterior tendonitis early consists of exercises, contrast baths, ultrasound therapy, NSAIDs, and shoe wedges. Steroid injections are contraindicated in active patients. Surgical therapy in severe cases (tenolysis of the tendon sheath and tenosynovectomy) may avert tendon rupture. Late (after rupture), nonoperative treatment may include the use of an orthotic (UCBL or AFO). Surgical treatment following rupture includes exploration and tibialis posterior **reconstruction with the FDL tendon** (the FDL tendon is rerouted through the tibialis posterior sheath and through a drill hole in the navicular from plantar to dorsal [**Mann**]; or by side-to-side anastomosis [**Jahss**]). More significant long-standing fixed deformities may require selective fusions (tarsonavicular) or triple arthrodesis (especially with limited subtalar motion).

    2. Flexor Hallucis Longus Tendonitis—Commonly has a similar presentation, and may cause triggering (stenosing tenosynovitis) within its tendon sheath. This disorder is very common in Ballet dancers. Nonoperative treatment is similar to that for tibialis posterior tendonitis. Surgical tenolysis for stenosing tenosynovitis may be required. Reconstruction is usually not necessary.

    3. Tibialis Anterior Tendon Rupture—Usually occurs between the extensor retinaculum and tendon insertion, resulting in weak dorsiflexion. Localized tenderness and drop foot gait may also be seen. If orthotic treatment fails, direct repair or use of a fifth toe extensor graft may be beneficial.

    4. Peroneal Tendonitis—Is unusual but can occur. Early treatment is similar to that outlined above. Attritional tears can be repaired by suturing peroneus brevis to peroneus longus (this can also be reinforced by peroneus tertius). Peroneus longus rupture can be associated with a disorder of the Os peroneum.

    5. Achilles Tendonitis—Usually caused by overuse, and conservative therapy is successful. Chronic inflammation can lead to stenosing tenosynovitis. This is associated with small tears, cysts, and nodules in an area of the tendon 2–5 cm proximal to its insertion, and a boggy peritenon. Surgical excision of the thickened peritenon and removal of granulation tissue and diseased tendon can be helpful.

  D. Peroneal Tendon Dislocation—These tendons are the most common tendons to dislocate, probably because of their poorly anchored location at the end of the fibula and weak retinaculum. Traumatic dislocation is associated with forced dorsiflexion of the ankle and contraction of the peroneals. The injury is seen often in skiers and paretics. Acute dislocations usually respond to closed reduction and casting. Surgical treatment may include direct repair acutely, or reconstructing the distal fibular groove and/or a new retinaculum for recurrent dislocation.

E. Open Tendon Lacerations—Occur usually on the plantar surface (e.g., patient who steps on glass). Surgical exploration is recommended in most cases in order to define the extent of the injury. FHL and EHL tendons should be repaired primarily. Tibialis anterior and posterior, extensor digitorum longus (EDL), and peroneal tendons should be repaired also (especially in children). FDL and flexor digitorum brevis (FDB) repair is probably not necessary because laceration of these tendons leaves only a mild deformity and no functional deficit. Isolated digital nerve injuries are left unrepaired. *Pseudomonas* osteomyelitis commonly follows puncture wounds of the foot. Early drainage, curettage when indicated, and antibiotics can help avoid disastrous results.

F. Acute Achilles Tendon Rupture—Usually occurs in a middle-age patient/athlete as a result of sudden ankle dorsiflexion, and is associated with a positive Thompson's test (squeezing the calf fails to produce dorsiflexion at the ankle). Treatment is controversial, but surgical treatment (primary repair through a posteromedial incision ± plantaris tendon augmentation) is favored in athletes because of decreased rerupture rates, but risks skin breakdown.

VII. Disorders of the Plantar Skin and Fascia

A. Plantar Warts (Verruca Plantaris; "Papillomas of the Sole)"—Caused by a DNA virus of the *Papovirus* group and are characterized by localized lesions **without a central core** with sharp margins and high vascularity (vigorous punctate bleeding with shaving) and pain with lateral compression. Three groups of plantar warts are commonly recognized: (1) solitary warts with surrounding callus, (2) multiple warts with a large "mother" and tiny "daughter" satellites, and (3) mosaic patches of coalescent cores. Treatment includes the use of salicylic acid plaster (± formalin), cryosurgery or liquid nitrogen application (for small warts), and blunt dissection/curettage. Deep electrosurgery or excision should be avoided because of associated scarring.

B. Skin Infections and Tumors
  1. Fungal Infections—Athlete's foot (tinea pedis) is caused by *Trichophytan rubrum* or *mentagrophytes*. These lesions can be wet or dry. Diagnosis is made by KOH preparation. Treatment include aeration of feet and antifungal agents.
  2. Bacterial Infections—Impetigo contegiosa, caused by staph or strep infections, can be treated with Burrow's solution and antibiotics. Infectious eczematoid dermatitis and other bacterial infections are best treated with antibiotics.
  3. Tumors—**Melanoma** is the **most common primary** of the foot, occurring most commonly on the plantar skin.

C. Plantar Fibromatosis—Locally aggressive idiopathic proliferative fasciitis of the plantar aponeurosis that is usually bilateral. Like Dupuytren's contractures in the hand, this disease (a.k.a. Ledderhosen syndrome) presents as discrete plantar nodules often seen in non–weight-bearing areas (especially medial plantar). Surgical excision is rarely successful but may be required for large,

painful nodules. Excision must include the entire slip of plantar fascia from origin to insertion in order to avoid recurrence rates of up to 90%.

D. Plantar Fasciitis—One of several causes of heel pain. Symptoms include gradual onset of pain at the origin of the plantar aponeurosis and 1 cm distal to this area. The pain is typically reproduced with dorsiflexion of the MTPs and palpation of the fascial band. Laboratory studies are often helpful (ESR, RF, serum uric acid) in order to rule out other etiologies of the pain (RA, Reiter's, etc.). Radiographs may demonstrate spurring of the medial calcaneal tuberosity. Treatment is nonoperative with NSAIDs, a soft shoe, limited injections (no more than two or three), taping the forefoot into adduction, and orthotics (flexible with $\frac{1}{8}$-inch medial wedge). Surgical treatment is controversial (spur removal, fascial release, etc.). Excision of a heel spur (which is located **at the origin of the FDB**, not the plantar fascia) may actually exacerbate heel pain by altering the mechanics of the heel pad. The differential diagnosis of heel pain should include stress fractures (identified on a 45-degree medial oblique radiograph or bone scan), inflammatory arthritides, and entrapment of the first branch of the lateral plantar nerve (discussed above).

VIII. Toenail Disorders

A. Ingrown Toenail (Onychocryptosis Unguis Incarnatus)—Caused by extrinsic pressure causing the nail fold to push into the sharp edge of an improperly cut nail (Fig. 4–6). Bacterial and fungal flora enter the wound, resulting in an abscess and later hypertrophic granulation tissue. Three stages are recognized: I Inflammatory, II Abscess, III Granulation. For all ingrown nails, the offending nail must be removed. This can be achieved with débridement of the nail spicule or partial nail excision (± matrixectomy).

B. Clubnail (Onychauxis)—Hypertrophied nail, usually on the great toe. Caused by systemic, or more commonly, local problems such as trauma or nail bed infection. Nail grinding or avulsion is usually required. Occasionally ablation may be required.

C. Subungual Exostosis—Bony projection that devel-

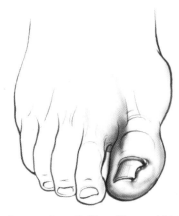

FIGURE 4–6. Ingrown toenail. (From Hoppenfeld, S.: Physical examination of the foot by complaint. In Disorders of the Foot, Jahss, M. H., ed., p. 114. Philadelphia, W. B. Saunders Company, 1982; reprinted by permission.)

ops on a distal phalanx, especially the great toe. May be related to trauma. Excision is indicated when elevation of the nail produces pain.

D. Fungal Infections (Onychomycosis)—Dermatophyte infection of the nails that usually begins with localized areas of discoloration beneath the nail. The nail plate becomes lusterless and gradually thickens; ultimately, the nail may become greatly distorted with marked thickening, cracking, and piling up of loose keratinous debris. Treatment includes oral griseofulvin for 8–12 months and an antifungal (e.g., clotrimazole) or gluteraldehyde applied beneath the nail bed. Nail removal may be required for nondermatophytic onychomycosis (e.g., *Scopulariopsis brevicaulis*).

IX. Pes Planus (Flatfoot)

A. Introduction—Loss of the normal medial longitudinal arch leads to pes planus, which can be flexible or rigid. Other associated abnormalities include valgus heel, mild subtalar subluxation, eversion of the calcaneus, abduction at the midtarsal joint, and supination of the forefoot. Radiographic evaluation includes both standing and nonstanding views (in order to differentiate flexible from rigid deformities) and oblique views for adolescents, which may show calcaneonavicular bar or synchondrosis.

B. Flexible Pes Planus—Usually seen in childhood, and most of the time will spontaneously correct. Use of orthosis may be of some help. Indications for surgery basically involve disabling pain following every effort at conservative treatment. Surgical procedures include the Miller (first MT–cuneiform and cuneiform-navicular arthrodesis), modified Hoke-Miller/Scottish Rite (cuneiform-navicular arthrodesis with opening wedge of the first cuneiform), Durham plasty (similar with tibialis posterior advancement), triple arthrodesis (calcaneocuboid, subtalar [talocalcaneal], and talonavicular), and calcaneal osteotomies. For flexible flatfoot caused by accessory navicular, the Kidner procedure was developed (remove accessory navicular and reroute the tibialis posterior tendon plantar). However, simple excision of the accessory navicular is equally effective.

C. Rigid Pes Planus—More frequently results in surgery than the flexible variety. Can be caused by congenital vertical talus, tarsal coalition (see Chapter 1, Pediatric Orthopaedics, Part XI: Lower Extremity Problems), and peroneal spastic flatfoot (correct with medially based closing wedge osteotomy of the calcaneus). Adult-acquired flatfoot can be secondary to tibialis posterior rupture, talonavicular arthritis, or neuropathic arthritis.

X. Ankle and Subtalar Injuries and Disorders

A. Ankle Sprains—The most common ligamentous injuries in the body and usually involve the lateral ankle ligaments (inversion injuries are the most common sports injury). The anterior talofibular ligament (ATFL) is the weakest and most commonly injured ligament, the posterior talofibular ligament (PTFL) is the strongest and least injured. Both the ATFL and the PTFL are intra-articular, whereas the other lateral ligament, the calcaneofibular ligament (CFL), is extra-articular. Mechanism of injury for acute injury is supination and plantar flexion

(ATFL injury) or dorsiflexion (CFL injury). Patients may describe a feeling of "giving way." Pain is increased with inversion stress. Complete evaluation should also include palpation of the individual ligaments, anterior drawer testing, and assessing amount of swelling. Sprains are graded as mild (grade I) when functional integrity is still present, moderate (grade II) where moderate functional loss is present and there is near complete ligamentous disruption, and severe (grade III) when there is ligament rupture. Anterior drawer testing in plantar flexion allows assessment of the ATFL; testing in dorsiflexion, the CFL. Radiographs are required to rule out fractures (lateral or posterior talar process, anterior process of the calcaneus, etc.), stress radiographs may also be helpful (drawer testing [>3 mm difference is consistent with ATFL injury] and talar tilt [>5 degrees is consistent with ATFL injury, >15 degrees with ATFL and CFL injury]); and arthrography, if done within 1 week of injury, is the most helpful. Treatment of grades I and II injuries consists of rest, ice, and elevation followed by exercises and rehab (balance board). Proprioception is usually the last function to return fully. Treatment of grade III injuries is controversial. Some feel that early operative repair is most beneficial. Studies have shown that late repair can be equally effective and therefore, most reserve surgery for chronic injury that fails conservative management.

B. Chronic Ligamentous Laxity—Follows severe or repeated ankle sprains or can be idiopathic (peroneal weakness). Nonoperative treatment includes the use of a lateral heel wedge, peroneal muscle strengthening, cast bracing, and activity modification. Surgical reconstruction usually involves peroneus brevis tenodesis through a drill hole in the fibula (Evans) or through several bones (Chrisman-Snook). Brösstrom reconstruction (primary repair of the ligaments with embrication of the capsule) is also successful in instability resulting from injuries within a year of the planned procedure.

C. Subtalar Instability—Can follow severe inversion ankle sprains. Stress radiographs including special subtalar stress views (Broden—45-degree internal rotation and 20-degree caudal tilt), and fluoroscopy can be helpful. Muscle strengthening, Achilles stretching, and proprioceptive reeducation can help. Lateral heel wedges, ankle braces to limit inversion, and subtalar bracing are helpful. Surgery can include the Chrisman-Snook procedure, which rebuilds both the ATFL and CFL, direct repair of the CFL and tightening of the inferior extensor retinaculum may be helpful.

D. Subtalar Degenerative Joint Disease—Commonly posttraumatic in origin. Advanced cases that do not respond to prolonged nonoperative management should be considered for selective subtalar fusion. Severe cases that involve calcaneocuboid and talonavicular joints may require triple arthrodesis (Fig. 4–7). Fusion of the subtalar joint should be in neutral or slight valgus. Excessive varus can lead to painful callosities under the fifth metatarsal head. The most common complication associated with a triple arthrodesis is pseudarthrosis of the talonavicular joint. Isolated subtalar fusions (e.g., talonavicular) result in nearly complete loss of sub-

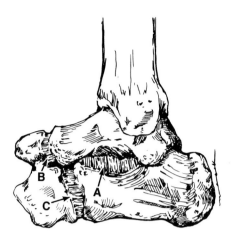

FIGURE 4–7. Triple arthrodesis: *A*, talocalcaneal; *B*, talonavicular; and *C*, calcaneocuboid. (From Gelman, M. I.: Radiology of Orthopedic Procedures, Vol. 24: Problems and Complications, p. 187. Philadelphia, W. B. Saunders Company, 1984; reprinted by permission.)

talar motion due to interdependence of the joints in the subtalar complex. However, isolated subtalar (i.e., talocalcaneal) fusion is indicated with posttraumatic arthritis of this joint, and results in a less rigid foot (does not tie up remainder of subtalar complex).

E. Tibiotalar Degenerative Joint Disease—The ankle is commonly injured, but rarely symptomatically degenerative. Osteochondrotic lesions can be treated with drilling of subchondral bone, and sometimes with pinning with bone grafting. Lateral lesions are usually flatter than the equally common medial lesions (cup shaped). Nonoperative treatment of ankle DJD includes rocker-bottom shoes with SACH heel, double upright AFOs, NSAIDS, etc. Early DJD is often limited to the anterior aspect of the joint, and anterior osteophyte excision may be helpful. For severe deformities, arthrodesis may be required, but is subject to a high complication rate. Fusion should be in 5–10 degrees of external rotation and 5 degrees of valgus. Many different fusion techniques have been described. Total ankle arthroplasty is rarely indicated (RA with limited demands).

F. Sinus Tarsi Syndrome—Pain and tenderness on the lateral side of the hindfoot originating from the area of the sinus tarsus (talocalcaneal sulcus—a "tunnel" between the talus and calcaneus). The sinus is filled with the interosseous talocalcaneal ligament, which, when injured (usually with lateral ankle sprains) or aggravated (e.g., with inflammatory arthritides), can lead to the characteristic pain. Arthrograms may show incomplete filling of the subtalar lateral recess and are helpful in equivocal cases. Injections into the sinus tarsi can be both diagnostic and therapeutic. Surgery may include excision of the tissue in this area, and, in refractory cases, subtalar fusion. It is important to note that this is a syndrome and not a disease; therefore, the clinician must search for an alternate source of pain (e.g., subtalar joint DJD, coalition, or peroneal tendon pathology) first.

XI. Rheumatoid Foot and Ankle

A. Rheumatoid Ankle—The ankle is one of the last joints to be affected by rheumatoid disease. Proliferative synovitis and recurrent effusions may cause swelling behind the mortises, recurrent effusions, and pain on weight bearing and motion. If conservative therapy fails, surgical synovectomy can significantly relieve pain. Arthrodesis is sometimes required in the rheumatoid ankle, but results are affected by involvement of the subtalar and midtarsal joints in ⅔ of patients. Ankle prostheses, although initially encouraging, often yield poor clinical results. High rates of loosening and wound problems have significantly limited their use.

B. Rheumatoid Hindfoot—The foot is almost universally affected in RA. The hindfoot (talus, calcaneus, and talonavicular, talocalcaneal [subtalar], and calcaneocuboid joints) is frequently involved. Most commonly, the disease affects the posterior tibial tendon sheath, leading to valgus deformity and subluxation of the talonavicular joint. Early features include synovitis, pain, and diffuse swelling. Hindfoot deformity should be measured, and a cavus foot may be present. Radiographs, including weight-bearing views, may show soft tissue swelling, subchondral bone erosions, osteopenia, joint space narrowing, and bony destruction. Measurement of the talocalcaneal angle (the first TMT angle) is important, as is obtaining other views. Special studies (MRI) and selective injections may be helpful. Treatment initially consists of optimization of drug therapy. Mobilization and limited steroid injections may be helpful later. Shoe modification and inserts (especially arch supports for posterior tibialis tendonitis) can also help. Operative intervention includes selective fusion (talonavicular—usually satisfactory, but has a high rate of nonunion), or triple arthrodesis if advanced (including realignment). Other hindfoot disorders in RA include tenosynovitis (esp. peroneals > post tibialis), which is best treated with drug therapy, steroid injection, splinting, and occasionally tenosynovectomy. Stress fractures, neuropathies, nodules, vasculitis, and other problems also are commonly present.

C. Rheumatoid Forefoot—Forefoot is the most commonly affected portion of the foot. Often involves claw toe or hammer toe of the lateral four toes, severe hallux valgus, and plantar keratosis beneath subluxed or dislocated MTP joints. If conservative therapy (extra depth shoes with inserts) fails for the latter problem, the Hoffman procedure (excision of the metatarsal heads through a plantar incision) or metatarsal head trimming or resection through a dorsal incision ± excision of all or part of the proximal phalanx may resolve symptoms. The Dwyer procedure (excision of lateral four MT heads with first MTP and second through fifth PIP fusions combined with interposition of divided extensor tendon at the second through fifth MTP joints) is very successful in rheumatoid feet. **First MTP fusion is the procedure of choice for hallux valgus in rheumatoid feet** because it buttresses the other toes. This is usually required before or in conjunction with lesser toe correction. IP joint involvement is addressed with resection arthroplasty (Keller) or replacement arthroplasty.

XII. Diabetic Foot

A. Introduction—Number of patients has greatly increased in recent years, probably due to increased survival of diabetics. There are three categories of problems: ischemia, soft tissue neuropathic changes, and neuropathic arthropathy. Infection is often a complication of any of these three.

B. Dysvascular Foot-Large vessel disease is largely responsible for ischemia in the diabetic foot. Usually the problem is a painful, nonhealing ulcer with decreased pulses, rubor, and hair loss. Ulcers begin as small necrotic foci and evolve into indolent ulcers, esp. on the dorsal toes, sides of feet, and heel. Causes may be shoewear or minor trauma. The following grading system (Wagner) is often used:

GRADE	FINDINGS
0	Intact skin
1	Superficial ulcer of skin or subcutaneous tissue
2	Ulcers extend into tendon, bone, or capsule
3	Deep ulcer with osteomyelitis, or abscess
4	Gangrene of toes or forefoot
5	Midfoot and/or hindfoot gangrene

Evaluation should include radiographs (often with calcification of arteries), and Doppler pressures to include the ankle-brachial index (ABI) (ankle pressure/brachial pressure). An ABI of >0.45 may indicate that healing is possible. Artificial elevation of the ABI (>1.0) may be due to atherosclerotic disease stiffening the arterial wall. Toe pressure measurements are also helpful. Treatment for grade I or II lesions with an ABI >0.45 includes wound débridement and management (saline irrigation), oral antibiotics (grade 3 or higher with cellulitis), and shoewear modifications (Plastazote). Total-contact casts also decrease weight-bearing stresses on ulcerated surfaces. Edema, from poor venous drainage, can be treated with ephedrine. Surgical correction of hallux valgus, hammer toes, etc may be helpful. Grade III or higher lesions require surgical débridement or amputation. With an ABI of <0.45, consideration of a bypass grafting should be addressed. Failing this, amputations are still often preferable to continued conservative care.

C. Neuropathic Ulceration—Caused by insensitivity and pressure, typically includes stocking distribution of sensory loss, beginning with pain and temperature, is characteristic. Combined later with motor loss to the intrinsic muscles of the foot, leads to clawing of the toes and malperforans ulcers beneath the metatarsal heads. These ulcers are painless, rimmed by callus, and typically less necrotic than vascular ulcers. Wound care, orthotics insoles, total-contact casting, and ultimately surgery may be required. Surgery includes proximal osteotomy through the metatarsal metaphysis for plantar ulcers, and PIP fusion with shortened extensor lengthening and dorsal MTP joint capsulotomy for claw toes. Grade 3 ulcers require hospitalization for débridement and Grade 4 antibiotics. Education on foot care is essential for both dysvascular and neuropathic ulcers.

D. Neuropathic Arthropathy—Usually affects the midtarsal joints and can lead to prolapse of the arch or valgus deviation of the forefoot. Often difficult to distinguish from infection. A Charcot joint can result with fragmentation of periarticular areas and subluxations and most commonly involves the midfoot. History and physical exam (nontender, and glucose under control), labs (ESR), and other studies (bone/gallium scan) may be helpful in ruling out osteomyelitis. Treatment includes protection from weight bearing, casts, splints, and later shoewear with a double upright PTB brace. Arthrodesis may be required in some instances, but often fails.

E. Diabetic Foot Infection—Diabetics may be at increased risk of infection because of altered chemotaxis and other considerations. Diabetic infections are more often associated with multiple organisms, often require hospitalization, last longer, and may require surgical intervention. Deep cultures to include anaerobic cultures are important. Broad spectrum antibiotics (third generation cephalosporins pending identification of an organism) and aggressive I&D is essential. Abscesses can be include necrotic as well as purulent material. Bone biopsy may be required for identification of organisms if osteomyelitis is suspected. Amputations may be required (discussed in chapter 8).

Selected Bibliography

Baxter, D.E., Pfeffer, G.B., and Thigpen, M.: Chronic heel pain: Treatment rationale. Orthop. Clin. N.A. 20:563–569, 1989.

Bordelon, R.L.: Evaluation and operative procedures for hallux valgus deformity. Orthopedics 10:38–44, 1987.

Chapman, M.W., ed.: Operative Orthopaedics. Philadelphia, J.B. Lippincott, 1988.

Coughlin, M.J.: Subluxation and dislocation of the second metatarsophalangeal joint. Orthop Clin. N.A. 20:535–551, 1989.

Crenshaw, A.H., ed.: Campbell's Operative Orthopaedics, 7th ed. St. Louis, C.V. Mosby Co., 1987.

Dee, R., Mango, E., and Hurst, L.C.: Principles of Orthopaedic Practice. New York, McGraw Hill Book Co., 1989.

Floyd, D.W., Heckman, J.D., and Rockwood, C.A., Jr.: Tendon lacerations of the foot. Foot Ankle 4:8–14, 1983.

Gould, J.S.: Metatarsalgia. Orthop. Clin. N.A. 20:553–562, 1989.

Harrelson, J.M.: Management of the diabetic foot. Orthop. Clin. N.A. 20:605–619, 1989.

Jahss, M.H.: Disorders of the Foot. Philadelphia, W.B. Saunders Company, 1982.

Johnson, K.A.: Surgery of the Foot & Ankle, New York, Raven Press, 1989.

Karpman, P.R., Chairman.: American Orthopaedic Foot and Ankle Review Course Syllabus. Surgery of the Foot and Ankle, Oct. 1991.

Kitaoka, H.B.: Rheumatoid hindfoot. Orthop. Clin. N.A. 20:593–604, 1989.

Kirby, E.J., Shereff, M.J., and Lewis, M.M.: Soft-tissue tumors and tumor-like lesions of the foot. An analysis of eighty-three cases. J. Bone Joint Surg. [Am.] 71:621, 1989.

Mann, R.A., ed.: Surgery of the Foot, 5th Ed. St. Louis, C.V. Mosby Co., 1986.

Mann, R.A.: Surgical implications of biomechanics of the foot and ankle. Clin. Orthop. 146:111–118, 1980.

Mann, R.A., and Clanton, T.O.: Hallux rigidus: Treatment by cheilectomy. J. Bone Joint Surg. [Am.] 70:400–406, 1988.

Mann, R.A., Coughlin, M.J, and DuVries, H.L.: Hallux rigidus: A review of the literature and a method of treatment. Clin. Orthop. 142:57–63, 1979.

Mann, R.A., and Coughlin, M.J: Hallux valgus: Etiology, anatomy, treatment and surgical considerations. Clin. Orthop. 157:31–41, 1981.

Mann, R.A.: Treatment of the bunion deformity. Orthopedics 10:49–55, 1987.

Mann, R.A.: The great toe. Orthop. Clin. N.A. 20:519–533, 1989.

Morgan, C.D., Henke, J.A., Bailey, R.W., and Kaufer, H.: Long-term results of tibiotalar arthrodesis. J. Bone Joint Surg. [Am.] 67:546–550, 1985.

Nistor, L.: Surgical and non-surgical treatment of Achilles tendon rupture. A prospective randomized study. J. Bone Joint Surg. [Am.] 63:394–399, 1981.

Orthopaedic Knowledge Update Home Study Syllabus I, II, and III. Chicago, American Academy of Orthopaedic Surgeons, 1984, 1987, 1990.

Snook, G.A., Chrisman, O.D., and Wilson, T.C.: Long-term results of the Chrisman-Snook operation for reconstruction of the lateral ligaments of the ankle. J. Bone Joint Surg. [Am.] 67:1–7, 1985.

Wu, K.K.: Surgery of the Foot. Philadelphia, Lea & Febiger, 1986.

CHAPTER 5

Hand

I. Anatomy and Pathophysiology (see also Chapter 10, Anatomy)

A. Dorsal Extensor Compartments of the Wrist

Comp.	Tendons	Associated Pathologic Conditions
1	EPB, APL	de Quervain's tenosynovitis
2	ECRL/B	Carpal boss
3	EPL	Rupture over Lister's tubercle
4	EDC, EIP	Extensor tenosynovitis
5	EDQ	Rupture in rheumatoids (Vaughn-Jackson syndrome)
6	ECU	Snapping at ulnar styloid

B. Joint Flexion and Extension

Joint	Flexion	Extension
MCP	IO, lumbricals	EDC (sagittal bands)
PIP	FDS, FDP	Lumbricals (lateral bands), EDC (central slip)
DIP	FDP	EDC (terminal tendon), ORL (Landsmeer's ligaments)

C. Relationships

1. Extensor indicis proprius (EIP) and extensor digiti quinti (EDQ) are ulnar to extensor digitorum communis (EDC) tendons.
2. Cleland's and Grayson's ligaments cover the digital neurovascular bundles. Cleland's ligament is above (dorsal; ceiling) and Grayson's (volar; ground) is below the nerve.
3. There are four dorsal interosseous (IO) Abductors (DAB) and the three palmar IO Adductors (PAD). The long finger is considered the central axis of the hand.
4. The lumbricals are the "workhorse of the hand" and insert radially into the extensor apparatus (lateral bands). The two radial lumbricals are supplied by the median nerve, and the two ulnar lumbricals are supplied by the ulnar nerve. Ulnar innervated muscles are multipenniform; median-innervated lumbricals are unipenniform. The **lumbrical** is the only muscle that **relaxes its own antagonist** (flexor digitorum profundus [FDP]).
5. The thenar and hypothenar abductors are superficial; the opponens muscles are deep. The flexor pollicis brevis (FPB) has a dual innervation (median supplies the superficial fibers, ulnar the deep fibers). The abductor pollicis brevis (APB), which is innervated by the Me-

dian nerve, is the key thenar muscle involved in opposition.

6. The superficial arch is distal and is supplied by the ulnar artery; the deep arch is proximal and is fed by the radial artery. However, the classic complete arch (codominant) is present in only $\frac{1}{3}$ of patients.
7. Digital arteries are volar to nerves in the palm but are dorsal to the digital nerves in the fingers.
8. Autogenous Zones of Sensory Nerves

Nerve	Zone
Ulnar	Small finger pulp
Median	Index finger pulp
Radial	Dorsal first web space

9. Carpal Tunnel—Nine tendons in tunnel: eight finger flexors and flexor pollicis longus (FPL; most radial structure) in canal.

D. Pathophysiology

1. Intrinsic Minus or Claw Hand—**Hyperextension of MCPs and flexion of PIPs**, with a flattened metacarpal arch (Fig. 5–1); results from ulnar ± median nerve palsies or Volkmann's ischemic contracture. This condition has decreased grip strength, a weak pinch (positive Froment's sign), asynchronous movement, and loss of abduction and adduction. Operative treatment includes tendon transfers (Bunnell, Zancolli).
2. Intrinsic Plus or Tight Hand—Presents with **MCPs flexed and IP joints in extension**. It results from ischemia or fibrosis of the intrinsics and other causes such as rheumatoid arthritis. It is associated with stiffness and weak grasp. Patients will typically have more flexion of the PIP when the MCP is flexed than when it is extended (intrinsic tightness or Bunnell's test).
3. Lumbrical Plus Hand—Occurs when the lumbricals are tighter than the extrinsics. It can be caused by a FDP laceration distal to the lumbrical origin leading to the quadriga effect, loose tendon grafts, amputations, etc. It presents with paradoxical extension: active flexion of the MCP joint causes extension of the PIP joint.
4. Swan Neck Deformity—Results in PIP hyperextension and DIP flexion (Fig. 5–1). It is caused by dorsal subluxation of the lateral bands following flexor digitorum superficialis (FDS) rupture, or entrapment (i.e., trigger finger and rheumatoid nodules), volar plate injuries, ex-

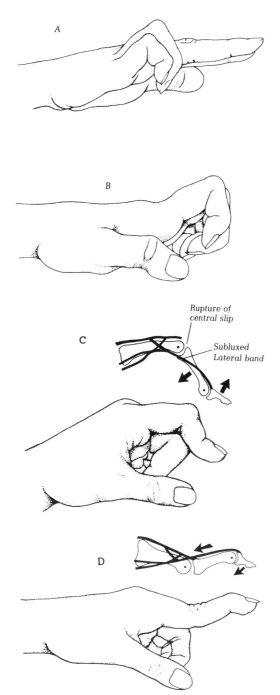

Rupture of
central slip

Subluxed
Lateral band

FIGURE 5–1. Anatomy of the hand. *A,* Ulnar claw hand. *B,* Ulnar and median claw hand. *C,* Boutonnière deformity. *D,* Swan neck deformity. (From The Hand, 2nd ed., pp. 67, 68, 69. Auroa, CO, American Society for Surgery of the Hand, 1983; reprinted by permission.)

trinsic adhesions, etc. Treatment must be individualized but includes central slip tenotomy (Fowler), or FDS tenodesis (Swanson).

5. Boutonnière Deformities—PIP flexion and DIP hyper- extension (Fig. 5–1); result from volar subluxation of the lateral bands usually following an unrecognized central slip rupture. Early diagnosis of central slip ruptures is important in avoiding this deformity. In addition to tenderness over the central slip, active extension

of the DIP with the PIP stabilized on the edge of a table (Elson test) can help in making the diagnosis. Boutonnière deformities are classically defined in four stages (Table 5–1). For established flexible boutonnière deformities with hyperextended DIP joints, an extensor tenotomy distal to the PIP is favored. Late reconstruction efforts may require central slip advancement or lateral band transfer.

6. The Quadriga Effect—Occurs when FDPs act as a single unit (i.e., individual finger flexion is not possible). This effect is caused by affected individual FDP tendons that share a common muscle belly. Usually presents with loss of maximum active flexion and decreased grip strength in adjacent digits. May be seen after digital amputation where flexors are sutured to the extensors or any time a FDP is tenodesed or lacerated (e.g., in replants, poor flexor tendon repairs, etc.).

II. Compressive Neuropathies

A. Introduction—The pathogenesis of compressive neuropathies is localized ischemia from mechanical entrapment of peripheral nerves (Fig. 5–2). This can be initiated by anatomic, postural, developmental, inflammatory, metabolic, neoplastic, iatrogenic, and idiopathic causes. Loss of vibratory sensation is typically the first manifestation. Indications for surgical decompression include failure of nonsurgical methods; acute, rapidly progressive symptoms; severe, chronic symptoms; recurrence; and the presence of motor weakness. ''Double crush'' syndrome (Upton and McComas) occurs when proximal compression interferes with axoplasmic flow and makes distal nerve function susceptible to mild compression.

B. Median Nerve

1. Pronator Syndrome—From entrapment of the nerve at the pronator teres or closely associated structures (**ligament of Struthers** [with supracondyloid process], lacertus fibrosis, FDS arch, etc.). Commonly associated with sensory findings (palmar cutaneous nerve distribution). Findings also include forearm muscle tenderness (positive Tinel's), pain with pronation and elbow flexion, and some weakness. The following provocative tests have been described:

Entrapment Location	Provocative Test
Lacertus/Struthers lig.	Elbow flexed 130°, resisted pronation
Pronator	Elbow extended, resisted supination
FDS arcade	Resisted flexion of middle finger FDS

EMGs are sometimes helpful. Avoidance of repetitive activity, NSAIDs, and temporary splinting are usually successful. Refractory symptoms in patients lasting more than 3 months may need exploration and release of all structures involved as listed above.

2. Anterior Interosseous Syndrome—Involves entrapment of this median nerve branch (usually at the origin of the deep head of the pronator

TABLE 5–1. STAGES OF BOUTONNIÈRE DEFORMITY

STAGE	DESCRIPTION	PRESENTATION	TREATMENT
1	Acute injury	Immediate	Splint in extension
2	Passively correctable	<2 weeks	Splint in extension
3	Retinacular contracture	2–4 weeks	Casting/joint jack
4	Articular stiffness	>8 weeks	Splint → capsulectomy

Nerves involved in common entrapment syndromes:

Median—5, 9, 10, 13
Ulnar—4, 6, 11
Radial—3, 7, 8, 12
Other—1, 2

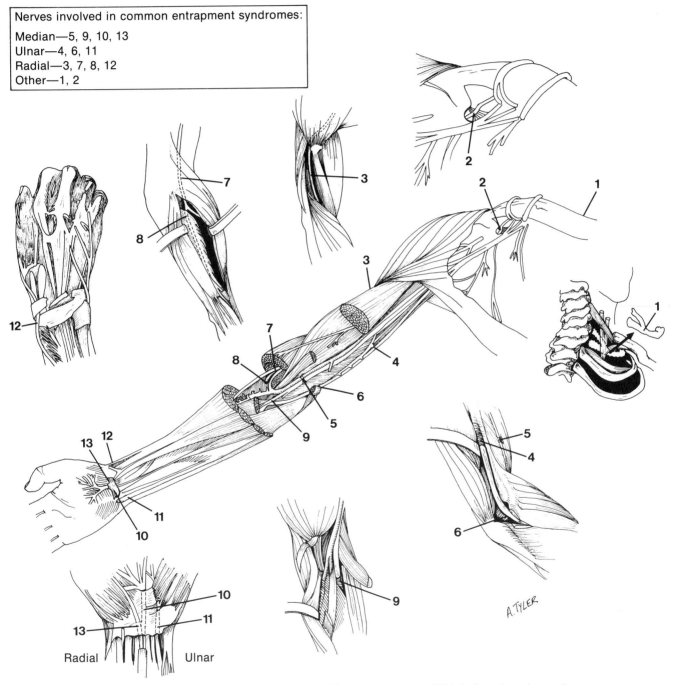

A. TYLER

FIGURE 5–2. Composite of upper extremity sites of nerve entrapment. *KEY: 1,* thoracic outlet syndrome; (lateral cord entrapment) *2,* suprascapular nerve entrapment; *3,* proximal humerus (radial nerve entrapment); *4,* arcade of Struthers (ulnar nerve entrapment); *5,* ligament of Struthers [off supracondylar process] (median nerve entrapment); *6,* cubital tunnel (ulnar nerve entrapment); *7,* radial tunnel (radial nerve entrapment); *8,* arcade of Froshe (posterior interosseous [deep radial] nerve entrapment); *9,* pronator syndrome (median nerve entrapment); *10,* carpal tunnel syndrome (median nerve entrapment); *11,* Guyon's canal ulnar tunnel syndrome (ulnar nerve entrapment); *12,* Wartenberg's syndrome (superficial radial nerve entrapment); *13,* flexor-retinaculum (palmar cutaneous branch of median nerve entrapment).

teres) that supplies motor innervation to the radial FDP, FPL, and pronator quadratus, causing forearm pain and **loss of precise pinch** (unable to make "OK sign"). Early, the patient may present with a "signpost" hand with poor flexion of the thumb and index finger. There are no sensory branches of this nerve and therefore there are **no sensory findings** with this syndrome. Important to rule out Mannerfelt syndrome (FPL rupture) in differential diagnosis. Failure of 3 months of conservative treatment is an indication for surgical exploration and release of accessory muscles, aberrant vessels, or tendinous bands that may be entrapping the nerve.

3. Carpal Tunnel Syndrome—The most common nerve entrapment syndrome. It results from compression of the median nerve within the carpal canal (under the transverse carpal ligament). Can be associated with diabetes, thyroid disease, alcohol abuse, amyloidosis, etc. Nerve compression most commonly is a result of flexor tenosynovitis. Diagnosis is confirmed with a classic history (night pain, paresthesias, clumsiness, etc.) as well as distribution of sensory complaints (median), APB weakness/atrophy, Tinel's sign, Phalen's sign, median nerve compression test, and diagnostic/therapeutic injections. As with all compressive neuropathies, nerve studies may be helpful (sensory conduction >3.5 ms) but are not always diagnostic. Activity modification, cock-up wrist splints, NSAIDs, and judicious use of steroid injections are often helpful. Carpal tunnel release using an ulnarly based incision to **avoid the palmar cutaneous branch** of the nerve is successful for treatment of refractory cases.

C. Ulnar Nerve
1. Cubital Tunnel Syndrome—From compression at the cubital tunnel (at flexor carpi ulnaris [FCU] origin) at the elbow. Findings include a positive Tinel's over the ulnar nerve and reproduction of symptoms with full elbow flexion. Grip weakness may also be present. Nerve conduction velocity studies are helpful (change in velocity across elbow). Compression can be secondary to trauma, deformity (cubitus valgus), subluxation of the nerve, bony spurs, tumors, aberrant muscles, etc. Activity modification and splinting are sometimes successful. Many procedures, including transposition, medial epicondylectomy and procedures that bury the nerve, have been devised but are not always successful. External and internal neurolysis can disrupt the blood supply to the nerve. The **arcade of Struthers** is a bridge of fibrous tissue beneath the medial intermuscular septum and medial head of the triceps (8 cm above medial epicondyle). It must be excised when the ulnar nerve is transposed.
2. Ulnar Tunnel Syndrome—From compression in Guyon's canal (ulnar and superficial to carpal tunnel). Usually caused by repetitive trauma (hypothenar hammer syndrome); arterial thrombosis or aneurysm may be present. Other offending structures include ganglia, lipomas, and fractures. Symptoms, if severe, may in-

clude intrinsic weakness and hypesthesias. Surgical release is occasionally indicated.

D. Radial Nerve
1. Proximal Entrapment—Rarely, the radial nerve can be entrapped as it crosses the lateral intermuscular septum in the arm (between the brachialis and brachioradialis). This is most commonly associated with humerus fractures and is addressed in Chapter 9, Trauma.
2. Posterior Interosseus Nerve (PIN) Syndrome—From entrapment of this main radial nerve branch in the arcade of Frohse (proximal supinator). Again, space-occupying lesions (lipomas, ganglia, displace fractures, etc.) may contribute to nerve entrapment. With the common presentation of "Saturday night" or "honeymoon" palsy from weight resting on forearm, classically the patient gives a history of awakening with a drop wrist. Patients may have increased pain with pronation and resisted supination of the forearm. The complete syndrome involves loss of extension to all digits and extensor carpi ulnaris (ECU); dorsiflexion of the wrist results in radial deviation. Distal PIN syndrome can cause dorsal wrist pain because the terminal branch of this nerve innervates the dorsal wrist capsule, but **cutaneous sensation is not affected**. The condition frequently spontaneously resolves, and treatment is observation. Surgical release through a dorsal (Thompson) approach is indicated for persistent symptoms.
3. Radial Tunnel Syndrome—From compression of the radial nerve. The radial tunnel is bounded by the brachioradialis and brachialis and extends distally to the distal border of the supinator. The radial nerve can be compressed at four levels within this tunnel: under the fibrous bands proximal to the supinator, under the radial recurrent vessels (leash of Henry), beneath the arcade of Frohse, and under the extensor carpi radialis brevis (ECRB) origin. **There are no motor or sensory deficits,** and it is often confused with tennis elbow. Typically, the pain is localized to an area 5 cm distal to the lateral epicondyle and is aggravated by stressing the extended middle finger (ECRB insertion is at the base of the third metacarpal [MC] or resisting forearm pronation. The mobile wad is intact and not affected by this syndrome. This may, in fact, be a mild PIN syndrome. Treatment includes activity modification, splinting, and often surgical exploration/release.
4. Superficial Radial Nerve Syndrome (Cheiralgia Paresthetica)—The superficial radial nerve can be compressed by tight fascial bands at the wrist as the nerve becomes superficial at the extensor carpi radialis longus (ECRL) and brachioradialis (BR) interval (Wartenberg's syndrome), leading to sensory disturbances. Exploration may reveal a pseudoneuroma.

E. Other Compressive Neuropathies
1. Thoracic Outlet Syndrome—From cervical ribs, anterior scalene muscle constriction, abnormal fibrous bands, or head of the sternocleidomastoid muscle compressing the lateral cord of the

brachial plexus. Typically affects young or middle-age females. Deficit is similar to ulnar nerve compression at the elbow combined with neck pain and paresthesias that are increased with overhead activities. Adson's test and hyperabduction stress test (3 minutes required) may be helpful in making the diagnosis. Radiographs should be examined for cervical ribs, pancoast tumors, and other problems. Arteriography is occasionally indicated (aneurysms are associated with cervical ribs). MRI can also be useful to rule out spinal disorders or soft tissue abnormalities. EMG/NCS studies may also be helpful to rule out other problems. Nonoperative treatment includes weight reduction and bracing-type exercises, and exercises with weights below chest level. Operative therapy includes rib resection ± scalenotomy.

2. Suprascapular Nerve—Entrapment of this nerve is uncommon and difficult to diagnose. Presents with deep diffuse pain in the posterolateral shoulder with radiation to neck and arm. Weakness and atrophy of the supraspinatus and infraspinatus are common. Symptoms are aggravated with arm adduction and palpation of the suprascapular notch. EMGs may be helpful; decompression is occasionally needed.

III. Tendon Injuries

A. Extensor Tendons—Pain may be the only symptom in proximal lacerations because junctura can function to extend digit. Partial lacerations (<50%) should not be repaired (actually weakens tendons). Treatment based on zones (Fig. 5–3).

1. Zone I (Central Slip Insertion Distal)—Repair lateral bands if they are injured. Mallet injuries (disruption of terminal tendon) can usually be treated closed with splinting of the DIP only (full time for 6–10 weeks then nighttime only for another 4–6 weeks). Classification is as follows: I, closed; II, laceration; III, deep abrasion; IV, epiphyseal. If there is bony involvement and the joint is subluxed >30–50%, some advocate ORIF.

2. Zone II (MCP to Central Slip)—Roll stitch (later pulled out) favored, especially over the MCP joint. Unrecognized/untreated injuries to the central slip can result in the development of a boutonnière deformity. The lateral bands displace volarly and create a tenodesis effect. Early diagnosis is best made with the Elson test (have patient extend PIP over edge of table). Early, nonoperative treatment includes splinting or casting in extension and use of a "reverse knuckle bender" orthosis. The senior editor feels that the best results are obtained with full-time use of a Capner splint for 8 weeks.

3. Zone III (Ext. retinaculum to MCP)—Permanent suture is acceptable in this zone.

4. Zone IV (Ext. Retinaculum)—Excise the overlying retinaculum after primary repair of the tendons. Some of the retinaculum should be left intact to prevent extensor tendon bowstringing.

5. Zone V (Proximal to Ext. Retinaculum)—Repair the musculotendinous unit.

6. Thumb Extensors—Treatment is similar. Late repair of the extensor pollicis longus (EPL) at the MCP joint may require rerouting the tendon around Lister's tubercle or EIP transfer.

7. Late repair of extensor tendon lacerations may require reconstruction. Tendon grafts using palmaris longus, plantaris, or toe extensors may be required. Postoperative splinting should allow 30–40 degrees of MCP motion.

B. Flexor Tendon Injuries—Repair also based upon zones: (Fig. 5–4). The **A2** (base of proximal phalanx) **and A4** (base of middle phalanx) flexor **pulleys should be preserved** or reconstructed if they are involved with these injuries.

1. Zone I (Distal to FDS insertion)—FDP avulsion is commonly seen with sports injuries (jersey finger—typically involves ring finger), and is best appreciated by having the patient flex their distal phalanx over the edge of a hard, flat surface with the proximal joints immobilized. Di-

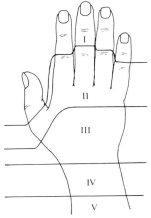

FIGURE 5–3. Extensor zones in the hand.

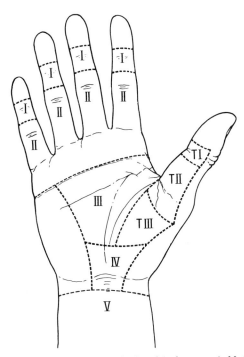

FIGURE 5–4. Flexor zones in the hand (refer to text). Note thumb zones (T). (From Tubiana, R.: The Hand, Vol. 3, p. 172. Philadelphia, W. B. Saunders, 1986; reprinted by permission.)

rect repair should be accomplished if possible, otherwise, advance to bone with pull-out suture if less than 1 cm of tendon remains. Repair volar plate if injured, and preserve A4 pulley. Zone I injuries can be repaired with graft if recognized late or retracted far, in a young patient, and if required for occupation (especially index finger). In older patients, DIP fusion is favored.

2. Zone II (Fibro-osseous Tunnel [MC Neck] to FDS Insertion)—"Bunnel's No man's land." Tendon lacerations will be distal to the skin laceration and at different levels in an injury to a flexed hand (e.g., by grasping a knife). Successful repairs are more difficult due to flexor sheath adhesion during healing. Repair both FDP and FDS and preserve both the A2 and A4 pulleys (over proximal and middle phalanx, respectively). One cm of tendon must be visible on each end for repair, which may require a distal window. With FDS be careful to recreate the normal anatomic spiral at Camper's chiasma. Late tenolysis is sometimes required.

3. Zone III (Transverse Carpal Ligament to Fibro-osseous Tunnel)—Repair all nerves and tendons through additional incisions if necessary. Late segmental grafting is helpful.

4. Zone IV (Transverse Carpal Ligament)—Although uncommon, repair through complete or incomplete transverse carpal ligament incision. Meticulous repair, Z-plasty or step-cut release with repair of the carpal ligament may avoid bowstringing. Immobilize postop with wrist at neutral and MCP joints more acutely flexed.

5. Zone V (Musculotendinous Junctions to Transverse Carpal Ligament)—accurate identification of the proximal and distal stump ["spaghetti wrist"] may be difficult. Look for hematoma in the tendon sheath or muscle belly. End to end repair is recommended.

6. Thumb—Similar guidelines apply, although cruciate pulleys are more important and should be preserved. Splint with 30 degrees of wrist flexion, and 15 degrees of MCP and IP flexion.

7. Principles—Core sutures should be palmar to the central axis of the tendon to preserve the dorsal blood supply. Supplementation with a running (Lembert) suture improves function and minimizes extrinsic healing. The strongest tendon repair is the Pulvertaft weave; the strongest suture is the Kirihmayer, a grasping suture later described by Kessler. The Kessler-Tajima stitch is popular. Sheath repair may improve gliding and initial nutrition. Repair is weakest at 7–10 days. Adhesions are best avoided with atraumatic technique, and a good postoperative program. Postoperatively only 5 mm of tendon excursion (passive) is required for 4 weeks. Begin active motion at this point; no full passive motion for 6 weeks. **Kleinert traction** allows controlled active extension and passive flexion with dorsal protective splint with flexed wrist and MCPs, and rubber bands under a roller bar from fingertip to forearm for 4 weeks, with wrist band traction for an additional 2–3 weeks if early motion is excellent. The **Duran program** is based on controlled passive motion with a dorsal block splint with full passive motion for the first 4 weeks, then weaning of the splint over the next 2 weeks and addition of active motion to wrist and composite digits. Late reconstruction techniques include the use of Silastic (Hunter) or silicone rods (the latter are preferred by the senior editor because of less synovitis) followed by staged tendon transfer (>3 months after rod insertion and after full passive ROM achieved).

IV. Infections

A. Overview—Infections are uncommon in the hand due to its good blood supply, but risk factors such as diabetes and fight bites should cause a high index of suspicion. Most hand infections involve *Staph. aureus* species, but polymicrobial infections are also common. Anaerobic species can be isolated in 30–40% of infections. Examination should include palpation of lymph nodes. Epitrochlear nodes drain the ring finger and small finger. Axillary nodes drain the radial digits. Cellulitis will resolve with antibiotics only, but pus under pressure requires surgical drainage (localized by the point of maximal tenderness). Initial IV antibiotics may resolve infection or localize area better.

B. Common Hand Infections—The following are some of the more common hand infections that are encountered.

1. Paronychia/Eponychia—Infection of the nail bed, the most common infection of the hand (Fig. 5–5). Best treated with I&D to include partial nail removal, loose packing, soaks, and oral antibiotics. An eponychia involves the entire eponychium and lateral fold.

2. Felon—Subcutaneous abscess of the distal pulp. I&D with lateral/dorsal incision and disruption of septae as well as antibiotics (usually IV antibiotics should be considered) is the treatment of choice. Avoid nerves, vessels, and flexor tendon sheath. Incisions should be placed lateral and ulnar (except in the thumb and small finger, where they should be radial).

3. Human Bite—Infections can be serious and, if they involve bone or joints, require formal I&D. Most commonly involves third and four-digit MCP joints. Although the most common organism involved is *Staph. aureus*, cover *Eikenella corrodens* (G−) with penicillin or Augmentin.

4. Dog and Cat Bite—Can also be very serious. Cover *Pasteurella multocida* (G− coccobacillus) with ampicillin (or, again, Augmentin). Early I&D required with any joint or flexor sheath penetration.

5. Suppurative Flexor Tenosynovitis—Infection of the flexor tendon sheath. If untreated, leads to tendon adhesions (decreased ROM) and necrosis. Presents classically with Kanavel's four cardinal signs: pain on passive extension (early), finger held in flexed position, *severe tenderness along the tendon sheath*, and symmetric swelling (sausage digit). Open I&D or closed irrigation is the correct treatment. Spread of infection into the deep spaces is as follows:

Index finger, thumb → thenar space
Middle, ring, small fingers → midpalmar space
Small finger → ulnar bursa

6. Radial and Ulnar Bursal Infections—FDP and

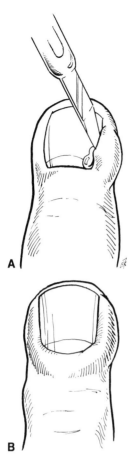

FIGURE 5–5. *A,* Paronychia. *B,* Eponychia. (From Bora, F. W.: The Pediatric Upper Extremity, pp. 362, 363. Philadelphia, W. B. Saunders, 1986; reprinted by permission.)

FDS (small finger) sheath infection with proximal extensions. Proximal extension requires I&D of these respective bursae. Ulnar bursa connects to small finger flexor sheath (Fig. 5–6).

7. Herpetic Whitlow—Seen especially in medical/dental personnel. Presents with pain, swelling, tenderness, and a vesicular rash. Usually involves thumb or index finger and may follow a viral illness. Splint, elevate, and restrict patient contact—**do not treat with I&D** for risk of systemic dissemination.

8. Deep Fascial Space Infections—Occur usually in the palm and may be limited to web space (**collar button** abscess). Treat with I&D both dorsally and volarly. Opening all deep spaces is required because the transverse MC ligament limits deep dissection; IV antibiotics to follow. With **midpalmar** infections (rare), there is loss of midline contour and pain on movement of the long, ring, and small fingers. With a **thenar space** infection there is thenar pain and pain on flexion of the thumb and index finger. Treatment for both includes I&D. Hypothenar space infections are rare.

9. Gangrene—**Necrotizing fasciitis** can be seen with streptococci (G+ cocci) (Meleny's) or with clostridia (G+ rod). Aggressive treatment is im-

mediate I&D or amputation and hyperbaric oxygen in some cases.

10. Sporotrichosis—From roses; lymphatic spread causing discoloration and small bumps on skin of hand/forearm. Treat with potassium iodine supersaturated solution (KISS).

11. Atypical *Mycobacterium* Infections—Include *Mycobacterium marinum* (seen in fishermen or pool workers), and *Mycobacterium kansasii* (in farmers). May present with chronic swelling and a nonhealing ulcer; biopsy and treat with appropriate antimicrobials. The specimens must be cultured at 30–32°C for identification. Oral rifampin and ethambutol or tetracyclene are often successful. Incision and drainage may be required.

12. Insect Bites—Brown recluse spider bite can cause areas of local necrosis and requires early wide local excision.

V. Vascular Occlusion/Disease

A. Compartment Syndrome—Increased tissue pressure within a limited space leads to decreased blood flow and function. Caused by fracture, soft tissue injury (classically ringer injury), arterial injury, drug/IV fluid infusion, burns, crush injuries, etc. Symptoms/findings include the "five Ps": pain, pallor, pulselessness, paresthesias, and paralysis. Pain (accentuated by passive stretching) is the most important and reliable parameter. Subacute compartment syndrome may not have classic signs but may develop late sequelae (progressive contractures, weakness). Recurrent compartment syndrome can occur in athletes with repetitive activities. Diagnosis is aided by measurement of compartment pressures. Myoglobinuria can lead to renal failure in severe cases. Fasciotomy is required if compartment pressures exceed 30 mm Hg or if there is any question. Compartments in the hand and digits frequently also must be released. Muscle viability can be determined by the "four Cs": color, consistency, contractility, and capacity to bleed.

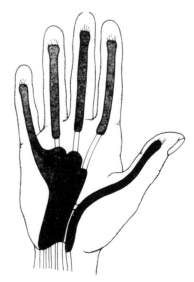

FIGURE 5–6. Tendon sheaths of the flexor tendon. Note communication of small finger sheath with ulna bursa. (From The Hand, 2nd ed., p. 96. Aurora, CO, American Society for Surgery of the Hand, 1983; reprinted by permission.)

B. Volkmann's Contracture—End result of compartment syndrome from injury to the deep tissues, usually the volar compartment. Can follow supracondylar or forearm fracture in children. Three varieties of established Volkmann's exist:

TYPE	AFFECTED MUSCLES	TREATMENT
Mild	Wrist flexors	Dynamic split, therapy, tendon lengthening/slide
Moderate	FDP/FDS, FPL, FCR/FCU	Tendon slide, neurolysis (M&U), extensor transfer
Severe	Flexors & extensors	Débridement, release, salvage procedures

C. Occlusive Disorders—Vascular occlusion can be caused by many factors, including:

1. Embolic Phenomena—Unusual in the upper extremity but can involve brachial artery from mural thrombi ± atrial septal defect.
2. Buerger's Disease—A paninflammatory arthritis in cigarette smokers characterized by development of tortuous digital arteries.
3. Hypothenar Hammer Syndrome—Ulnar artery spasm or thrombosis. Symptoms include pain, cold intolerance, numbness, and ulceration. Often seen in smokers, heavy alcohol users, and patients with hypertension, heart disease, or blood dyscrasias. It can be verified with Doppler studies ± angiogram, and treated with microvascular surgery (resection and grafting).
4. Frostbite—Can be treated with intra-arterial reserpine if warming is not sufficient.
5. Raynaud's...
   a. *Phenomenon*—Pallor of the digits, triple color changes (hyperemia, pallor, and cyanosis—red, white, and blue) with exposure to the cold.
   b. *Syndrome*—When Raynaud's phenomenon occurs in conjunction with a disease such as a connective tissue disorder, neurologic disorder, occlusive disorder, or blood dyscrasia.
   c. *Disease*—When Raynaud's phenomenon occurs without any underlying disease. Usually occurs in young females (often black) without clinical occlusion and peripheral arteries with *distal* trophic changes/gangrene.
   d. Treatment is based on addressing the underlying disease (if known), smoking cessation, avoiding cold weather, digital protection, calcium channel blockers, α blockers, calcitonin or serotonin antagonists, and sympathetic blockade. Digital sympathectomy may sometimes be indicated.

D. Reflex Sympathetic Dystrophy—Neurologic dysfunction following trauma, surgery, or disease characterized by intense/exaggerated burning pain, vasomotor disturbances, delayed functional recovery, and trophic changes of the extremity. Caused by sustained efferent activity from sympathetic fibers. If associated with a known nerve trunk injury it is termed "causalgia." Related to shoulder-hand syndrome.

1. Stages (Lankford and Evans):

STAGE	ONSET	FINDINGS
1—Acute	0–3 mos	Localized pain, swelling, warmth, decreased ROM, radiographs negative, triple-phase bone scan positive
2—Dystrophic	3–6 mos	Change in pain, glossy skin, cool, atrophy, contracture
3—Atrophic	6–9 mos +	Tight skin, flexion contractures, decr. temp, diffuse osteoporosis on radiographs (Sudek's atrophy)

2. Diagnosis—Four cardinal signs (pain out of proportion, swelling, stiffness, discoloration), endurance testing, and relief with sympathetic blockade are diagnostic. ESR, thermography, radiographs, and triple-phase bone scan (increased in both early and late phase) are also helpful.

3. Treatment—Splinting and physical therapy (TENS and fluidotherapy) are essential early. Later sympathetic block (stellate ganglion) can be curative. Sympathectomy considered if six to eight blocks provide initial relief, but with recurrence of signs and symptoms. Sympatholytic medications (guanethidine and reserpine) and steroids are sometimes helpful. Prevention (protecting nerves, avoiding tight dressings and casts, early treatment, etc.) is most effective.

VI. Replantations and Microsurgery

A. Traumatic Amputation

1. Replantation-Reattachment of a body part totally severed from the body; requires revascularization to restore viability. Attempted for all thumb amputations, patients with multiple digits amputated, all children, all amputations proximal to digits, and single digits **distal to FDS insertion** (Fig. 5–7). Thumb amputations

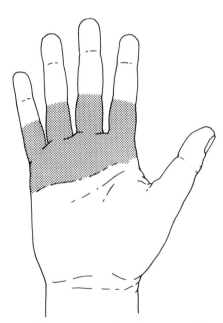

FIGURE 5–7. "No man's zone" is also a zone where single-digit replantation is not recommended. (From Magee, D. J. Orthopedic Physical Assessment, p. 109. Philadelphia, W. B. Saunders, 1987; reprinted by permission.)

should be salvaged or reconstructed (index pollicization or toe transfer) whenever possible. Contraindicated for mangled/crushed digits, with other life-threatening injuries, for individual digits proximal to FDS, for prolonged warm ischemia time, for severe ring avulsion (degloving) injuries, with arteriosclerotic vessels, and in mental patients. Maximum warm ischemia time is 6 hours; maximum cold ischemia time is 12–18 hours. Later repairs can lead to renal damage from muscle breakdown. High-volume diuresis and alkalization of urine (pH >6.5) will help. Sequence: Isolate nerves and vessels, débride, **shorten and fix Bone, repair Extensor tendon, repair Flexor tendon, anastomose Artery, then Nerve repair, and finally anastomosis of Veins [BEFANV].** Postop care includes anticoagulation, rest, monitoring (keep >30°C). Early failure is from thrombosis, which usually responds only to vascular revision. Results best in children (85% viable). Adults can usually expect 10–12 mm two-point discrimination, 50% total active motion (TAM), and cold intolerance for up to 2 years.

2. Ring Avulsion Injuries—Classified based on extent of injury (Urbaniak):

   I: Circulation is intact
   IIA: Arterial compromise but no bone, tendon or nerve injury
   IIB: Arterial compromise and bone, tendon and/or nerve injury
   III: Complete degloving or amputation

   Treatment is selective. Types I and IIA can be salvaged, but types IIB and III may not be salvageable and, if so, should undergo skeletal shortening and closure (injury proximal to FDS—see above).
3. Fingertip Amputations—Usually require only rongeuring of the exposed distal phalanx and allowing the wound to heal by secondary intention. Simple flaps (volar advancement flaps are useful for thumb tuft avulsions) and split-thickness skin grafting are alternative treatment options.

B. Elective Amputations—May be required because of infection, tumors, trauma, etc. Function is of primary importance, but cosmesis should be considered. Distal tuft amputations can be managed with rongeuring of bone to allow soft tissue coverage, and wound care to allow granulation tissue to cover the digit. Skin grafts may also be used. For more proximal amputations, contour the condyles, allow tendons to retract, and use generous volar flaps. For ray amputation, particularly with the long finger, suture the intermetacarpal ligaments or perform a transposition. Index ray amputations should include digital nerve transposition to lower the incidence of painful dysfunction. In crush injuries, bony defects should be stabilized before soft tissues are addressed. Late problems with digital amputations can be caused by adherence of tendons.

C. Microsurgery
1. Vessels and Nerves—Repair is limited to structures >0.3 mm diameter. Reversed vein graft patency can be improved with papaverine (with

cold heparinized blood), atraumatic technique, and controlled distention. Arterial repair with magnification requires exacting technique. Experimental mechanical coupling devices, thermic sleeves, and laser techniques may improve results in the future. Patency may be improved with topical agents (thorazine) and heparin infusion. Use of streptokinase is reserved for salvage procedures. Nerve repair should be primary when possible and done with 10-0 or 11-0 nylon suture under microscopic control. Poor prognosis is associated with intra-articular fractures, vascular impairment, and immediate precise loss of function. Other factors include patient age and condition, delay, level, and experience of the surgeon. Treatment should be delayed 4 months in the presence of intra-articular fractures, and 9 months following gunshot wounds. Key areas for digital nerve repair are ulnar thumb and radial index finger (pinch) and ulnar small finger. Fascicular matching (electrically or histochemically) improves results. Tube grafts may have future use. Nerve grafting may be required if primary repair is not possible (e.g., under tension). Lateral (LABC) or medial antibrachial cutaneous (MABC) nerve can be used to fill a segmental defect in a digital nerve; sural nerve grafts are used for larger defects. Again, best results are with younger patients. Specific guidelines for some nerves follow:

NERVE	REPAIR
Superficial branch radial n.	Resect proximally, avoiding a neuroma
Dorsal branch ulnar n.	Can repair at wrist
Ulnar n. at wrist	Match bundles for correct rotation
Median n. at wrist	Resect proximal neuroma and distal glioma
Digital n.	Primary repair using MABC nerve graft
Cranial n. XI (iatrogenic)	Neurolysis early (6 mos), reconstruction (Eden Lange—rhomboid and levator transfer) late

Differential motor and sensory staining may be of value in repairing chronic defects of mixed nerves.
2. Monitoring is done with transcutaneous oxygen monitors (requires precise temperature regulation and patient cooperation), tissue pH monitors (abrupt decline signifies arterial occlusion; slow decline is consistent with venous occlusion), or laser Doppler velocimetry (measures moving RBCs; less effective).
3. Flaps—If done for injury, are usually best accomplished within 72 hours (less scar, infection, and necrosis), but can be effective up to 1 week postinjury. **Flaps can also be very helpful in treatment of osteomyelitis after the wound is clean.** In the presence of dorsal hand burns, immediate escharotomy is preferred. The following types of skin flaps have been described (Fig. 5–8):

Type	Vessels	Example
Random pattern cutaneous	Random vessel supply	Abdominal
Axial pattern cutaneous	A + V supply	Scapular
Fasciocutaneous	Vessels in fascia	Radial forearm
Myocutaneous (pedicle)	Muscle w/ A + V	Plantar island
Free	Reattach vessels	Latissimus dorsi

Myocutaneous flaps can significantly reduce bacterial infection in tissues. Free muscle flaps, including latissimus dorsi and rectus abdominus muscles, have the advantage of being a one-stage procedure: they close the wound, enhance mobilization, and improve vascularity to the recipient area. The disadvantages of these flaps include the risk of flap loss, and they require extensive surgery. Local heel flaps include the instep flap (provides padding and innervation), FDB, abductor hallucis, and abductor digiti minimus flaps. **Gastrocnemius flaps are used for wounds in the proximal 1/3 of the leg (medial head for medial and *midline* defects, lateral head for lateral defects); soleus flaps for wounds in the middle 1/3 of the leg; and free myocutaneous (latissimus) flaps are used for the distal 1/3 of the leg and to cover large defects.** Expanded flaps have increased vascularity and may be useful. Newer indications for flaps include coverage of fourth-degree burns, peripheral vascular disease, and chronic osteomyelitis.

4. Other Tissue Transfers—Include free bone as an osteomyocutaneous free flap (e.g., vascularized fibula grafts), vascularized nerve graft (sural vascularized graft under investigation), and free functional muscle graft (e.g., gracilis and pectoralis major). Temporoparietal free flaps, dorsalis pedis flaps, and back fascial flaps can also be used.

5. Other Microsurgical Procedures in Hand Surgery—include digital sympathectomy for digital ischemia that improves with local anesthetic block.

D. Reconstruction of Bony Defects
1. Thumb

Location	Procedure
Proximal to MCP	Pollicization or toe transfer
Distal to MCP	Pollicization, toe transfer, or osteoplastic lengthening

2. Joints—Reconstruction with second toe joint transfer may be an alternative in children.

3. Bone—Allografts for metacarpal segmental defect may be useful.

VII. Wrist Pain/Instability

A. Introduction—Wrist instability often leads to wrist pain. Functional ROM of the wrist is 5 degrees of palmar flexion, 30 degrees of dorsiflexion, 10 degrees of radial deviation, and 15 degrees of ulnar deviation. Evaluation of wrist pain requires accu-

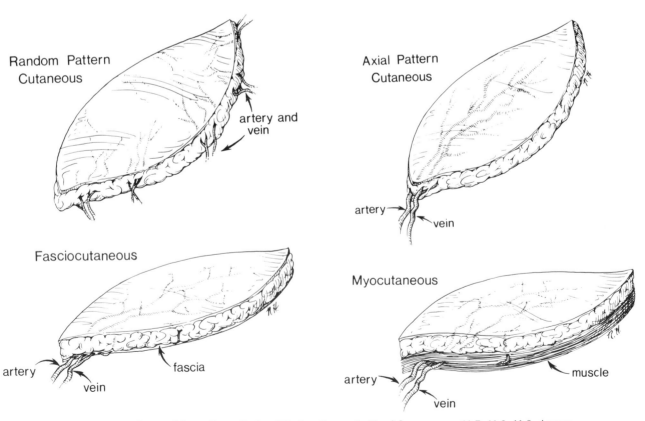

FIGURE 5–8. Types of flaps. (From Regional Review Course in Hand Surgery, pp. 11-7, 11-8, 11-9. Aurora, CO, American Society for Surgery of the Hand, 1990; reprinted by permission.)

rate history, documentation of motion, and localization of pain. Key tools in this effort include exam (PMT and provocative tests [e.g. Watson]), diagnostic injections, plain x-rays, bone scan, cineradiograms (for carpal instability), polytomograms, arthrograms (ligament injection), CT (structural abnormalities), MRI (avascular necrosis, [AVN], soft tissue tumors), and arthroscopy. The proximal row of carpal bones dorsiflex with ulnar deviation and palmar flex with radial deviation. The volar intercarpal ligaments (particularly the radioscaphocapitate and radioscapholunate) are important stabilizers of the wrist.

B. Wrist Instability—Many classifications have been developed, but most are based on the scapholunate angle (normal: 30–60 degrees) (Linscheid and Dobyns). Further classified based on dissociation (presence or absence of separation [gap]).

  1. Carpal Instability, Dissociative (CID)—Includes the following.

    a. Dorsal Intercalcated Segment Instability (DISI)—Can result from scaphoid fracture or scapholunate dissociation (usually secondary to disruption of the scapholunate interosseous and radioscaphoid ligaments, best seen with PA clenched fist view showing a gap >3 mm [Terry Thomas sign]). The disorder is also characterized by an **increased scapholunate angle** on lateral radiographs (>60 degrees) and an abnormal radiolunate angle. Rotary subluxation of the scaphoid decreases contact area and increases pressure at the radioscaphoid articulation. Acute injuries (within 3–6 weeks) should be immobilized or (if ligaments are 100% torn) repaired through a dorsal approach and stabilized with K-wires. Late reconstruction (>6 weeks) usually results in a salvage procedure (limited fusion, scaphoid-trapezium-trapezoid [STT] or scaphocapitate, proximal row carpectomy, or wrist fusion). Late repair is unpredictable.

    b. Volar Intercalated Segment Instability (VISI)—May result from disruption of the radial carpal ligaments on the ulnar side of the wrist and is characterized by a decreased scapholunate angle (<30 degrees). Exam should include a ballottement test (Reagan). Early treatment with closed reduction and casting (± percutaneous K-wires) may avert the need for difficult late ligamentous reconstruction or limited arthrodesis.

    c. Other types of CID can involve the distal row or be a combination of proximal and distal rows.

  2. Carpal Instability, Nondissociative (CIND)—Includes the following.

    a. Radiocarpal—From ligament injuries or deformity (e.g., Madelungs).

    b. Midcarpal (Triquetrohamate [TQH])—Disruption of this "helicoid" joint often presents with painful click (Lichtman) and ulnar tenderness. Triquetrohamate or four-bone arthrodesis may be indicated if conservative options fail.

    c. Combined Radiocarpal and Midcarpal—May result in wrist arthrodesis.

  3. Limited Arthrodesis—May be successful in some disorders with severe decreases in ROM (55% decrease with radiocapitate fusion, 27% decrease with intercarpal fusion between rows).

C. Diagnosis based on location.

  1. Radial—Can be scaphoid (fracture, dissociation, arthritis, or AVN), tendonitis, or other problems.

    a. Scaphoid Fracture—May not be seen on plain films until 10–21 days postinjury. Due to a precarious blood supply that enters the scaphoid predominately distally; nonunion and AVN are common in fractures of the scaphoid. The majority of fractures involve the middle third, and if there is no displacement or carpal instability, they heal with nonoperative treatment >90% of the time. Treatment should proceed by assuming a scaphoid fracture is present (with anatomic snuff box tenderness) until proven otherwise. Prolonged immobilization (up to 5 months) may be required. Displaced fracture requires ORIF and bone grafting. Bone grafting and internal fixation of nonunions is important to avoid progressive degenerative joint disease (DJD). Silastic implants should be avoided because of late development of cystic lesions. Although controversial, some authors (Watson) suggest that silicone disease will not occur if the wrist is adequately stabilized. Bone scan may have a role in early diagnosis. Polytomography is also helpful.

    b. Proximal Scaphoid Avascular Necrosis (Preiser's Disease)—Can be a late result of a scaphoid fracture because the blood supply enters the scaphoid distally. MRI may be helpful, but the presence of punctate bleeding when the proximal fragment is curetted is most prognostic. Russé bone grafting provides the best results.

    c. Perilunar Instability/Scapholunate Dissociation—Findings include history of injury (usually wrist extension and supination) and positive Watson test (clunk [dorsal displacement of proximal pole with radial deviation] with passive radioulnar wrist movement when scaphoid is immobilized volarly). X-rays may show widening of the scapholunate interval, scaphoid "ring" sign, and lack of parallelism on AP fist view; definitive study is wrist cinearthogram with radial and ulnar deviation. Four stages have been described (Mayfield). See also fig. 9–25.

STAGE	CHARACTERISTICS
I	Scapholunate diastasis
II	Perilunar dislocation
III	Lunotriquetral diastasis
IV	Lunate dislocation (volar)

Treatment includes ligament reconstruction and pinning (early), or intercarpal arthrodesis (STT fusion [Watson]) proximal row carpectomy or fusion (late).

d. Scapholunate Advanced Collapse (SLAC Wrist)—Can follow scaphoid fracture or scapholunate dissociation and is manifested by degeneration of the radioscaphoid and capitolunate joints (**radiolunate joint is spared**). Four stages are described (Fig. 5–9):

STAGE	INVOLVEMENT
1	Radial styloid and scaphoid
2	Radioscaphoid articulation
3	Capitolunate ± scaphocapitate joint
4	Scapholunate dissociation and migration of the capitate proximally

Treatment options include scaphoid excisional arthroplasty with capitolunate fusion, proximal row carpectomy, and wrist fusion. The first two options preserve motion but are associated with pain and decreased grip strength. Fusion allows maximum grip strength and no pain, but at the sacrifice of motion. Proximal row carpectomy requires

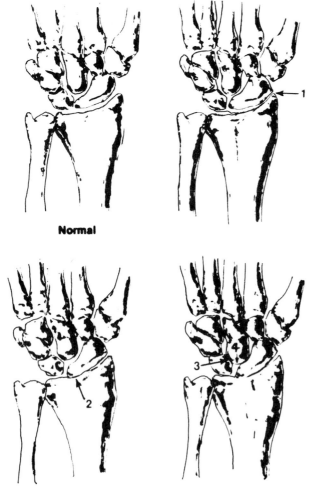

Normal

FIGURE 5–9. SLAC Wrist. Note the four stages of progression to proximal migration of the capitate. (From Watson, H. K., and Ryu, J. Evolution of wrist arthritis. Clin. Orthop. 202:61, 1986; reprinted by permission.)

good lunate fossae of the radius and proximal capitate articular surfaces. Fusions available include dorsal fusion with iliac crest bone graft to second and fourth MC, and AO plate (8–10 hole).

e. Triscaphe Degeneration (Trapezium-Trapezoid-Scaphoid)—Second most common degenerative pattern in the wrist. Treatment options include triscaphe (STT) fusion, trapeziectomy with soft tissue, or (rarely) silicone arthroplasty with trapezoid-scaphoid fusion and soft tissue interposition.

f. Lunotriquetral Sprain—Can be diagnosed with the "shear test" (Kleinman; shear force applied at this joint while stabilizing lunate dorsally and pisotriquetral plane volarly). Shuck test (Reagan) is similar but less specific. The compression test (Linscheid) applies axial load to this joint and is also less specific of lunotriquetral pathology. Treatment of lunotriquetral injuries is usually nonoperative. Occasionally, limited arthrodesis is required.

g. Tendonitis—Includes de Quervain's, tenosynovitis, flexor carpi radialis (FCR) tendonitis, and intersection syndrome.

(1) De Quervain's tenosynovitis involves the first dorsal wrist compartment. Most common in 30–50-yo females engaged in repetitive actions. Diagnosis is confirmed with the Finkelstein test (ulnar deviation of wrist with passive flexion of thumb causes maximum pain). Rule out CMC DJD with grind test and radiographs. Treatment includes injection, splinting, and first compartment release. Postoperative pain can be caused by neuromas of the superficial branch of the radial nerve (positive Tinels, hypesthesia) or inadequate decompression of the involved tendons. (Extensor pollicis brevis [EPB] usually lies in a separate compartment, and is often overlooked because both EPB and abductor pollicis longus [APL] can have several tendinous slips.)

(2) FCR Tendonitis—Similar to de Quervain's, with localized pain and tenderness on stretch. Splinting and injection are also helpful. Surgical treatment is rarely required.

(3) Intersection Syndrome—Caused by irritation at the intersection of the outrigger muscles (APL, EPB) and ECRL/ECRB. Supportive therapy, splinting and injections are helpful.

2. Ulnar—Includes instability, tendonitis, abutment, pisiform pathology, and TFCC injuries.

a. Ulnar—Carpal instability is less common but includes lunotriquetral instability CID (*VISI*) (point tenderness and positive ballottement test are diagnostic), and triquetral-hamate instability (CIND—midcarpal). Treatment may include lunotriquetral or triquetral-hamate fusion.

b. Tendonitis—Involves ECU or FCU.

(1) ECU Subluxation—Can palpate snap-

ping out of groove. Treatment involves operative stabilization.

(2) FCU Calcific Tendonitis—Represents a chemical process. Treatment is splinting and NSAIDs; aspiration/steroid injection is also useful. This is usually a self-limited process.

c. Ulnar-Carpal Abutment—Diagnosed radiographically (lytic lunate ± triquetrum [chondromalacia], and ulnar plus variant), and positive bone scan. Treatment is ulnar shortening. This and other distal radioulnar problems may benefit from a "matched" distal ulna resection (Bower's hemiresection arthroplasty), which preserves the ulnar styloid and TFCC.

d. Pisiform Pathology—Includes fractures (immobilize), and pisotriquetral DJD (inject or, if it persists, remove pisiform).

e. TFCC Tears—TFCC consists of the articular disc (triangular fibrocartilage), meniscus homologue (lunocarpal), ulnocarpal ligament, dorsal and volar radioulnar ligament, and ECU sheath. The TFCC is important in loading and stabilizing of the distal radioulnar joint. History of a twisting injury with palmar rotation and positive bone scan helpful. May be associated with ulnar plus variance. Arthrogram will demonstrate leakage of dye proximally. Treatment can be difficult but includes casting in supination, injections, joint leveling procedures, and arthroscopic débridement or repair.

3. Dorsal Wrist Problems—Include AVN of the lunate and capitate (very rare), distal PIN syndrome, occult ganglion, and abutment syndrome.

a. Kienbock's Disease (AVN of the Lunate)—Associated with ulnar minus variance and is described as having four stages (Lichtman):

STAGE	RADIOGRAPHIC	TREATMENT
I	Sclerosis	Conservative/splinting
II	Fragmentation	Joint leveling (radial shortening or ulnar lengthening)
III	Collapse	Controversial (most treat like stage II ± scaphocapitate or triscaphe (STT) and capitohamate fusion)
IV	Radiocarpal, intercarpal DJD	Salvage (fusion or proximal row carpectomy)

Radiographs, bone scan (positive before plain radiograph), and MRI all may have a role in diagnosis.

b. AVN of the Capitate—Rare; can follow a transverse fracture. Treatment is curettage/fusion.

c. Distal PIN Syndrome—See Section II: Compressive Neuropathies.

d. Occult Ganglion—Can cause dorsal wrist pain. Ganglions result from cystic degeneration within the dorsal scapholunate ligament and may be related to scapholunate pathology.

4. Palmar Wrist Problems—Can include carpal tunnel syndrome (discussed in Section II: Compressive Neuropathies), and volar carpal ganglion, which arises from the scaphotrapezial ligament.

VIII. Arthritis—Pain relief and increasing function are the primary considerations in dealing with the arthritic hand. Many arthritides affect the hand; some of the more common forms are discussed in this section.

A. DJD—Typically females are affected more than males. Joints commonly involved include the CMC joint of the thumb (diagnose with grind test, decreased pinch strength, and characteristic radiographs) and DIP joints of the digits (Heberden's nodes and mucous cysts), and less commonly the PIP joints (Bouchard's nodes). Treatment includes splinting, therapy, paraffin (digits), injections (CMC), and NSAIDs. Surgical options include mucous cyst and osteophyte excision, arthroplasty (PIP), arthrodesis (DIP), and interposition arthroplasty (CMC). Occasionally, DJD of the radial sesamoid of the thumb can cause pain at the CMC joint with narrowing of the space between the radial sesamoid and radial condyle of the metacarpal and osteophytes. Excision is usually helpful. Wrist DJD is discussed in Section VII: Wrist Pain/Instability.

B. Rheumatoid Arthritis (RA)—Systemic and soft tissue disease that affects the bones secondarily. Hypertrophic synovitis, if not controlled adequately medically, can destroy cartilage, compress or rupture tendons, affect nerves, and result in erosion and often dislocation of joints. Compensatory deformities often develop. Joints of the wrist and the MCP joints are most often affected. PIP joints can be involved with Sjögren's syndrome (associated with dry eyes/mouth). Synovitis can also lead to de Quervain's syndrome, carpal tunnel, trigger finger/thumb, and tendon ruptures.

STAGE	CLINICAL FINDINGS	TREATMENT
I	Early synovitis	Nonoperative medical management/splinting
II	Persistant synovitis	Synovectomy
III	Specific deformation	Reconstructive
IV	Severe crippling	Salvage

Splinting and therapy are important early. Surgery is often directed at correcting the specific problem (synovectomy—limited, use when isolated; preserve collateral ligaments). Surgical indications include pain, chronic synovitis not responsive to adequate medical therapy for 6 months, nerve entrapment, tendon rupture, and deformities resulting in decreased function. Tenosynovectomy is universally acceptable and prevents tendon rupture. This must be done early; however, because tenosynovitis is relatively painless, patients typically present late. A helpful axiom for surgical procedures in RA is to start proximally and work distally alternating fusion with motion-sparing procedures. Begin with predictable procedures. Staged procedures are usually favored, but the thumb is frequently addressed (usually with fusion) at the same time as other procedures (e.g., MCP arthroplasties). Deformity alone is not an indication for surgery. The procedure must be tailored to the individual's needs. The simplest, most successful procedure should be tried first. Goals of treatment should be (1) pain relief, (2) improved function, (3) preventing further damage, and (4) cosmesis. Severe, progressive deformities (arthritis mutilans, end-stage disease with a characteristic "opera-glass" hand) should be fused early to avoid progressive bone loss. Specific deformities and their management follow.

1. Intrinsic Plus Deformity—Results from intrinsic stiffness (diagnosed by Bunnel test—hold the MCP in extension and flex the PIP joint). Corrected with therapy or, if that fails, sometimes by intrinsic release/transfer (Littler distal, Zancolli proximal, especially later).
2. PIP Swan Neck Deformity—Dysfunctional disorder caused by muscle imbalance, (including FDS tenosynovitis), intrinsic tightness, and ligamentous/capsular relaxation at PIP leading to hyperextension. Treatment includes splinting early, PIP synovectomy, mobilization of lateral bands ± intrinsic release, and lengthening of the central slip; or tenodesis of the FDS proximal to the PIP (Swanson). The MCP joint must be addressed at the same time (arthroplasty) to balance the extensor mechanism. There is a high incidence of recurrence.
3. PIP Boutonnière—Functional deformity caused by extensor imbalance at MCP resulting in hyperextension or PIP synovitis leading to volar subluxation of the lateral bands. Patients may be unable to actively flex their DIP joints. Treatment includes injection early, release or reconstruction of the lateral bands distal to the PIP (lateral bands can be transfered to the attenuated or ruptured central slip), and release of the terminal tendon at the DIP. Later, salvage procedures or fusion are used. Soft tissue procedures commonly fail and are indicated only if the DIP can be passively flexed. PIP arthroplasties fail frequently, so arthrodesis is often favored at this joint for severe deformities. Fusion should be at 25–50 degrees of flexion at PIP (more flexion for ulnar digits).
4. MCP Ulnar drift—Occurs at the MCPs due to stretching of soft tissues and ulnar shift of the extensor tendons (exact etiology is obscure). Nonsurgical treatment includes rest, injection, splinting, and synovectomy—and results are unpredictable. Surgery includes realignment of extensor tendons and intrinsic balancing. If the deformity is severe (possibly including MCP dislocation—arthritis mutilans), MCP Silastic implants ± PIP fusion may be required. This often results in pain relief, improved function, cosmesis, and delayed progression. Patients should expect only limited improvement in motion—and no change in grip strength. Complications include recurrence, implant failure, infection (rare), and Silastic synovitis (very rare).
5. Tendon rupture—Can occur due to tenosynovitis.
   a. **Vaughn-Jackson Syndrome—Rupture** of the **EDC of the ring and small finger** secondary to caput ulna. This disorder is an attritional rupture that must be differentiated from subluxation (patient can maintain extension achieved passively), PIN palsy (tenodesis effect present [not present with rupture]), and locked trigger finger (no passive movement possible). Prior to rupture, extensor tenosynovectomy and ulnar resection (Darrah) can be done when the symptomatic wrist is unresponsive to medical management. The "tuck sign" (synovitis tucks under the skin with movement) is helpful. Wrist prosthesis implantation after a Darrah is contraindicated. Primary tendon repair may be possible early (within 4–6 weeks). Later, grafting (EIP to EDQ and ring finger EDC to long finger) and synovectomy are possible, but tendon grafts may become adherent, and therefore tendon transfer may be a better alternative.
   b. EPL—Related to avascularity of the tendon with subsequent rupture at Lister's tubercle. EPL rupture is best reconstructed with EIP transfer.
   c. **Mannerfelt Syndrome—FPL rupture** from carpal irregularities, volar synovitis, or volar carpal subluxation at the carpal tunnel. Patients typically have passive but not active flexion of the thumb at the IP joint. Treatment includes rerouting of the tendon or arthrodesis of the PIP joint and synovectomy after anterior interosseous nerve compression is first ruled out. FDP rupture is uncommon and surgery is less successful.
6. Thumb Deformities—Classified by Nalebuff into six common types (although several less common types were also noted) (Table 5–2; Fig. 5–10). MCP thumb fusion is the single most helpful hand procedure for RA.
7. Synovitis—Usually controlled by appropriate rheumatologic management. Synovectomy is indicated if synovitis is uncontrolled after 6 months of excellent conservative management, including medications and splinting. Surgical synovectomy must be meticulous and remove all synovium from the affected joint. Synovium will regenerate initially with normal synovium; however, this usually degenerates into rheumatoid synovium later. Tenosynovitis may present with difficulty with active PIP flexion, carpal tunnel symptoms, trigger finger, and de Quervain's; and is best managed with NSAIDs, splinting, selective injections, and ultimately release of the affected soft tissue. Persistent pain following de Quervain's release can be from a neuroma of the superficial radial nerve (hypesthesias, positive Tinel's) or inadequate release of the EPB tendon (numerous tendinous slips of APL can be deceiving). Careful surgical technique can avert these complications. Flexor synovectomy, as on the extensor side, can be of benefit in patients with boggy flexor synovium. Unlike in conventional triggering, the A1 pulley should be preserved in rheumatoids. MCP/PIP synovectomy (combined with intrinsic release at MCP) and extensor tendon relocation may allow temporary correction.
8. Wrist Involvement—Begins with synovitis at distal ulna, can lead to dorsal subluxation of the ulna (supination of hand on wrist) and carpal

TABLE 5–2. TYPES OF THUMB DEFORMITIES

TYPE	DEFORMITY	1MC	JOINT POSITION MCP	IP	INIATING FEATURE	COMMENTS
I	Boutonnière	Abd.	Flex.	Hyperext.	MCP synovitis	Arthroplasty, *MCP* (or IP) *fusion*, ± extensor realignment
II	Boutonnière and swan neck	Add.	Flex.	Hyperext.	MCP and CMC synovitis	Same as type I uncommon
III	Swan neck	Add.	Hyperext.	Flex.	CMC synovitis, MCP volar plate attenuation	CMC arthroplasty
IV	Gamekeeper's	Add.	Abd.	—	Ulnocarpal ligament destruction	Ligament reconstruction/ MCP fusion
V	—	Neutral	Hyperext.	Flex.	Stretching of MCP volar plate	MCP fusion
VI	Arthritis mutilans	Short	unstable	unstable	Bone destruction	Fusion

shift. Resection of the distal ulna (Darrah) and soft tissue procedures may help initially. Indications include pain at the distal radioulnar joint ± tendon rupture. Distal ulna resection can lead to carpal migration and ulnar snapping; therefore some favor preserving the distal ulnar buttress and TFCC with a hemiresection arthroplasty or a Lauenstein procedure (distal arthrodesis with proximal resection). Later, arthrodesis (in neutral or slight dorsiflexion) or wrist arthroplasties (Swansons can be successful in RA, especially with opposite side fused) are required. Fusion is often favored because of frequent failure of arthroplasties. The Nalebuff technique for wrist arthrodesis includes placing a Steinman pin through the third MC or interspace. AO fusion is preferred for younger patients. Concurrent distal ulnar resection is often necessary in rheumatoids.

9. Elbow—See Section XIII: Elbow Reconstruction.

C. Other Forms of Arthritis of the Hand—Include **systemic lupus erythematosus** (SLE), which causes ligamentous laxity affecting the MCPs, and **psoriasis,** which can involve the DIP joints with fu-

siform swelling of the digits and nail changes (it is also associated with a "gull wing" deformity). **Reiter's syndrome** and **gout** more commonly affect the lower extremity. **Scleroderma** or progressive systemic sclerosis is associated with skin and GI manifestation and calcinosis; ulcerations can lead to spontaneous fingertip amputations.

IX. Dupuytren's Disease—Proliferative fibrodysplasia of subcutaneous palmar connective tissue; can lead to contractures from nodules and cords that progressively develop. Associated with myofibroblast proliferation and increased quantities of type III collagen. Typically patients are >40 yo, males, of northern European ancestry, with positive family history, alcohol use, smoking, diabetes mellitus, or seizure history. Can be bilateral in 45%, and can be associated with similar fibrosis of the feet (Ledderhosen syndrome) in 5%, the penis (Peyronie's disease) in 3%, and the knuckle pads. Most frequently involves the ulnar digits. Dupuytren's diathesis is a more aggressive disease with early involvement. Dupuytren's typically involves the palmar aponeurosis and digital prolongations (not the superficial transverse ligament) in the palm; and involves the lateral digital sheet, Gray-

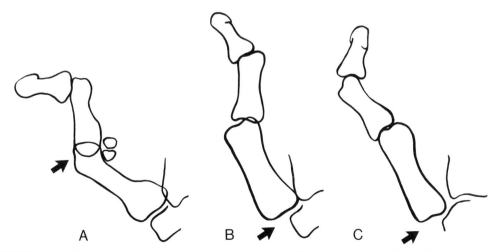

FIGURE 5–10. Nalebuff classification of common rheumatoid thumb disorders. *A*, Type I (boutonnière). *B*, Type II (boutonnière and swan neck). *C*, Type III (swan neck). (From Wiessman, B. N., and Sledge, C. B., eds.: Orthopaedic Radiology, p. 103. Philadelphia, W. B. Saunders Company, 1986; reprinted by permission.)

son's ligament (not Cleland's ligament), **pretendi-nous bands, natatory ligaments,** and **spiral bands** in the digits (Fig. 5–11). Typically, the digits develop central (pretendinous) and spiral cords. Surgical intervention is usually reserved for significant MCP involvement (30–45 degrees) and any PIP involvement. Careful dissection is necessary to preserve neurovascular structures as spiral cords can displace them. Selective subtotal palmar fasciectomy (STPF) is usually the recommended procedure. Leaving incisions open (open palm technique [McCash]) is favored for advanced disease, especially in diabetics. Dermofasciectomy (Hueston) may be required for recurrent cases. Postop complications include recurrence hematoma, skin loss, infection (treated with early débridement), joint stiffness, and occasionally RSD. Salvage options for severe PIP contractures include fusion, skeletal shortening, interpositional arthroplasty, and amputation.

X. Nerve Injury/Paralysis/Tendon Transfers—Paralysis can be at any level and from a variety of causes. Tendon transfers are helpful in allowing function when return of normal function has not occurred after the appropriate time period (classically regeneration of nerves can occur about 1 mm/day or 1 inch/month after a 1-month latent period following an injury). Principles of tendon transfers include first correcting all contractures and ensuring that there is adequate power and amplitude in the transfer. Muscle expendability and synergistic group of the donor muscle are also important. Amplitude of tendons can generally be considered in four groups:

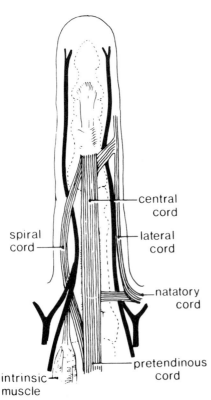

FIGURE 5–11. Pathoanatomy of Dupuytren's disease. (From Chiu, H. P., and McFarlane, R. M.: Pathogenesis of Dupuytren's contracture. J. Hand Surg. 3:9, 1978; reprinted by permission.)

TENDONS	AMPLITUDE
Wrist flexors/extensors, EPB, APL	30 mm
BR, lumbricals, Thenar muscles	40 mm
EDC, FPL, EPL	50 mm
FDS, FPL	60–70 mm

Muscle power can also be considered in groups:

MUSCLE(S)	RELATIVE POWER
FDP/FDS	4.5
FCU, BR, EDC	2
PT, FPL, ECU, ECRL	1.1
ECRB, FCU, FCR	0.9
PL, APL	0.1

One grade decrease of muscle strength with tendon transfer can be expected (5 = full, 4 = resistance, 3 = resistance against gravity, 2 = movement with gravity eliminated, 1 = trace of movement, 0 = no contraction). A straight line of pull for transferred tendons is best. Pulleys may be required if this is not possible. Synergistic muscle transfer and integrity (one transfer, one function) should be preserved if possible. Individual levels/nerves are considered below.

A. C-Spine Paralysis—Divided into three classes based on highest functioning level:

CLASS	LEVEL	FUNCTIONING MUSCLES	TRANSFERS
1	C5	BR only	BR → wrist ext. (Moberg)
2	C6	BR, ECRB/L	ECRL → FDP, BR → FPL
3	C7	BR, ECRB/L, FCR	FCR → thumb opposition

As a general rule, surgery should follow a year of observation. In partial/incomplete quadriplegia spasticity should be considered.

B. Brachial Plexus Injuries—Elbow flexion (biceps, C5 dysfunction) can be restored with latissimus dorsi flexoroplasty (Zancolli) or pectoralis major and minor transfer. Elbow extension can be restored with transfer of the posterior $\frac{1}{3}$ of the deltoid to the trapezius. Free functioning muscle transfer (gracilis, pectoralis major, latissimus) sometimes useful.

1. Anatomic Considerations—Root-level avulsions involve both anterior (plexus) and posterior (dorsal sensory) regions, whereas plexus injuries spare posterior areas. C4–C7 nerve roots are well secured to their respective vertebrae and are less prone to avulsion injuries; C8 and T1 roots are not. T1-level preganglionic injuries often include a Horner's syndrome due to disrupting the first sympathetic ganglion. Traction injuries are most common at C5 and C6 levels. Proximal cord lesions will injure supraclavicular branches as well as distal plexus and will lead to winging of the scapula (long thoracic nerve).

TABLE 5–3. DEGREES OF NERVE INJURY

DEGREE	DISCONTINUITY	DAMAGE	TREATMENT	PROGNOSIS
First	None; conduction block (neurapraxia)	Distal nerve fibers remain intact	Observation	Excellent
Second	Axon (axonotmesis)	Based on fibrosis	Observation	Good
Third	Axon and endoneurium	Based on fibrosis	Lysis	OK
Fourth	Axon, endoneurium, and perineurium	Fibrotic connective tissue connects	Nerve grafts	Marginal
Fifth	Complete (neurotmesis)	Complete	Graft/transfer	Poor

2. *Leffert Classification*

CLASS	DESCRIPTION
I	Open (usually from stabbing)
II	Closed (usually from motorcycle accident)
IIA	Supraclavicular
	1. Preganglionic—Avulsion of nerve roots, usually from high-speed injuries with other injuries and LOC. No proximal stump, no neuroma formation (negative Tinel's sign), pseudomeningocele, denervation of dorsal neck muscles are common sequelae. Horner's sign (ptosis, miosis, anhydrosis).
	2. Postganglionic—Roots remain intact; usually from traction injuries. There are proximal stump and neuroma formation (positive Tinel's), deep dorsal neck muscles are intact, and pseudomeningoceles will not develop.
IIB	Infraclavicular—Usually involves branches from the trunks (suprascapular). Function is affected based on trunk involved:

Trunk Injured	Functional Loss
Upper	Biceps, shoulder muscles
Middle	Wrist and finger extension
Lower	Wrist and finger flexion

III	Radiation therapy induced
IV	Obstetric (see Chapter 1, Pediatric Orthopaedics)
IVA	Erb's (upper root)—waiter's tip hand
IVB	Klumpke (lower root)
IVC	Mixed

The nerve injury can be classified into five degrees (Sunderland) (Table 5–3; Fig. 5–12).

3. Treatment—Controversial, but most closed injuries are treated with observation, usually for 3 months with passive ROM and bracing. If no progress or halted progress is noted, neurolysis and nerve grafting may be indicated. Fibrosis, which is subclassified based on extent, is common, and treatment is based on overcoming this problem. Nerve transfer (usually with neurotization of intercostal nerves) and muscle/tendon transfers are also helpful in some cases. Prognosis is guarded but is better with C5, C6 injuries. Open injuries (especially from lacerations) should be repaired primarily.

C. Upper Extremity Peripheral Nerve Paralysis—**Tendon transfers** (Table 5–4) and fusions should be considered as the final step in the rehabilitation of the hand following maintenance of full passive ROM, adequate soft tissue coverage, appropriate bony work, and adequate sensation. FDS tendons are often used in transfers because they are the most important expendable tendons, and they are best for motion, opposition, and strength.

D. Cerebral Palsy (CP)—The hand in CP is usually palmar flexed, and may have a thumb-in-palm de-

TABLE 5–4. TENDON TRANSFERS

TRANSFER	LOSS	RECONSTRUCTION
Low radial	EDC	FCU → EDC
	EPL	PL—(reroute) → EPL
	APL	PT → APL
High radial (Jones)	EDC	FCU → EDC
	EPL	PL—(reroute) → EPL
	APL	
	ECRB/L	PT (insertion) → ECRB
	BR	
Low ulnar	Adductor pollicis	BR—reroute around third MC → add. pollicis (Boyes); or FDS → add. pollicis (Royle-Thompson, Brand)
	IO (and ulnar Lumbricals)	Stabilize MCP (Zancolli capsulotomy, tenodesis, or bone block); or split transfers (FDS, EIP, etc.) to radial dorsal extensor apparatus
High ulnar	Adductor pollicis	BR—(reroute) → APL
	IO	As for low ulnar transfer
	FDS (RF, SF)	Suture to other tendons ± ECRL for power
	FCU	
Low median	Thumb opposition	FDS (ring finger) → FCU pulley → APB (Riordan); EIP → APB (opponensplasty); or muscle transfer (ADQ → APB) (Huber)
	Decreased sensation	Neurovascular island graft (ulnar ring finger → thumb)
	Radial first, second lumbricals	No significant deficit if ulnar nerve intact
High median	Pronation of forearm	
	Wrist flexion	
	Index and middle finger flexion	Suture to FDP of index and middle fingers ± ECRL transfer (adds power)
	Thumb flexion	BR → FPL
	Thumb opposition	EIP transfer to APB + EPL (Burkhalter)
	Decreased sensation	Neurovasclar island graft
Low median and ulnar	Palm sensation	Correct contractures, fuse IP if required
	Intrinsics	ECRB—tendon graft—intrinsics (Brand)
	Thumb opposition	FDS (ring finger) → FCU pulley → EPL (Riordan)
	Thumb adduction	EIP → adductor
High median and ulnar	Hand anesthesia	Arthrodesis of thumb MCP, (Zancolli)
	Flexors, intrinsics	Capsulodesis of MCP joints, ECRL → FDP, BR → FPL, ECU (with graft) → EPB

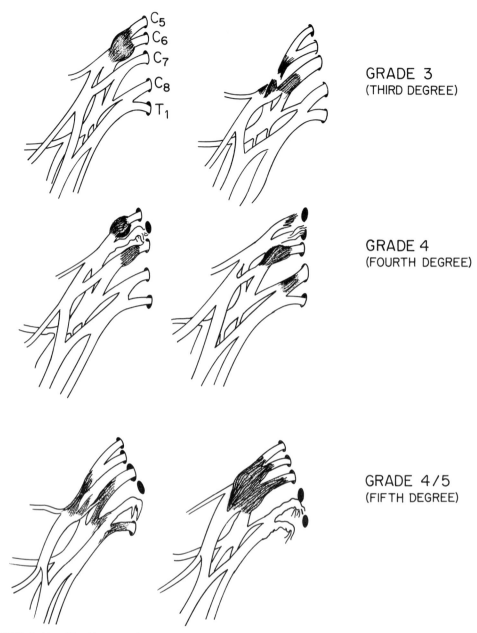

GRADE 3
(THIRD DEGREE)

GRADE 4
(FOURTH DEGREE)

GRADE 4/5
(FIFTH DEGREE)

FIGURE 5–12. Classification of nerve injuries. Grades 1 and 2 (not shown) have no macroscopic changes. (From Bora, F. W.: The Pediatric Upper Extremity, p. 250. Philadelphia, W. B. Saunders, 1986; reprinted by permission.)

formity, a flexed elbow, and a pronated forearm. Patients may also demonstrate mirror movements of the upper extremities and poor sensation. Usually surgery is indicated only for spastic hemiplegia with a reasonable IQ. Nonoperative treatment includes splinting in extension and with thumb out of palm. Surgery includes early myotomies after 7 yo (APB and FPB release); later tendon transfers (pronator teres for pronation deformities; FPL radial and proximal for thumb-in-palm; FCU to EDC for finger extension and release, or FCU to ECRB/L if finger extension is possible with an extended wrist—used in patients with a weak grasp); and finally arthrodesis (fuse wrist only if fingers can extend in fixed position and patient is at least 12 yo). Elbow flexion contractures may be present

with normal pronation and supination. Early treatment is observation. Later, musculocutaneous neurectomy or biceps/brachialis release may be effective for contractures <30 degrees caused by increased biceps tone.

E. Neuromas—Usually result from disorderly growth of resected nerves; become sensitive to mechanical stimulation and develop spontaneous activity. Usually responsive to treatment with anticonvulsants and local injection with local anesthetics ± steroids.

XI. Congenital Hand Disorders

A. Introduction—Genetic cause in 30%, nongenetic (environmental) in 10%, and unknown in 60%.

Goals of surgery in these disorders are to preserve or improve function and appearance. Timing of surgery should be immediate if extremity is threatened (e.g., constriction band), within the first year if disorder has a tethering growth effect (e.g., club-hand), before age 3 if development patterns are influenced (e.g., pollicization), and delayed until past 4 years in cases that require cooperation of the child (e.g., tendon grafts).

B. Digits

1. Syndactyly (Joined Phalanges)—One of the most common congenital hand deformities, and is the most common anomaly in the United States. **More common in white males** and most frequently involves the ring and long fingers. Can be simple (skin only), complex (bony involvement), complete (entire length of digits), or incomplete/partial (Fig. 5–13). Release should be done at 18 months to 5 yo and usually requires a skin graft. Can be associated with many different anomalies, including Poland's syndrome (also associated with chest wall anomalies), Streeter's dysplasia, and Apert's. **Apert's syndrome** (acrocephalosyndactyly) is a severe form of syndactyly involving all of the

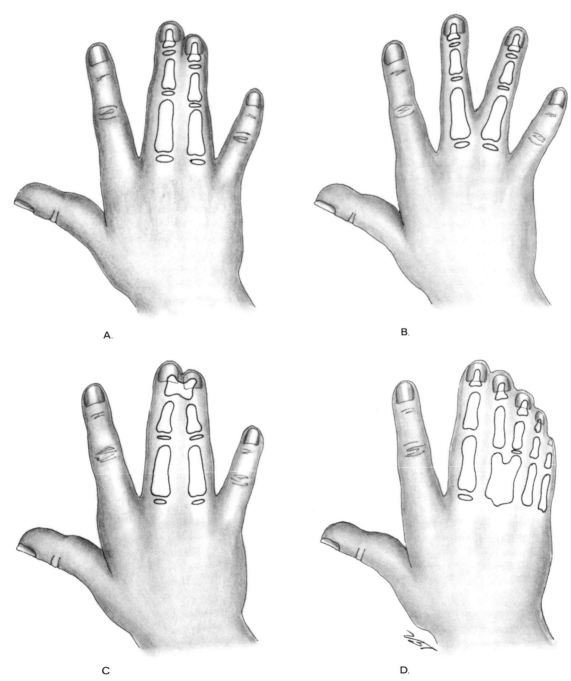

A.

B.

C

D.

FIGURE 5–13. Classification of syndactyly. *A*, Complete simple syndactyly. *B*, Incomplete simple syndactyly. *C*, Complex syndactyly. *D*, Complex syndactyly and polydactyly. (From Tachdjian, M. O.: Pediatric Orthopaedics, 2nd ed., p. 223. Philadelphia, W. B. Saunders, 1990; reprinted by permission.

digits, which also have limited interphalangeal motion, and sometimes is associated with mental retardation, visceral abnormalities, and grotesque facies. Surgery is indicated earlier in this case, and should initially address the thumb and small finger. Web space contractures following release are common (decreased incidence with large zigzag incisions and dorsal flaps). Skin graft is required, and careful neurovascular dissection is necessary.

2. Polydactyly (Duplicated Phalanges)—The most common congenital hand abnormality, **more common in blacks**. Usually involves ulnar digits (postaxial), especially in blacks. Can be one of three types based on development: I—extra soft tissue only, can be treated in nursery with ligation; II—includes bone, tendon, and cartilage; and III—completely developed with own metacarpal (rare). Involvement of radial digits (preaxial), usually only the thumb, is more common in whites, and is often associated with a generalized syndrome. Wassel classification (Fig. 5–14) commonly used: I = bifid distal phalanx (DP), II = duplicated DP, III = bifid proximal phalanx (PP), IV = duplicated PP (most common type), V = bifid metacarpal (MC), VI = duplicated MC, VII = triphalangism. Surgical excision of least developed digit (preserving the ulnar collateral ligament), or a combination of bifid portions (Bilhaut-Cloquet) is recommended. Postaxial (ulnar) is more common in blacks and orientals and is isolated.

3. Brachydactyly (Short Digits)—Highly variable presentation. Amputation of useless tiny nubbins is recommended. If empty digital skin sleeve is of sufficient size, a nonvascularized toe proximal phalanx transfer to fill the skin sleeve and to create an MCP joint is favored prior to 12 months of age. Vascularized second toe transfer has limited indications.

4. Macrodactyly—Involves enlargement of all structures, especially the nerves of one or more digits. Can be isolated or **associated with** generalized disorders such as **neurofibromatosis**. Two types based on proportionate increase with growth. Osteotomy or physeal arrest may be helpful. Digital nerve resection does not diminish growth.

5. Deviated Digits
   a. Clinodactyly—Skeletal abnormality with deviation in the *lateral* plane, usually involves the small finger at the joint; often seen in mentally retarded patients. It is usually caused by a trapezoid-shaped middle phalanx. Closing wedge osteotomy may be done, but only for cosmesis.
   b. Camptodactyly—Familial soft tissue abnormality with deviation in the *AP* plane. May be secondary to aberrant lumbrical insertion, abnormal FDS, or an abnormal extensor apparatus. Commonly involves the small finger with a flexion contracture of the PIP joint and may be associated with a PIP flexion deformity. There are two peaks in presentation (3 and 13 yo). Passive stretching or static splinting may correct the deformity. Few good surgical options exist. FDS transfer to

the extensor hood, if the deviated digit is passively correctable, is acceptable.
   c. Kirner's Deformity—Incurling of small finger DP in prepubertal females. Treatment usually is observation. Hemiephysiodesis is required for early deformities, osteotomies are required late.
   d. Symphalangism—Stiff PIPs secondary to congenital ankylosis of the joint. Often associated with Apert's syndrome and brachydactyly. Treatment is observation, especially in children.
   e. Delta Phalanx—Triangular phalanx and physis, usually the proximal phalanx of thumb and small finger with deviation toward the middle digit. Realignment procedures are indicated with severe deformation.

6. Thumb Anomalies (Hypoplastic Thumb)—Generally are best corrected at about 1 year of age and are classified as follows (Bauth):

Grade	Description	Treatment
I	Short thumb, hypoplastic thenar muscles	Augment intrinsics
II	Like grade I with adducted thumb MCP	Soft tissue Z-plasty
III	Deficient metacarpal abducted thumb	Augment/bone graft or pollicization
IV	Floating thumb	Pollicization
V	Absent thumb	Pollicization

   a. Congenital Flexion/Adduction of Thumb (Thumb-in-Palm or "Clasped Thumb" Disorder)—EPB weakness or absence, XR inheritance, usually bilateral. Passive correction early, EIP transfer late.
   b. Anomalous FPL Insertion—Reroute insertion of FPL around APB for better function.
   c. Congenital Hypoplasia of Thumb—Absent EPL and APL. Treated by tendon transfers (EIP to EPL, PL to APL) and MCP arthrodesis.
   d. Floating Thumb—Attached to radial surface of hand by a slender pedicle with skeletal support, usually containing a single neurovascular bundle and no intrinsic or extrinsic structures. Treatment is ablation of the pouce flottant.

7. Congenital Trigger Finger/Thumb—Congenital stenosing tenosynovitis at A1 pulley. Often bilateral, with fixed flexion contractures at presentation. Up to 30% may resolve spontaneously by 1 year of age. Attempt splinting early and correct surgically before 2–3 yo to avoid permanent flexion contractures.

8. Constriction Band/Ring (Streeter's Dysplasia)—Most commonly involves digits, especially central fingers and toes, but can be more proximal. Fibrous amniotic bands can cause intrauterine constriction of extremities. Associated with syndactyly, club feet, and neurologic abnormalities. Treatment includes Z-plasties and avoidance of amniocentesis with future children.

9. Congenital Amputation—Can be due to constriction bands or failure of development. Most

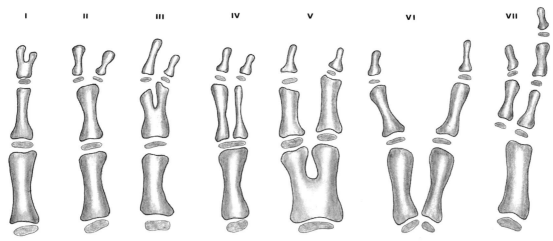

FIGURE 5–14. Wassel classification of thumb polydactyly. (From Tachdjian, M. O.: Pediatric Orthopaedics, 2nd ed., p. 243. Philadelphia, W. B. Saunders, 1990; reprinted by permission.)

common form is very short below-elbow amputation, usually with radial head dislocation. Treatment can include lengthening of digits, toe transfers, index finger pollicization, or prosthesis if more proximal. **Passive terminal devices are indicated as early as 3–6 months** of age (when the child is able to sit upright) in the upper extremity. With complete absence of the hand, a Krukenberg procedure (creation of a radial-ulnar claw) may be indicated in blind children.

C. Hand, Wrist, and Forearm
   1. Clubhand (Hemimelia)
      a. Radial Clubhand (Radial Aplasia [Preaxial])—Disorder of radial development leading to radial deviation of the hand, absent scaphoid, stiff fingers, and sometimes hypoplastic thumb. It is most common in the right hand (bilateral in 50%) of males. Any radial deformity can have concomitant heart or GI/GU abnormalities. These children usually have symptoms that can be discovered at the same time. Can be **associated with aplastic anemia** (Fanconi's syndrome [AR] with pancytopenia, brown skin pigment, aplastic thumb, hip dislocation, and poor prognosis); **thrombocytopenia** (TAR—thrombocytopenia absent radius, which is always bilateral, AR, and often with lower limb anomalies [especially knee dysplasia]); **heart anomalies** (Holt-Oram-Lewis); *VATER* (*V*ertebral anomalies, imperforate *A*nus, *T*racheal-*E*sophageal aplasia, and *R*enal [and cardiac] anomalies); and chromosomal abnormalities (trisomy 17). Classified I–IV based on amount of radius present (Bayne) (Table 5–5). Intercalary variety includes an absent radius with normal carpus and first ray. Longitudinal type has a normal ulna. Treatment initially may involve early splinting, manipulation ± soft tissue releases (median nerve may be radially displaced and immediately subcutaneous!). Later, centralization of the distal wrist/hand over

the ulna with a "shish kebab" procedure within the first year of life is favored. Newer centralization procedures (radialization) do not disrupt the carpal bones and require less immobilization time. Contraindications to surgery include severe associated medical problems and stiff, nonfunctional elbow.
      b. Ulnar Clubhand (Postaxial)—Much less common. Also classified into four subtypes (Miller):

TYPE	ULNA	ELBOW	TREATMENT
A	Anlage	Radial head dislocated	None
B	Absent	Radial head dislocated, cubital webbing	Radical release; amputation
C	Anlage	Synostosis	Humeral osteotomy
D	Neutral	Synostosis	None

Ulnar clubhand is not associated with systemic disorders, as is radial hand, but can be associated with other musculoskeletal (esp. digital) disorders. Treatment of digital disorders (syndactyly release, web deepening) often requires surgical intervention.
      c. Central Deficiencies (Cleft Hand)—Often AD, bilateral, and may have foot deformities. Classified as follows (Blauth and Falliner):

TYPE	CATEGORY	FEATURES	TREATMENT
I	Typical	Bilateral, familial, syndactyly	Close defect
II	Atypical	Severe, lobster claw	Krukenberg
III	Absent rays	Best function	Syndactyly release

   2. Reduplication of the Ulna (Mirror Hand)—Ulna and carpus are reduplicated, leaving seven or eight digits and no thumb. Treatment includes

TABLE 5–5. CLASSIFICATION OF RADIAL CLUBHAND

Type	Characteristics	Radiographic Findings	Clinical Findings	Treatment
I	Short distal radius	Delayed distal epiphyses	Hypoplastic thumb	Address thumb
II	Hypoplastic radius	Defective proximal and distal epiphyses, short radius, bowed ulna	Short forearm	Individualized
III	Partially absent radius	Usually medial/distal ⅓; thick, bowed ulna	Short and bowed deviation	Centralization†
IV	Totally absent radius*	Radius absent, forearm deviated	Marked deviation, elbow stiffening	Centralization†

* Most common; † contraindicated with stiff elbow.

removing the most abnormal digit and pollicization of a digit to create a five-digit hand and correct radial deviation of the hand.

3. Congenital Radial-Ulnar Synostosis—Union of the forearm bones, usually proximally, placing the forearm in pronation; most often bilateral. Associated with developmental dysplasia of the hip, clubfoot, and chromosomal abnormalities. Two types exist: (1) medullary canals of both bones are joined, creating a large radius with anterior bowing; and (2) proximal radius dislocation with less extensive fusion, usually unilateral. Both types are difficult to treat. Consider osteotomies for disabling pronation deformities. If bilateral, leave the dominant arm pronated and osteotomize the nondominant arm at the distal portion of the fusion mass, for 20–30 degrees of supination. Can be associated with fetal alcohol syndrome (associated also with brachydactyly and camptodactyly). Surgical release should be considered if motion, function, and potential growth of interconnected segments are interfered with. Classified based on location of synostosis and the position of the radial head.

Type	Synostosis	Radial Head
I	Fibrous	Normal
II	Osseous	Normal
III	Osseous	Hyperplastic Posteriorly dislocated
IV	Short/osseous	Anteriorly dislocated

4. Congenital Dislocation of the Radial Head—Abnormally formed head on a long radius with a bowed ulna. Often associated with a connective tissue disorder. Abnormal shape of capitellum differentiates this condition from traumatic dislocations. Treatment includes therapy and late head resection (after growth is complete). This will relieve pain but will not correct abnormality/ROM.

5. Madelung's Deformity (AD, Female > Male)—Abnormal growth of the distal radial epiphysis with premature fusion of the ulnar half of the distal radius. Can cause progressive ulnar and volar angulation. Early treatment includes observation, especially in the asymptomatic patient. Operative treatment includes ulnar shortening ± dorsal radial closing wedge osteotomy

for severe cases. Epiphysiolysis of the ulnar/palmar aspect of the radius may also be successful.

6. Congenital Pseudarthrosis of the Forearm—Rare disorder associated with neurofibromatosis. Can be cystic (leads to fractures and pseudarthrosis and is refractory to treatment) or associated with diaphyseal narrowing (more destructive with proliferative fibrous tissue). Vascularized bone graft may be helpful.

7. Lipofibromatous Hematoma of the Median Nerve—Rare enlargement of median nerve at the wrist; can present as a progressive macrodactyly. Microvascular excision is difficult.

8. Congenital Webbing of the Elbow (Pterygium Cubitale)—Characterized by a broad skin web spanning the elbow, a flexion deformity, and pronated forearm. Can be associated with other webbing disorders and underlying muscle abnormalities (esp. biceps and BR). Surgery is difficult and usually hazardous and, since it sometimes requires vessel and nerve lengthening, it may not be helpful.

XII. Hand Tumors (See Also Chapter 7, Orthopaedic Pathology)

A. Benign Tumors

1. Giant Cell Tumor of the Tendon Sheath (Fibroxanthoma)—A benign but highly recurrent lesion that may originate in tendon sheaths or joint synovium. It is usually seen on the palmar surface of digits, especially at PIP of index and long fingers. It is slow growing, and recurs in 10% of excisions. Second most common hand mass (next to ganglions).

2. Vascular Tumors/Abnormalities
   a. False Aneurysm—Does not include all layers of the arterial wall. Can follow trauma late but may not have a bruit.
   b. True Aneurysms—May be difficult to differentiate. Will have all layers of arterial wall on pathologic exam.
   c. A-V Fistula—May have thrill or bruit with decreased distal filling.
   d. Glomus Tumor—Tumor that frequently involves the nail bed with classic triad of pain, **tenderness, and cold sensitivity**. Nail **bed** ridging ± a small blue spot at base of nail can be seen. Radiographs may show a shelled out dorsal lesion. Treatment is excision; usually a normal nail matrix can be preserved.

e. Kaposi's Sarcoma—Vascular tumor associated with AIDS.
3. Neural Tumors—Traumatic neuromas are usually iatrogenic from prior operative procedures, and treatment includes excision and transfer to a deeper, padded area. Neurofibromas are less common, and rarely require excision (only if irritating). Neurilemmomas are also uncommon, but should be excised while protecting the involved nerve.
4. Enchondroma—Most destructive benign lesion of bone, usually in proximal phalanx. Frequently a cause of pathologic fractures. Radiographs show lytic lesion. Curettage and bone grafting may be required **after fracture healing**.
5. Lipomas-Common in 30–60-yo females, can be mistaken for ganglions. Mobile, nontender. Excision may be required.

B. Tumorous Conditions
1. Ganglion—The most common hand mass. Usually dorsal carpal ganglion (over scapholunate ligament) but can be volar (from ST interval) or elsewhere. Lesions are soft, nontender, and transilluminant. Treatment includes aspiration or rupture and surgical excision (with a portion of the wrist capsule) if it recurs and is symptomatic.
2. Epidermoid (Inclusion) Cyst—Implantation of epithelioid tissues into deeper areas as a result of penetrating trauma. Mildly painful palmar bulboid deformity that transilluminates. Mass is nontender and subcutaneous. Radiographs may show a cystic lesion. Excision and curettage requires preserving very little overlying adherent skin.
3. Mucous Cyst—Usually at dorsal DIP joint in adult females these cysts are actually ganglias that originate from the DIP joint. Frequently associated with Heberden's nodes, osteophytes that should be removed at surgery.
4. Volar Retinacular Cyst—Located at volar A1 pulley. These often disappear spontaneously. Treatment includes aspiration and removal of a window of the pulley if it recurs.
5. Foreign Body Granuloma—Firm, fibrous capsule and deep granuloma; resolves with resection.
6. Calcinosis—May be secondary to degeneration. Symptoms include pain, tenderness, and erythema. Commonly occurs near FCU insertion. Treatment includes heat, rest, injection/aspiration, and surgery for larger deposits. Calcinosis circumscripta can be seen in SLE, RA, and scleroderma, usually in the fingers, and may be associated with Raynaud's phenomenon. Treatment may include partial excision.
7. Déjérine-Sottas Disease—Localized swelling of a peripheral nerve from hypertrophic interstitial neuropathy. Usually involves median nerve and may require carpal tunnel release. Resection of the pathology is not possible without resecting the nerve.
8. Turret Exostosis—Traumatic subperiosteal hemorrhage that follows trauma. Extracortical bone beneath the extensor mechanism can be excised after the bone matures.
9. CMC Boss—Bony growth at bases of second and third metacarpal. Special radiographs can demonstrate the osteophytes, which may be resected if symptoms warrant. Associated with ganglia at least 30% of the time, and often associated with os styloideum (accessory ossicle).

C. Malignancies—Extremely rare in the hand. Most common primary malignancy of the hand is squamous cell carcinoma. This tumor in the hand requires aggressive treatment (usually amputation). The most common bony malignancy in the hand is chondrosarcoma. Most common metastasis in the hand is from lung (and may involve DP).

XIII. Elbow Reconstruction

A. Introduction—The medial collateral ligament is a more important stabilizer than the lateral collateral ligament. Functional ROM 30–130 degrees with 50 degrees of pronation and supination.
B. Distal Biceps Tendon Rupture—rare. Presents with painful swollen elbow usually in a 30–50-yo active male. If treated nonoperatively, supination and flexion strength affected (35–40%) and patients complain of prolonged pain. Repair with two-incision approach (Boyd and Anderson anterior and posterior incisions) to decrease incidence of radial nerve injury, but may be associated with increased incidence of synostosis.
C. Tennis Elbow
1. Lateral Epicondylitis—Common degeneration at extensor origin, usually ECRB. Conservative treatment: strap, wrist extension stretching exercises, NSAIDs, injections (peritendinous, *not* intratendinous), etc. Surgical treatment: release of origin (slide) or excision of fibrinous tissue at ECRB origin. This disorder is often difficult to distinguish from posterior interosseous nerve compression.
2. Medial Epicondylitis—Less common (10%) in tennis players; may be seen more commonly in golfers and baseball players. Usually responds to conservative treatment (injections, casting, bracing, etc.). It is commonly associated with ulnar nerve neurapraxia. Rarely, surgery (pathology usually localized to EDC origin) is indicated.
D. Rheumatoid Elbow—Three primary methods of treatment.
1. **Synovectomy—With radial head excision** if secondary change present; useful if done early in the disease process. Radial head implant is not required. Also useful in hemophiliacs with refractory hemarthrosis. Arthrodesis rarely indicated, because of increased incidence of failure.
2. Total Elbow Arthroplasty—Greater constraint leads to loosening, lower constraint leads to instability. Has evolved to semi-constrained design. Increased complications (esp. infection) with revisions.
3. Excisional Arthroplasty with Interposition of Various Substances—Good motion but unstable (esp. in rheumatoids).
E. Contractures—If arthrosis is absent, anterior capsulotomy is often effective to regain some extension in a posttraumatic patient.

Selected Bibliography

Allen, B.N., Frykman, G.K., Unsell, R.S., et al.: Ruptured flexor tendon tenorrhaphies in zone II: Repair and rehabilitation. J. Hand Surg. [Am.] 12:18–21, 1987.

American Society for Surgery of the Hand: Regional Review Courses in Hand Surgery, San Antonio, Texas, October 13–14, 1990.

Badalamente, M.A., Stern, L., and Hurst, L.C.: The pathogenesis of Dupuytren's contracture: Contractile mechanisms of the myofibroblasts. J. Hand Surg. 8:235–243, 1983.

Bayne, L.G., and Klug, M.S.: Long-term review of the surgical treatment of radial deficiencies. J. Hand Surg. [Am.] 12:169–179, 1987.

Beckenbaugh, R.D.: Total joint arthroplasty: The wrist. Mayo Clin. Proc. 54:513–515, 1979.

Bieber, E.J., Weiland, A.J., and Volenec-Dowling, S.: Silicone-rubber implant arthroplasty of the metacarpophalangeal joints for rheumatoid arthritis. J. Bone Joint Surg. [Am.] 68:206–209, 1986.

Bora, F.W.: The Pediatric Upper Extremity. Philadelphia, W.B. Saunders, 1986.

Brumfield, R.H., Jr., and Resnick, C.T.: Synovectomy of the elbow in rheumatoid arthritis. J. Bone Joint Surg. [Am.] 67:16–20, 1985.

Burke, F., and Flatt, A.: Clinodactyly. A review of a series of cases. Hand 11:269–280, 1979.

Chapman, M.W., ed.: Operative Orthopaedics. Philadelphia, J.B. Lippincott, 1988.

Chow, S.P., and Ho, E.: Open treatment of fingertip injuries in adults. J. Hand Surg. 7:470–476, 1982.

Cooney, W.P., Linscheid, R.L., Dobyns, J.H., et al.: Scaphoid nonunion: Role of anterior interpositional bone grafts. J. Hand Surg. [Am.] 13:635–650, 1988.

Crenshaw, A.H., ed.: Campbell's Operative Orthopaedics, 7th ed., St. Louis, C.V. Mosby Co., 1987.

Daniel, R.K., and May, J.W., Jr.: Free flaps: An overview. Clin. Orthop. 133:122–131, 1978.

Daniel, R.K., and Weiland, A.J.: Free tissue transfer for upper extremity reconstruction. J. Hand Surg. 7:66–76, 1982.

Dee, R., Mango, E., and Hurst, L.C.: Principles of Orthopaedic Practice. New York, McGraw Hill Book Co., 1989.

Eaton, R.G., Glickel, S.Z., and Littler, J.W.: Tendon interposition arthroplasty for degenerative arthritis of the trapeziometacarpal joint of the thumb. J. Hand Surg. [Am.] 10:645–654, 1985.

Epps, C.H., ed.: Complications in Orthopaedic Surgery, 2nd ed. Philadelphia, J.B. Lippincott Company, 1986.

Ewald, F.C., and Jacobs, M.A.: Total elbow arthroplasty. Clin. Orthop. 182:137–142, 1984.

Failla, J.M., Amadio, P.C., and Morrey, B.F.: Post-traumatic proximal radio-ulnar synostosis. Results of surgical treatment. J. Bone Joint Surg. [Am.] 71:1208, 1989.

Fatti, J.F., Palmer, A.K., and Mosher, J.F.: The long-term results of Swanson silicone rubber interpositional wrist arthroplasty. J. Hand Surg. [Am.] 11:166–175, 1986.

Flatt, A.E.: The Care of Congenital Hand Anomalies. St. Louis, C.V. Mosby, 1977.

Gelberman, R.H., Van de Berg, J.S., Lundborg, G.N., and Akeson, W.H.: Flexor tendon healing and restoration of the gliding surface: An ultrastructural study in dogs. J. Bone Joint Surg. [Am.] 65:70–80, 1983.

Gelberman, R.H., Wolock, B.S., and Siegal, D.B.: Current concepts review. Fractures and non-unions of the carpal scaphoid. J. Bone Joint Surg. [Am.] 71:1560, 1989.

Goldberg, V.M., Figgie, H.E., III, Inglis, A.E., and Figgie, M.P.: Current concepts review. Total elbow arthroplasty. J. Bone Joint Surg. [Am.] 70:778, 1988.

Green, D.P., ed.: Operative Hand Surgery, 2nd ed. New York, Churchill Livingstone, 1988.

Green, D.P.: Proximal row carpectomy. Hand Clin. 3:163–168, 1987.

Jaeger, S.H., Tsai, T., and Kleinert, H.E.: Upper extremity replantation in children. Orthop. Clin. North Am. 12:897–907, 1981.

Kleinert, H.E., Kutz, J.E. and Cohen, M.: Primary repaired zone 2 flexor tendon lacerations. AAOS Symposium on Tendon Surgery in the Hand, pp 115–124, C.V. Mosby, 1975.

Kleinert, J.M., Stern, P.J., Lister, G.D., and Kleinhans, R.J.: Complications of scaphoid silicone arthroplasty. J. Bone Joint Surg. [Am.] 67:422–427, 1985.

Kleinman, W.B., Steichen, J.B., and Strickland, J.W.: Management of chronic rotary subluxation of the scaphoid by scapho-trapezio-trapezoid arthrodesis. J. Hand Surg. 7:125–136, 1982.

Kudo, H., and Iwano, K.: Total elbow arthroplasty with a non-constrained surface-replacement prosthesis in patients who have rheumatoid arthritis. A long-term follow-up study. J. Bone Joint Surg. [Am.] 72:355, 1990.

Levinsohn, E.M., Palmer, A.K., Coren, A.B., et al.: Wrist arthrography: The value of the three compartment injection technique. Skeletal Radiol. 16:539–544, 1987.

Lichtman, D.M., Noble, W.H., and Alexander, C.E.: Dynamic triquetiolunate instability. J. Hand Surg. 9:185, 1984.

Linscheid, R.L., Dobyns, J.H., Beckenbaugh, R.D., Cooney, W.P.: Instability patterns of the wrist. J. Hand Surg. 8:682–686, 1983.

Lister, G.D., Kalisman, M., and Tsai, T.M.: Reconstruction of the hand with free microneurovascular toe-to-hand transfer: Experience with 54 toe transfers. Plast. Reconstr. Surg. 71:372–384, 1983.

McCash C.R.: The open palm technique in Dupuytren's contractions. Br. J. Plastic Surg. 17:271, 1964.

McFarlane R.M.: The current status of Dupuytren's disease. J. Hand Surg. 8:703, 1983.

Mackinnon, S.E., and Holder, L.E.: The use of three-phase radionuclide bone scanning in the diagnosis of reflex sympathetic dystrophy. J. Hand Surg. [Am.] 9:556–563, 1984.

Miller, J.K., Wenner, S.M. and Kruger, L.M.: Ulnar deficiency. J. Hand Surg. 11A:822–829, 1986.

Morrey, B.F.: The Elbow and Its Disorders. Philadelphia, W.B. Saunders, 1985.

Morrey, B.F., and An, K.N.: Functional anatomy of the ligaments of the elbow. Clin. Orthop. 201:84–90, 1985.

Morrey, B.F., and Bryan, R.S.: Revision total elbow arthroplasty. J. Bone Joint Surg. [Am.] 69:523–532, 1987.

Nalebuff, E.A.: Surgical treatment of the Swan Neck deformity in rheumatoid arthritis. Orthop. Clin. N.A. 15:369, 1984.

Nirschl, R.P., and Pettrone, F.A.: Tennis elbow: The surgical treatment of lateral epicondylitis. J. Bone Joint Surg. [Am.] 61:832–839, 1979.

Omer, G.E., and Spinner, M., eds.: Management of Peripheral Nerve Problems. Philadelphia, W.B. Saunders, 1980.

Orthopaedic Knowledge Update Home Study Syllabus I, II, and III. Chicago, American Academy of Orthopaedic Surgeons, 1984, 1987, 1990.

Palmer, A.K., and Werner, F.W.: The triangular fibrocartilage complex of the wrist: Anatomy and function. J. Hand Surg. 6:153–162, 1981.

Reagan, D.S., Linscheid, R.L., and Dobyns, J.H.: Lunotriquetral sprains. J. Hand Surg. [Am.] 9:502–514, 1984.

Simmons, B.P., Southmayd, W.W., and Riseborough, E.J.: Congenital radioulnar synostosis. J. Hand Surg. 8:829–838, 1983.

Smith, R.J., ed.: Symposium on congenital deformities of the hand. Hand Clin. 1:371–596, 1985.

Smith, R.J., Atkinson, R.E., and Jupiter, J.B.: Silicone synovitis of the wrist. J. Hand Surg. [Am.] 10:47–60, 1985.

Strickland, J.W.: Flexor tendon repair. Hand Clin. 1:55–68, 1985.

Sunderland, S.: Nerves and Nerve Injuries, 2nd ed. Edinburgh, Churchill Livingstone, 1978.

Swanson, A.B., Swanson, G.D., and Tada, K.: A classification for congenital limb malformation. J. Hand Surg. 8:693–702, 1983.

Taleisnik, J.: Current concepts review. Carpal instability. J. Bone Joint Surg. [Am.] 70:1262, 1988.

Tolego, L.C., and Ger, E.: Evaluation of the operative treatment of syndactyly. J. Hand Surg. 4:556–564, 1979.

Upton, A.R.M., and McCames, A.J.: The double crush in nerve entrapment syndromes. Lancet 1:359, 1973.

Urbaniak, J.R., Evans, J.P., and Bright, D.S.: Microvascular management of ring avulsion injuries. J. Hand Surg. 6:25–30, 1981.

Urbaniak, J.R., Hansen, P.E., Beissinger, S.F., and Aitken, M.S.: Correction of post-traumatic flexion contracture of the elbow by anterior capsulotomy. J. Bone Joint Surg. [Am.] 67:1160–1164, 1985.

Urbaniak, J.R., Roth, J.H., Nunley, J.A., Goldner, R.D., and Koman, L.A.: The results of replantation after amputation of a single finger. J. Bone Joint Surg. [Am.] 67:611–619, 1985.

Vicar, A.J., and Burton, R.I.: Surgical management of the rheumatoid wrist: Fusion or arthroplasty. J. Hand Surg. [Am.] 11:790–797, 1986.

Watson, H.K., and Ballet, F.L.: The SLAC wrist: Scapholunate advanced collapse pattern of degenerative arthritis. J. Hand Surg. [Am.] 9:358–365, 1984.

Weiland, A.J., Kleinert, H.E., Kutz, J.E., and Daniel, R.K.: Free vascularized bone grafts in surgery of the upper extremity. J. Hand Surg. 4:129–144, 1979.

Weissman, B.N., and Sledge, C.B., eds.: Orthopaedic Radiology. Philadelphia, W.B. Saunders, 1986.

Wood, V.E.: Polydactyly and the triphalangeal thumb. J. Hand Surg. 3:436–444, 1978.

Zancolli, E.A., and Zancolli, E.J.: Surgical management of the hemiplegic spastic hand in cerebral palsy. Surg. Clin. North Am. 61:395–406, 1981.

Zancolli, E.: Structural and Dynamic Basis of Hand Surgery, 2nd ed. Philadelphia, J.P. Lippincott, 1979.

CHAPTER 6

Spine

I. Differential Diagnosis

A. Congenital Anomalies and Deformities—Discussed in detail in Chapter 1, Pediatric Orthopaedics.

B. Back Pain—A ubiquitous complaint. Standard work-up, beginning with history taking (most important) and progressing to physical examination (Table 6–1). Radiographic and laboratory studies can help in diagnosis. Some important considerations in the evaluation of back pain are presented below.

1. Age—Children may be affected by congenital or, more commonly, developmental disorders, infection, or primary tumors. Younger adults are more likely to suffer from disc disease, spondylolisthesis, or acute fractures. In older adults, spinal stenosis, metastatic disease, and osteopenic compression fractures are more common.

2. Radicular Signs and Symptoms—Often associated with disc herniation or spinal stenosis. Intraspinal pathology or other entities associated with cord or root impingement may be responsible. Herpes zoster is a rare cause of lumbar radiculopathy with pain preceding the skin eruption.

3. Systemic Symptoms—Careful history taking can lead to the diagnosis of metabolic disease, ankylosing spondylitis, or infection (confirmed with laboratory studies). Associated signs and symptoms may be essential to the diagnosis (e.g., ophthalmologic symptoms with spondyloarthropathies; other joint involvement—rheumatoid arthritis [RA], osteoarthritis [OA]; etc).

4. Referred Pain—"Back pain" can often be viscerogenic, vascular, or related to other skeletal areas (especially with hip arthritis). Careful history and physical exam are essential.

5. Psychogenic—Psychological disturbances play an important role in some patients with chronic low back pain disorders. Evidence of secondary gain (especially compensation or litigation) and inappropriate (Wadell) signs and symptoms can help identify these patients. Nevertheless, one must be wary of real pathology, even in such patients.

6. Prior History of Back Pain—Perhaps the most important risk factor for future pain, especially with frequent disabling episodes and short intervals between episodes. Compensation work situations, smoking, and age >30 years are also associated with development of persistent disabling lower back pain. The incidence of disabling pain actually declines after age 60.

II. Cervical Spine

A. Cervical Spondylosis—Chronic disc degeneration and associated facet arthropathy. May lead to myelopathy (cord compression), radiculopathy (root compromise), or both. Cervical spondylosis typically begins to be seen at age 40–50, is seen in men > women, and most commonly occurs at the C5–C6 > C6–C7 levels. Risk factors include frequent lifting, cigarette smoking, and a history of excessive diving.

1. Pathoanatomy—Involves the disc and four other articulations: the two facet joints and two false uncovertebral joints (of Lushka). The cervical cord becomes impinged when the diameter of the canal (normally about 17 mm) is reduced to less than 13 mm. In hyperextension, the cord increases in diameter and it and the roots are pinched between the discs and adjacent spondylitic bars anteriorly, and the hypertrophic facets and infolded ligamentum flavum posteriorly. In hyperflexion, the cord narrows and the neural structures are tethered anteriorly across the discs or spondylitic bars. Progressive collapse of the normally lordotic cervical discs results in loss of normal lordosis of the cervical spine and chronic anterior cord compression. Spondylotic changes in the foramina primarily from chondro-osseous spurs of the joints of Luschka may restrict motion and may lead to nerve root compression. Soft disc herniation is usually posterolateral, between the posterior edge of the uncinate process and the lateral edge of the posterior longitudinal ligament, resulting in acute radiculopathy. Myelopathy may be seen occasionally with large central herniation, or spondylotic bars with a congenitally narrow canal. Ossification of the posterior longitudinal ligament (OPLL), resulting in cervical stenosis and myelopathy, is common in Orientals and may occasionally be seen in non-Orientals.

2. Signs and Symptoms—One of the earliest symptoms of neural compression is pain, which may be ischemic in origin. **Myelopathy** may be characterized by weakness (upper > lower extremity), ataxic broad-based suffling gait, sensory changes, and rarely urinary retention. "Myelopathy hand" has recently been described, with the "finger escape sign" (small finger spontaneously abducts due to weak intrinsics) indicating cervical myelopathy. Upper motor neuron findings such as hyperreflexia, clonus, or Babinski's sign may be

TABLE 6–1. DIFFERENTIAL DIAGNOSIS OF DISORDERS IN THE L-SPINE[a]

Evaluation	Back Strain	HNP	Spinal Stenosis	Spondylo-listhesis/ Instability	Tumor	Spondylo-arthropathy	Metabolic	Infection
Predominant pain (leg versus back)	Back	Leg	Leg	Back	Back	Back	Back	Back
Constitutional symptoms					+	+		+
Tension sign		+						
Neurologic examination		+	+ after stress					
Plain x-ray studies			+	+	±	+	+	±
Lateral motion x-ray studies				+				
CT scan		+	+		+			+
Myelogram		+	+					
Bone scan					+	+	+	+
ESR					+	+		+
Ca/P/alk phos					+			

[a] From Weinstein, J.N., and Wiesel, S.W.: The Lumbar Spine, p. 360. Philadelphia, W.B. Saunders, 1990; reprinted by permission.

present. Funicular pain, characterized by central burning and stinging ±Lhermitte's phenomenon (radiating lightning-like sensations down the back with neck flexion) may also be present with myelopathy. **Radiculopathy**, often associated with myelopathy, can involve one (monoradicular) or multiple (polyradicular) roots, and symptoms include neck, shoulder, and arm pain, paresthesias, and numbness. Findings may overlap because of intraneural intersegmental connections of sensory nerve roots. Mechanical stress, such as excessive vertebral motion, may exacerbate these symptoms. The lower nerve root at a given level is usually affected (Table 6–2).

3. Diagnosis—Largely based on history and physical. Plain radiographs, including oblique views, should be studied for changes in Lushka (apophyseal) joints, osteophytes (bars), and disc space narrowing (Fig. 6–1). However, radiographic changes of the degenerated cervical spine may not correlate with symptoms. Myelography combined with CT or MRI demonstrates neural compressive pathology well in the cervical spine. Discogram use is controversial and it is rarely used in cervical spine disorders. MRI is also useful for detecting intrinsic changes in the spinal cord, as well as disc degeneration. Electrodiagnostic studies have a high false-negative rate, but may be helpful in select cases for differentiating peripheral nerve compression from more central

compression and diseases such as Amyotrophic lateral sclerosis.

4. Treatment—Analgesics, exercises, use of a cervical collar, cervical traction, and pain clinic modalities will be helpful in the majority of cases. Indications for surgery include myelopathy with progressive motor/gait impairment, or radiculopathy with persistent disabling pain and weakness. Surgery usually involves an anterior approach. Smith Robinson discectomy and block fusion is preferred over the Cloward dowel for involvement of one or two interspaces. For multilevel spondylosis and myelopathy, with more extensive anterior decompression involving excision of osteophytes and multiple vertebrectomies, a strut graft fusion is indicated. Posterior approaches include canal-expansive laminoplasty (commonly used in OPLL), which can help decrease the incidence of instability associated with multilevel laminectomy. Foraminotomy is useful for single-level radiculopathy. Multilevel laminectomy may fail due to failure to adequately relieve anterior compression, or secondary to progressive kyphosis, which may require anterior decompression and fusion with a strut graft to correct the deformity. Complications of the anterior approach include neurologic injury (<1%), pseudarthrosis, or injury to other neck structures, including the recurrent laryngeal nerve if the right-sided approach is used. Complications of

TABLE 6–2. FINDINGS IN NERVE ROOT COMPRESSION

Level	Root	Muscles Affected	Sensory Loss	Reflex
C3–C4	C4	Scapular	Lateral neck, shoulder	None
C4–C5	C5	Deltoid, biceps	Lateral arm	Biceps
C5–C6*	C6	Wrist extensors, biceps, triceps (supination)	Radial forearm	Brachioradialis
C6–C7	C7	Triceps, wrist flexors (pronation)	Middle finger	Triceps
C7–C8	C8	Finger flexors, interossei	Ulnar hand	None
C8–T1	T1	Interossei	Ulnar forearm	None

* Most common.

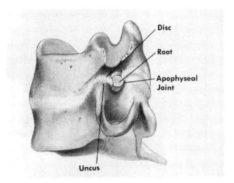

FIGURE 6–1. Cervical root impingement. (From Rothman, R. H., and Simeon, F. A.: The Spine, 2nd ed., p. 452. Philadelphia, W. B. Saunders Company, 1982; reprinted by permission.)

laminectomy include subluxation if facets are sacrificed, leading to a swan neck deformity, muscle ischemia, and direct spinal cord injury with quadriparesis. Radicular symptoms may improve following decompression but gait damages may not.

B. Cervical Stenosis—Absolute (AP canal diameter <10 mm) or relative (10–13 mm canal diameter) stenosis predisposes the patient to the development of myelopathy, radiculopathy, or both due to relatively minor soft or hard disc pathology or trauma. Absolute canal width of <13 mm is abnormal, but may not be reliable. Pavlov's ratio (canal–vertebral body width) should be 1.0, with <0.85 indicative of stenosis. A ratio <0.80 is considered a significant risk factor for later neurologic injury. This is more reliable in identifying a congenitally narrow canal. Symptoms in absolute stenosis may include progressive weakness (distal > proximal) and spasticity. Minor trauma such as hyperextension may lead to a central cord syndrome, even without overt injury. In relative stenosis, radicular symptoms usually predominate. Evaluation may include somatosensory evoked potentials, which help identify cord compromise in absolute stenosis. MRI, including flexion and extension studies, is also very helpful. Surgery may serve a prophylactic function, but is usually reserved for patients who develop myelopathy or radiculopathy. Surgical approaches are similar to those described above.

C. Rheumatoid Spondylitis—Cervical spine involvement is common in rheumatoids (up to 90%) and is more common with long-standing disease and multiple joint involvement. Neurologic impairment in patients with RA usually occurs very gradually and may cause decreased pain sensation and hyperreflexia early. However, neck pain, decreased range of motion, crepitation, or occipital headaches are the most common complaints. Surgery may not be successful in reversing significant neurologic deterioration, so it is essential to look for subtle signs of early neurologic involvement or myelopathy. Surgical indications for stabilization are when the spinal cord becomes compressed with less than 13 mm of room either at the upper or lower cervical spine or with basilar invagination.

1. Atlantoaxial Subluxation—Usually a result of pannus formation at the synovial joints between the dens and the ring of C1, and the dens and the transverse ligament, resulting in destruction of the transverse ligament, the dens, or both. Anterior subluxation of C1 on C2 is most common, but posterior and lateral subluxation can also occur. Findings on examination may include limitation of motion, upper motor neuron signs, and detection of a "clunk" with neck flexion (Sharp and Purser sign [not recommended]). Plain radiographs to include patient-controlled **flexion and extension views** are evaluated to determine the anterior atlantodens interval (ADI). Instability is present with a 3.5-mm ADI difference on flexion and extension views, but radiographic instability in RA is common and is not an indication for surgery. A 7-mm difference may imply disruption of the alar ligaments. A difference of >9–10 mm is associated with an increase in neurologic injury and will usually require posterior fusion and wiring. Progressive neurologic impairment and/or instability are indications for surgical stabilization. (Halo realignment and posterior C_1C_2 fusion). Ranawat has classified these deficits as follows:

Grade	Characteristics
I	Subjective paresthesias
II	Subjective weakness UMN findings
III	Objective weakness UMN findings (A = Ambulatory; B = Non-Ambulatory)

Surgery is less successful in patients with severe (Ranawat IIIB) neurologic deficits. Complications include pseudarthrosis and recurring myelopathy. The pseudarthrosis rate may be lessened by extending the fusion to the occiput with wire fixation. An ADI of >7–10 mm or a posterior space of < 13 mm is a contraindication to surgery in other areas, and the spine should be stabilized first.

2. Atlantoaxial Impaction (Basilar Invagination)—Cranial migration of the dens from erosion and bone loss between the occiput and C1/C2. McGregor's line (hard palate–occipital curve) is useful in evaluating impaction. Diagnosis is based on the tip of the dens being >8 mm above this line in men and >10 mm above the line in women. Ranawat's line (center of C2 pedicle to the C1 arch—a distance of <13 mm is consistent with impaction) and Chamberlain's line (anterior foramen to the top of the C1 posterior arch—dens >6 mm above line consistent with impaction) are helpful measurements (Fig. 6–2). Progressive cranial migration or neurologic compromise may require operative intervention (occiput-C2 fusion). SSEPs may be helpful in evaluation. When brain stem compromise is significant, with functional impairment, transoral or anterior retropharangeal odontoid resection may be required.

3. Lower Cervical Spine—May also be involved, because the joints of Lushka and facet joints are affected by RA. Subluxation may occur at multiple levels. The lower cervical spine is more common in males, with steroid use, with seropositive RA, in patients with rheumatoid nodules, and in patients with severe RA. Posterior fusion and wiring

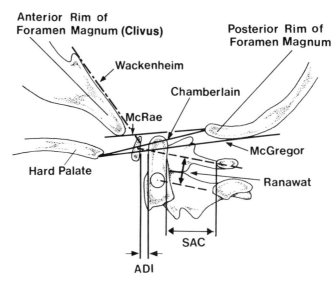

FIGURE 6–2. Composite illustration showing common measurements in C1–C2 disorders.

Criteria for Atlantoaxial Impaction:

McGregor: Males—Tip of odontoid >8 mm above line
                    Females—Tip of odontoid >9.7 mm above line
Ranawat: Males—Distance >19 mm
                    Females—Distance >17 mm
Wackenheim: Protrusion of odontoid process posterior to line
Chamberlain: Tip of odontoid >6 mm above line
McRae: Tip of odontoid superior to line

Atlantodens Interval (ADI):

Normally <3 mm in adults and <4 mm in children

Space Available for the Cord (SAC):

≥18 mm—no cord compression
15–17 mm—cord compression possible
≤14 mm—always cord compression

Steel's Rule of Thirds: At the level of the axis, there is 1 cm available for the cord, 1 cm for the odontoid, and 1 cm of free space.

is sometimes required for subluxation > 4 mm with intractable pain and neurologic compromise.

D. Cervical Spine and Cord Injuries

   1. Introduction—Spinal cord injuries (SCIs) occur most commonly in young males involved in motor vehicle accidents, falls, and diving accidents. Findings are often very subtle; the significant morbidity and mortality associated with missed injuries has led to current emphasis on cervical spine protection in polytrauma. Missed cervical spine injuries are most common in the presence of decreased level of consciousness, alcohol intoxication, head injury, or in patients with multiple injuries. Facial injuries, hypotension, and localized tenderness or spasm should be sought. Careful neurologic exam to document the lowest remaining functional level and to assess for the possibility of sacral sparing, or sparing of posterior column function indicating an incomplete SCI, is essential. Drug and alcohol intoxication may obscure the exam. **Initial treatment with large doses of methylprednisolone** (30 mg/kg initially and 5.4 mg/kg per hour for the first 24 hours) has been shown to slightly improve neurologic recovery if initiated within the first 8 hours after injury. Spinal shock (spinal cord concussion) usually involves a 24–72-hour period of paralysis, hypotonia, and areflexia, and at its conclusion there may be hyperreflexia, hypertonicity, and clonus. The return of the **bulbocavernosus reflex** (anal sphincter contraction in response to squeezing the glans penis or tugging on the Foley catheter) **signifies the end of spinal shock,** and, for complete injuries, **further neurologic improvement will be minimal.** Neurogenic shock (secondary to loss of sympathetic tone) can be differentiated from hypovolemic shock based on the presence of relative bradycardia in neurogenic shock, as opposed to tachycardia and hypotension with hypovolemic shock. Swan-Ganz monitoring is helpful in this setting as neurogenic and hypovolemic shock often occur concurrently.

   2. Prognosis—The Frankel classification is useful to consider functional recovery for spinal cord injury:

FRANKEL GRADE	FUNCTION
A	Complete paralysis
B	Sensory function only below injury level
C	Incomplete motor function below injury level
D	Fair to good motor function below injury level
E	Normal function

Another system developed by the ASIA group, based on a 100-point scale that assigns 0–5 points for each muscle group, may be more accurate in grading spinal cord injury.

3. Radiographic Evaluation—Includes complete cervical spine series (C1–T1, multiple-level injuries are common [10–20%]), as well as obliques, tomograms (especially in dens fractures and facet joint fractures/dislocations), CT, myelography, and MRI. CT scanning is useful to evaluate C1 fractures and assess bone in the canal. Myelography may be used in patients with an otherwise unexplained neurologic deficit. MRI has advantages in demonstrating posterior ligamentous disruption, disc herniation, and canal compromise, and actually demonstrating the status of the spinal cord.

4. Cord Injuries—May be complete (no function below a given level, or incomplete (with some sparing of distal function). In complete injuries, an improvement of one nerve root level can be expected in 80% of patients, and approximately 20% will recover two additional function levels. Several categories of incomplete lesions exist. These syndromes are classified based upon the area of the spinal cord that has been the most severely damaged. The **central cord** syndrome is the **most common** and is seen most often in patients with preexisting cervical spondylosis who sustain a hyperextension injury. The cord is compressed by anterior osteophytes and posteriorly by the infolded ligamentum flavum. The cord is injured in the central gray matter, which results in proportionately greater loss of motor function to the upper extremities than the lower extremities with variable sensory sparing. The second most common cord injury is the **anterior cord** syndrome, in which the damage is primarily in the anterior two thirds of the cord (related to vascular insufficiency), sparing the posterior columns (position sense, proprioception, and vibratory sensation). This patient demonstrates greater motor loss in the legs than the arms. CT scans may demonstrate bony fragments compressing the ante-

rior spinal cord. The anterior cord syndrome has the worst prognosis. The rare Brown-Séquard syndrome damages half of the cord, causing ipsilateral motor loss and position/proprioception loss and contralateral pain and temperature loss (usually two levels below the insult). This injury carries the best prognosis. Posterior cord syndrome spares only a few tracts anteriorly (with only crude touch sensation remaining). It is very rare, in fact some authors do not believe that it exists. **Single-root** lesions can occur at the level of the fracture, most commonly C5 or C6, leading to deltoid or biceps weakness, and are usually unilateral. A summary of the syndromes is presented in Table 6–3.

5. Specific Cervical Spine Injuries—The reader is referred to Chapter 9, Trauma, for classification and treatment of cervical spine injuries.

6. Treatment—Discussed in Chapter 9, Trauma, but basically includes immobilization (collar for undisplaced fractures; skeletal traction, halo vest, or surgery for unstable fractures), and the immediate application of skeletal traction to realign the spine in the presence of a displaced fracture with or without neurologic injury. If necessary, anterior decompression for incomplete injuries with persistent cord compression (can lead to improvement of one to three levels even in complete injuries), and stabilization may be indicated. **Laminectomies are contraindicated except in the rare patient with ankylosing spondylitis** and massive epidural hemorrhage, or in the rare case of posterior compression from a fractured lamina. Gunshot wounds are treated closed except with esophageal perforation.

7. Complications—Numerous and include neurologic injury, nonunion, malunion, etc. **Autonomic dysreflexia** can follow cervical and upper thoracic spinal cord injuries. It is commonly related to bladder overdistention or fecal impaction and manifests with pounding **headache (from severe hypertension), anxiety, profuse head and neck sweating, nasal obstruction, and blurred vision.** Urinary catheterization or rectal disimpaction and supportive treatment will usually relieve symptoms. If not, nifedipine (10 mg) is given sublingually immediately, followed by Dibenzylene (10 mg) administered daily for prophylaxis. Instability in the cervical spine can occur late and is associated with >3.5 mm of subluxation and >11 degrees of angulation.

E. Other Cervical Spine Problems—Ankylosing Spondylitis (AS) and neuromyopathic conditions can cause severe flexion deformities of the cervical spine.

TABLE 6–3. SPINAL CORD INJURY SYNDROMES

SYNDROME	MOI/PATHOLOGY	CHARACTERISTICS	PROGNOSIS
Central	>50 yo, extension injuries	Affects upper > lower extremities, motor and sensory loss	Fair
Anterior	Flexion-compression (vertebral A)	Incomplete motor and some sensory loss	Poor
Brown-Séquard	Penetrating trauma	Loss of ipsilateral motor function, contralateral pain and temp. sensation	Best
Root	Foramina compression/herniated nucleus pulposis	Based on level—weakness	Good
Complete	Burst/canal compression	No function below injury level	Poor

Patients with AS must be carefully evaluated for silent fractures because of the problem of pseudarthrosis and progressive kyphotic deformity. Traction, surgical release of contracted sternocleidomastoid muscles, and posterior fusion are sometimes required for severe neuromyopathic conditions. Severe chin-on-chest deformity in AS, with the inability to look straight ahead, occasionally represents a major functional limitation. The kyphosis is treated with cervicothoracic laminectomy, osteotomy, and fusion for correction of the flexion deformity. This procedure is performed under local anesthesia with brief general anesthesia, and immobilization postoperatively is carried out in a halo-cast.

III. Thoracic/Lumbar Spine

    A. Herniated Nucleus Pulposus (HNP)

        1. Introduction—Disc degeneration with aging includes loss of water content, annular tears, and myxomatous changes, resulting in herniation of nuclear material. Changes in proteoglycan metabolism, secondary immunologic factors, and structural factors also play a role. Discs can **protrude** (bulging nucleus, intact annulus), **extrude** (through annulus but confined by posterior longitudinal ligament [PLL]), or be **sequestrated**

(disc material free in canal) (Fig. 6–3). HNP is usually a disease of younger and middle-age adults, because the disc nucleus dessicates and is less likely to herniate in older populations.

        2. Thoracic Disc Disease—Relatively uncommon and produces pain and/or paralysis. Usually involves the mid- to lower thoracic levels, and is divided equally between central and lateral herniations. Central disease can cause chest, low back, or even leg pain, paraparesis, and sphincter/sexual dysfunction. Lateral discs can cause radicular pain and sensory changes with numbness, paresthesias, or midabdominal band-like discomfort. Physical findings may be difficult to elicit, but may include localized tenderness, sensory pinprick level, upper motor neuron signs with leg hyperreflexia, weakness, and abnormal rectal exam. Radiographs may show disc narrowing and calcification or osteophytic lipping. Underlying Scheuermann's disease may predispose patients to develop HNP. Myelo-CT or MRI should demonstrate thoracic HNP, and MRI is useful to rule out cord pathology. Immobilization, analgesics, and nerve blocks are sometimes helpful for radiculopathy. Surgery, usually through an anterior transthoracic approach or

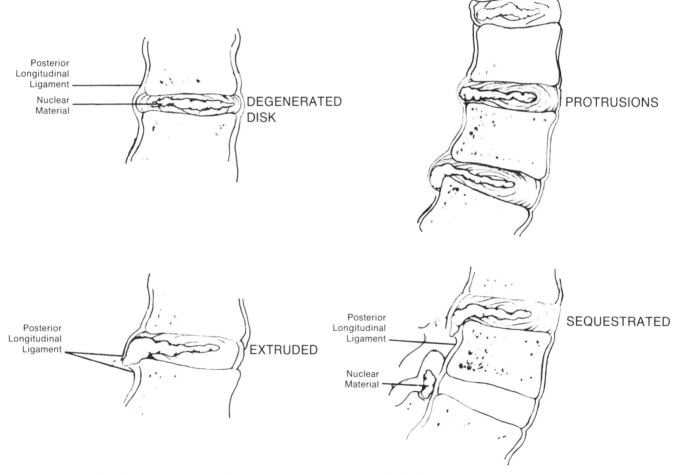

FIGURE 6–3. Nomenclature for disc pathology. (From Wiltse, L. L.: Lumbosacral spine reconstruction. In Orthopaedic Knowledge Update I, p. 247. Chicago, American Academy of Orthopaedic Surgeons, 1984; reprinted by permission.)

costotransversectomy (including anterior discectomy and hemicorpectomy as needed), is recommended in the presence of neurologic dysfunction or persistent unremitting pain with documented pathology. Posterior approach to a thoracic HNP is contraindicated due to the high rate of neurologic injury.

3. Lumbar Disc Disease—Major cause of increased morbidity and financial impact in the United States. Most often involves the L4–L5 disc (the "backache disc"), followed closely by L5–S1. Most herniations are posterolateral (where the PLL is the weakest) and may present with back pain and nerve root pain/sciatica involving the lower nerve root at that level. Central prolapse is usually associated with back pain only; however, acute insults may precipitate a **cauda equina compression syndrome** (Fig. 6–4). This is a surgical emergency that presents with bowel or bladder dysfunction (usually urinary retention), saddle anesthesia, and varying degrees of loss of lower extremity motor or sensory function. Immediate myelography (or MRI) and surgery (if the tests are positive) are indicated to arrest progression of neurologic loss.

   a. History and Physical Exam—An acute injury or precipitating event should be sought, and location of symptoms (especially pain radiating to the extremity), the character of pain, night pain (rule out spinal tumor), postural changes (neurogenic claudication), effect of increased intrathecal pressures, and a complete review of symptoms (including psychiatric history) should be elicited. Occupational risks, such as a job requiring prolonged sitting that creates increased pressure in the nucleus

pulposus, and repetitive lifting are also important factors. Referred pain in mesodermal tissues of the same embryologic origin, often to the buttocks or posterior thighs, must be differentiated from true radicular pain from nerve root impingement, with symptoms that typically reach distal to the knee. Psychosocial evaluation, pain drawings, and psychological testing can also be helpful in some cases. The findings of an "inverted V" triad of hysteria, hypochondriasis, and depression on MMPI has been identified as a major negative risk factor in lumbar disc surgery. Physical examination should include observation (change in lordosis or a list—sciatic scoliosis [away from side with sciatica = lateral prolapse, towards side with sciatica = axillary prolapse]); palpation of the posterior spine (spasm, localized tenderness); measurement of range of motion (decreased flexion); hip examination vascular exam (distal pulses); abdominal and rectal exam; and neurologic exam—all are important. Tension signs (straight leg raising, bowstring sign, femoral nerve stretch test) are important findings suggesting HNP. Specific findings, by level are presented in Table 6–4. A central disc herniation at one level may impinge on more than one nerve root. Inappropriate signs and symptoms (Wadell) are also important to note. Inappropriate symptoms include pain at the tip of the "tailbone"; pain, numbness, or giving way of the whole leg; inappropriate reactions such as moaning, and emergency admissions. Nonorganic physical signs include tenderness with light touch in nonanatomic areas, light axial loading, dis-

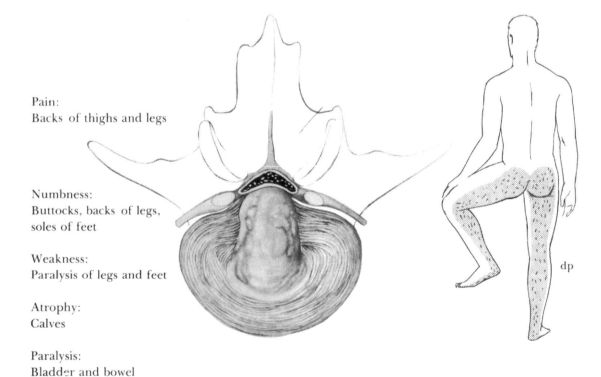

Pain:
Backs of thighs and legs

Numbness:
Buttocks, backs of legs, soles of feet

Weakness:
Paralysis of legs and feet

Atrophy:
Calves

Paralysis:
Bladder and bowel

FIGURE 6–4. Cauda equina syndrome. (From DePalma, A. F., and Rothman, R. H.: The Intervertebral Disc, p. 194. Philadelphia, W. B. Saunders, 1970; reprinted by permission.)

TABLE 6–4. FINDINGS IN LUMBAR DISC DISEASE

LEVEL	NERVE ROOT	SENSORY LOSS	MOTOR LOSS	REFLEX LOSS
L1–L3	L2, L3	Anterior thigh	Hip flexors	None
L3–L4	L4	Medial calf	Quadriceps, tibialis anterior	Knee jerk
L4–L5	L5	Lateral calf, dorsal foot	EDL, EHL	None
L5–S1	S1	Posterior calf, plantar foot	Gastrocnemius/soleus	Ankle jerk
S2–S4	S2, S3, S4	Perianal	Bowel/bladder	Cremasteric

traction testing, pain with pelvic rotation, negative sitting (and positive supine) straight leg raising test, regional nonanatomic disturbances, and overreaction.

b. Diagnostic Tests—Plain radiographs are indicated before proceeding with special tests to rule out other pathology, such as isthmic defects. However, most plain radiographic findings are nonspecific. Myelography, CT, and MRI studies are effective when used as a confirming study. While there is no clear-cut advantage to any one of these modalities, CT is noninvasive and helpful for demonstrating bony stenosis and for identifying lateral pathology, including far-lateral disc herniations. MRI is superior for identifying neural compression and neural tumors. It is noninvasive, involves no ionizing radiation, and has the advantages of demonstrating lateral disc pathology, of giving a "myelogram" effect on the T_2 images, and helping to identify spinal stenosis. In addition, it demonstrates the state of hydration of the discs and visualizes the marrow of the vertebral bodies, thus representing an excellent modality to screen for tumor or infection. Myelography, unless combined with CT, has few advantages and limited indications. EMG studies (which demonstrate fibrillations 3 weeks after nerve root pressure) are not usually helpful and rarely provide more information than a good physical exam. Thermography does not have proven efficacy in the evaluation of disc disease.

c. Treatment—Short-term bed rest (3–7 days) with support beneath the knees and neck, NSAIDs or aspirin, and progressive ambulation is successful in returning most patients to their normal function. Over half of patients who present with low back pain will recover in 1 week and 90% will recover within 1–3 months. One half of patients with sciatica will recover in 1 month. This treatment is followed by a back rehabilitation program and a fitness program. Aerobic conditioning and education are the most important factors in avoiding missed work days due to disc disease and in returning patients to work. Instruction should include avoiding rotation and flexion due to increased disc pressure associated with these activities. If patients fail to improve with up to 6 weeks of conservative care, then further evaluation is indicated. Those patients with predominately low back pain should receive a bone scan and medical work-up (to rule out spinal tumors or infection). If these studies are normal, then back rehabilitation is continued.

In patients failing conservative therapy who have predominately leg pain (sciatica), a trial of lumbar epidural steroids may be helpful, but has not been proven effective in controlled studies. Additional studies (myelogram [± CT] or MRI) are undertaken in patients who, after 6–12 weeks, continue to be symtomatic with neurologic deficit or positive nerve tension signs. These studies should be done only to confirm clinical suspicions because up to 25–35% of asymptomatic patients will have positive myelo-CT or MRI studies. Patients with positive studies, neurologic findings, tensions signs, and predominately sciatic symptoms without mitigating psychosocial factors are the best candidates for surgical discectomy. Standard partial laminotomy and discectomy is most commonly performed. With proper indications, 95% of patients will have initially good or excellent results, although as many as 30% of patients have significant backache on long-term follow-up. Microdiscectomy is of limited value because the keyhole incision significantly decreases visualization of herniated or extruded disc fragments and lateral root stenosis. Percutaneous discectomy may have limited indications in the treatment of protruded discs in the future, but at this time there are no long-term follow-up studies proving its efficacy. It is contraindicated in the presence of a sequestered fragment or spinal stenosis. Intradiscal enzyme therapy has fallen out of favor due to questionable efficacy and serious complications (anaphylaxis and transverse myelitis). Indications for its use for disc herniations are similar to those for surgery (leg pain, tension signs, neurologic deficits, and positive studies).

d. Complications—Fortunately are rare, but can be devastating.
   1. Vascular Injury—May occur during attempts at disc removal if curettes are allowed to penetrate the anterior longitudinal ligament. Intraoperative pulsatile bleeding from deep penetration is treated with rapid wound closure, IV fluids and blood, repositioning the patient, and a transabdominal approach (by a vascular surgeon) to find and stop the source of bleeding. Mortality may exceed 50%. Late sequelae of vascular injuries may include delayed hemorrhage, false aneurysm, or A-V fistula formation.
   2. Nerve Root Injury—More common with anomalous nerve roots. Dural tears should be repaired primarily when they occur to

avoid the development of a pseudomeningocele or spinal fluid fistula. Adequate hemostasis, lighting, magnification, and careful surgical technique are important to diminish the incidence of the "battered root syndrome."

3. Failed Back Syndrome—Often may be the result of poor patient selection, but other causes include recurrent herniation (usually acute recurrence of signs/symptoms following 6–12-month pain-free interval), herniation at another level, discitis (occurs 4–6 weeks post operatively with onset of severe back pain) unrecognized lateral stenosis (may be most common), or vertebral instability. Epidural fibrosis occurs at about 3 months postoperatively, may have associated leg pain, is related to hemorrhage and surgical trauma, and responds poorly to reexploration. Scar can best be differentiated from recurrent HNP with a gadolinium-enhanced MRI.

4. Dual Tear—More common in revision surgery and should be repaired immediately if it is recognized. Fibrin adhesive sealant may be a useful adjunct for effecting dural closure. Bed rest is advocated if it is suspected postoperatively. If symptoms persist, a subarachnoid drain may be indicated.

5. Infection—Similar to infection elsewhere, I & D and removal of loose graft may be required.

B. Lumbar Segmental Instability—Present when normal loads produce abnormal spinal motion. Degenerative lumbar disc disease is indicated by disc space narrowing. A combination of annulus damage and disc space narrowing may cause reduction in the disc's ability to resist rotatory forces. Continuing degeneration or facet subluxation may then lead to rotary instability. The most consistent clinical sign is the "instability catch" (sudden, painful snapping with extension). Radiographically, traction spurs (horizontal and below disc margin [vs. syndesmophyte]), angular changes >10 degrees (20 degrees at L5–S1) on flexion films, and translatory motion >3–4 mm (6 mm at L5–S1) with flexion-extension views are all characteristic of lumbar instability, but are difficult to quantify and may not correlate with clinical symptoms. Iatrogenic instability can occur following removal of one or more facet joints during lumbar procedures. Surgical treatment options do not have clearly defined indications, but include posterolateral fusion, posterior lumbar interbody fusion (PLIF—iliac crest graft is "keyed" into the intervertebral space), and anterior interbody fusion. These procedures are associated with a high incidence of pseudarthrosis and neurologic injury. Internal fixation, utilizing pedicle screw fixation in rod or plate constructs, is gaining popularity as an adjunct in lumbar spine fusion surgery, but the efficacy of these implants remains unproven. Additionally, the increased operating time and morbidity are important considerations.

C. Spinal Stenosis

1. Introduction—Spinal stenosis is narrowing of the spinal canal or neural foramina producing root ischemia and neurogenic claudication. Central stenosis produces compression of the thecal sac and lateral stenosis involves compression of individual nerve roots, and is more common. Lumbar spinal stenosis usually does not become symptomatic until patients reach late middle age, affecting males twice as often as females.

2. Central Stenosis

a. Introduction—Can be congenital (idiopathic or developmental in achondroplastic dwarfs) or acquired. Acquired stenosis, the most common type, is degenerative due to enlargement of osteoarthritic facets with medial encroachment, and can be secondary to spondylolisthesis, posttraumatic, postsurgical, or from various disease processes (Paget's, fluorosis, etc.). Preexisting "trefoil" canal shapes or a congenitally narrow canal may limit the ability to tolerate minor acquired encroachment (Fig. 6–5). Central stenosis represents compression of the thecal sac (usually to <100 mm^2 or <10 mm of AP diameter as seen on CT cross section), causing symptoms of neurogenic claudication. Soft tissue (ligamentum flavum and disc) may contribute as much as 40% to dural sac compression. Central stenosis is more common in males because their spinal canal is smaller at the L3–L5 levels than females.

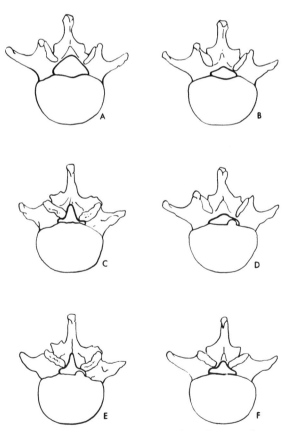

FIGURE 6–5. Spinal stenosis. *A,* Normal. *B,* Congenital stenosis. *C,* Degenerative stenosis. *D,* Congenital stenosis with disc herniation. *E,* Degenerative stenosis with disc herniation. *F,* Congenital and degenerative stenosis. (From Arnoldi, C. C., et al.: Lumbar spinal stenosis and nerve root entrapment syndromes. Clin. Orthop. 115:4, 1976; reprinted with permission.)

b. Symptoms include insidious pain and paresthesias with ambulation and extension, relieved by lying supine or with flexion of the spine. Patients commonly complain of lower extremity pain, numbness, or "giving way." A history of radiating leg pain in a dermatomal distribution, while typical in patients with HNP, is relatively uncommon in spinal stenosis. Neurogenic claudication, which occurs in less than half of patients with stenosis, usually can be differentiated from vascular claudication by history:

Activity	Vascular Claudication	Neurogenic Claudication
Walking	Distal → proximal pain, calf pain	Proximal → distal pain, thigh pain
Uphill walking	Symptoms develop sooner	Symptoms develop later
Rest	Relief with standing	Relief—sitting or bending
Bicycling	Symptoms develop	Symptoms do not develop
Lying flat	Relief	May exacerbate symptoms

Physical examination is also important. Patients with stenosis may have pain with extension, have normal pulses, and may have neurologic findings (weak extensor hallucis longus [EHL]). However, abnormal neurologic findings or positive tension signs are seen in less than one half of patients. Neurologic findings not otherwise obvious may sometimes be demonstrated with a "stress test" (walking until symptoms occur).

c. Imaging—Further work-up may include plain radiographs on which disc degeneration, interspace narrowing, and flattening of the lordotic curve are commonly seen; subluxation and degenerative changes of the facet joints may be seen. EMGs or SSEPs may be used but sensitivity is variable and depends on the examiner. Bone scan or MRI may be helpful to rule out malignancy. Myelography, followed by CT, or MRI are standard imaging modalities. Careful inspection of these studies is necessary to assess lateral nerve root entrapment by medial hypertrophy of the superior facet, the tip of the superior facet, osteophyte formation of the posterior vertebral body (uncinate spur), or a combination of these. Central stenosis is a diminution in the area of the thecal sac and is produced by thickening of the ligamentum flavum and/or posterior protrusion of the disc; this soft tissue component to stenosis can be responsible for up to 40% of thecal sac compromise and must be identified. Simply looking for the "bony" measurements will result in underestimating the degree of stenosis.

d. Treatment—Rest, isometric abdominal exercises, pelvic tilt, Williams' flexion exercises, and weight reduction are important in management of patients with stenosis. Lumbar epidural steroids may be helpful for short-term relief, but have not shown efficacy in controlled studies. Surgery is indicated in patients with positive studies and persistent impairment in quality of life. Adequate decompression of the identified pathology should include laminectomy and partial faceteotomy of the lateral recess, which can be done without destabilizing the spine, thus avoiding fusion. Fusion is indicated in patients with surgical instability (bilateral facet joint removal), neural arch defects with disc disease, symptomatic radiographic instability (>4–6 mm horizontal translation or reversal of the intervertebral angle), degenerative or isthmic spondylolisthesis, and degenerative scoliosis.

3. Lateral Stenosis—Impingement of nerve roots lateral to the thecal sac, as they pass through the neural foramen. Often associated with facet joint arthropathy (superior articular process enlargement) and disc disease (Fig. 6–6). The three-joint complex (disc and both facets) must be considered when evaluating lateral stenosis. Nerve root compression can occur at more than one level, and must be completely decompressed to relieve symptoms. Compression can be subarticular (lateral recess stenosis), which consists of compression between the medial aspect of a hypertrophic superior articular facet, made worse at times with hypertrophy of the ligamentum flavum and/or joint capsule, and vertebral body osteophyte/disc. Foraminal stenosis can be produced by intraforaminal disc protrusion, impingement of the tip of the superior facet, or uncinate spurring. Subarticular stenosis, which is more common, affects the traversing (lower) nerve root. Foraminal stenosis affects the exiting (upper) nerve root. Lateral stenosis in general usually involves middle-aged patients (but can also be seen in younger adults) with symptoms of radicular pain unrelieved by rest and without tension signs. Lower lumbar areas are most commonly involved because the foramina size decreases as the nerve root size increases. Pain may be the result of intraneural edema and demyelination. Substance P

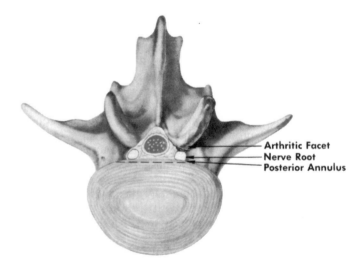

FIGURE 6–6. Lateral stenosis. Note nerve root entrapment laterally on the right by arthritic facet and bulging posterior annulus. (From Rothman, R. H., and Simeon, F. A.: The Spine, 2nd ed., p. 520. Philadelphia, W. B. Saunders, 1982; reprinted by permission.)

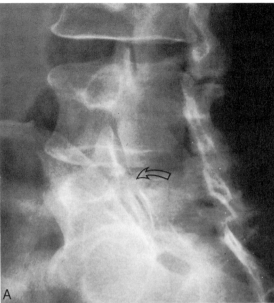
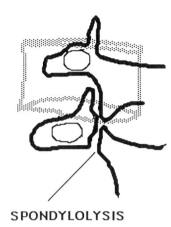

SPONDYLOLYSIS

FIGURE 6–7. Spondylolysis; note disruption of "collar" on Scottie dog. (From Helms, C. A.: Fundamentals of Skeletal Radiology, p. 101. Philadelphia, W. B. Saunders Company, 1989; reprinted by permission.)

may be released as a response to spinal nerve root irritation. After failure of nonoperative regimen, decompression of the hypertrophied lamina and ligamentum flavum and partial facetectomy are usually successful. Fusion may be necessary if instability is present or created.

4. Extraforaminal Lateral Root Compression ("Far Out Syndrome" ([Wiltse])—Involves L5 root impingement between the sacral ala and the L5 transverse process and is usually seen in degenerative scoliosis; isthmic spondylolisthesis, or with extraforaminal herniated discs. It must be specifically sought on special radiographs (25-degree caudocephalic [Ferguson] view), or CT. Treatment is decompression.

D. Spondylolysis and Spondylolisthesis
1. **Spondylolysis**—A defect in the pars interarticularis, and the most common cause of low back pain in children and adolescents. The defect in the pars is felt to be a fatigue fracture from repetitive hyperextension stresses (more common in gymnasts, football lineman), to which there may be a hereditary predisposition. Oblique radiographs may show a defect in the "neck" of the "Scottie dog" as described by Lachapelle (Fig. 6–7). Bone scan may be helpful in patient evaluation because increased uptake is more compatible with acute lesions that have the potential to heal, and bracing or casting (a single thigh pantaloon spica) might be indicated. Treatment is usually aimed at symptomatic relief, however, rather than fracture healing and includes activity restriction, flexion exercises, and bracing. Nonunion is common and may have normal scans.
2. **Spondylolisthesis**—Forward slippage of one vertebra on another. Can be classified into six types (Newman, Wiltse, McNab) (Table 6–5; Figs. 6–8 and 6–9). Severity of slip in spondylolisthesis is based on the amount or degree (as compared to S1 width): I = 0–25%; II = 25–50%; III = 50–

75%; IV = >75%, V = >100% (spondyloptosis). Other measurements, including the sacral inclination (normally >30°), and the lumbosacral joint angle (normally >0°), are also useful (Fig. 6–10).
3. Childhood Spondylolisthesis—Usually at L5–S1, is typically type II, and usually presents with back pain (instability), deformities, or alteration in gait ("pelvic waddle" and hamstring spasm). While the onset of symptoms may occur at any time of life, screening studies identify the occurrence of the slippage as being most common at 5–8 years. Spondylolisthesis is most common in whites, boys, and youngsters involved in hyperextension activities. It is remarkably common in Eskimos (>50%). It is thought to result from shear stress at the pars intra-articularis. Severe slips may be associated with radicular findings (L5) and kyphosis of the lumbosacral junction ± a palpable step-off and a "heart-shaped" buttocks. Spina bifida occulta, thoracic kyphosis, and Scheuermann's disease are associated with spondylolisthesis.

TABLE 6–5. TYPES OF SPONDYLOLISTHESIS

CLASS	TYPE	AGE	PATHOLOGY/OTHER
I	Congenital	Child	Congenital dysplasia of S1 superior facet
II	Isthmic*	5–50	Predisposition leading to elongation/fracture of pars (L5–S1)
III	Degenerative	Older	Facet arthrosis leading to subluxation (L4–L5)
IV	Traumatic	Young	Acute fracture/other than pars
V	Pathologic	Any	Incompetence of bony elements
VI	Postsurgical	Adult	Excessive resection of neural arches/facets

* Most common.

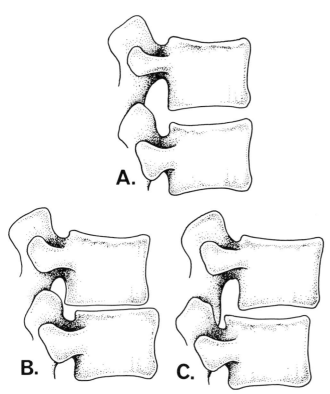

FIGURE 6–8. Degenerative spondylolisthesis. *A*, Normal. *B*, Retrolisthesis—disc narrowing is greater than posterior joint degeneration. *C*, Anterolisthesis—posterior joints are more degenerated than the disc. (From Weinstein, J. N., and Wiesel, S. W.: The Lumbar Spine, p. 84. Philadelphia, W. B. Saunders Company, 1990; reprinted by permission.)

a. Low-Grade Disease (<50% Slip)—Spondylolysis or mild spondylolisthesis may require bone scan or tomograms for diagnosis, and usually responds to nonoperative treatment consisting of bracing and exercise. Adolescents with a grade I slip may return to normal activities, including contact sports, once they are asymptomatic. Those with asymptomatic grade II spondylolisthesis should be restricted from activities such as gymnastics. Progression is uncommon, but risk factors include young age at presentation, female sex, a slip angle of >10 degrees [angle formed by intersection of lines parallel to the inferior border of the body of L5 and the top of the sacrum on a lateral radiograph (Fig. 6–10)], a high-grade slip, and a domed-shaped or significantly inclined sacrum (>30 degrees beyond vertical). Furthermore, patients with type I or congenital spondylolisthesis are at higher risk for slip progression and the development of cauda equina dysfunction because the neural arch is intact. Surgery for patients with a low-grade slip generally consists of L5–S1 posterolateral fusion in situ, and is usually reserved for patients with intractable pain who have failed nonoperative treatment, or for those demonstrating progressive slippage. Wiltse has popularized a paraspinal splitting approach to the lumbar transverse processes and sacral alae that is frequently utilized in this setting. L5 radiculopathy is uncommon in children with low-grade slips, and rarely, if ever, requires decompression. Repair of the pars de-

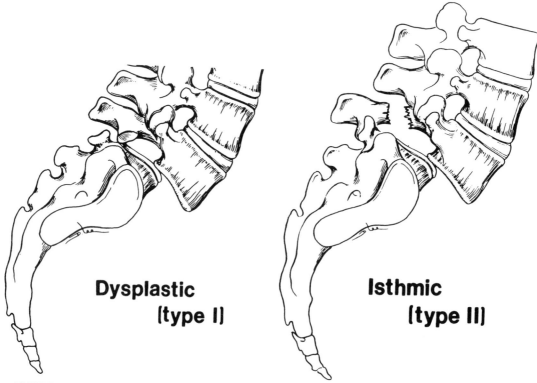

**Dysplastic
(type I)**

**Isthmic
(type II)**

FIGURE 6–9. Spondylolisthesis. (From Rothman, R. H., and Simeon, F. A.: The Spine, 2nd ed., p. 264. Philadelphia, W. B. Saunders Company, 1982; reprinted by permission.)

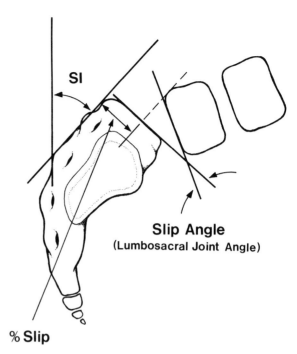

SI

Slip Angle
(Lumbosacral Joint Angle)

% Slip

FIGURE 6–10. Composite of measurements used in evaluation of spondylolisthesis. (Modified from Wiltse, L. L., and Winter, R. B.: Terminology and measurement of spondylolisthesis. J. Bone Joint Surg. [Am.] 65:768–772, 1983; reprinted by permission.)

fect, utilizing a lag screw (Buck) or tension band wiring (Bradford) with bone grafting, has been reported. This may be indicated in younger patients with slippage less than 25%, and a pars defect at L4 or above.

b. Grades III and IV Spondylolisthesis and Spondyloptosis (Grade V)—More commonly causes neurologic abnormalities. Prophylactic fusion in children with slippage greater than 50% is recommended. This usually requires bilateral posterolateral fusion in situ, usually at L4–S1 without instrumentation. Nerve root exploration is reserved for cases with persistent weakness. Reduction of spondylolisthesis has been associated with a 20–30% incidence of L5 root injuries, and should be utilized cautiously with a cosmetically unacceptable deformity, or when the L5 kyphosis is so severe that the posterior fusion mass from L4 to the sacrum would be under tension without reversal of the kyphosis. Close neurologic monitoring should be done during the procedure and for several days afterward to identify postoperative neuropathy. A posterior decompression, fibular interbody fusion, and posterolateral fusion without reduction has been reported with excellent long-term results (Bohlman). "Spondylolisthesis crisis" is seen in patients with severe slips, increasing pain, and hamstring tightness. The Gill procedure, consisting of removal of the loose elements without fusion, is contraindicated in children and is rarely performed in adults.

4. Adult Degenerative Spondylolisthesis—More commonly involves blacks, diabetics, and women over the age of 40 and is most commonly at the L4–L5 level (Fig. 6–8). It is reported to be more common in patients with transitional L5 vertebrae. Degenerative spondylolisthesis frequently causes L4 and L5 radiculopathy due to compres-

sion of the roots under the hypertrophic facets and in the foramina at L4–L5. The operative treatment of degenerative spondylolisthesis involves decompression of the nerve roots as well as stabilization by posterolateral floating fusion.

5. Adult Isthmic Spondylolisthesis—While the significance of isthmic spondylolisthesis in an adult is controversial, it remains a common indication for surgery. Nonoperative treatment includes rest, corset, NSAIDs, and flexion exercises. It is essential to assess for other more common sources of adult low back pain before assuming that spondylolisthesis is the cause; MRI scanning is a useful tool in this setting. Isthmic L5–S1 spondylolisthesis frequently causes radicular symptoms in the adult, resulting from compression of the exiting L5 root in the L5–S1 foramen; compression may involve hypertrophic fibrous repair tissue at the pars defect or posterior L5 body and bulging of the L5–S1 disc. Operative treatment is favored with the presence of radicular symptoms and usually involves thorough foraminal decompression and fusion, with or without pedicular screw fixation. Compromised results in workers' compensation patients have been reported.

E. Thoracolumbar Injuries

1. Introduction—Although the classification and treatment of these injuries is included in Chapter 9, Trauma, some points need to be emphasized here. The upper thoracic spine (T1–T10) is stabilized by the ribs and the facet orientation, and is less susceptible to trauma. At the T12–L1 junction, however, there is a fulcrum of increased motion and this area is more commonly affected with spine trauma. Two anatomic points also bear repeating: (1) the middle T-spine is a vascular "watershed" area, and vascular insult can lead to cord ischemia; and (2) the spinal cord ends and the

cauda equina begins at the level of L1–L2, so lesions below the L1 level carry a better prognosis because nerve roots and not cord are affected.

2. Stable vs. Unstable Injuries—The three-column system (Denis) is helpful in evaluating spinal injuries and determining which are stable or unstable. The anterior column is composed of the anterior longitudinal ligament and the anterior ⅔ of the annulus and vertebral body. The middle column consists of the posterior ⅓ of the body and annulus, and the posterior longitudinal ligament. The posterior column is comprised of the pedicles, facets, spinous processes, and the posterior ligaments, including interspinous and supra spinous ligaments, ligamentum flavum, and facet capsules. Disruption of the middle column (seen as widening of the interpedicular distances on AP radiographs or a change in height of the posterior cortex of the body) results in an unstable injury that may require operative fixation. In addition, disruption of the posterior ligamentous complex in the face of anterior fracture or dislocation is a strong indication of instability and of the potential necessity of surgical stabilization. Exceptions may include the upper thoracic spine, which is inherently more stable, and with bony Chance fractures. Compression fractures of three sequential vertebrae leads to an increase in risk of posttraumatic kyphosis.

3. Treatment—Anterior decompression and fusion is felt by many to favorably affect neurologic recovery and decrease residual pain, deformity, and length of hospitalization. Decompression of the canal is indicated emergently in the presence of a progressive neurologic deficit (rare). Decompression can be accomplished by posterior instrumentation via ligamentotaxis, or posterolaterally (through the pedicle using the ''eggshell'' technique or after pedicular resection), or anteriorly under direct vision followed by strut grafting. Posterior instrumentation is indicated following anterior decompression and strut grafting when the posterior ligament complex is torn. Instrumentation for two levels above and two levels below the affected fracture is the standard for fractures at the thoracolumbar junction. The potential harmful effect of ''rodding long and fusing short'' with prolonged immobilization of normal facets has been cited as a drawback to this technique. Adjuncts (or alternatives) to standard Harrington rod instrumentation of spine fractures include the use of spinous process or sublaminar wires, the Cotrel-Dubousset system utilizing multiple hooks or screws, or the use of pedicle-screw implants. The latter two implants provide more rigid fixation and may allow shorter fusions. Rehabilitation following spinal injury is discussed in Chapter 8, Rehabilitation.

F. Other Thoracolumbar Disorders

1. Destructive Spondyloarthropathy—Seen in hemodialysis patients with chronic renal failure and typically involves three adjacent vertebrate with two intervening discs. Changes include subluxation, degeneration, and narrowing of the disc height. Although the process may resemble infection, it probably represents crystal or amyloid deposition.

2. Facet Syndrome—Inflammation or degeneration of the lumbar facet joints may cause pain that is characteristically in the low back with radiation down one or both buttocks and posterior thighs, and is worse with extension. Selective injections of local anesthetic can be helpful in diagnosis of this condition but anesthetic/steroid injections into the facet joint as a treatment modality are less effective (<20% with excellent pain relief).

3. Diffuse Idiopathic Skeletal Hyperostosis (DISH)—Also known by the eponym Forestier's disease, this entity is defined by the presence of nonmarginal syndesmophytes (differentiated from ankylosing spondylitis, with marginal syndesmophytes [Fig. 6–11]) at three successive levels. DISH can occur anywhere in the spine, but is most common in the thoracic spine and is more often seen on the right side. DISH is associated with chronic lower back pain and is more common in patients with diabetes and gout. The prevalence of DISH has been found to be as high as 28% in autopsy specimens. While there does not appear to be any relationship between DISH and spinal pain, DISH is associated with extraspinal ossification at several joints, including an increased risk of heterotopic ossification following total hip surgery.

4. Ankylosing Spondylitis—HLA-B27–positive patients are usually young males who present with insidious onset of back and hip pain in the third or fourth decade. Sacroiliac joint obliteration and marginal syndesmophytes allow radiographic differentiation from DISH. Ankylosing spondylitis may result in fixed cervical, thoracic, or lumbar hyperkyphosis. It occasionally causes marked functional limitation, primarily due to the inability of affected patients to face forward. Extension osteotomy and fusion of the lumbar spine with compression instrumentation can successfully balance the head over the sacrum. Assessment for hip flexion contractures or cervicothoracic kyphosis is mandatory; these conditions require correction. The cervical spine may be corrected by a C7–T1 osteotomy and fusion under local anesthesia. Complications of osteotomies include nonunion, loss of correction, and neurologic and aortic injury.

5. Adult Scoliosis—Usually defined as scoliosis in patients >20 yo, it is more symptomatic than its childhood counterpart (discussed in Chapter 1, Pediatric Orthopaedics). Etiology is usually idiopathic, but can also be neuromuscular, senes-

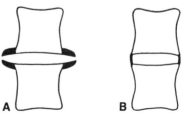
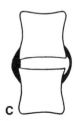

FIGURE 6–11. Differential diagnosis of *A*, osteophytes (DJD), *B*, marginal syndesmophytes (ankylosing spondylitis), and *C*, nonmarginal syndesmophytes (DISH). (From Rothman, R. H., and Simeon, F. A.: The Spine, 2nd ed., p. 924. Philadelphia, W. B. Saunders, 1982; reprinted by permission.)

cent (secondary to degenerative disease or osteoporosis), posttraumatic, and postsurgical. Curves are usually thoracic (secondary to unrecognized adolescent scoliosis), or lumbar/thoracolumbar (senescent). While the association between pain and scoliosis is controversial, back pain is the most common presenting complaint and appears to be related to curve severity and location (lumbar curves are more painful). Pain usually begins in the convexity of the curve and later moves to the concavity, reflecting a more refractory condition. Radicular pain and stenosis can occur and may require surgical decompression. Other complaints may include cosmetic deformity, cardiopulmonary problems (thoracic curves >60–65 degrees may alter pulmonary function tests; [PFTs]; curves >90 degrees affect mortality), and neurologic symptoms (secondary to stenosis). There is no demonstrated association between curve progression and pregnancy. Progression is unlikely in curves <30 degrees. Right thoracic curves >50 degrees are at highest risk for progression (usually 1 degree/year) followed by right lumbar curves. Myelography with CT or MRI is useful for the evaluation of nerve root compression in stenosis. Facet injections and/or discography may be utilized to evaluate symptoms in the lumbar spine. Nonoperative treatment includes NSAIDs, weight reduction, back school, muscle strengthening, facet joint injections, and orthotics (used with activity). The uncertain correlation between adult scoliosis and back pain makes conservative management, including a thorough evaluation for other more common causes of back pain, essential. Surgery is usually reserved for symptomatic curves >50–60 degrees in young adults and up to 90 degrees and beyond in older patients, for progressive curves, in patients with cardiopulmonary compromise (worsening PFTs in severe curves) and patients with refractory spinal stenosis. Operative risk is high (up to 25% complication rate in older patients), and complications include pseudarthrosis (15% with posterior fusion only), UTI, instrumentation problems, infection (up to 5%), and neurologic deficits. Additionally, long convalescence is usually required. Combined anterior release and fusion and posterior fusion and instrumentation may be beneficial for larger (>70-degree), more rigid curves (as determined on side-bending films), or curves in the lumbar spine. Preservation of the normal spinal kyphosis and lordosis with fusion is critical. Fusion to the sacrum is associated with more complications (pseudarthrosis, instrumentation failure, loss of normal lordosis, and pain), and should be avoided when possible. Achieving a successful result, including fusion to the sacrum, is enhanced by combined anterior and posterior fusion. The ideal implant for instrumentation in these cases has not been found; commonly used instrumentation for sacral fixation includes Galveston fixation and sacral pedicle or alar screw constructs.

6. Postlaminectomy Deformity—Progressive deformity (usually kyphosis) from prior wide laminectomy. Laminectomy in children is followed by a high risk (90%) of deformity. Fusion ± internal fixation may be considered as prophylactic

for younger patients who require extensive decompression. Fusion utilizing pedicular screw fixation is best for reconstruction in the adult lumbar spine.

7. Idiopathic Vertebral Sclerosis—Narrowing of the L4–L5 interspace and sclerosis of the L4 vertebral body seen on radiographs aids in the diagnosis of this disorder, which is yet to be fully understood. It may be related to degenerative disc disease or trauma. Idiopathic vertebral sclerosis occurs more commonly in females and is best treated nonoperatively.

G. Kyphosis

1. Introduction—Kyphosis in adults may be posttraumatic, congenital, secondary to trauma or ankylosing spondylitis, or a result of metabolic bone disease. Progressive kyphosis secondary to multiple osteoporotic compression fractures is usually treated with exercises, bracing, and medical management of the underlying bone disease. Surgical attempts at correction and stabilization are marked by a high complication rate. Consideration of an underlying malignancy as a cause of osteopenia should be made; evaluation with MRI is sensitive for determination of the presence of tumor.

2. Nontraumatic Adult Kyphosis—Severe idiopathic (old Scheuermann's) or congenital kyphosis may be a source of back pain in the adult, particularly when present in the thoracolumbar or lumbar spine. When the symptoms fail to respond to nonoperative management (see Adult Scoliosis above), posterior instrumentation and fusion of the entire kyphotic segment, utilizing a compression implant, may be indicated. Anterior fusion in conjunction is performed in curves not correcting to 55 degrees or less on hyperextension lateral radiographs.

3. Posttraumatic Kyphosis—May be seen following fractures of the thoracolumbar spine treated nonoperatively, particularly when the posterior ligamentous complex has been disrupted, in fractures treated by laminectomy without fusion, and in fractures in which fusion has been performed unsuccessfully. Progressive kyphosis may produce pain at the fracture site, occasionally with radiating leg pain and/or neurologic dysfunction if there is associated neural compression. Operative options include posterior fusion with compression instrumentation for more mild deformities; combined anterior and posterior osteotomies, instrumentation, and fusion for more severe deformities; and anterior spinal cord or cauda equina decompression combined with posterior instrumentation and fusion for cases involving neurologic dysfunction.

IV. Sacrum and Coccyx

A. Sacroiliac Joint Pain—Elicited with the patient lying on the affected side without support (Gaenslen's test), direct compression, or Flexion, ABduction and External Rotation (FABER or Patrick test). Local injections may have a diagnostic and therapeutic role. Orthotic management (trochanteric cinch) can be helpful. Fusion is not indicated unless an infection is present.

B. Idiopathic Coccygodynia—Painful coccyx is frequently associated with psychological conditions.

Four types of cocci have been identified (Postacchini and Massobrio):

Type	Coccyx Morphology	Coccygodynia
I	Slight forward curve, apex dorsal	Rare
II	Marked curve, apex ventral	Common
III	Sharp angulation between coccyx segments	Common
IV	Ventral subluxation of segments (sacrococcxygeal or coccycoccygeal)	Common

Treatment of coccygodynia should be conservative, with a donut pillow and NSAIDS. Complete or partial coccygectomy may relieve symptoms in type III or IV cocci, but is a last resort and is associated with a high complication and failure rate.

V. Spine Tumors and Infections

A. Introduction—The spine is a frequent site of metastasis, and certain tumors with a predilection for the spine have unique manifestations in vertebrae. These will be discussed in this section. **Tumors of the vertebral body include histiocytosis X, giant cell tumor, chordoma, osteosarcoma, hemangioma, metastatic disease, and marrow cell tumors. Tumors of the posterior elements include aneurysmal bone cysts, osteoblastoma, and osteoid osteoma**. Radiographic changes include absent pedicles, cortical erosion or expansion, and vertebral collapse. Bone scans can be helpful in cases of protracted back pain and night pain. MRIs are also useful—malignant tumors will have decreased T_1 and increased T_2 intensity. Malignant tumors occur more commonly in lower (lumbar>thoracic>cervical) spinal levels and in the vertebral body. Complete surgical excision is difficult and usually consists of tumor debulking and stabilization. Adjuvant therapy is essential. For more details on these tumors, please refer to Chapter 7, Orthopaedic Pathology.

B. Metastasis—The most common tumors of the spine, with spread to the vertebral body first and later invade the pedicles. Most tumors are osteolytic, and are not demonstrated on plain films until >30% destruction of the vertebral body has occurred. Breast, lung, and prostate metastases are most common, the latter being blastic. CT-guided needle biopsy is often possible, and surgery for diagnosis can be avoided. Poor prognosis is associated with neurologic dysfunction, proximal lesions, long duration of symptoms, and rapid growth. **Radiation therapy and chemotherapy are the mainstays of treatment** unless the tumor is destabilizing and progressive, or causes spinal cord or cauda equina dysfunction. In cases of neurologic deficit and/or spinal instability, anterior decompression and stabilization (preserving intact posterior structures) has a role and may result in recovery of neurologic function. Posterior stabilization is indicated in cases without anterior cord compression, in which there is persistent pain, or in which radiation therapy cannot be used. Life expectancy should play an important role as to whether surgical treatment is performed. Methylmethacrylate may be useful as an anterior strut, but should only be utilized as an adjunct because of the high complication rate. Iliac crest graft is favored if life expectancy is

>6 months. Anterior internal fixation may be indicated.

C. Primary Tumors

1. Osteoid Osteoma and Osteoblastoma—Common in the spine, and may present with painful scoliosis in a youngster. Scoliosis (the lesion is typically at the apex of the convexity) will resolve with early resection (within 18 months) in a child <11 yo. Osteoblastomas typically occur in the posterior elements in older patients, with neurologic involvement in over half. This presentation typically requires resection and posterior fusion.

2. Aneurysmal Bone Cyst (ABC)—May represent degeneration of other, more aggressive tumors. ABCs typically occur in the second decade of life. They occur in the posterior elements but may also involve the anterior elements. Treatment is excision and/or radiation therapy.

3. Hemangioma—Typically seen in asymptomatic patients. Symptomatic patients over 40 years old may present following small spine fractures. Classically has "jailhouse striations" on plain films and "spikes of bone" demonstrated on CT. Vertebrae are typically normally sized and not expanded (as in Paget's disease). Treatment is observation, and radiation therapy in cases of persistent pain after pathologic diagnosis. Anterior resection and fusion are reserved for refractory cases or pathologic collapse and neural compression.

4. Eosinophilic Granuloma—Seen more often in the thoracic spine; may present with progressive back pain. Classically may cause vertebral flattening (vertebra plana) seen on lateral radiographs. Biopsy may be required for diagnosis unless the radiographic picture is classic or histiocytosis has already been diagnosed. Chemotherapy is useful for the systemic form. Bracing may be indicated in children to prevent progressive kyphosis. Low-dose radiation therapy may be indicated in the face of neurologic deficits; otherwise symptoms are usually self-limited. At least 50% reconstitution of vertebral height may be expected.

5. Giant Cell Tumor—Destroys the vertebral bodies. Surgical excision and bone grafting are the usual recommended treatment. High recurrence rate is reported. Radiation therapy should be avoided because of the possibility of malignant degeneration of the tumor.

6. Plasmacytoma/Multiple Myeloma—Also common in the spine, causing osteopenic, lytic lesions. Pain, pathologic fractures, and diffuse osteoporosis are common. Increased calcium and decreased hematocrit are common, as well as abnormal protein studies. Treatment is radiation therapy (3,000–4,000 centigrays) ± chemotherapy. Surgery is reserved for instability and patients with refractory neurologic symptoms.

7. Chordoma—Classically a slow growing lytic, anterior sacral, or cervical lesion. These tumors may present with intra-abdominal complaints and a presacral mass. Radiation therapy and surgery are favored. Surgical excision can include up to half of the sacral roots (i.e., all roots on one side) and still maintain bowel and bladder function. Recurrence rate is high, but aggressive attempts at surgical excision are indicated. While a "cure"

is rare, patients typically survive 10–15 years following diagnosis.

8. Osteochondroma—Arises in the posterior elements. It is seen commonly in the cervical spine. Treatment is excision, which may be necessary to rule out sarcomatous changes.

9. Neurofibroma—Can present with enlarged intervertebral foramina seen on oblique radiographs.

10. Malignant Primary Skeletal Lesions—Osteosarcoma, Ewing's, and chondrosarcoma are uncommon in the spine. When they do occur they are associated with a poor prognosis. Chemotherapy and radiation therapy are the mainstays of treat-

ment, but aggressive surgical excision may have a role. Lesions may actually be metastases which are treated palliatively.

11. Lymphoma—Can present with "ivory" vertebrae. Usually associated with a systemic disease, lymphoma is treated after histologic diagnosis by radiotherapy and/or chemotherapy.

D. Spine Infections

1. Disc Space Infection—Osteomyelitis of the vertebral end plates can secondarily invade the disc space in children. *Staph. aureus* is the most common offender, but other gram-negative organ-

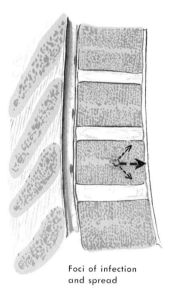
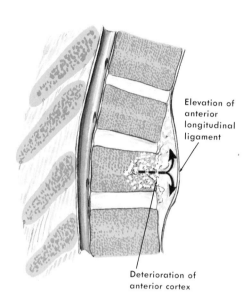

Foci of infection and spread

Elevation of anterior longitudinal ligament

Deterioration of anterior cortex

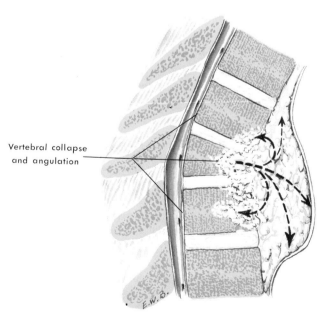

Vertebral collapse and angulation

FIGURE 6–12. Pathogenesis of spinal tuberculosis. (From Tachdjian, M. O.: Pediatric orthopaedics, 2nd ed., p. 1450. Philadelphia, W. B. Saunders, 1990; reprinted by permission.)

isms are common in older patients. Children (mean age 7, although all age groups are affected) commonly present with inability to walk, stand, or sit, back pain/tenderness, and restricted spine ROM. Lab studies may be normal except for an elevated ESR and WBC count. Radiographic findings include disc space narrowing and end plate erosion, but these findings do not occur until 10 days to 2 weeks, and their absence is unreliable. Bone scan is the diagnostic test of choice, and its use should not be delayed when a disc space infection is suspected. MRI is also useful in diagnosis, and may eventually supplant bone scanning. Treatment includes bed rest (traction, however, is contra-indicated), immobilization, and antibiotics.

2. Pyogenic Vertebral Osteomyelitis—Seen with increasing frequency, but still associated with a significant (6–12-week) delay in diagnosis. Older debilitated patients and IV drug addicts are at increased risk. A history of pneumonia, UTI, skin infection, or immunologic compromise is common. The organism is usually hematogenous in origin. A history of unremitting spine pain at any level is characteristic, and tenderness, spasm, and loss of motion are seen. Neurologic deficits are seen in 40% and are increased in older patients, with infections at higher levels in the spine, in patients with debilitating systemic illness (diabetes or RA), and with a marked delay in diagnosis. Plain radiographic findings include osteopenia, paraspinous soft tissue swelling, erosion of the vertebral end plates, and disc destruction. **Disc destruction, seen on plain radiographs or MRI, is atypical of neoplasms.** Bone scanning is sensitive for a destructive process, and MRI is both sensitive for detecting infection and specific in differentiating infection from tumor. Tissue diagnosis via blood cultures or aspirate of the infection is mandatory and, when made, 6–12 weeks of IV antibiotics is the treatment of choice. Bracing may be used adjunctively. Open biopsy is indicated when a tissue diagnosis has not been made, and anterior approaches or costotransversectomy are utilized. Anterior débridement and strut grafting are reserved for refractory cases, typically associated with abscess formation, or cases involving neurologic deterioration extensive bony destruction, or marked deformity.

3. Spinal Tuberculosis (TB; Pott's Disease)—The most common extrapulmonary location of TB is in the spine. Originating in the metaphysis of the vertebral body and spreading under the anterior longitudinal ligament, spinal TB can cause destruction of several contiguous levels or can result in skip lesions (15%) or abscess formation (50%) (Fig. 6–12). About 2/3 of patients will have abnormal chest x-rays. Severe kyphosis, sinus formation, and (Pott's) paraplegia are all late sequelae. Spinal cord injury may occur secondary to direct pressure from the abscess, bony sequestra (good prognosis), or rarely due to meningomyelitis (poor prognosis). Radical anterior débridement of the infection followed by iliac strut grafting (Hong Kong procedure) is the accepted surgical treatment in most centers. Advantages include less progressive kyphosis, earlier healing, and decrease in sinus formation. Adjuvant chemotherapy beginning 10 days before surgery is essential. In cases without severe kyphosis or neurologic deficit, ambulant chemotherapy and bracing remain a viable treatment option, particularly in centers not equipped for major anterior spinal surgery.

Selected Bibliography

Albrand, O.W., and Corkill, G.: Thoracic disc herniation: Treatment and prognosis. Spine 4:41–46, 1979.

Allen, B.L., and Ferguson, R.L.: The Galveston technique for L-rod instrumentation of the scoliotic spine. Spine 7:276–284, 1982.

Andersson, G.B., Jr.: Epidemiologic aspects of low-back pain in industry. Spine 6:53–60, 1981.

Bell, G.R., and Rothman, R.H.: The conservative treatment of sciatica. Spine 9:54–56, 1984.

Boachie-Adjei, O., Lonstein, J.E., Winter, R.B., et al.: Management of neuromuscular spinal deformities with Luque segmental instrumentation. J. Bone Joint Surg. [Am.] 71:548, 1989.

Bohlman, H.H., and Eismont, F.J.: Surgical techniques of anterior decompression and fusion for spinal cord injuries. Clin. Orthop. 154:57–67, 1981.

Bohlman, H.H., Sachs, B.L., Carter, J.R., et al.: Primary neoplasms of the cervical spine: Diagnosis and treatment of twenty-three patients. J. Bone Joint Surg. [Am.] 68:483–494, 1986.

Boxall, D., Bradford, D.S., Winter, R.B., and Moe, J.H.: Management of severe spondylolisthesis in children and adolescents. J. Bone Joint Surg. [Am.] 61:479–495, 1979.

Bradford, D.S., and Boachie-Adjei, O.: Treatment of severe spondylolisthesis by anterior and posterior reduction and stabilization. A long-term follow-up study. J. Bone Joint Surg. [Am.] 72:1060, 1990.

Bradford, D.S., Ganjavian, S., Antonious, D., et al.: Anterior strut-grafting for the treatment of kyphosis. Review of experience with forty-eight patients. J. Bone Joint Surg. [Am.] 64:680–690, 1982.

Bradford, D.S., Lonstein, J.E., Ogilvie, J.W., and Winter, R.B., eds.: Moe's Textbook of Scoliosis and Other Spinal Deformities, 2nd ed. Philadelphia, W.B. Saunders Company, 1987.

Brain, L., and Wilkinson, M.: Cervical Spondylosis. Philadelphia, W.B. Saunders, 1967.

Cain, J.E., Dryer, R.F., and Barton B.R.: Evaluation of dural closure techniques—suture methods, fibrin adhesive sealant, and cyanodcrylate polymer. Spine 13:720–725, 1988.

The Cervical Spine Research Society: The Cervical Spine, 2nd ed. Philadelphia, J.B. Lippincott, 1989.

Cervical Spine Research Society: Cervical spondylotic myelopathy. Spine 13:828–880, 1988.

Chapman, M.W., ed.: Operative Orthopaedics. Philadelphia, J.B. Lippincott, 1988.

Clark, C.R., Goetz, D.D., and Menezes, A.H.: Arthrodesis of the cervical spine in rheumatoid arthritis. J. Bone Joint Surg. [Am.] 71:381–392, 1989.

Cotrel, Y., Dubousset, J., and Guillaumat M.: New universal instrumentation in spine surgery. Clin. Orthop. 227:10–23, 1988.

Crawshaw, C., Frazer, A.M., Merriam, W.F., Mulholland, R.C., and Webb, J.K.: A comparison of surgery and chemonucleolysis in the treatment of sciatica: A prospective randomized trial. Spine 9:195–198, 1984.

Crenshaw, A.H., ed., Campbell's Operative Orthopaedics, 7th ed., St. Louis, C.V. Mosby Co., 1987.

Cummine, J.L., Lonstein, J.E., Moe, J.H., Winter, R.B., and Bradford, D.S.: Reconstructive surgery in the adult for failed scoliosis fusion. J. Bone Joint Surg. [Am.] 61:1151–1161, 1979.

D'Ambrosia, R., ed.: Musculoskeletal Disorders: Regional Examination and Differential Diagnosis, 2nd ed. Philadelphia, J.B. Lippincott Company, 1986.

Dee, R., Mango, E., and Hurst, L.C.: Principles of Orthopaedic Practice. New York, McGraw Hill Book Co., 1989.

DeLaTorre, J.C.: Spinal cord injury: Review of basic and applied research. Spine 6:315–335, 1981.

Ducker, T.B., Bellegarrigue, R., Salcman, M., and Walleck, C.: Timing of operative care in cervical spinal cord injury. Spine 9:525–531, 1984.

Dupuis, P.R., Yong-Hing, K., Cassidy, J.D., and Kirkaldy-Willis, W.H.: Radiologic diagnosis of degenerative lumbar spinal disability. Spine 10:262–276, 1985.

Eismont, F.J., Bohlman, H.H., Soni, P.L., Goldberg, V.M., and Freehafer, A.A.: Pyogenic and fungal vertebral osteomyelitis with paralysis. J. Bone Joint Surg. [Am.] 65:19–29, 1983.

Eismont, F.J., and Currier, B.: Current concepts review. Surgical management of lumbar intervertebral-disc disease. J. Bone Joint Surg. [Am.] 71:1266, 1989.

Epps, C.H., ed.: Complications in Orthopaedic Surgery, 2nd ed. Philadelphia, J.B. Lippincott Company, 1986.

Farey, I.D., McAfee, P.C., Davis, R.F., et al.: Pseudarthrosis of the cervical spine after anterior arthrodesis. Treatment by posterior nerve-root decompression, stabilization, and arthrodesis. J. Bone Joint Surg. [Am.] 72:1171, 1990.

Farfan, H.: The pathological anatomy of degenerative spondylolisthesis. A cadaver study. Spine 5:412–418, 1980.

Farfan, H., and Kirkaldy-Willis, W.: The present status of spinal fusion in the treatment of lumbar intervertebral joint disorders. Clin. Orthop. 158:198–214, 1981.

Fredrickson, B.E., Baker, D., McHolick, W.J., Yuan, H.A., and Lubicky, J.P.: The natural history of spondylolysis and spondylolisthesis. J. Bone Joint Surg. [Am.] 66:699–707, 1984.

Freeman, B.L., III, and Donati, N.L.: Spinal arthrodesis for severe spondylolisthesis in children and adolescents. A long-term follow-up study. J. Bone Joint Surg. [Am.] 71:594, 1989.

Frymoyer, J.W., Pope, M.H., Clements, J.H., Wilder, D.G., MacPherson, B., and Ashikage, T.: Risk factors in low-back pain: An epidemiological survey. J. Bone Joint Surg. [Am.] 65:213–218, 1983.

Frymoyer, J., Pope, M., Costanza, M., Rosen, J., Goggin, J., and Wilde, D.: Epidemiologic studies of low-back pain. Spine 5:419–423, 1980.

Gore, D.R., and Sepic, S.B.: Anterior cervical fusion for degenerated or protruded discs: A review of one hundred forty-six patients. Spine 9:667–671, 1984.

Griswold, D.M., Albright, J.A., Schiffman, E., Johnson, R., and Southwick, W.O.: Atlanto-axial fusion for instability. J. Bone Joint Surg. [Am.] 60:285–292, 1978.

Grubb, S.A., Lipscomb, H.J., and Coonrad, R.W.: Degenerative adult onset scoliosis. Spine 13:241–245, 1988.

Hales, D.D., Dawson, E.G., and Delamarter, R.: Late neurological complications of Harrington-rod instrumentation. J. Bone Joint Surg. [Am.] 71:1053, 1989.

Harris, I.E., and Weinstein, S.D.: Long-term follow-up of patients with grade-III and IV spondylolisthesis: Treatment with and without posterior fusion. J. Bone Joint Surg. [Am.] 69:960–969, 1987.

Helms, C.A.: Fundamentals of Skeletal Radiology. Philadelphia, W.B. Saunders, 1989.

Hensinger, R.N.: Current concepts review. Spondylolysis and spondylolisthesis in children and adolescents. J. Bone Joint Surg. [Am.] 71:1098, 1989.

Herkowitz, H.N., and Rothman, R.H.: Subacute instability of the cervical spine. Spine 9:348–357, 1984.

Herron, L.D., and Turner, J.: Patient selection for lumbar laminectomy and discectomy with a revised objective rating system. Clin. Orthop. 199:145–152, 1985.

Kelsey, J., and White, A.A., III: Epidemiology and impact of low-back pain. Spine 5:133–142, 1980.

Kirkaldy-Willis, W.H.: The relationship of structural pathology to the nerve root. Spine 9:49–52, 1984.

Kirkaldy-Willis, W., Wedge, J., Yong-Hing, K., Tchang, S., deKorompay, V., and Shannon, R.: Spinal nerve lateral entrapment. Clin. Orthop. 169:171–178, 1982.

Klein, B.P., Jensen, R.C., and Sanderson, L.M.: Assessment of workers' compensation claims for back strains/sprains. J. Occup. Med. 26:443–448, 1984.

Lauerman, W.C., Bradford, D.S., Transfeld, E.E., and Ogilvie, J.W.: Management of pseudoarthrosis after arthrodesis of the spine for idiopathic scoliosis. JBJS [Am] 73:222–236, 1991.

Lipson, S.J.: Rheumatoid arthritis of the cervical spine. Clin. Orthop. 182:143–149, 1984.

Lonstein, J.E., Winter, R.B., Moe, J.H., Bradford, D.S., Chou, S.N., and Pinto, W.C.: Neurologic deficits secondary to spinal deformity. Spine 5:331–355, 1980.

Lucas, J.T., and Ducker, T.B.: Motor classification of spinal cord injuries with mobility, morbidity and recovery indices. Am. Surg. 45:151–158, 1979.

Luque, E.R.: Segmental spinal instrumentation of the lumbar spine. Clin. Orthop. 203:126–134, 1986.

McAfee, P.C., and Bohlman, H.H.: One-stage anterior cervical decompression and posterior stabilization with circumferential arthrodesis. A Study of twenty-four patients who had a traumatic or a neoplastic lesion. J. Bone Joint Surg. [Am.] 71:78, 1989.

McAfee, P.C., Bohlman, H.H., and Yuan, H.A.: Anterior decompression of traumatic thoracolumbar fractures with incomplete neurological deficit using a retroperitoneal approach. J. Bone Joint Surg. [Am.] 67:89–104, 1985.

McKenzie, R.: The Lumbar Spine: Mechanical Diagnosis and Therapy. New Zealand, Spinal Publications, 1981.

Nachemson, A.: Adult scoliosis and back pain. Spine 4:513–517, 1979.

Nachemson, A.: The lumbar spine: An orthopaedic challenge. Spine 1:59–71, 1976.

Nachemson, A.L.: The Natural Course of Low Back Pain. St. Louis, C.V. Mosby Company, 1982.

Nachemson, A.: Recent advances in the treatment of low back pain. Int. Orthop. 9:1–10, 1985.

Nachemson, A.: Work for all: For those with low back pain as well. Clin. Orthop. 179:77–85, 1983.

Nash, C.L., Jr., and Brown, R.H.: Current concepts review. Spinal cord monitoring. J. Bone Joint Surg. [Am.] 71:627, 1989.

Ogilvie, J.W., and Sherman, J.: Spondylolysis in Scheuermann's disease. Spine 12:251–253, 1987.

Orthopaedic Knowledge Update Home Study Syllabus I, II, and III. Chicago, American Academy of Orthopaedic Surgeons, 1984, 1987, 1990.

Pedersen, A.K., and Hagen, R.: Spondylolysis and spondylolisthesis. Treatment by internal fixation and bone-grafting of the defect. J. Bone Joint Surg. [Am.] 70:15, 1988.

Peek, R.D., Wiltse, L.L., Reynolds, J.B., et al.: In situ arthrodesis without decompression for grade-III or IV isthmic spondylolisthesis in adults who have severe sciatica. J. Bone Joint Surg. [Am.] 71:62, 1989.

Postacchini, F., and Massobrio, M.: Idiopathic coccygodynia: Analysis of fifty-one operative cases and a radiographic study of the normal coccyx. J. Bone Joint Surg. [Am.] 65:1116–1124, 1983.

Ransford, A.O., Pozo, J.L., Hutton, P.A.N., and Kirwan, E.O'G.: The behaviour pattern of the scoliosis associated with osteoid osteoma or osteoblastoma of the spine. J. Bone Joint Surg. [Br.] 66:16–20, 1984.

Rothman, R.H., and Simeone, F.A.: The Spine, 2nd ed. Philadelphia, W.B. Saunders Co., 1982.

Santavirta, S., Slatis, P., Kankaanpaa, U., Sandelin, J., and Laasonen, E.: Treatment of the cervical spine in rheumatoid arthritis. J. Bone Joint Surg. [Am.] 70:658, 1988.

Siegal, T., Tiqva, P., and Siegal, T.: Vertebral body resection for epidural compression by malignant tumors: Results of forty-seven consecutive operative procedures. J. Bone Joint Surg. [Am.] 67:375–382, 1985.

Simmons, E.H.: Flexion deformities of the neck and ankylosing spondylitis. J. Bone Joint Surg. [Br.] 51:193, 1969.

Simmons, E.H.: Kyphotic deformity of the spine in ankylosing spondylitis. Clin. Orthop. 128:65–77, 1977.

Simmons, J.W., Chairman: The Challenge of the Lumbar Spine '88, Conference, November 9–13, 1988, San Antonio, Texas.

Slatis, P., Santavirta, S., Sandelin, J., et al.: Cranial subluxation of the odontoid process in rheumatoid arthritis. J. Bone Joint Surg. [Am.] 71:189, 1989.

Smith, M.D., and Bohlman, H.H.: Spondylolisthesis treated by a single-stage operation combining decompression with in situ posterolateral and anterior fusion. An analysis of eleven patients who had long-term follow-up. J. Bone Joint Surg [Am.] 72:415, 1990.

Sponseller, P.D., Cohen, M.S., Nachemson, A.L., et al.: Results of surgical treatment of adults with idiopathic scoliosis. J. Bone Joint Surg. [Am.] 69:667–675, 1987.

Veidlinger, O.F., Colwill, J.C., Smyth, H.S., and Turner, D.: Cervical myelopathy and its relationship to cervical stenosis. Spine 6:550–552, 1981.

Weber, H.: Lumbar disc herniation: A controlled prospective study with ten years of observation. Spine 8:131–140, 1983.

Weinstein, J.N., and Wiesel, S.W.: The Lumbar Spine. Philadelphia, W.B. Saunders, 1990.

Weinstein, J.N., and McLain, R.F.: Primary tumors of the spine. Spine 12:843–851, 1987.

Weinstein, P.R., Karpman, R.R., Gall, E.P., and Pitt, M.: Spinal cord injury, spinal fracture, and spinal stenosis in ankylosing spondylitis. J. Neurosurg. 57:609–616, 1982.

Weinstein, S.L., and Ponseti, I.V.: Curve progression in idiopathic scoliosis. J. Bone Joint Surg. [Am.] 65:447–455, 1983.

White, A.A., Johnson, R.M., Panjabi, M.M., and Southwick, W.O.: Biomechanical analysis of clinical stabilization in the cervical spine. Clin. Orthop. 109:85–96, 1975.

Zdeblick, T.A., and Bohlman, H.H.: Cervical kyphosis and myelopathy. Treatment by anterior carpectomy and strut-grafting. J. Bone Joint Surg. [Am.] 71:170, 1989.

CHAPTER 7

Orthopaedic Pathology

I. Introduction

A. Nomenclature—**Sarcomas** are malignant neoplasms of connective tissue (mesenchymal) origin, and are the least common of all tumors. Spindle cell tumors form solid lesions that grow centrifugally and may be surrounded by a capsule in benign lesions or a pseudocapsule (fibrovascular zone of reactive tissue) in malignant tumors (sarcomas). Sarcomas generally remain within anatomic borders and compartments, but can expand into adjacent compartments as they mature. Malignant tumors can destroy the overlying cortex and go directly into the adjacent soft tissue. Musculoskeletal tumors can be classified as benign (subclassified as latent, active, or aggressive) or malignant (subclassified as low or high grade) based on their behavior. Tumor spread, unlike carcinomas, is almost exclusively by the hematogenous route. **Satellite lesions** represent local spread of tumor that remains within the pseudocapsule or reactive zone and do not represent metastases. **Skip metastases** are tumor nodules located within normal tissue outside the reactive zone, and represent true metastatic disease (Fig. 7–1). Both of these entities may be responsible for local recurrences after incomplete tumor resection.

B. Staging—Based on the GTM system (grade, tumor site, and metastases [Enneking]).

1. Grade—Tumors can be benign (G_0), or malignant (subclassified as low [G_1] or high [G_2] grade). Although newer methods of grading are being developed (including determining nuclear DNA concentration [ploidy] with flow cytometry), grade is usually assigned based on histologic, radiographic, and clinical parameters. G_0 lesions are clearly differentiated, have benign cytology, and have distinct margins on radiographs without satellite or skip lesions. They can be subdivided into latent (stage 1), active (stage 2), and aggressive (stage 3) forms. G_1 lesions have frequent mitoses, moderate differentiation, and may be indolently invasive but do not have satellite lesions. G_2 lesions have more frequent mitoses, are poorly differentiated, and are **anaplastic** (loss of structural differentiation), **pleomorphic** (variable size and shape), and **hyperchromatic** (increased nuclear staining). Sarcoma grading systems used by pathologists are based on three or four grades. In the four-grade system, grades 1 and 2 are considered Enneking G_1, and grades 3 and 4 are considered Enneking G_2. In the three-

grade system, grade 1 is considered Enneking G_1, and grade 3 is considered Enneking G_2. Grade 2 lesions in the three-grade system are evaluated individually.

2. Tumor Site—Determined by using specialized procedures, including radiography, tomography, nuclear studies, CT, and MRI. Compartments are used to describe the tumor site. Usually compartments are easily defined based upon fascial borders in the extremities. Of note, the skin and subcutaneous tissues are classified as a compartment, and the periosseous potential space between cortical bone and muscle is often considered as a compartment as well. T_0 lesions are confined within the capsule and within its compartment of origin. T_1 tumors have extracapsular extension into the reactive zone around it, but both the tumor and the reactive zone are confined within the compartment of origin. T_2 lesions extend beyond the anatomic compartment of origin by direct extension or otherwise (trauma, surgical seeding, etc.). Tumors that involve major neurovascular bundles are almost always classified as T_2 lesions.

3. Metastases—Regional and distal metastases both have an ominous prognosis; therefore the distinction is simply between no metastases (M_0) or the presence of metastases (including "skip" metastases) (M_1).

4. Staging of sarcomas is based on these parameters:

STAGE	GTM	DESCRIPTION
IA	$G_1T_1M_0$	Low grade, intracompartmental, no mets
IB	$G_1T_2M_0$	Low grade, extracompartmental, no mets
IIA	$G_2T_1M_0$	High grade, intracompartmental, no mets
IIB	$G_2T_2M_0$	High grade, extracompartmental, no mets
IIIA	$G_{1/2}T_1M_1$	Any grade, intracompartmental, with mets
IIIB	$G_{1/2}T_2M_1$	Any grade, extracompartmental, with mets

C. Evaluation

1. History—Night or rest pain of an aching or unrelenting character is classic in patients with sar-

167

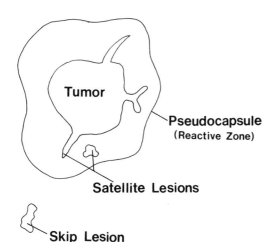

FIGURE 7–1. Satellite versus skip lesion—terminology.

comas. Detailed history of onset, symptoms, location, prior treatment, previous malignancies, injuries, exposure to noxious agents, family history, and other pertinent information is sought.
2. Physical Examination—Location, depth, attachment of masses, lymph node involvement, skin changes, tenderness, neurovascular status, effusion/pain/decreased range of motion of adjacent joints, and potential sites of occult primary carcinomas are all evaluated carefully.
3. Radiographs—Orthogonal views of the involved area are carefully reviewed. A concerted effort must be made to obtain any old films for comparison. At least 40% bone loss is required before lytic lesions can be detected on plain radiographs. A chest x-ray should be done with any potential malignancy. Radiographic characterization is based on the following parameters (**Enneking's four questions**).
   a. **Anatomic Location** and Site (Fig. 7–2)

LOCATION/SITE	TYPICAL PATHOLOGY
Epiphyseal	Chondroblastoma, chondrosarcoma, giant cell tumor, infection
Metaphyseal	Any lesion
Diaphyseal	Osteoblastoma, Ewing's, eosinophilic granuloma, lymphoma, adamantinoma, fibrous dysplasia
Pelvis	Mets, myeloma, Ewing's, chondrosarcoma, Paget's
Proximal humerus	Chondroid lesions
Knee	Osteosarcoma, adamantinoma, chondromyxoid fibroma
Ribs	Mets, myeloma, Ewing's, chondrosarcoma, fibrous dysplasia
Spine (Vertebral body)	Mets, myeloma, eosinophilic granuloma, chordoma, Paget's, hemangioma
Spine (Posterior elements)	Aneurysmal bone cyst, osteoid osteoma, osteoblastoma
Parosteal	Myositis, osteosarcoma, chondrosarcoma, chondroma
Multiple lesions	Mets, myeloma, hemangioma, fibrous dysplasia, osteochondromas, enchondromas, histiocytosis X

b. **Effect of the Lesion on the Bone**—Malignancies are more often associated with larger lesions with destruction of normal cortices, soft tissue masses, and irregular margins. Local extension into adjacent tissues is of importance in prognosis; MRI is very helpful in evaluation of this.
c. **Response of Bone to the Lesion**—Internal margins can be geographic (well circumscribed [either sclerotic or nonsclerotic] or ill defined); moth eaten (multiple staggered holes); or permeative (multiple oval cortical lucencies). Well-defined geographic internal margins are more characteristic of benign lesions. Certain lesions (e.g., aneurysmal bone cyst [ABC], fibrous dysplasia, and enchondromas) may expand bone, but are still contained by it. Lodwick has classified bony response to lesions as follows:

CLASS	DESCRIPTION	TUMOR
IA	Thick rim of reactive bone	Benign
IB	Thin rim of reactive bone	Benign
IC	Indistinct margin	Benign or malignant
II	Motheaten	Malignant
III	Permeative	Malignant

Periosteal reaction is a measure of intensity and aggressiveness. It is classified as continuous (either destructive [shelled] or exaggerated [onion skinning]); interrupted (common with malignancy—Codman's triangle); or complex (e.g., sunburst pattern with osteosarcoma).
d. **Unique Characteristics** (Matrix)—Based on the extracellular substance appearance: osteoid is cloud-like, chondroid calcification can give a "rings and arcs" appearance, and fibroid may look like ground glass. Distinctive features: vertebra plana (eosinophilic granuloma [EG]), "jail house" vertebrae (hemangioma), "picture frame" vertebrae (Paget's), "ivory" vertebrae (lymphoma, Paget's, and osteoblastic metastasis), "shepherd's crook" proximal femur (fibrous dysplasia), nidus in oval lesion (osteoid osteoma), "fallen leaf" (fracture through a bone cyst), fluid-fluid levels on CT (ABC), and eccentric "soap bubble" appearance (nonossifying fibroma). There are five diagnoses that can look like almost anything and should always be considered: metastases, infection, cartilage tumors, fibrous dysplasia, and eosinophilic granuloma.
4. Laboratory Studies—Are often nonspecific; but can be helpful. Elevated WBC and ESR is common, and Ca/Phos, Alk. Phos, liver function tests, BUN, Cr, and urinalysis can help. Thyroid function tests (TFTs) may help identify a thyroid carcinoma or thyroid dysfunction. Serum/urine protein electrophoresis (SPEP/UPEP) or immunoelectrophoresis (IEP) is required if myeloma is within the differential diagnosis.
5. Nuclear Medicine Studies—Whole-body bone scan assists in determining metastatic disease,

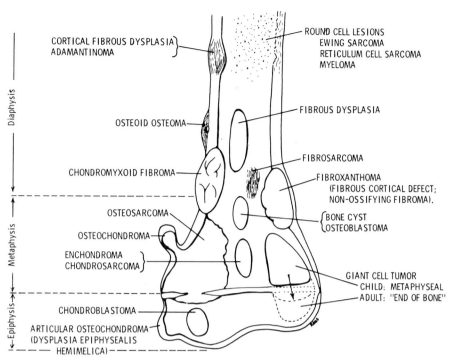

FIGURE 7–2. Location of common bone tumors. (From Madewell, J.E., Ragsdale, B.D., and Sweet, D.E.: Radiologic and pathologic analysis of solitary bone lesions—part I: Internal margins. Radiol. Clin. North Am. 19:715–748, 1981; reprinted by permission.)

polyostotic involvement, intraosseous extension of the tumor, and relation of underlying bone to a soft tissue sarcoma. Magnification imaging is often helpful in evaluating satellite lesions. High-grade lesions frequently have increased uptake beyond radiographic limits. "Cold" scans can be seen with tumors that stimulate little reaction, such as multiple myeloma, EG, lymphoma, and anaplastic sarcomas, and with thyroid, renal, and neuroblastoma metastases. Gallium scan can help identify malignant soft tissue lesions and can pick up subtle metastases (mets).

6. Computerized Tomography (CT)/Magnetic Resonance Imaging (MRI)—CT is very useful in evaluating bony lesions, including subtle cortical destruction, fractures, and calcification. Chest CT is also essential to evaluate lung mets with established bony malignancies. MRI is especially useful for soft tissue lesions and evaluating medullary extent, extraosseous extension, joint involvement, and "skip" lesions. **Malignant neoplasms have high intensity on T$_2$-weighted images** (edematous/myxoid) and are often heterogeneous (areas of hemorrhage and necrosis). Marrow extent is best seen on T$_1$ imaging.

7. Angiography—Useful for surgical planning when tumors are near neurovascular structures or possibly to identify neoangiogenesis to predict chemotherapy efficacy preoperatively. Can also be used to administer intra-arterial chemotherapy, and to embolize extremely vascular tumors preoperatively. Angiography can differentiate neovasculature versus normal vasculature and vascular "pooling" in the late venous phase of soft tissue sarcomas.

8. Biopsy—Done only after all staging studies are obtained. It must be in line with anticipated incisions and intramuscular (**longitudinal**). Care must be taken not to contaminate potential tissue planes. Needle or core biopsy can often be sufficient, especially with homogeneous tumors with characteristic radiographs. Diagnostic accuracy of needle biopsies is 70–80%. Careful marking of the needle track is important for later excision. Surgical biopsies should be carefully planned, and the capsule, if present, is closed. Biopsy of the bone should be avoided if possible, but if required, oval bone windows and elliptical soft tissue excisions are done. Bone cement (PMMA) can be used to "plug" holes to reduce tumor spread. Hemostasis and tight closure are important. Most biopsies are incisional. Excisional biopsies are reserved for obviously benign lesions, lesions of dubious malignancy where the pathologist is likely to require the entire tumor to establish a diagnosis, and small superficial lesions where excision does not compromise subsequent wide resection, if necessary. If autogenous bone graft is to be used, care must be taken not to contaminate the donor site. Frozen sections are most helpful for confirming intraoperatively that diagnostic tissue has been obtained as well as for establishing intraoperative diagnosis to guide immediate surgical decisions. Electron microscopic ultrastructural analysis and the newer DNA ploidy measurements may help establish tissue diagnosis and grade. Stains for monoclonal antibodies can also identify tumor types. Fresh tissue is required. The following are commonly tested immunohistochemical tumor markers:

MARKER	TUMOR
Leukocyte common antigen	Lymphoma
Cytokeratins	Synovial, epithelioid sarcomas
Desmin	Muscle tumors
S 100 protein	Neural tumors and myeloma
Vimentin, keratin	Carcinomas

Flow cytometry may be useful in determining if soft tissue lesions are malignant.

D. Surgical Procedures—In general, one centimeter of tissue on each side of the biopsy incision should be removed. Classification of surgical procedures is based on the surgical plane of dissection in relation to the tumor (Fig. 7–3).

1. Intracapsular—Through the capsule/pseudocapsule and directly into the lesion. Gross tumor is left, and the entire operative field is potentially contaminated.

2. Marginal—The entire lesion is removed in one piece. The plane of dissection passes through the capsule/pseudocapsule, leaving microscopic disease.

3. Wide—En bloc resection including the entire tumor, the reactive zone, and a cuff of normal tissue. May leave skip lesions in high-grade tumors.

4. Radical—Extracompartmental removal of the entirety of all tissue compartments that contain tumor. Usually curative in lesions that have not metastasized. Previously radial resection mandated amputation, but **limb salvage is possible if the oncologic result is similar** and anticipated function is acceptable. Significant neurovascular involvement, extensive disease, skeletal immaturity, and inadequate soft tissue coverage are all relative contraindications. Osseous resection can be intercalary (diaphysis), intra-articular (metaphysis), or extra-articular (both sides of a joint—

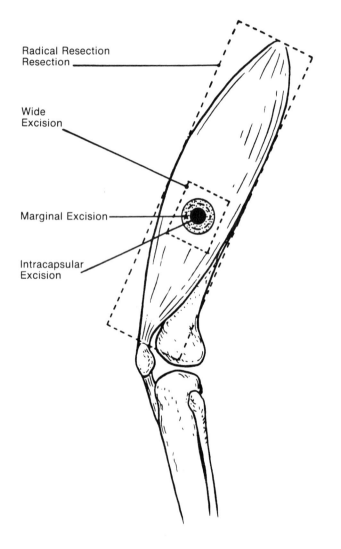

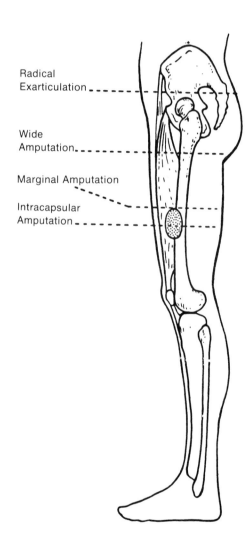

A   B

FIGURE 7–3. Tumor margins. (From Enneking, W.F.: A system of staging musculoskeletal neoplasms. Instr. Course Lect. 37:8, 9, 1988; reprinted by permission.)

usually involves arthrodesis). The entire compartment(s) is/are removed and a prosthesis or allograft is rigidly fixed to the adjacent bone. Limb salvage surgery is associated with numerous potential complications, but has established important new possibilities in tumor surgery.

E. Adjuvant Therapy—Chemotherapy and radiation therapy (XRT) have become increasingly important in the management of musculoskeletal tumors.

1. Chemotherapy—Has had a positive impact on disease-free survival in bony malignancies. Effective agents include doxorubicin, methotrexate (usually with leucovorin rescue), *cis*-platinum, and others. Neoadjuvant chemotherapy (preop) may also play an important role in some tumors. Chemotherapy may delay the onset of metastases and reduce local recurrence. Chemotherapy-induced secondary malignancies include leukemias (cyclophosphamides and melphalan), bladder cancer, and skin cancer.

2. Radiation Therapy (XRT)—Also efficacious, especially in the treatment of round cell and soft tissue tumors. It can be combined with surgery and sometimes allows less resection. It may also

be helpful preoperatively in some cases (creates a firm rind from reactive zone/pseudocapsule). Postirradiation sarcoma (usually osteosarcoma) is well recognized, extremely rare, and associated with a poor prognosis. Diagnosis requires a history of >5000–6000 cGys [centi-Greys] of therapy in the field of the lesion at least 5 years previously.

II. Soft Tissue Tumors (Table 7–1)

A. Introduction—Tumors of mesenchymal origin, can be benign or malignant (sarcoma).

1. Benign Soft Tissue Tumors—Important to differentiate from malignant counterparts, and often can be symptomatic in and of themselves (based on size or location). Benign soft tissue lesions are 100 times more common than their malignant counterparts.

2. Sarcomas—Arise from the supporting extraskeletal tissue of the body (muscle, fibrous tissue, fat) and are rare (<1% of all malignancies). They are typically a disease of adulthood (except for rhabdomyosarcoma), and are found most commonly in the lower extremity (especially the anterior thigh). They usually present as a painless

TABLE 7–1. SOFT TISSUE TUMORS

Tumor	Common Sites	Clinical Presentation	Histology	Treatment	Prognosis
Fibrous Tumors					
Juv. aponeurotic fibroma	Hands & wrists	Painful masses	Disorganized fibrous tissue, cartilage islands	En bloc excision	Mod. recurrence
Aggressive fibromatosis	Trunk	Infiltrative, aggressive spread	Spindle cells Dense collagen	Wide excision	High recurrence
Nodular fasciitis	Volar forearm	Tender, rapidly growing nodules	Fibroblasts, myxoid; inflammatory cells	Excision	Mod. recurrence
MFH	Thigh	Mass	Spindle cells/histiocytes, storiform pattern	Wide/radical excision ± XRT, ± chemo	Poor
Fibrosarcoma	Thigh/arm	Lobulated deep mass	Spindle cells, herringbone pattern	Wide/radical excision ± XRT, ± chemo	Poor
Fatty Tumors					
Lipoma	Shoulder, prox. thigh	Well defined, painless mobile mass	Mature lipocytes, myxoid	Marginal excision	Low recurrence (except angiolipoma)
Liposarcoma	Shoulder, prox. thigh	Large painful mass	Lipoblasts, myxoid or pleomorphic	Wide/radical excision ± XRT, ± chemo	Poor
Neural Tumors					
Neurilemmoma	Peripheral nerve (UE > LE)	Enlarged nerve	Antoni A & B areas	Marg. excision (shell out)	Good
Neurofibroma	Multiple	Multiple nodules	Nodules (Verocay bodies)	Excision if painful	Malig. degeneration
Neurofibrosarcoma	Multiple	Multiple painful nodules	Palisading pleomorphic spindle cells	Wide/radical excision ± XRT, ± chemo	Poor
Muscle Tumors					
Leiomyoma	Multiple	Subcutaneous mass	Normal smooth muscle cells	Excision	OK
Leiomyosarcoma	Deep	Painful mass	Wavy mitotic cells	Wide/radical	Mod. poor
Rhabdomyosarcoma	Extremities	Painful mass	Pleo: spindle cells parallel bundles, giant cells	Wide excision, chemo, ± XRT	Poor

(continued)

TABLE 7–1. SOFT TISSUE TUMORS (*Continued*)

TUMOR	COMMON SITES	CLINICAL PRESENTATION	HISTOLOGY	TREATMENT	PROGNOSIS
Vascular Tumors					
Hemangioma	Thigh, intramuscular	Purple mass, thrill	Epithelium-lined vessels	Observation	Good
Glomus tumor	Hands & feet	Blue-red skin discoloration, nail changes	Abundant vessels	Marginal excision	Good
Angiosarcoma	Extremities	Painful, purple mass	Vessels, pleomorphic cells	Wide/radical excision ± XRT, ± chemo	Poor
Kaposi's sarcoma	Hands & feet	Like pyogenic granuloma, AIDS	Spindle cells, vasc. spaces, phagocytic cells	Chemotherapy/excision	High recurrence
Synovial Tumors					
Ganglia	Wrist	Painless, cystic nodule	Collagenous tissue with few cells, myxoid fluid	Aspiration/excision	Good
PVNS	Knee	Painful boggy joint	Vascular villi, hemosiderin-stained giant cells	Synovectomy	High recurrence
Synovial chondromatosis	Large joints	Painful, swelling, stiffness	Nests of cartilge, stalks, free bodies	Synovectomy	Mod. recurrence
GCTTS	Hands & feet	Firm nodules, flexor surface	Round cells, spindle cells, giant cells, xanthoma cells	Marginal excision	Good
Synovial sarcoma	Long bone joints	Multinodular, radiographic calcification	Biphasic: spindle & epithelioid	Wide/radical excision ± XRT, ± chemo	Poor-moderate
Lymphatic Tumors					
Lymphangioma	Skin, subcutaneous	Subcutaneous masses	Lymph, vessels, smooth muscles	Avoid excision	Moderate
Lymphangiosarcoma	Skin, subcutaneous	Painful subcutaneous masses	Like angiosarcoma	Wide/radical excision ± XRT, ± chemo	Poor
Other					
Epithelioid sarcoma	Hand	Firm multinodular mass	Granulomatous, focal necrosis, inflammatory	Wide excision	High recurrence
Clear cell sarcoma	Foot & ankle	Multinodular mass near tendons	Nests of round cells with clear cytoplasm ± pigment	Wide/radical excision, chemo, ± XRT	Poor-moderate
Alveolar cell sarcoma	Skeletal muscle	Multiple nodules	Glandular nest of PAS + cells	Wide/radical excision	Moderate-poor

mass without systemic signs or laboratory changes. Soft tissue sarcomas commonly present with a firm, fixed mass with a history of weeks to months of steady growth. Approximately 25% are subcutaneous. They have a tendency to remain intracompartmental. They are frequently highly vascular and have a reactive zone surrounding them that may develop a pseudocapsule. Radiographs usually demonstrate a soft tissue mass. Bone scans must be studied carefully, including tangential views, to determine if the cortex is within the reactive rim of the lesion (and therefore must be included within the surgical margin). CT scan and/or MRI demonstrates a heterogeneous mass deep to the fascia. Microscopic extensions are common, emphasizing the need for wide excision of most tumors. Sarcoma cells are easily transplantable (vs. carcinoma), and require increased care in preserving surgical margins. Prognosis is based largely on size (**masses >5 cm require more aggressive work-up because they are more likely to be malignant**), histologic grade, and the presence of metastases. Small (<5-cm) lesions that are superficial, soft, and cystic may be observed initially. Surgery (wide local resection), chemotherapy (may prevent pulmonary dissemination and for rhabdomyosarcoma in younger patients), and XRT (5000–6500 cGys) to decrease local recurrence) all have a role in treatment. Preoperative XRT will allow easier resection because it allows the reactive zone to solidify into a rind.

B. Tumors of Fibrous Tissue—Like all categories, has benign (fibroma, aggressive fibromatosis) and sarcomatous (malignant fibrous histiocytoma [MFH], fibrosarcoma) members.

1. Fibroma—May in fact be a diffuse group of reactive lesions such as nodular fascitis, fibromatoses (Dupytrens, Desmoids, keloids, etc.), and

other lesions composed of benign fibrous tissue. Juvenile aponeurotic fibromas can occur in the hands and wrists of children and consist of fibrous tissue with islands of cartilage. Treatment includes en bloc resection.

2. Fibromatosis
   a. Palmar (Dupuytren's) and Plantar (Ledderhosen) Fibromatosis—Firm nodules that develop in the palmar or plantar fascia enlarge and the fascia hypertrophies, producing thickening and contractures. Increased amounts of benign fibrous tissue are commonly seen histologically.
   b. Aggressive Fibromatosis (Extra-Abdominal Desmoid)—The most serious of all benign soft tissue tumors occurring in adolescents and young adults. This lesion can infiltrate into multiple compartments and can result in death (from intrathoracic or retroperitoneal extension). The lesions can often be multiple (usually symmetrical). Staging studies are often inaccurate and usually underestimate the lesion's extent. Grossly, they are dense, white, firm lesions with poorly defined capsules and deep intertwining "roots." Histology demonstrates numerous thick strands of parallel collagen bundles that infiltrate adjacent normal tissue without destroying it. Uniform spindle cells in a regular pattern give a false impression of benignity. Wide resection is required for cure. Recurrence is common and difficult to differentiate from local scar tissue. Wide resection is necessary to avoid this complication. XRT may help control disease that cannot be surgically removed.
3. Nodular Fasciitis—Presents with tender, rapidly growing subcutaneous nodules, most commonly on the volar forearm. Tightly packed fibroblasts with a myxoid background are seen with inflammatory cells and relatively frequent mitoses on histology.
4. Malignant Fibrous Histiocytoma (MFH)—Most common soft tissue sarcoma of late adulthood. Can be solitary or multinodular and most commonly is seen in the thigh, with higher grade lesions occurring in deeper areas. Histologic features include spindle and histiocytic cells arranged in a **storiform** (cartwheel) **pattern**. Pleomorphism, chronic inflammatory cells, and varying degrees of myxomatous areas may be present. Histocytes demonstrating erythrophagocytosis are also common. Pleomorphic MFH is more common than myxoid MFH, but has a worse prognosis. The giant cell variant (giant cell sarcoma of soft parts) is similar to pleomorphic MFH but has scattered giant cells seen histologically. Surgery and XRT are effective in treatment; chemotherapy has not been shown to increase long-term survival.
5. Fibrosarcoma—Rare tumor arising from connective tissues. Can be seen in any age and in any location (proximal > distal). Most commonly occurs in the deep tissues of the thigh or arm, and can be near neurovascular structures. Grossly, the tumor may be lobulated or rounded. Microscopic features include intersecting fascicles of uniform spindle cells with sparse mitotic features and collagen arranged in interlacing bundles (**"herringbone" pattern**).
6. Dermatofibrosarcoma Protuberans—A less aggressive fibrous tissue tumor that appears in the subcutaneous tissues and skin. It typically presents as a purplish, elevated, firm mass firmly fixed to the skin. Cells are hyperchromatic, anaplastic, and pleomorphic but with few mitoses. The collagen is arranged in a storiform pattern (in fact, more so than in MFH!). Some consider this lesion to actually represent a subcutaneous MFH.

C. Tumors of Fatty Tissue—Benign lesions are lipomas, malignancies are liposarcomas.
   1. Lipoma—*The most common tumor of mesenchymal origin*, these tumors arise from fat and can be subcutaneous or deep. They are commonly found around the shoulder girdle and proximal thigh as painless, well-circumscribed, mobile, round or oval yellow masses. Histologically, mature fat cells and small vessels ± areas of myxoid tissue are present. Spindle cell lipomas, found most commonly around the neck and shoulder, also have clusters of spindle cells within the fat tissue. Intramuscular and intermuscular varieties also exist, and must be distinguished from liposarcoma. Angiolipomas are more aggressive, painful lesions that are poorly encapsulated, invasive, and highly vascular. Histologically, mature fat cells surround a proliferation of endothelial cells and cavernous sinuses. Recurrence after excision is common.
   2. Liposarcoma—Relatively common soft tissue sarcoma that usually occurs in middle age with a wide range of malignant potential. Radiographs may demonstrate radiolucency, and bone scans show more uptake than most other sarcomas. Liposarcomas are typically large, well circumscribed, and multilobulated, white-gray, and firm or rubbery. Identification of typical lipoblasts with fat droplets (signet-ring cells) are required for the diagnosis. Other histologic features may include mature fat cells, collagen, myxoid tissue, and poorly differentiated round cells. Two varieties of liposarcoma are commonly recognized:

TYPE	GROSS	HISTOLOGY
Myxoid	Red color, a well encapsulated, large reactive zone	Loose, poorly differentiated, small capillaries, round cells, mucinous background
Pleomorphic	Poor encapsulation, large reactive zone	Immature, disorganized cells, high mitotic rate; giant cells

The pleomorphic variety typically is higher grade and has a higher recurrence rate. Treatment includes wide resection for low grades, and radical resection and chemotherapy for higher grades.

D. Tumors of Neural Tissue—Benign neural tumors include neurilemmomas and neurofibromas; neurofibrosarcoma (malignant schwannoma) is the primary sarcoma in this group.
   1. Neurilemmoma—Encapsulated, fusiform growth

from a peripheral nerve. Verocay bodies with a central area of amorphous eosinophilic fibrillar material ringed by oval-shaped cells are the hallmark of this lesion. These lesions can usually be "shelled out" surgically without recurrence.

2. Neurofibroma—Unencapsulated tumor of Schwann cells that can occasionally degenerate into sarcoma. Histologically, slender bundles of wavy spindle cells with interposed dense collagen fibers predominate. Diagnosis requires identification of two microscopically distinct areas: **Antoni A** (pallisading/whirling groups of spindle cells), and **Antoni B** (fewer cells in a myxoid matrix). Verocay bodies are also seen in some areas.

3. Neurofibrosarcoma (Malignant Schwannoma)—Malignant tumor that arises from peripheral nerves, and most often is seen in patients with neurofibromatosis (10%). It may present with fusiform or bulbous enlargement of a large nerve. Histologically, intersecting wavy spindle cells in a pallisading pattern are common. Nuclear atypia and mitosis differentiate this lesion from benign neural tumors.

E. Tumors of Muscular Tissue—Include the benign leiomyoma (smooth muscle) and rhabdomyoma (striated muscle), and the malignant leiomyosarcoma and rhabdomyosarcoma.

1. Leiomyoma—Benign tumor of smooth muscles found usually in the uterus and GI tract. Occasionally seen in the subcutaneous tissues, usually originating from blood vessels. Normal smooth muscle predominates on histologic sections.

2. Rhabdomyoma—Benign tumor of striated muscle; very rare and may actually be a hamartoma.

3. Leiomyosarcoma—Rare smooth muscle tumor usually found in the deeper tissues, originating from blood vessels. It appears encapsulated grossly, and microscopically the cells have elongated nuclei with increased mitotic figures and a wavy undulating pattern. Treatment is similar to liposarcoma.

4. Rhabdomyosarcoma—Malignant tumor of striated muscle. The most common soft tissue sarcoma of childhood and young adulthood. Can be embryonal, botryoid, alveolar, or the more rare **pleomorphic** type (which appears in the large muscles of the extremities) based on histology. Histologically, rhabdomyosarcomas are composed of spindle cells in parallel bundles, multinucleated giant cells, and **racquet-shaped cells**, and are sometimes confused with MFH. The histologic hallmark is the appearance of **cross-striations** within the tumor cells (seen best on electron microscopy or with special stains, but may not be present in the adult form). This tumor can be very malignant, and treatment is wide resection if possible, or marginal excision with XRT and chemotherapy if not possible. Chemotherapy (Vincristine-Adriamycin-Cytoxan–VAC) is very effective in the treatment of rhabdomyosarcoma.

F. Vascular Tumors—Include benign hemangiomas and glomus tumor and malignant hemangiopericytoma, angiosarcoma, and Kaposi's sarcoma. Vascular tumors typically have only one arterial supply (seen on angiography) versus other tumors.

1. Hemangioma—Benign tumors of blood vessels. Can be generalized or (more commonly) localized. Classified based upon gross and histologic characteristics as capillary (most common), cavernous, venous, or arteriovenous. A diffuse variety (angiomatosis) can involve an entire limb. Grossly, the tumors are red-purple, and histologically, numerous epithelium-lined vascular channels predominate. They are usually intramuscular and are seen most commonly in the thigh. Most tumors occur during childhood, and surgery is only rarely indicated.

2. Glomus Tumor (Glomangioma)—A rare, painful lesion of the hands and feet that develops subungually, especially in women. **Small blue-red skin discoloration** and nail changes may be present. Uniform epithelial cells lining abundant vessels are seen. Surgical excision is curative.

3. Hemangiopericytoma—Benign tumor of blood vessels may originate from pericyte (of Zimmerman) cells (adventitia), and has a variable presentation/course.

4. Angiosarcoma—Malignant tumor of blood vessels. It is highly vascular and can occur at any age. Normal vascular channels are seen with other vascular channels made directly from malignant cells. Preoperative XRT may allow limb salvage. Infiltration and metastasis are common.

5. Kaposi's Sarcoma—Multiple hemorrhagic nodules that develop on the hands and feet resembling pyogenic granulomas on gross exam and microscopically consisting of spindle cells, vascular spaces, and hemosiderin-laden phagocytic cells. Commonly associated with AIDS; XRT, chemotherapy, and sometimes surgery can help temporarily control these lesions.

G. Tumors of Synovial Tissues—Include benign ganglion, pigmented villonodular synovitis (PVNS), and synovial chondromatosis, and malignant synovial sarcoma.

1. Ganglia—Cystic outpouching of a synovium-lined cavity, frequently about the wrist, and consisting of myxoid degeneration of synovial fluid. Histologically, the cyst wall is made up of dense paucicellular collagenous tissue without a true epithelial or synovial lining. Ganglia may erode into underlying bone (by external pressure). Intraosseous ganglia are sometimes seen in the medial malleolus and the scapular neck.

2. Pigmented Villonodular Synovitis (PVNS)—Exuberant proliferation of synovial villi and nodules characterize this disease, which occurs in adolescence and early adulthood. Pain, thickened synovium, and a brownish/serosanguineous effusion are common. Large, grape-like nodules protrude into cavities of joints, bursae, or tendon sheaths. Erosions into adjacent bone and cystic cavities occur in up to 1/3 of cases. Radiographs also demonstrate involvement of both sides of the joint (differential: tuberculosis and vascular lesions). The knee is the most common location. Grossly, a pannus-like projection of tissue can cover the joint surface. Histologically, highly vascular **villi** lined with plump hyperplastic synovial cells, **hemosiderin-stained multinucleated giant cells**, and sheets of heterogeneous cells are present. Treatment is with marginal excision via synovectomy through anterior and posterior ap-

proaches or arthroscopically (high recurrence rate). Treatment of diffuse or recurrent forms is more difficult and may include radiation therapy or intra-articular radiation synovectomy (yttrium-90).

3. Giant Cell Tumor of Tendon Sheath (GCTTS)—A benign tumor that usually occurs about the flexor tendons of the hands and feet. These are well-circumscribed, discrete lesions that arise from synovial tissue. They are well encapsulated, firm, fibrous lesions. Histologically, whirling connective tissue and sheets of round, oval, and spindle cells are common. Multinucleated giant cells of various sizes and shapes are seen around the edges of the lesions, often containing cholesterol slits. **Xanthoma** (foam) **cells** with hemosiderin staining and bland mesenchymal stromal cells are commonly seen. This tumor is considered by some to be a late stage of PVNS.

4. Synovial (Osteo-) Chondromatosis—Results from cartilaginous or osteocartilaginous metaplasia within the synovial membrane of joints, bursae, or tendon sheaths of the larger joints, especially the knee. Occurs in young adults who present with pain, swelling, and stiffness. Radiographs show multiple loose bodies. Grossly, large numbers of cartilaginous loose bodies may be seen. Some of the cartilage may undergo enchondral ossification in situ. **Arthrography** is often helpful to identify this disorder. Histologically, loose bodies with central necrosis and peripheral viable cartilage are seen. The joint capsule may have minute nests of cartilage that may protrude by a stalk of synovial cells into the joint. These often break off to form the loose bodies. Total synovectomy and removal of loose bodies is recommended but frequently is not curative.

5. Synovial Sarcoma—Malignant tumor with histologic similarities to synovium but rarely directly arising from a joint. Virtually all are high grade, and the histologic appearance is deceiving. The well-circumscribed, multinodular mass gives the appearance of synovium, but these tumors do not arise from a joint and are rarely connected to actual synovial tissue. **Soft tissue calcification** within the mass (occurs in about 25%) is an important radiographic feature of this tumor. Microscopically, a **biphasic pattern** of spindle cells (form an interlacing fascicular pattern) and epithelioid cells (nests of gland-like structures) is classic, but monophasic varieties are common. Lymphatic or vascular metastatic spread is common and carries a poor prognosis.

H. Tumors of Lymphatic Tissue—Include the benign lymphangioma and the malignant lymphangiosarcoma.

1. Lymphangioma—A benign tumor that develops in the skin, subcutaneous tissues, and sometimes bone. Histologically, lymph, blood vessels, and sometimes smooth muscle (lymphangiomyomas) are present. Excision should be avoided because of the high incidence of recurrence, hypertrophic scars, and persistence of symptoms.

2. Lymphangiosarcoma—May develop in chronically edematous extremities and consists of areas that resemble angiosarcoma on histology. Radical surgical resection and XRT are seldom curative.

I. Other Tumors

1. Epithelioid Sarcoma—Occurring more frequently in young adults, it is the **most common sarcoma of the hand**. The tumor arises in the deep soft tissues and presents as a firm, multinodular mass. Histologically, a granulomatous pattern with central areas of focal necrosis and chronic inflammation (leading to misdiagnosis in some cases) is common. Nodules of epithelioid cells with angulated, hyperchromatic nuclei predominate. Local recurrence and metastasis to regional lymph nodes are common.

2. Clear Cell Sarcoma—A small, unusual tumor that arises in conjunction with tendons or aponeuroses, especially around the foot and ankle of young adults. May be related to malignant melanoma. Usually it is a solitary or multinodular mass attached to tendons or aponeuroses. Microscopically, distinct fascicles and nests of large round cells with central nuclei and clear cytoplasm and collagenous trabeculae are present. Fine, granular pigmentation (melanin) may be seen. Lung metastases are often fatal.

3. Alveolar Cell Sarcoma—Aggressive tumor occurring within skeletal muscle. It is poorly encapsulated and may present with multiple nodules. Microscopically, it has a glandular appearance, thin-walled vascular spaces, and separate nests of round tumor cells that stain PAS positive.

J. Pseudotumors

1. Hematoma—Can occur following trauma and later become organized, simulating a tumor. Treatment is observation.

2. Myositis Ossificans (Stener's Tumor)—Extraskeletal ossification that occurs in muscles and other soft tissues. Can be traumatic (75%), nontraumatic, or progressive (rare). Typically, the lesions are distant from joints, have decreasing pain with time, are associated with an intact cortex, and demonstrate a zonal pattern—all of which help differentiate these lesions from osteosarcomas. Radiographically, soft tissue ossification not attached to bone is common. Microscopically, hypercellular spindle cells, peripheral woven bone, surrounding diseased and often "trapped" muscle, and normal osteoblasts making bone are typical. The **zonation from central immature fibrous tissue to peripheral mature bone** is characteristic, and helps distinguish myositis ossificans from osteosarcoma, where the central bone is likely to be most mature.

III. Bone Tumors

A. Introduction—Each tumor is discussed based upon its clinical, radiographic, gross, and microscopic characteristics, followed by a brief description of variants and current treatment options.

B. Osteogenic Lesions

1. Osteoid Osteoma (Fig. 7–4)—Usually are intracortical lesions of any bone, especially the femur, tibia, and vertebra (posterior elements), with a characteristic "**nidus**" and associated pain. The classic **pain** is worse at night, **relived by salicylates** (not narcotics), and exacerbated by alcohol. This tumor typically presents in the lower extremity of males in their second decade. If the lesion is in the vertebrae, the patient may present

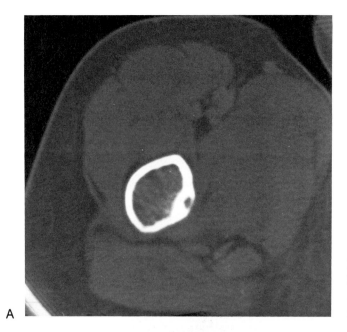

A

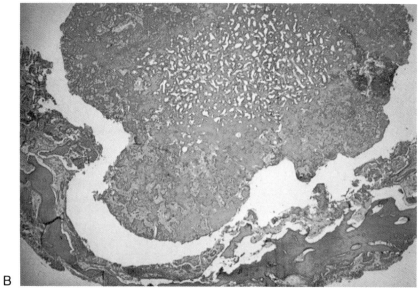

FIGURE 7–4. Typical osteoid osteoma. *A*, CT scan. *B*, Low-magnification micrograph. *C*, High-magnification micrograph. (From Wold, L.E., McLeod, R.A., Sim, F.H., and Unni, K.K.: Atlas of Orthopedic Pathology. Philadelphia, W.B. Saunders, 1990; reprinted by permission.)

B

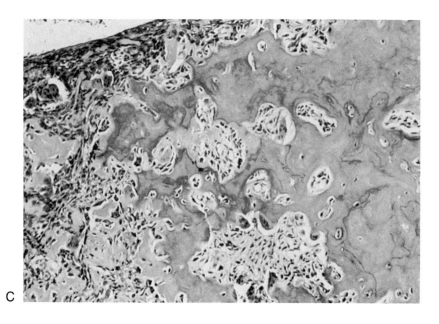

C

TABLE 7–2. BONE TUMORS

TUMOR	DECADE	COMMON SITE	LOCATION[a]	RADIOGRAPHS	HISTOLOGY	TREATMENT	PROGNOSIS
Osteogenic							
Osteoid osteoma	2	Proximal femur	M/D	Nidus with sclerotic rim	Trabeculae, giant cells, fibrovascular stroma	Observation, marginal excision	Rare recurrence
Osteoblastoma	2	Vertebrae (post. elements)	(P)V	Lucent, thin reactive rim >2 cm size	Trabeculae, giant cells, fibrovascular stroma	Marg. excision ± cryosurgery	Rare recurrence
Osteoma	2–5	Mandible, maxilla tibia	Flat	Ossified protrusion	Lamellar bone	Observation	Rare recurrence
Ossifying fibroma	2	Tibia, fibula	D(Ec)	Bowing	Fibrous tissue, bone, giant cells	Observation	Good
Paget's	3–5	Sacrum, spine, femur	Flat	Ivory vertebrae, cotton wool, bowing	Incr. blasts & clasts mosaic appearance	Calcitonin, diphosphonates	6% malig. degeneration
Osteosarcoma:							
Central	2	Knee, prox. humerus	M	Lytic and/or blastic, ST mass	Hypercellular, anaplastic spindle cells making osteoid	Radical/wide excision/adjuvant chemotherapy	Poor
Parosteal	3	Distal posterior femur	M	Lobulated ossified mass	Low-grade, fibroblastic stroma	Wide excision	Good
Periosteal	2	Femur, tibia	D	"Scooped out," partial calcification	Chondroid with osteoid spicules	Wide local excision, reconstruction	Moderate
High-grade surface	2	Femur	M/D	Cortical destruction	Chondroid, spindle osteoid, pleomorphic, freq. mitosis	Radical/wide excision, adjuvant chemotherapy	Poor
Chondrogenic							
Enchondroma	2–5	Hands, feet	IM	Medullary, punctate, calcification	Hypocellular cartilage	Observation, curretage, bone graft	Rare recurrence
Periosteal chondroma	2–4	Prox. humerus	M/D	Shallow cortical defect <3 cm in size	Cartilage lobules	En bloc excision	Rare recurrence
Osteochondroma	2	Distal femur, tibia, humerus	M	Contiguous proj., calcification cartilage cap	Marrow connects to bone, disorg. epiphyseal cartilage	Observation, excision at maturity	Rare recur., 1% malig. degeneration
Chondromyxoid fibroma	2–3	Prox. tibia	M(Ec)	Eccentric, elongated, radiolucent	Chondroid (stellate cells), myxoid & fibrous areas	Curettage, graft, or marg. excision	Rare recurrence
Chondroblastoma	2	Prox. humerus, knee	E	Lucent, small, sharp margins	Fibrochondroid islands, giant cells, chicken wire calcification	Curettage, bone graft	10% recurrence
Chondrosarcoma							
Central	4–6	Pelvic/shoulder girdle	M/D	Partial calcif., cortical erosion	Chondroid, cellular, pleomorphic binucleation	Wide excision	Histology dependent
Peripheral	3–4	Ilium, humerus, femur	M	Osteochondroma with change, lytic	Cytologic atypia, stringing of matrix	Wide excision	Histology dependent
Mesenchrymal	3	Pelvis, ribs, jaw	D	Poor marg., cortical destr., calcif.	Bimorphic: hyaline cartilage, round/spindle cells	Wide excision	Poor
Dedifferentiated	5–7	Femur, pelvis	M/D	Like central with aggressive area	Bimorphic: hyaline cartilage, high-grade spindle cells	Radical/wide excision ± chemo, ± XRT	Poor
Clear cell	3–4	Prox. femur	E	Epiphyseal, ± marginated	Lobulated, mononuclear clear cell, giant cells	En bloc resection	Good
Fibrogenic							
Simple cyst	1–2	Prox. humerus/femur/tibia	M	Sharply marg., "fallen leaf"	Thin fibrous lining, macrophages, giant cells	MPA injections, curettage & bone graft	40–50% recurrence
ABC	2	Vertebrae, femur, tibia	M	Cystic expansion, sclerotic rim	Cavernous space, fibrous walls giant cells	Curettage & bone graft	15% recurrence
Fibrous dysplasia	2–3	Skull, ribs, femur	M/D	Ground glass, expansile, bowing	Fibrous tissue, irregular woven bone	ASX: observation; SX: curettage & bone graft	Variable recurrence
Fibrous cortical defect	2	Distal femur, tibia	M(Ec)	Oval, sharp marg., multilocular	Fibrous tissue, clusters of giant cells, lipophages & macrophages	Observation	Rare recurrence
MFH	2–7	Distal femur, tibia	M/D	Lytic, cortical destr., soft tissue mass	Spindle cell, storiform pattern, giant cells	Radical/wide excision ± chemo, ± XRT	Poor
Fibrosarcoma	2–7	Knee, humerus	M/D(Ec)	Lytic, cortical destr., soft tissue mass	Spindle cell, herringbone pattern, giant cells	Radical/wide excision ± chemo, ± XRT	Poor
Hematopoietic							
Eosinophilic granuloma	1–2	Pelvis, femur, spine	D	Lytic, vertebra plana	Histiocytes + eosinophils, giant cells	Observation, chemotherapy	Rare recurrence
Myeloma	5–7	Spine, pelvis, ribs	(B)V	Multiple lytic lesions	Plasma cells, amyloid	Chemo ± XRT, prophylatic stabilization	Solitary:Moderate
Malignant lymphoma	3–7	Femur	D	Permative, lytic, poor marg.	Lymphocytes, cleaved nucleus strands	XRT ± chemo	Poor
Vascular							
Hemangioma	3–7	Skull, spine	(B)V	"Jailhouse" vertebrae	Cavernous, vascular spaces	ASX: observation; SX: curettage & bone graft	Rare recurrence
Angiosarcoma	2–7	Long bones, vertebrae	(B)V	Lytic, multifocal	Atypical endothelial cells	Wide/radical resection ± chemo, ± XRT	Unknown
Hemangiopericytoma	3–6	Pelvis	Flat	Lytic ± honeycomb	Incr. oval cells, thin "staghorn" vessels	Wide resection	Unknown
Neurogenic							
Chordoma	5–7	Sacrum/skull	(B)V	Asym destruction, soft tissue mass	Lobulated cords of physaliferous cells, chondroid	Wide excision	High recurrence
Neurilemmoma	2–7	Mandible	Flat	Discrete, erosive	Hypocellular spindle cells, verocay bodies	Marginal excision	Protracted

(continued)

TABLE 7–2. BONE TUMORS (*Continued*)

TUMOR	DECADE	COMMON SITE	LOCATION[a]	RADIOGRAPHS	HISTOLOGY	TREATMENT	PROGNOSIS
Other/Unknown:							
Giant cell	3–4	Knee, distal radius	E	Expansive lytic lesion	Giant cells w/nuclei = mononuclear cells	Excision ± cryosurgery/ phenol bone graft vs. PMMA	30% recurrence, 5% malig. degeneration
Adamantinoma	2–3	Tibia	D	Multicentric lucency, expansion	Epithelial nests w/nuclear palisading (spindle)	Wide local excision	Good
Ewing's	1–2	Pelvis, fibula, femur	D	Perm., lytic, onion skin	Small blue cell, fibrous strands, pseudorosettes	Chemo, wide excision vs. XRT	Poor
Metastases	4–7	Proximal	D/M	Multiple lucencies	Glandular (breast, prostate, lung, kidney, thyroid) or squamous	Tailored to patient	Poor

[a] M, metaphyseal; D, diaphyseal; (P)V, posterior vertebral; IM, intramedullary; E, epiphyseal; M(Ec), metaphyseal (eccentric); M/D(Ec), metaphyseal/diaphyseal (eccentric); (B)V, vertebral body.

with painful scoliosis. Radiographically, the nidus that represents the lesion is intracortical and is surrounded by dense reactive bone, giving the characteristic target appearance. Bone scans, tomograms, and CT are often helpful. Grossly, the nidus is usually red, granular, and surrounded by dense cortical bone. Histologically, the nidus has an interlacing network of osteoblast-lined, haphazardly arranged trabeculae, giant cells, and a fibrovascular stroma. It may be difficult to differentiate histologically from an osteoblastoma, except for its size (<1–2 cm). The natural history is thought to be self-limited, with spontaneous resolution over a period of years if the pain can be controlled (based on case reports). Treatment ordinarily consists of surgical removal of the nidus with a marginal excision. Radiographs of the specimen should be taken to ensure complete removal.

2. Osteoblastoma (Fig. 7–5)—Characterized by immature osteoid production and found commonly in the cancellous bone of the spine (posterior elements) and skull. It is typically seen in the second decade in males with a long history of pain. Radiographically, osteoblastomas are large, faintly radiodense lesions with thin reactive rims. Grossly, the lesions are reddish and granular, can be quite large (**must be at least 2 cm** large), and are well circumscribed. Histologically, an interlacing network of irregular, partially calcified bony trabeculae is characteristic, and often identical to the appearance of the nidus in osteoid osteoma. There are usually more giant cells and vascularity than in the nidus of the osteoid osteoma. It is an aggressive benign lesion with a high recurrence rate following curettage. Cryosurgery may help decrease this rate.

3. Osteoma—Osseous overgrowth of dense cortical bone usually occurring in the skull and mandible. It is occasionally seen in long bones like the tibia. A dome-like outcropping of encapsulated dense bone that is confluent with the periosteum is typically seen. Bone scans are intensely hot early and may be "spotty" later (because of areas of necrosis). Histologically, dense cancellous bone with small-diameter haversian canals is seen. Multiple osteomas may be seen in Gardner's syndrome.

4. Paget's Disease—This disease, which affects about 3% of men and women, is characterized by increased bony turnover. Increased osteoclastic bone resorption with irregular bone formation

leads to focally deficient bone. Paget's disease typically involves the sacrum, spine, femur, and cranium of older patients. Some have hypothesized a viral etiology. Paget's is usually described as having three stages: (1) osteoclastic (2) osteoblastic, and (3) sclerotic.

STAGE	RADIOGRAPHS	HISTOLOGY
Osteoclastic	Advancing "flame" of lucency	Incr. osteoclasts & vascularity
Osteoblastic	Thickened trabeculae, bowing	Osteoblasts > osteoclasts, fibrous tissue
Sclerotic	Dense, sclerotic bone	Mosaic, irregular trabeculae

Features of Paget's include deformities (bowing), pain, change in size of bones (increased hat size), kyphosis, and systemic features like cranial nerve impingement, bruits, and **high-output cardiac failure**. Lab studies are notable for increased alkaline phosphatase (osteoblasts) and urinary hydroxyproline (osteoclasts). Radiographic features vary with the stage of the disease but include cortical thickening, coarse trabeculae, sclerotic "ivory" or enlarged "picture frame" vertebrae, "cotton wool" appearance of the femur and pelvis, and "osteoporosis circumscripta" of the calvarium. Late radiographic hallmarks include enlarged bone, thickened cortices, and prominent trabeculae. Bone scans are also helpful for screening purposes. Histologically, there is "mosaic"-appearing bone with numerous random intersecting cement lines, overly active osteoclasts and/or osteoblasts (depending on the stage), and fibrous tissue replacement of marrow. Widened osteoid seams are also common. Fractures occur commonly, are usually transverse, and frequently require internal fixation; total hip arthroplasty is often required for stabilization of proximal femur fractures. Available treatment for symptomatic patients (with significant deformity or impending fracture) includes calcitonin (directly inhibits osteoclastic bone resorption); diphosphonates (EHDP, a pyrophosphate analogue that indirectly inhibits bone resorption by incorporating into bone and decreases turnover); and cytotoxic agents (mithramycin—works at the DNA level; limited indications, can cause paraplegia). Malig-

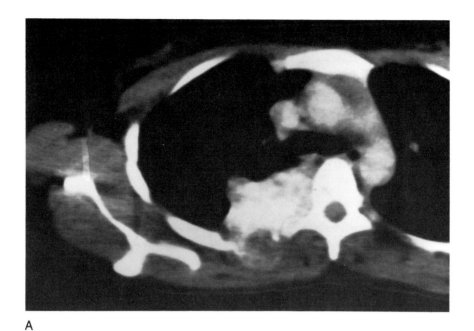

A

B

C

FIGURE 7–5. Typical osteoblastoma. *A,* CT scan. *B,* Low-magnification micrograph. *C,* High magnification micrograph. (From Wold, L.E., McLeod, R.A., Sim, F.H., and Unni, K.K.: Atlas of Orthopedic Pathology. Philadelphia, W.B. Saunders, 1990; reprinted by permission.)

nant degeneration (usually to osteosarcoma, chondrosarcoma, or MFH) has been reported in up to 6% of cases and is usually heralded with an increase in pain. Nuclear medicine studies are useful in evaluation of patients with known Paget's who are symptomatic. Bone scans show decreased uptake in areas of malignant degeneration and gallium scans demonstrate increased uptake. Malignant degeneration of Paget's disease usually carries a poor prognosis.

5. Ossifying Fibroma (Osteofibrous Dysplasia, Campanacci's Tumor)—Sometimes considered to be a variant of fibrous dysplasia, this rare tumor is typically seen eccentrically in the tibial and/or fibular diaphyses of children around 5 years old. Histologically, central fibrous tissue is surrounded by bony trabeculae that are rimmed with osteoblasts. Giant cells are common. Surgery is contraindicated for this lesion except with rapid progression, recurrent pathologic fracture, or persistence beyond skeletal maturity. The literature supports an unclear association with adult adamantinoma.

6. Osteosarcoma—The most common primary bone malignancy in children (boys > girls), occurs most commonly in the second and third decades of life. It is characterized by the **production of osteoid directly from malignant spindle cell stroma**. The knee and proximal humerus are common sites, and early diagnosis is difficult. A relatively painless mass is a frequent presentation. Osteosarcomas are classified as primary or secondary (following a preexisting lesion such as Paget's or a result of XRT, and usually seen in older patients). Primary tumors are further classified as central or juxtacortical.

   a. Central Osteosarcomas (Fig. 7–6)—Originate within bone and include conventional, telangiectatic, small cell, and fibrohistiocytic varieties. Conventional osteosarcoma (most common) can be further subdivided into osteoblastic, chondroblastic, and fibroblastic varieties based upon the predominant cell type. Telangiectatic osteosarcoma has one of the worst prognoses and typically is a lytic lesion with pools of RBCs and giant cells on histologic exam. Small cell osteosarcoma is histologically similar to Ewing's sarcoma but the cells are more "spindly." Fibrohistiocytic osteosarcoma is usually seen in older patients, and the microscopic appearance is similar to MFH. Radiographically, increased radiodensity, areas of radiolucency, and permeative destruction and soft tissue extension/ossification is common. Thickening of areas of bone and elevated periosteum may produce a "Codman's triangle" on radiographs. Grossly, the tumor begins from an intramedullary focus and is bony, with areas of necrosis and hemorrhage. Skip lesions are relatively common (20%). Microscopically, identification of malignant osteoid-producing stroma is required. Highly cellular areas contain microscopic trabeculae of bone between the cells. The spindle cells are pleomorphic, with hyperchromatic nuclei and often with atypical mitotic figures. Tetracycline labeling before biopsy will help identify osteoid production and skip lesions.

Adjuvant chemotherapy (pre- and/or postoperatively) has profoundly improved survival. Limb-sparing resection (contraindicated with major neurovascular involvement, pathologic fractures, inappropriate biopsies, infection, significant skeletal immaturity, or extensive muscle involvement) has helped improve quantity and quality of life. Patients who are "good responders" to chemotherapy will have 95% tumor necrosis, will have a good tumor "rind," and are better candidates for limb salvage procedures. Even in the best candidates, however, recurrence is greater (10%) than with radical amputation.

   b. Juxtacortical Osteosarcomas—Do not communicate with the medullary canal, occur typically in older patients (30–40 years old), and have a better prognosis (with the exception of the rare high-grade surface osteosarcoma).

      (1) Parosteal Osteosarcoma (Fig. 7–7)—Arises from the periosteum or adjacent soft tissues, especially around the **distal posterior femur**, the proximal humerus medially, and the proximal tibia laterally, and is not usually associated with pain. Radiographically, large, lobulated, broad-based lesions with dense, homogeneous new bone are commonly seen. Typically, there is a delineation between the tumor and the adjacent cortex. Small satellites can be seen as the lesion progresses. Grossly, there is **increased fibrous tissue**, there may be a cartilaginous cap, and the tumor at least partially encircles, but does not invade, normal bone. Histologically, the neoplasm is usually low grade. Parallel osteoid trabeculae lie in a hypocellular fibrovascular stroma. Occasionally tissue will invade adjacent trabeculae. The spindle cells are all strikingly similar and directly produce bone. Cement lines are typically irregular. Treatment is wide excision; 10% of these lesions dedifferentiate into high-grade osteosarcoma, and dedifferentiation is greater with recurrence after excision.

      (2) Periosteal Osteosarcoma (Fig. 7–8)—Arises from the superficial cortex of bone, usually the tibial shaft. It is more aggressive and more **chondrogenic** than parosteal osteosarcoma. Radiographs demonstrate a small radiolucent lesion with bone spiculation. A "scooped out" cortex and Codman's triangle are common. It is often associated with a large soft tissue mass arising from a cortical defect. The tumor is well-circumscribed and may have a chondroid consistency. Microscopically, cartilaginous lobules with atypical chondrocytes and peripheral osteoid producing spindle cells is common. Treatment consists of wide excision when possible, and sometimes requires amputation.

      (3) High-Grade Surface Osteosarcoma (Fig. 7–9)—A rare variant that is more aggressive, destructive, and carries a worst prognosis. It is best considered a conventional osteosarcoma that begins on the cortex

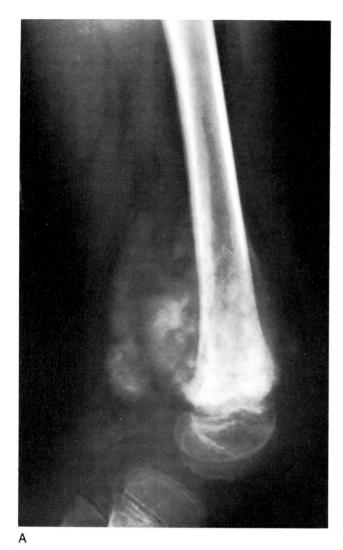

A

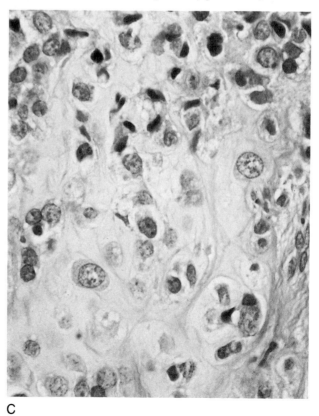

FIGURE 7–6. Osteosarcoma of the distal femoral metaphysis. *A*, Radiograph. *B*, Low-magnification micrograph. *C*, High-magnification micrograph. (From Wold, L.E., McLeod, R.A., Sim, F.H., and Unni, K.K.: Atlas of Orthopedic Pathology. Philadelphia, W.B. Saunders, 1990; reprinted by permission.)

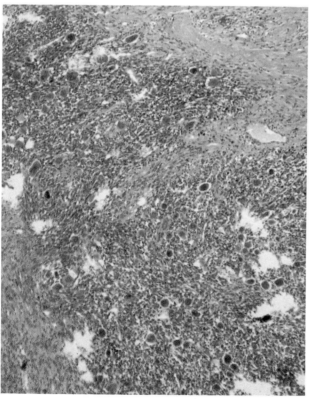

B

C

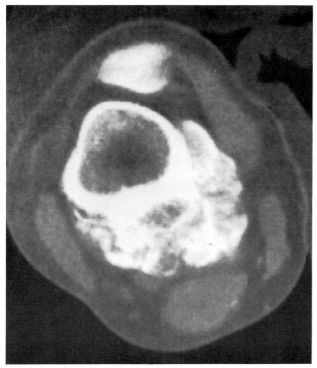

A

FIGURE 7–7. Typical parosteal osteosarcoma. *A*, CT scan. *B*, Low-magnification micrograph. *C*, High-magnification micrograph. (From Wold, L.E., McLeod, R.A., Sim, F.H., and Unni, K.K.: Atlas of Orthopedic Pathology. Philadelphia, W.B. Saunders, 1990; reprinted by permission.)

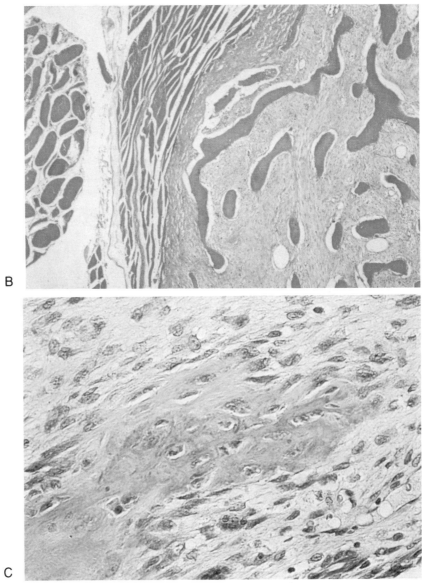

B

C

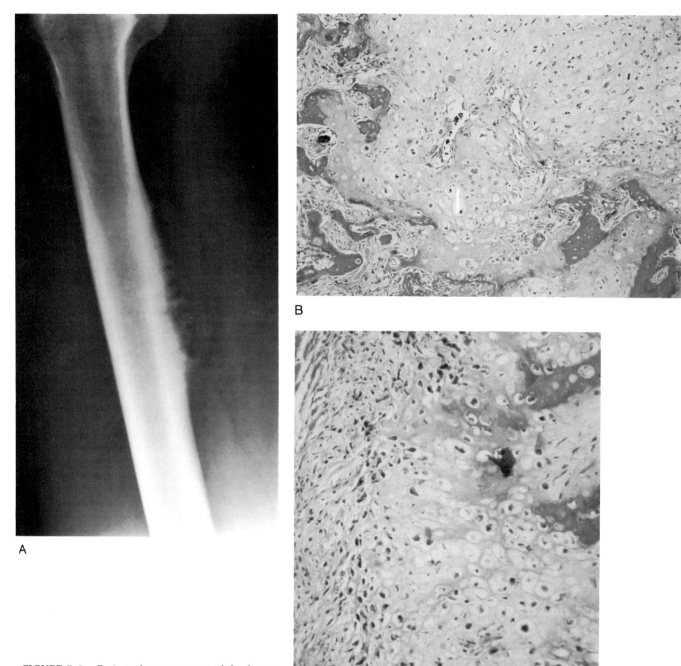

FIGURE 7–8. Periosteal osteosarcoma of the femur. *A,* Radiograph. *B,* Low-magnification micrograph. *C,* High-magnification micrograph. (From Wold, L.E., McLeod, R.A., Sim, F.H., and Unni, K.K.: Atlas of Orthopedic Pathology. Philadelphia, W.B. Saunders, 1990; reprinted by permission.)

and usually involves the femur. Histology is similar to central osteosarcoma. Treatment is also similar.

C. Chondrogenic Lesions
  1. Chondromas—Benign tumors of mature hyaline cartilage usually located within bone (enchondroma), but occasionally on the bony surface (periosteal chondroma).
     a. Enchondroma (Fig. 7–10)—Benign cartilaginous neoplasm arising in diaphyseal medullary cavities of long bones, possibly from epi-

physeal plate remnants. Can be solitary or multiple (Ollier's disease [alone] and Maffucci's syndrome [with skin hemangiomata]—both with higher rates of malignant transformation [up to 30% in Ollier's]). Enchondromas are asymptomatic and can be located in any bone, especially in the hands and feet. Radiographic scalloping, endosteal buttressing, cortical destruction, and soft tissue masses are signs of local aggressiveness, as enchondromas can undergo malignant transformation. Lesions that appear radiographically benign

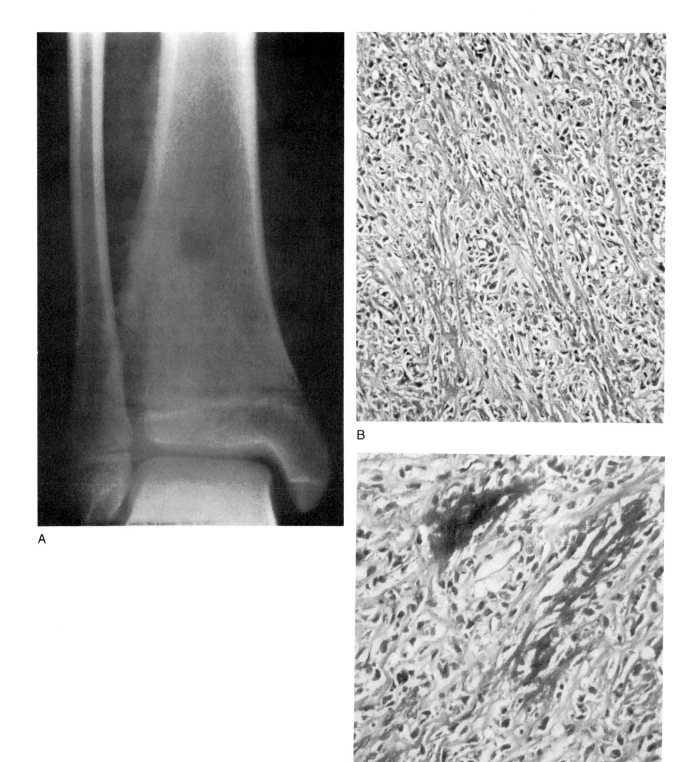

FIGURE 7–9. High-grade surface osteosarcoma. *A*, Radiograph. *B*, Low-magnification micrograph. *C*, High-magnification micrograph. (From Wold, L.E., McLeod, R.A., Sim, F.H., and Unni, K.K.: Atlas of Orthopedic Pathology. Philadelphia, W.B. Saunders, 1990; reprinted by permission.)

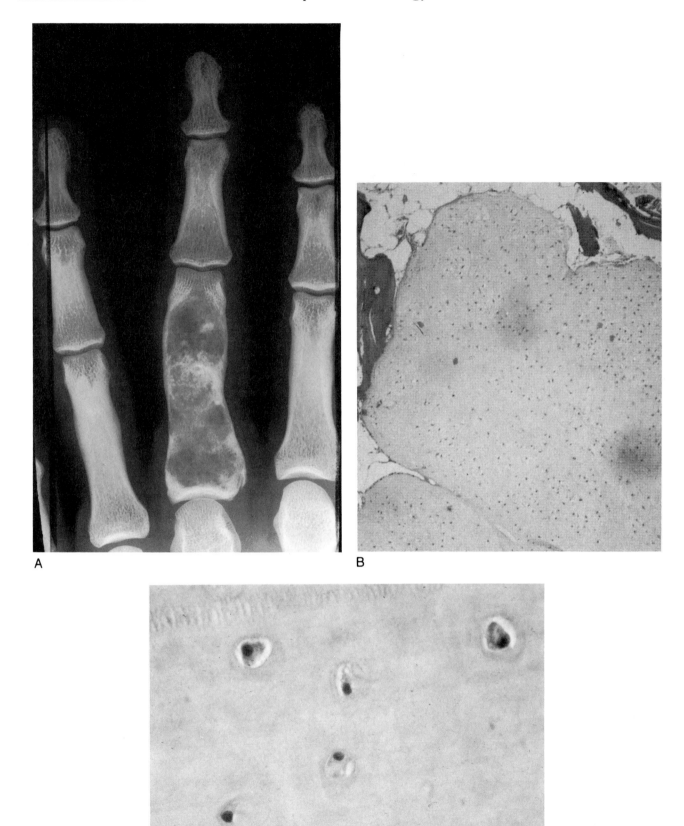

FIGURE 7–10. Typical enchondroma. *A*, Radiograph. *B*, Low-magnification micrograph. *C*, High-magnification micrograph. (From Wold, L.E., McLeod, R.A., Sim, F.H., and Unni, K.K.: Atlas of Orthopedic Pathology. Philadelphia, W.B. Saunders, 1990; reprinted by permission.)

can actually be malignant, especially in the pelvis or shoulder girdle. Grossly, the lesions consist of lobules of gray hyaline cartilage and are well circumscribed. Microscopically, nodules of normal hyaline cartilage with small, uniform chondrocytes and minimal atypia help to differentiate this from chondrosarcoma. Enchondromatosis (Ollier's or Maffucci's) can lead to bony deformities, pathologic fractures, and malignant transformation (best followed by bone scan). Malignant transformation is more likely in older patients with larger (>4–5-cm) lesions that do not involve the hands and feet. A change in sequential bone scans (cold to hot) is most indicative of malignant transformation.

b. Periosteal Chondroma (Fig. 7–11)—Benign cartilage lesions arising from the metaphyseal cortex of long bones, **especially the proximal humerus** and femur. They are typically oval masses of cartilage located near the periphery of the cortex. These tumors are usually seen in the second through fourth decade. Radiographs demonstrate a well-defined, shallow, **"scalloped" cortical defect** with occasional small flocculent foci of calcification outlined by a thin rim of mature bone. Histologically, lobules of cellular immature cartilage, with small immature nuclei, some with double nuclei and hypercellularity, are seen. Typically, there is a marrow zone of enchondral ossification at the interface of the lesion and the underlying cortex. Treatment is en bloc excision of the lesion with an intact rim of normal bone.

c. Extraskeletal Chondromas—Unusual lesions that can occur in the hands and feet.

2. Osteochondroma (Osteocartilaginous Exostosis) (Fig. 7–12)—One of the most common benign bone tumors. These lesions represent a disorder of normal enchondral bone growth, and are usually sessile or pedunculated lesions arising from the cortex of a long bone adjacent to the epiphyseal plate. They are usually solitary except in the disorder multiple hereditary exostosis. Tumor enlargement is common and ceases after maturity. Deformities of the forearm occur in about half of patients with forearm lesions. Ulnar bowing and radial head dislocation can occur, requiring distal hemiradial epiphysiodesis. Radiographically, a protuberant bony lesion on a stalk that arises adjacent to an epiphyseal plate and with marrow spaces contiguous with the normal bone is diagnostic. Pathologically, cartilage (<1–2 cm thick) resembling a disorganized epiphyseal plate caps irregularly shaped (unremodeled) trabecular bone. Calcified cartilage matrix may appear throughout the lesion, including within trabeculae and organized frequently within lobules. **Malignant transformation** (to low-grade chondrosarcoma) is possible, and is more common with multiple osteochondromas and more proximal lesions and growth with skeletal maturity. Angiography may show neovasculature, and bone scans are "hot," allowing differentiation from symptomatic bursae (although aspiration is probably more useful). CT is useful to follow **increased thickness of the cartilaginous cap**. In benign lesions, surgical excision is reserved for

symptomatic lesions or those arising from the axial skeleton and pelvic or shoulder girdle. Lesions in the forearm and ankle should also be considered for early removal if they adversely affect motion. Osteochondromas should rarely be removed prior to skeletal maturity due to the risk of growth disturbance and local recurrence. Care should be taken to avoid violating the overlying perichondrium and cartilage cap. **Multiple hereditary exostosis** (Ehrenfried's disease) is an autosomal dominant disorder with a mild decrease in stature, normal intelligence, and multiple osteochondromas. It is commonly accompanied by leg length discrepancy, knee and elbow angular deformities, and other skeletal abnormalities. Osteochondromas develop in multiple metaphyses of affected children and they continue to increase in size and number until skeletal maturity. Problems include nerve compression (especially peroneal nerve), ankle diastasis, angular deformities, and malignant transformation (2%). Evaluation should include baseline examination, bone scan, and plain radiographs of all identified lesions. Annual bone scan and exam can be used to follow patients, with further evaluation of lesions that show change or are symptomatic.

3. Chondromyxoid Fibroma (Fig. 7–13)—Metaphyseal eccentric lesion occurring typically in the **proximal tibial metaphysis** in the second and third decades. Radiographs show a sharply circumscribed, eccentric, radiolucent lesion. Other studies demonstrate that the lesion is partially in and partially out of bone. Histologically, chondroid (with stellate cells), myxomatous tissue, and fibrous areas are present. Treatment includes curettage and bone grafting or marginal excision. Recurrence rates are low.

4. Chondroblastoma (Fig. 7–14)—Benign chondroid production in the **epiphyses** of a skeletally immature child is characteristic of this lesion. Most commonly seen in the humerus (Codman's tumor), the lesions are lytic and radiolucent with faint calcification occurring about half of the time. Grossly, these tumors are small, gray-brown, and firm. Histologically, large numbers of polygonal chondroblasts with large nuclei, scattered mitotic figures, and some giant cells are present in a bland stroma with "lace-like" strands or islands of chondroid matrix. Sometimes described as a "bird's-eye view of a cobblestone street." Among the cartilage islands, areas of **"chicken wire" calcification** may be seen. Secondary ABCs may also be present with these lesions. Like osteoblastomas, chondroblastomas are aggressive benign lesions that tend to recur. Metastasis can occur. Again, cryosurgery may have a role in treatment.

5. Chondrosarcoma—Second to osteosarcoma in prevalence of bony sarcomas. Chondrosarcomas can arise from preexisting lesions (osteochondromas, chondromas) or they can be primary. They are usually associated with dull, deep pain. Radiographs may show invasiveness and soft tissue extension. Classically, osteochondromas with cartilage caps larger than 2 cm may have undergone malignant change to a secondary chondrosarcoma. However, secondary chondrosarcoma more commonly occurs in patients with multiple enchondromas. Scalloping and periosteal reac-

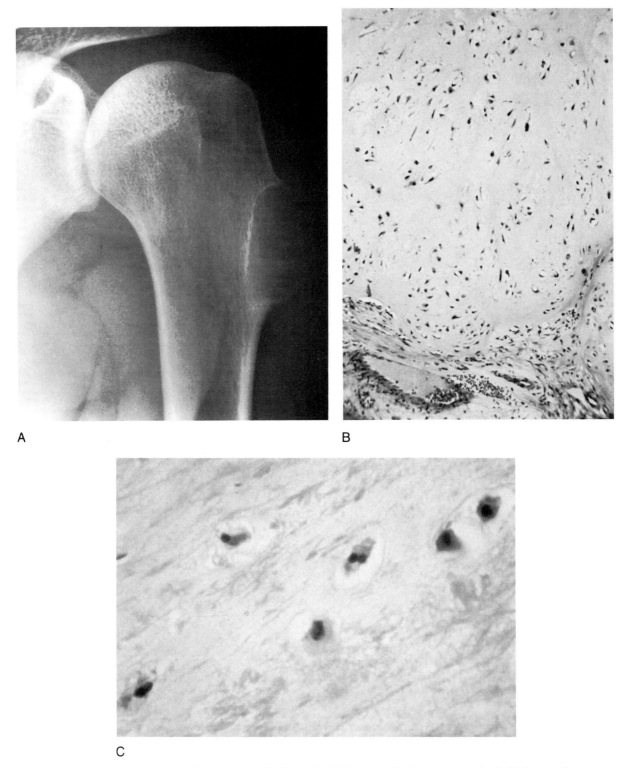

FIGURE 7–11. Periosteal chondroma. *A*, Radiograph. *B*, Low-magnification micrograph. *C*, High-magnification micrograph. (From Wold, L.E., McLeod, R.A., Sim, F.H., and Unni, K.K.: Atlas of Orthopedic Pathology. Philadelphia, W.B. Saunders, 1990; reprinted by permission.)

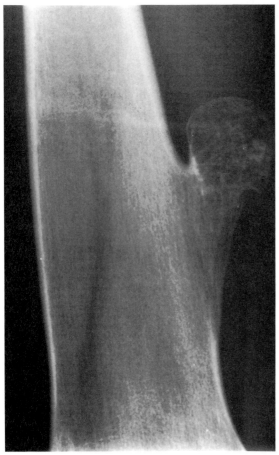

A

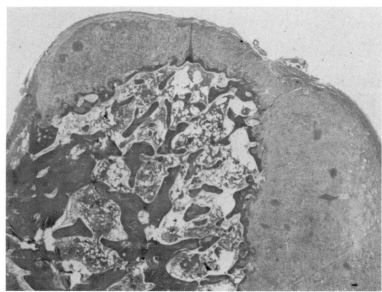

B

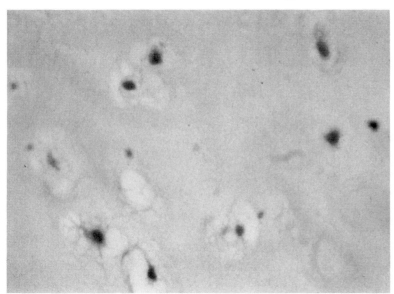

C

FIGURE 7–12. Osteochondroma of the distal femur. *A*, Radiograph. *B*, Low-magnification micrograph. *C*, High-magnification micrograph. (From Wold, L.E., McLeod, R.A., Sim, F.H., and Unni, K.K.: Atlas of Orthopedic Pathology. Philadelphia, W.B. Saunders, 1990; reprinted by permission.)

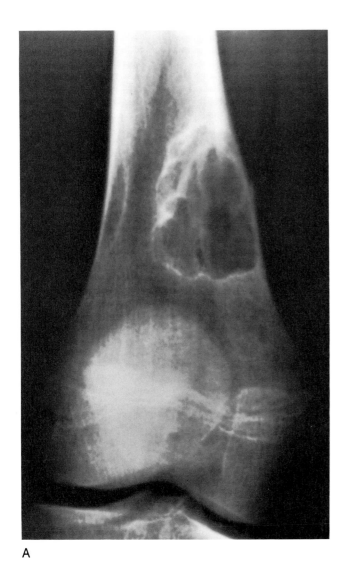

A

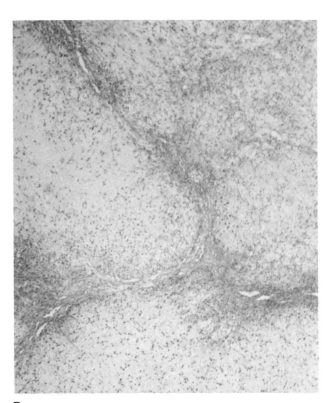

B

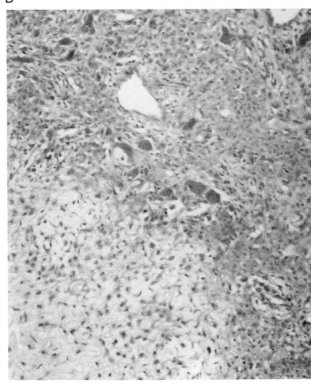

C

FIGURE 7–13. Chondromyxoid fibroma. *A*, Radiograph. *B*, Low-magnification micrograph. *C*, High-magnification micrograph. (From Wold, L.E., McLeod, R.A., Sim, F.H., and Unni, K.K.: Atlas of Orthopedic Pathology. Philadelphia, W.B. Saunders, 1990; reprinted by permission.)

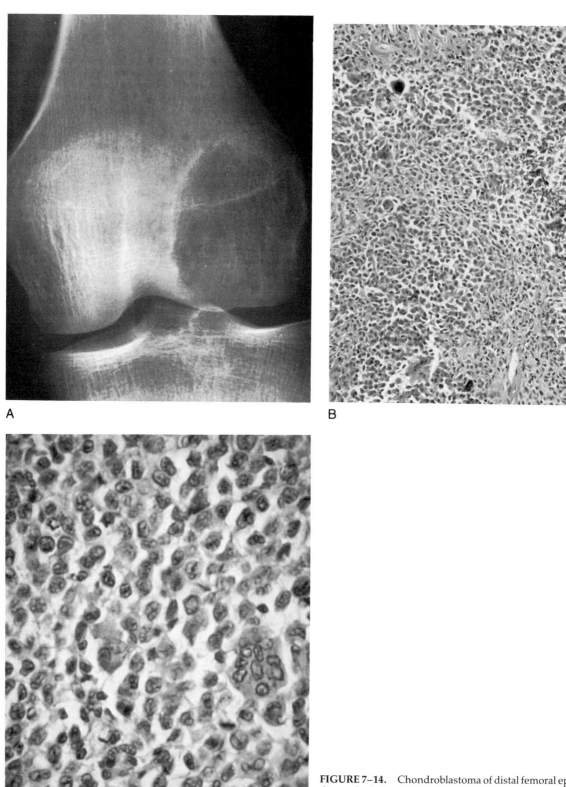

FIGURE 7–14. Chondroblastoma of distal femoral epiphysis. *A*, Radiograph. *B*, Low-magnification micrograph. *C*, High-magnification micrograph. (From Wold, L.E., McLeod, R.A., Sim, F.H., and Unni, K.K.: Atlas of Orthopedic Pathology. Philadelphia, W.B. Saunders, 1990; reprinted by permission.)

tion is consistent with chondrosarcomatous change. Secondary chondrosarcomas have a good prognosis but are frequently associated with other carcinomas. Primary, central, and appendicular chondrosarcomas all have a worse prognosis. Chondrosarcomas are commonly divided into five types:

TYPE	SITE	GRADE	OTHER
Central	Intramedullary	Mod.	Little calcification
Peripheral	Cortical	Low	Calcification, secondary
Mesenchymal	Intramedullary	High	Small round cells
Dedifferentiated	Medullary	High	Osteosarcoma/ MFH
Clear cell	Epiphyseal	Low	Like chondro- blastoma

a. Central Chondrosarcoma (Fig. 7–15)—Most chondrosarcomas are the central type, and they usually occur in middle-age patients in the pelvis, femur, and shoulder girdle. Pain is common and indicates growth. Painful "benign" cartilaginous tumors should arouse suspicion. Radiographically, these lesions are lytic ± with a sclerotic border, and have endosteal scalloping and calcification. Grossly, central lesions are expansile cauliflower-shaped masses with a fibrous pseudocapsule, and with cortical destruction and soft tissue extension. Fused nodules of gray hyaline tissue and areas of calcification are common. Microscopically, atypical cartilage is present with increased cellularity and nuclear atypia, as well as mitotic figures and multiple nuclei within individual cells. Touch preps are sometimes helpful in demonstrating these findings. More calcification and less cellularity and atypia are present in the center of the lesion. **Low-grade lesions are difficult to differentiate from enchondromas**, and clinical behavior (and bone scan changes) may distinguish these two diagnoses. Treatment is surgical removal, and is similar to osteosarcoma for high-grade lesions. Wide local resection is generally successful for treatment. Removal without initial biopsy is often indicated in obvious lesions to decrease recurrence rates (which can be high). Curettage ± cryosurgery or phenolization has been used for low-grade lesions, but this treatment may be hazardous.

b. Peripheral or Periosteal Chondrosarcoma—Less common and similar to periosteal osteosarcoma. Chondrosarcoma can also develop in osteochondromas. Older age, pain, and increase in size are more consistent with chondrosarcoma change.

c. Mesenchymal Chondrosarcoma—Rare, aggressive variant with biphasic small, compact, round spindle cells and islands of cartilaginous matrix. It is said to have a hemangiopericytoid appearance. More common in flat bones in younger patients. Treatment, including surgical removal, XRT, and chemotherapy, is rarely curative.

d. Dedifferentiated Chondrosarcoma—Presents as a lesion made up primarily of mature cartilage but with areas of malignant fibrosarcomatous components. Metaplasia of chondrosarcoma into osteo- or fibrosarcoma is often fatal. Treatment is like that for other high-grade sarcomas. Limb salvage is usually not a possibility.

e. Clear Cell Chondrosarcoma—Rare, slow-growing, locally recurrent tumor easily confused with chondroblastoma but malignant. Microscopically, sheets of cartilaginous cells in a lobular arrangement are mixed with scattered giant cells. This radiolucent lesion is often misdiagnosed and undertreated.

D. Fibrogenic Lesions

1. Simple (Unicameral) Bone Cyst (Fig. 7–16)—Benign lesions that occur during growth. Commonly located immediately beneath the epiphyseal plate in the proximal humerus > proximal femur, these lesions are usually asymptomatic until a pathologic fracture (which are common) occurs. Radiographs show the radiolucent lesion with well-defined margins, and sometimes a **"fallen leaf" sign** that occurs with pathologic fractures. Bone scan shows decreased uptake in the area if the diagnosis is in doubt. The lesion contains clear or bloody fluid, thin septae, and a thin cyst lining. Histologically, the fibrocollagenous cuboidal cell lining encloses variable amounts of loose mesenchymal cells, giant cells, chronic inflammatory cells, and macrophages with hemosiderin. Treatment includes observation, curettage, or aspiration and injection with methylprednisolone acetate (MPA) if they persist after pathologic fractures heal. Active cysts, which typically occur in children <10 years old, are associated with increased intralesional pressure, are immediately adjacent to the physis with a thin wall, and have increased numbers of osteoclasts and increased recurrence (50%).

2. Aneurysmal Bone Cyst (ABC) (Fig. 7–17)—Cystic cavities lined by a thick brown membrane containing blood. Half are primary and half secondary (to another benign lesion such as chondroblastoma) and they can occur in any bone. Commonly seen in flat bones and the metaphyses of long bones as well as the spine. Radiographs demonstrate expansile eccentric lesions with septation and a thin surrounding "eggshell" ring of bone. This ring is also well demonstrated on angiography and bone scans. **CT scans may demonstrate a fluid-fluid level** within the cyst. Microscopically, giant cells and endothelial cells lining cystic cavities containing extravasated RBCs are common. Stromal cell nuclei are more elongated than those of the giant cell. Intervening tissue is composed of loose mesenchymal tissue with giant cells, fibroblasts and fatty areas. Treatment of ABCs is usually liberal curettage and bone grafting.

3. Fibrous Dysplasia (Fig. 7–18)—Benign tumor of metaphysis/diaphysis that affects bone remodeling. May be a result of a developmental disorder

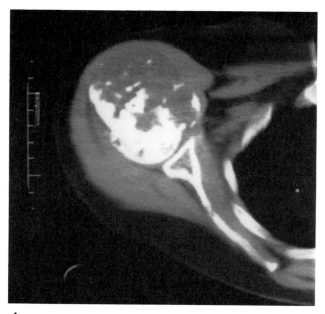

A

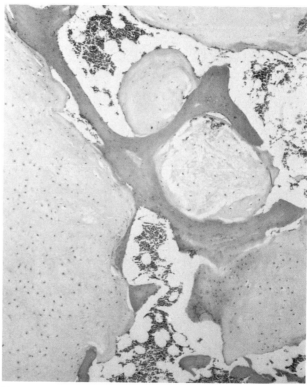

B

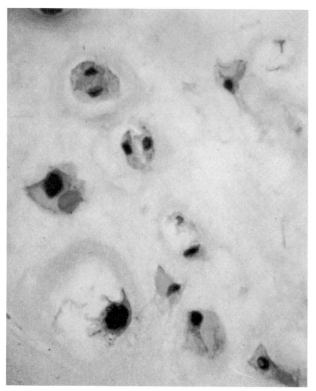

C

FIGURE 7–15. Chondrosarcoma of the humeral head. *A*, CT scan. *B*, Low-magnification micrograph. *C*, High-magnification micrograph. (From Wold, L.E., McLeod, R.A., Sim, F.H., and Unni, K.K.: Atlas of Orthopedic Pathology. Philadelphia, W.B. Saunders, 1990; reprinted by permission.)

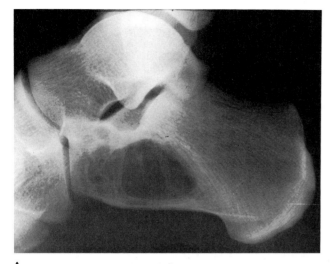

A

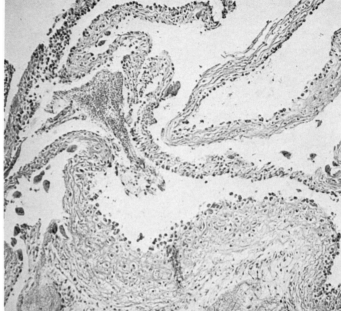

B

C

FIGURE 7–16. Unicameral (simple) bone cyst. *A*, Radiograph. *B*, Low-magnification micrograph. *C*, High-magnification micrograph. (From Wold, L.E., McLeod, R.A., Sim, F.H., and Unni, K.K.: Atlas of Orthopedic Pathology. Philadelphia, W.B. Saunders, 1990; reprinted by permission.)

of skeletal maturation. It can present in monostotic or polyostotic forms. Fractures and bowing are common. The "shepard's crook" deformity of the proximal femur is a result of bowing and multiple fractures, and can be associated with leg length discrepancies. Fibrous dysplasia is also common in the skull, ribs, and tibia. Radiographs also show a typical **ground glass appearance** and "scalloping from within." Histologically, woven bone, often in unusual shapes (**"Chinese letters"**) is surrounded by benign fibrous tissue. Fibrous tissue also replaces the marrow. Like Paget's, osteoblasts and osteoclasts can be seen in the same field. Café-au-lait spots in fibrous dysplasia differ

from those in neurofibromatosis because they are more irregular (described as similar to the rough "coast of Maine" in contrast to the smooth "coast of California" appearance in neurofibromatosis). **Albright's syndrome** includes polyostotic fibrous dysplasia, café-au-lait spots, and **precocious puberty**. Polyostotic fibrous dysplasia can also be associated with hyperthyroidism, vitamin D–resistant rickets, and Cushing's syndrome. Fractures occur commonly in this disease and heal by dysplastic callus, and therefore recur commonly. Treatment of these lesion often requires internal fixation and structural (cortical) bone grafting. Allografts may last longer than autografts. Al-

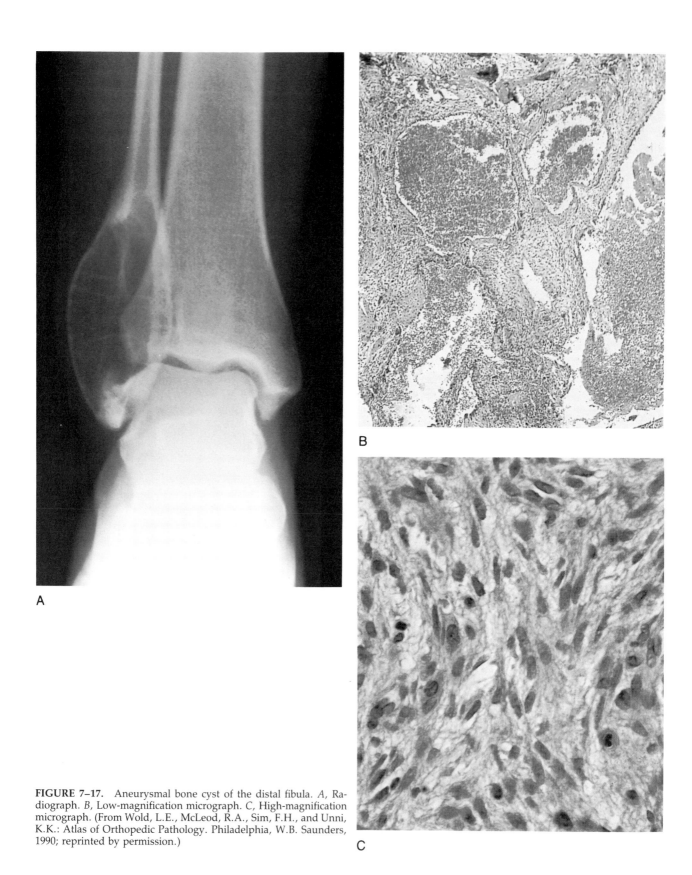

FIGURE 7–17. Aneurysmal bone cyst of the distal fibula. *A*, Radiograph. *B*, Low-magnification micrograph. *C*, High-magnification micrograph. (From Wold, L.E., McLeod, R.A., Sim, F.H., and Unni, K.K.: Atlas of Orthopedic Pathology. Philadelphia, W.B. Saunders, 1990; reprinted by permission.)

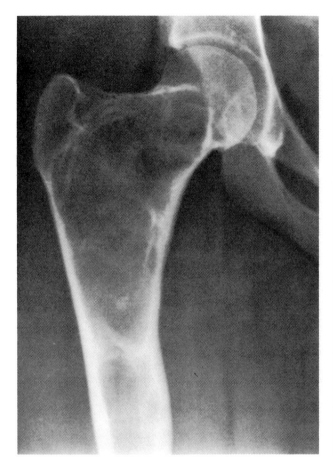

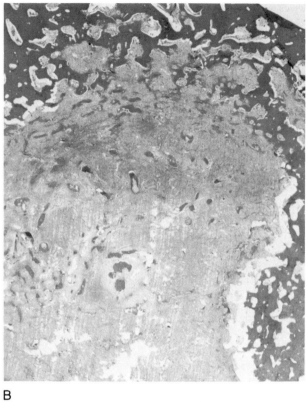

A

B

C

FIGURE 7–18. Fibrous dysplasia of the proximal femur. *A*, Radiograph. *B*, Low-magnification micrograph. *C*, High-magnification micrograph. (From Wold, L.E., McLeod, R.A., Sim, F.H., and Unni, K.K.: Atlas of Orthopedic Pathology. Philadelphia, W.B. Saunders, 1990; reprinted by permission.)

though the disease usually regresses at puberty, sarcomatous change has been very rarely reported.

4. Nonossifying Fibroma (Fibrous Cortical Defect) (Fig. 7–19)—Localized defect in the cortex of long bones usually occurring in the metaphyses around the knee. According to Enneking, it is the **most common skeletal lesion**. It represents a localized area (usually <⅓ of bone diameter) where bone fails to form. Radiographs show eccentric bulging and a well-defined cortical outline with scalloped sclerosis. When present in the distal radius, it is almost always on the radial side of the bone. Bone scan is usually positive early and normal later. Histology shows whirling fibrous tissue and smaller giant cells, with a thin shell of reactive bone. Most lesions are **self-limited** and ossify by the middle of the third decade. Management is by serial observation. Overhealing of these lesions may be the cause of bone islands seen commonly in adulthood. Surgery should be reserved for large lesions causing actual or impending pathologic fracture.

5. Desmoplastic Fibroma—Benign fibrous lesion of bone seen in adolescence and young adulthood that uncommonly occurs in diaphyseal bone as large defects filled with encapsulated, thick, rubbery tissue. This lesion is similar to soft tissue aggressive fibromatosis. Histologically, dense fibrous tissue with few cells is surrounded by an incomplete capsule and reactive bone. The lesion may "percolate" through the reactive bone around it. The radiographic appearance is like a simple cyst, but frequently with septation. CT scans may show microbroaching of the reactive rim. This is a benign aggressive lesion and should be treated with aggressive curettage and grafting. Recurrences may require wide excision.

6. Malignant Fibrous Histiocytoma (MFH) (Fig. 7–20)—High-grade tumor of adulthood. Occurs commonly in the metaphyses about the knee. Radiographs show a moth-eaten osteolytic lesion, cortical disruption, minimal periosteal reaction, and no bone formation. Histologically, there are spindle cells in a **storiform** (cartwheel or pinwheel) **pattern** with bizarre, giant foamy histiocytes and occasional erythrophagocytosis. Can be associated with bone infarcts and Paget's, and can be post-XRT. Adjuvant chemotherapy is favored, and prognosis is guarded.

7. Fibrosarcoma (Fig. 7–21)—Unusual tumor of middle-aged patients that occurs most commonly in long bones. Radiographically, a lytic lesion with variable margins (correlates with grade); and occasional pathologic fractures are seen. Fascicles of spindle cells with tapered nuclei arranged in a **"herringbone" pattern** are the most striking histologic feature. Giant cells are also commonly scattered throughout the lesion. Can follow XRT, Paget's disease, bone infarcts, and chondrosarcoma (dedifferentiation).

E. Hematopoietic Lesions
   1. Histiocytosis (Fig. 7–22)—One of the reticuloendothelioses with an unknown etiology. **Eosinophilic granuloma** is a solitary lesion that arises from the reticuloendothelial system in young children. The long bones, periacetabular pelvis, ribs, and vertebrae are common sites, and it can be multiple. Radiographs typically show a lytic, "punched out" lesion in long bones and **"vertebra plana"** in the spine. Periosteal thickening is also common. The tissue is usually yellow or pink when curetted and microscopically consists of sheets of Langerhans type histiocytes and eosinophils. On electron microscopy these cells have racquet-shaped inclusions (Birbeck bodies) in their cytoplasm. Treatment usually is simple observation, as many of these lesions will spontaneously heal and may reconstitute affected bone. Treatment of persistent lesions may require curettage or excision. The other two syndromes comprising histiocytosis are Hand-Schüller-Christian (develops in 20% of patients with EG and presents with widespread visceral [liver and spleen] and bony involvement and diabetes insipidus [from pituitary involvement]; lesions do not heal spontaneously and may destroy large areas of bone), and Letterer-Siwe (typically with less skeletal involvement but is associated with hepatosplenomegaly, adenopathy, CNS involvement, fever, anemia, thrombocytopenia, and fulminant fatal clinical course).

   2. Myeloma (Fig. 7–23)—Uncontrolled proliferation of marrow plasma cells (highly differentiated B lymphocytes) leads to the development of this tumor, **the most common primary malignant tumor in bone**. Common presentations include bone pain and anemia in a 50–60-year-old patient. SPEP and UPEP demonstrate a monoclonal gammopathy with an elevated M spike. Bence Jones proteins may be demonstrated in the urine of affected patients as well. Radiographically, multiple "punched out" lesions in ribs, vertebrae, skull, and pelvis are common. Bone scans may be falsely negative, and skeletal survey should be used for screening if myeloma is suspected. MRI can often identify subtle lesions. Solitary lesions (plasmacytomas) can present in bone (commonly vertebrae) or soft tissue. Histology demonstrates sheets of **plasma cells** ("clock faced" eccentric nuclei, perinuclear clear area, and increased RER on electron microscopy). Of note, the lesion lacks any background stroma. Myeloma can be associated with systemic amyloid disease, immunologic alterations, and hypercalcemia. Aggressive treatment is mandated. Systemic therapy with an alkylating agent plus a corticosteroid is combined with XRT and surgical stabilization of pathologic fractures. Some authors suggest wide excision of solitary lesions.

   3. Lymphoma of Bone (Histiocytic Lymphoma) (Fig. 7–24)—Usually a sign of disseminated disease, only rarely a primary tumor. The tumor typically presents in the third through fifth decades and fills the marrow cavity and extends through the cortex. It frequently involves the diaphyses of long bones and may be associated with a localized soft tissue mass. Radiographs may show a moth-eaten appearance. In the spine, "ivory" vertebrae of normal size (vs. Paget's—enlarged) may be seen. Bone scan is typically "hot." Histologically, large "foamy" tumor cells with indistinct cytoplasmic borders and eosinophilic cytoplasm with folded nuclei predominate. Silver staining highlights reticulum surrounding individual cells (also

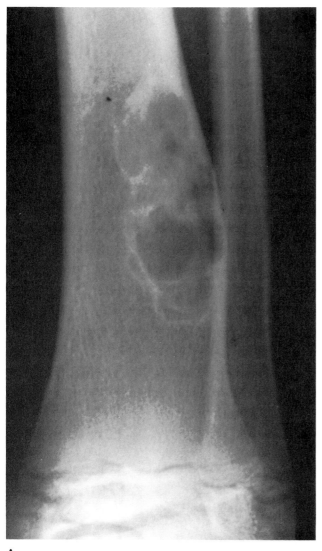

A

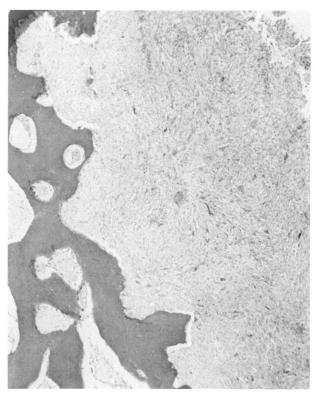

B

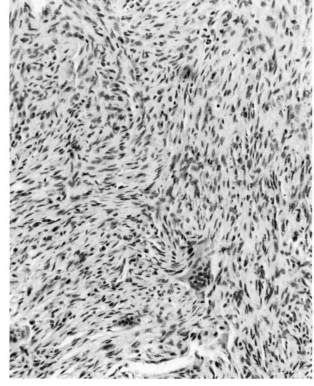

C

FIGURE 7–19. Nonossifying fibroma (metaphyseal fibrous defect). *A*, Radiograph. *B*, Low-magnification micrograph. *C*, High-magnification micrograph. (From Wold, L.E., McLeod, R.A., Sim, F.H., and Unni, K.K.: Atlas of Orthopedic Pathology. Philadelphia, W.B. Saunders, 1990; reprinted by permission.)

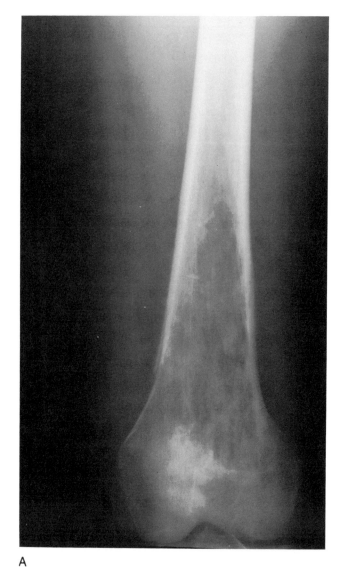

A

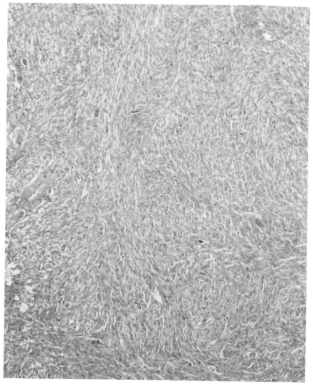

B

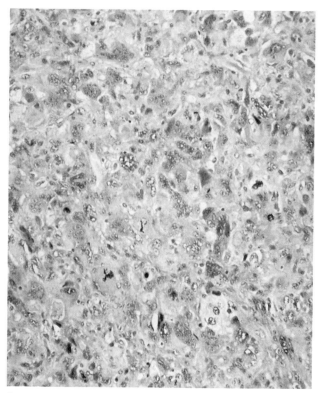

C

FIGURE 7–20. Femoral malignant fibrous histiocytoma. A, Radiograph. B, Low-magnification micrograph. C, High-magnification micrograph. (From Wold, L.E., McLeod, R.A., Sim, F.H., and Unni, K.K.: Atlas of Orthopedic Pathology. Philadelphia, W.B. Saunders, 1990; reprinted by permission.)

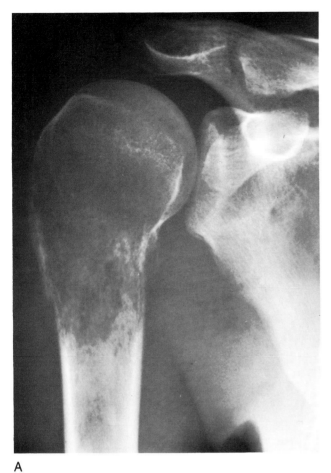

A

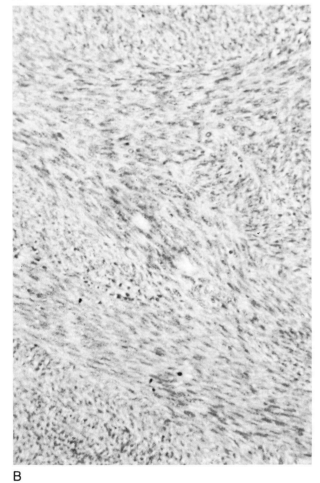

B

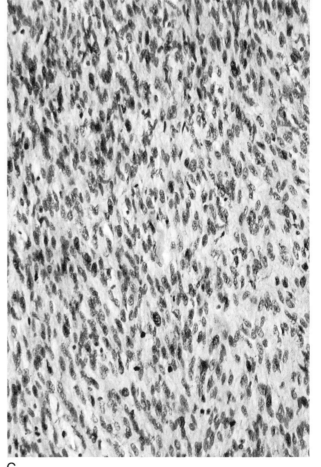

C

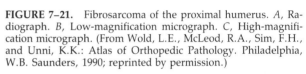

FIGURE 7–21. Fibrosarcoma of the proximal humerus. *A*, Radiograph. *B*, Low-magnification micrograph. *C*, High-magnification micrograph. (From Wold, L.E., McLeod, R.A., Sim, F.H., and Unni, K.K.: Atlas of Orthopedic Pathology. Philadelphia, W.B. Saunders, 1990; reprinted by permission.)

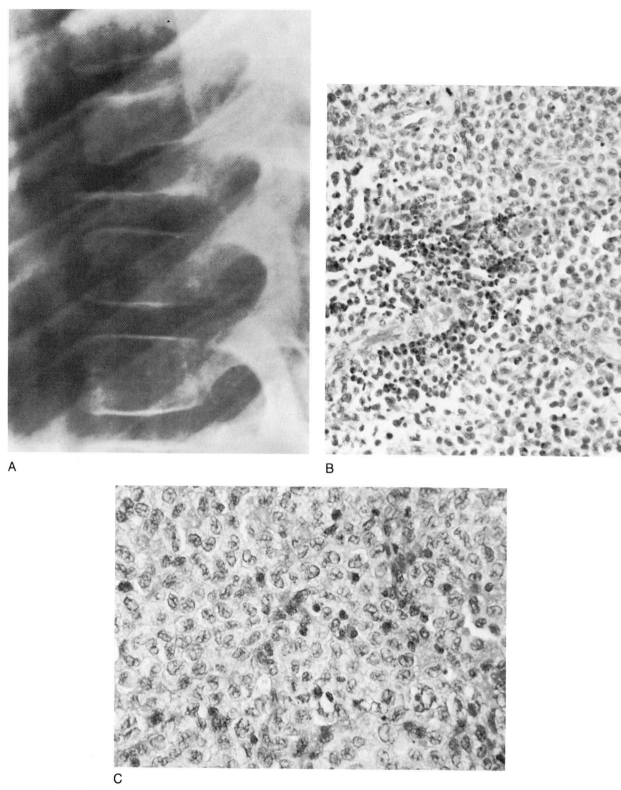

FIGURE 7–22. Vertebra plana in eosinophilic granuloma. *A,* Radiograph. *B,* Low-magnification micrograph. *C,* High-magnification micrograph. (From Wold, L.E., McLeod, R.A., Sim, F.H., and Unni, K.K.: Atlas of Orthopedic Pathology. Philadelphia, W.B. Saunders, 1990; reprinted by permission.)

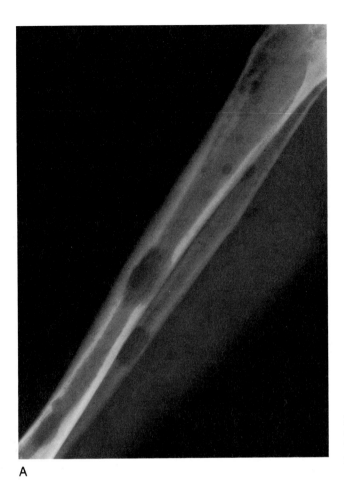

A

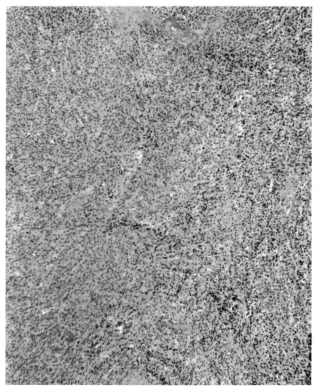

B

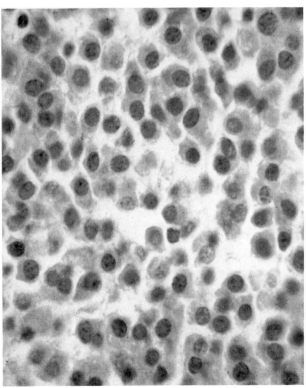

C

FIGURE 7–23. Multiple myeloma in the tibia and fibula. *A*, Radiograph. *B*, Low-magnification micrograph. *C*, High-magnification micrograph. (From Wold, L.E., McLeod, R.A., Sim, F.H., and Unni, K.K.: Atlas of Orthopedic Pathology. Philadelphia, W.B. Saunders, 1990; reprinted by permission.)

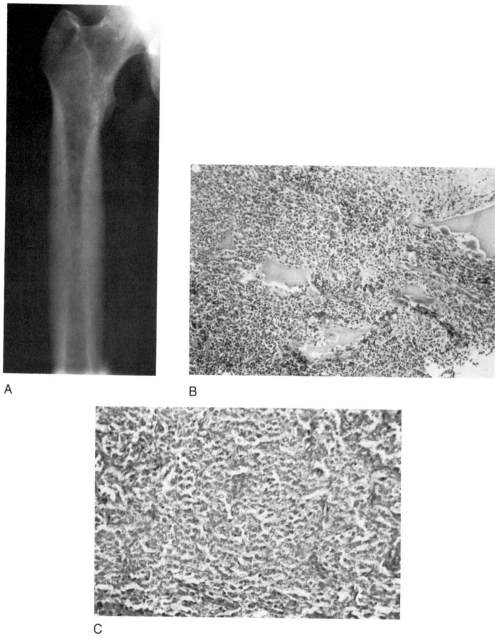

FIGURE 7–24. Diaphyseal lymphoma. *A*, Radiograph. *B*, Low-magnification micrograph. *C*, High-magnification micrograph. (From Wold, L.E., McLeod, R.A., Sim, F.H., and Unni, K.K.: Atlas of Orthopedic Pathology. Philadelphia, W.B. Saunders, 1990; reprinted by permission.)

seen in Ewing's and lymphosarcoma). Lesions can be rapidly progressive. Staging is based on solitary vs. multiple involvement, visceral involvement, and its location in relation to the diaphragm. Treatment is primarily XRT, and prognosis is generally poor.

F. Vascular Lesions—Discussed under soft tissue tumors; rarely involve bone. Most common is **hemangioma** (Fig. 7–25), which involves the vertebral body or skull. Vertebral involvement is usually found incidentally, and radiographs demonstrate a typical **"jailhouse"** vertical **striation**. Weaker, horizontally placed trabeculae are removed but larger weight-bearing trabeculae are spared, causing this appear-ance. Histologically, large vascular lakes lined by flattened endothelial cells form cavernous hemangiomas most commonly. Very little reactive bone surrounds the lesions. Treatment is nonoperative. **Angiosarcomas** of bone are rare and may be multifocal. Osteolytic lesions are seen on radiographs. Treatment includes a combination of surgery, chemotherapy, and XRT. Prognosis is poor. **Hemangiopericytomas**, like angiosarcomas, present with osteolytic destruction of large long bones. They can occur as multiple lesions in one bone or in adjacent areas of two bones. Histologically, sheets of tissue with abnormal capillaries and pericytes of Zimmerman (large cells with clear cytoplasm and small nuclei) are seen with proliferating vascular channels.

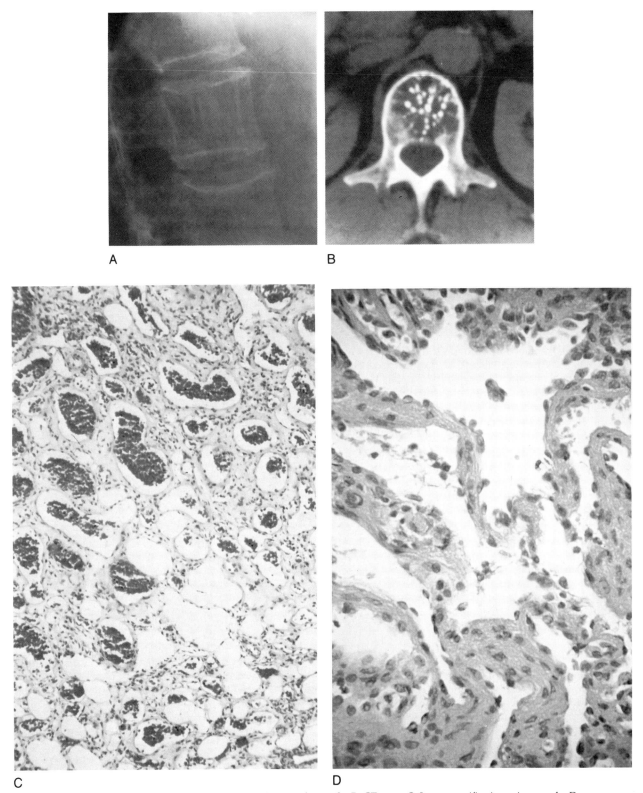

A

B

C

D

FIGURE 7–25. Spinal hemangioma. *A*, Classic radiograph. *B*, CT scan. *C*, Low-magnification micrograph. *D*, High-magnification micrograph. (From Wold, L.E., McLeod, R.A., Sim, F.H., and Unni, K.K.: Atlas of Orthopedic Pathology. Philadelphia, W.B. Saunders, 1990; reprinted by permission.)

G. Lipogenic Lesions
  1. Lipoma—Intraossseous lipomas are rare, and are often found incidently. Treatment includes curettage and bone grafting. Parosteal lipomas are also rare, and may be associated with bony exostoses. Surgical removal for symptomatic lesions is usually curative.
  2. Liposarcoma—Extremely rare in bone. Wide excision is needed. Chemotherapy may be appropriate for high-grade tumors.

H. Neurogenic/Notochordal Lesions
  1. Chordoma (Fig. 7–26)—Rare, slow-growing tumor arising from remnants of the notochord in the axial skeleton of middle-aged adults. Most occur **midline** at the base of the **skull** and in the **sacrococcygeal** area (it is the most common primary bone tumor of the sacrum). Neurologic symptoms are possible (including bladder and bowel dysfunction), and the finding of a mass on rectal exam is also characteristic. Radiographically, destruction of vertebrae and soft tissue expansion (seen best on MRI) are common. Grossly, they appear as a gelatinous, grayish, vascular tumors encased in pseudocapsules. Satellites and skip lesions are common. Histologically, a lobular framework of **physaliferous** cells, with large, vacuolated, "bubbly" pink cytoplasm and a central "bull's-eye" nucleus, is common. Vascular fibrous septae run throughout the lesion. Mucinous matrix and chondroid production are also seen. Presentation is usually late, and resection is difficult, with frequent recurrence. Two-stage anterior and posterior approach is required for lesions above the S3 level. XRT is used when complete resection is not possible, but is of limited use.
  2. Neurilemmoma (Fig. 7–27)—Very rare in bone. Discrete lytic lesions are seen on x-rays.

I. Other Tumors—Undetermined Etiology
  1. Giant Cell Tumor (Fig. 7–28)—Aggressive, locally recurrent tumor with a low metastatic potential. Represents about 20% of primary bone tumors. Most lesions **occur in closed epiphyses** around the knee joint and distal radius of 20–40-year-old female > male patients. Radiographically, the lesions are eccentric, lytic lesions with well-defined borders with some sclerosis. They are often juxtaposed to articular cartilage, which can be violated by the tumor, and can be in more than one location. Pathologic fracture is common. Microscopically, a uniform distribution of giant cells in a benign stroma with occasional mitotic figures is present. Prominent vascularity is also seen. Spontaneous necrosis with "ghosts" of giant cells may be seen in some areas. Characteristically, the stromal **cell nuclei are similar to those of the giant cells**, with round vesiculated nuclei. Giant cell nuclei are numerous and are scattered throughout the cell. Most (60%) present as active (stage 2) tumors, although up to 30% present as aggressive (stage 3) lesions. Treatment includes surgical removal (usually curettage and bone grafting), ± phenol, cryosurgery, **methacrylate**, or XRT. Aggressive, stage 3 lesions will do better with wide en bloc excision. Recurrence is common, and malignant transformation is seen. **Giant cell sarcoma** is a more aggressive giant cell

lesion, occurring in unusual sites with increased mitoses, and must be treated more aggressively: Metastatic disease is rare and usually is not fatal.
  2. Adamantinoma (Fig. 7–29)—Rare tumor found predominately eccentrically in the diaphyses of the **tibia** of young adults. Radiographs show involvement of a large section of the bone with irregular lucent zones and surrounding sclerosis. Histology demonstrates epithelial nests and peripheral **pallisading of biphasic cells** (epithelial and spindle cells). Wide resection and bone grafting are favored.
  3. Ewing's Sarcoma (Fig. 7–30)—Second (to osteosarcoma) most common malignant bone tumor of childhood. Etiology is obscure, but may be from neuroectodermal cell lines. Occurs in young (white >> black) children in the flat and axial bones (pelvis), and in the diaphyses of long bones (**fibula**, femur). Often associated with systemic signs (**fever**, weight loss) and local tenderness with **erythema** and induration, and can be confused with osteomyelitis. It is typically rapidly growing and frequently associated with a large soft tissue mass. Radiographs demonstrate a highly destructive radiolucency without bone formation. Bone scan is very hot and extends beyond the radiographic margins of the lesion. Periosteal "onion skin" reaction is common. The lesion may involve large areas of the diaphysis and may appear to skip areas. Lymphatic and visceral spread is also common, and metastasis may be present at initial presentation. Microscopically, large nests and **sheets of uniform round cells** with scant cytoplasm and indistinct borders are seen. It typically is seen spread throughout muscle tissue. "Geographic necrosis" and "pseudorosettes" (several cells surrounding a central area of necrosis) may be seen. Large vascular lakes and capillaries are also prominent. Silver stains show reticulum surrounding these clumps of cells. Glycogen staining is also helpful (PAS-positive/Diastase-negative cells). Electron microscopy shows prominent intracellular glycogen storage deposits. Treatment includes chemotherapy and XRT (occasionally produces secondary osteosarcoma). Surgery (usually after induction chemotherapy) is reserved for expendable bones. With current treatment 60% of patients can expect to survive at least 5 years.
  4. Squamous Cell Carcinoma—Can occur in bone as a complication of chronic osteomyelitis (spread of tumor developing in a sinus tract). Metastasis is via lymphatics. Histologically, malignant squamous cells (with frequent mitoses) invade and destroy adjacent bone. Keratin "pearls" may be scattered throughout the reactive tissue.

J. Metastatic Tumors (Fig. 7–31)—**The most common bony malignancies** are metastatic carcinomas. With improved treatment regimens, which has prolonged survival, the skeleton is involved in over half of all metastatic carcinomas through hematogenous spread. Spread can be arterial or venous (retrograde venous spread is though the veins of Batson in the spine). Metastatic lesions represent the most common cause of pathologic fractures due to a neoplasm. Classically, they are lytic lesions in the axial skeleton and long bone diaphyses of older adults. Usually are multiple, but can be solitary. Most common primar-

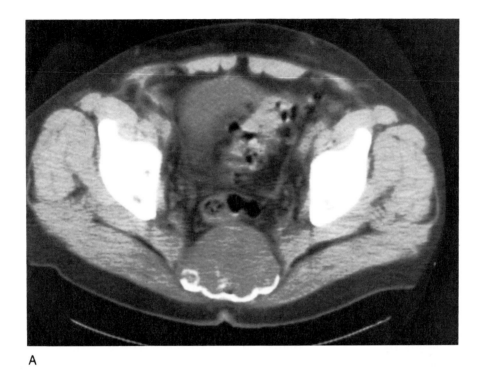

A

B

C

FIGURE 7–26. Sacral chordoma with anterior extension. *A*, CT scan. *B*, Low-magnification micrograph. *C*, High-magnification micrograph. (From Wold, L.E., McLeod, R.A., Sim, F.H., and Unni, K.K.: Atlas of Orthopedic Pathology. Philadelphia, W.B. Saunders, 1990; reprinted by permission.)

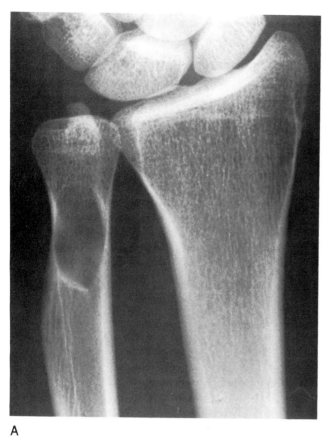

A

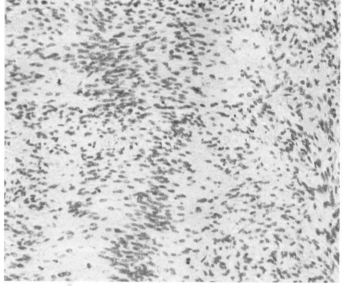

B

FIGURE 7–27. Intraosseous neurilemmoma. *A*, Radiograph. *B*, Low-magnification micrograph. *C*, High-magnification micrograph. (From Wold, L.E., McLeod, R.A., Sim, F.H., and Unni, K.K.: Atlas of Orthopedic Pathology. Philadelphia, W.B. Saunders, 1990; reprinted by permission.)

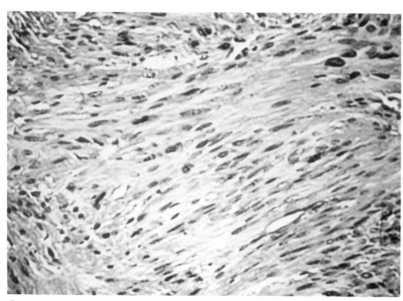

C

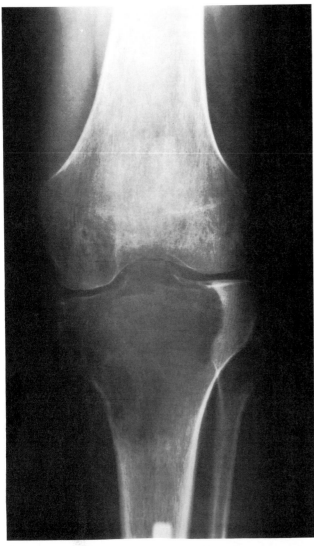

A

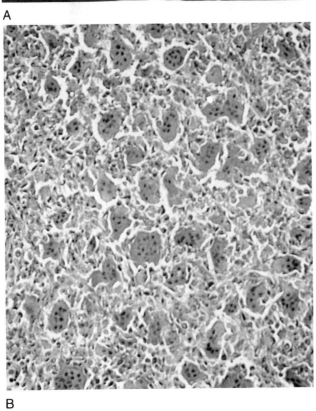

B

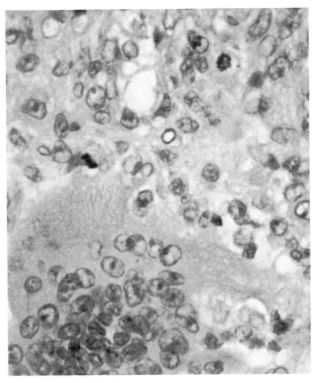

C

FIGURE 7–28. Proximal tibial giant cell tumor. *A*, Radiograph. *B*, Low-magnification micrograph. *C*, High-magnification micrograph. (From Wold, L.E., McLeod, R.A., Sim, F.H., and Unni, K.K.: Atlas of Orthopedic Pathology. Philadelphia, W.B. Saunders, 1990; reprinted by permission.)

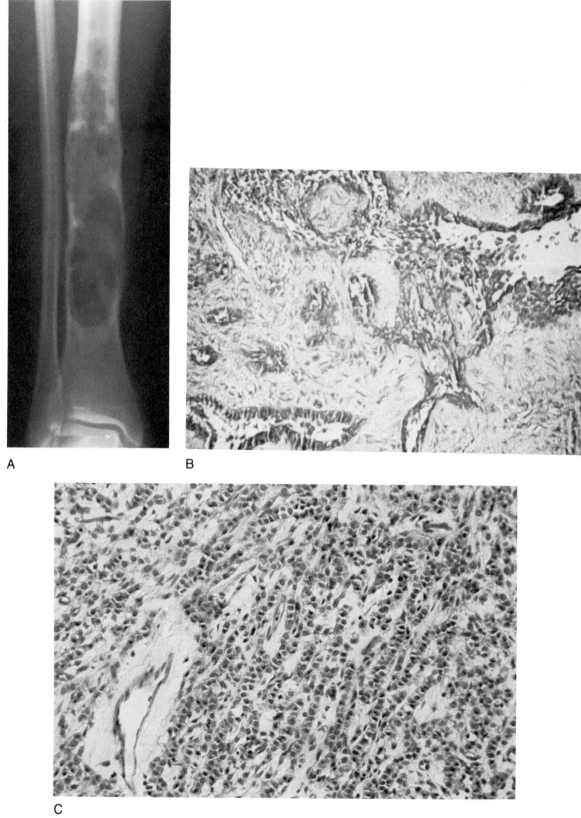

FIGURE 7–29. Adamantinoma. *A*, Classic radiograph. *B*, Low-magnification micrograph. *C*, High-magnification micrograph. (From Wold, L.E., McLeod, R.A., Sim, F.H., and Unni, K.K.: Atlas of Orthopedic Pathology. Philadelphia, W.B. Saunders, 1990; reprinted by permission.)

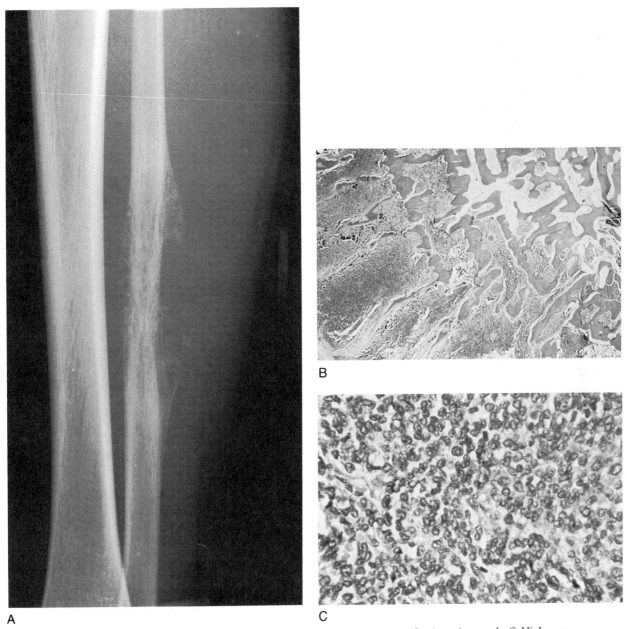

FIGURE 7–30. Diaphyseal Ewing's sarcoma. *A*, Radiograph. *B*, Low-magnification micrograph. *C*, High-magnification micrograph. (From Wold, L.E., McLeod, R.A., Sim, F.H., and Unni, K.K.: Atlas of Orthopedic Pathology. Philadelphia, W.B. Saunders, 1990; reprinted by permission.)

ies are breast, prostate, lung, kidney and thyroid (Hürthle cell), in that order. Renal mets are quite vascular and have "cold" bone scans, and histology may demonstrate clear cells that are PAS positive. Prostate and breast mets are typically osteoblastic. Wilms's tumor and neuroblastoma (rosettes) are the most common metastatic lesions in childhood. **Prophylactic fixation** of weight-bearing bones (often with PMMA supplementation) is recommended for **lesions >2.5 cm in** diameter or **involving >50% of the cortex**, or in patients having **pain**. XRT is often helpful for tumors metastatic to bone (it is administered preop in patients with thyroid and kidney mets). Work-up should include labs (increased calcium common but nonspecific), bone scan (looking for multiple lesions), CT (axial lesions, and chest CT), angiography (preop for thyroid and hypernephroma mets), and biopsy. In general, 50% of patients with bony mets will survive 6 months and 30% will survive 1 year. Shorter survival periods can be anticipated with lung cancer, and longer periods with thyroid mets.

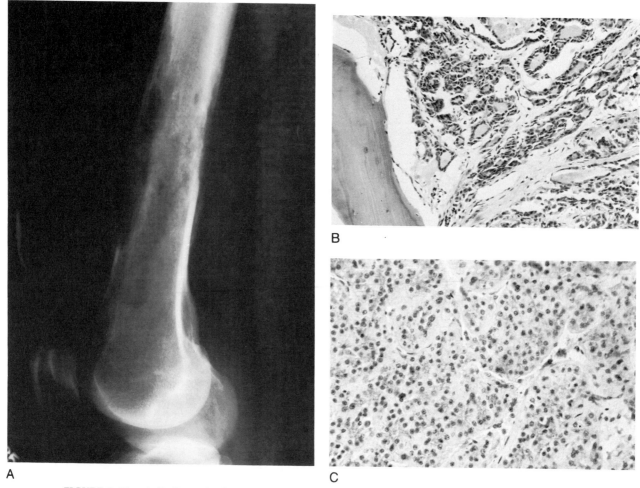

FIGURE 7–31. *A*, Radiograph of metastatic lesion to the distal femur. *B*, Low-magnification micrograph of typical features of thyroid and hepatic metastases. *C*, High-magnification micrograph of undifferentiated renal cell tumor metastasis. (From Wold, L.E., McLeod, R.A., Sim, F.H., and Unni, K.K.: Atlas of Orthopedic Pathology. Philadelphia, W.B. Saunders, 1990; reprinted by permission.)

Selected Bibliography

Bell, R.S., O'Sullivan, B.; Liu, F.F., et al.: The surgical margin in soft-tissue sarcoma. J. Bone Joint Surg. [Am.] 71:370, 1989.

Berrey, B.H., Jr., Lord, C.F., Gebhardt, M.C., et al.: Fractures of allografts. Frequency, treatment, and end-results. J. Bone Joint Surg. [Am.] 72:825, 1990.

Chapman, Michael W., ed.: Operative Orthopaedics. Philadelphia, J.B. Lippincott, 1988.

Crenshaw, A.H., ed.: Campbell's Operative Orthopaedics, 7th ed. St. Louis, C.V. Mosby Co., 1987.

Dee, R., Mango, E., and Hurst, L.C.: Principles of Orthopaedic Practice. New York, McGraw Hill Book Co., 1989.

Dollahite, H.A., Tatum, L., Moinuddin, S.M., et al.: Aspiration biopsy of primary neoplasms of bone. J. Bone Joint Surg. [Am.] 71:1166, 1989.

Eilber, F.R., Eckhardt, J., and Morton, D.L.: Advances in the treatment of sarcomas of the extremity: Current status of limb salvage. Cancer 54:2695–2701, 1984.

Enneking, W.F.: Clinical Musculoskeletal Pathology, 3rd rev. ed. Gainesville, FL, University of Florida Press, 1990.

Enneking, W.F., Eady, J.L., and Burchardt, H.: Autogenous cortical bone grafts in the reconstruction of segmental skeletal defects. J. Bone Joint Surg. [Am.] 62:1039–1058, 1980.

Enneking, W.F., Spanier, S.S., and Goodman, M.A.: A system for the surgical staging of musculoskeletal sarcoma. Clin. Orthop. 153:106–120, 1980.

Enneking, W.F., Spanier, S.S., and Malawer, M.M.: The effect of the anatomic setting on the results of surgical procedures for soft parts sarcoma of the thigh. Cancer 47:1005–1022, 1981.

Enzinger, F.M., and Weiss, S.W.: Soft Tissue Tumors, 2nd ed. St. Louis, C.V. Mosby, 1987.

Gitelis, S., Bertoni, F., Picci, P., and Campanacci, M.: Chondrosarcoma of bone. The experience at the Istituto Ortopedico Rizzoli. J. Bone Joint Surg. [Am.] 63:1248–1257, 1981.

Goldenberg, R.R., Campbell, C.J., and Bonfiglio, M.: Giant-cell tumor of bone: An analysis of two hundred and eighteen cases. J. Bone Joint Surg. [Am.] 52:619–663, 1970.

Goorin, A.M., Abelson, H.T., and Frei, E., III: Osteosarcoma: Fifteen years later. N. Engl. J. Med. 313:1637–1643, 1985.

Goorin, A.M., Frei, E., III, and Abelson, H.T.: Adjuvant chemotherapy for osteosarcoma: A decade of experience. Surg. Clin. North Am. 61:1379–1389, 1981.

Heare, T.C., Enneking, W.F., and Heare, M.J.: Staging techniques and biopsy of bone tumors. Orthop. Clin. North Am. 20:273, 1989.

Levy, R.N.: Symposium on metastatic disease of bone. Clin. Orthop. 169:15–114, 1982.

Lodwick, G.S.: Solitary malignant tumors of bone. The application of predictor variables and diagnosis.

Mankin, H.J., Doppelt, S.H., Sullivan, T.R., and Tomford, W.W.: Osteoarticular and intercalary allograft transplantation in the management of malignant tumors of bone. Cancer 50:613–630, 1982.

Mankin, H.J., Lange, T.A., and Spanier, S.S.: The hazards of biopsy in patients with malignant primary bone and soft-tissue tumors. J. Bone Joint Surg. [Am.] 64:1121–1127, 1982.

Medsger, T.A., Jr., et al.: Twenty-fifth rheumatism review: Paget's disease. Arthritis Rheum. 26:281–283, 1983.

Merkow, R.L., and Lane, J.M.: Current concepts of Paget's disease of bone. Orthop. Clin. North Am. 15:747–764, 1984.

Miller, M.D., Yaw, K.M., and Foley, H.T.: Malpractice maladies in the management of musculoskeletal malignancies. Contemporary Orthop. 23:577–584, 1991.

Mindell, E.R.: Chordoma. J. Bone Joint Surg. [Am.] 63:501–505, 1981.

Mirra, J.H.: Bone Tumors, Clinical, Radiographic, and Pathologic Correlations. Philadelphia, Lea & Febiger, 1989.

O'Connor, M.I., and Sim, F.H.: Salvage of the limb in the treatment of malignant pelvic tumors. J. Bone Joint Surg. [Am.] 71:481, 1989.

Orthopaedic Knowledge Update Home Study Syllabus I, II, and III. Chicago, American Academy of Orthopaedic Surgeons, 1984, 1987, 1990.

Pritchard, D.J., Lunke, R.J., Taylor, W.F., Dahlin, D.C., and Medley, B.E.: Chondrosarcoma: A clinicopathologic and statistical analysis. Cancer 45:149–157, 1980.

Schajowicz, F.: Tumors and Tumor-Like Lesions of Bone and Joints. New York, Springer-Verlag, 1981.

Sim, F.H., Beauchamp, C.P., and Chao, E.Y.: Reconstruction of musculoskeletal defects about the knee for tumor. Clin. Orthop. 221:188–201, 1987.

Simon, M.A.: Biopsy of musculoskeletal tumors. J. Bone Joint Surg. [Am.] 64:1253–1257, 1982.

Simon, M.A.: Current concepts review: Limb salvage for osteosarcoma. J. Bone Joint Surg. [Am.] 70:307–310, 1988.

Simon, M.A., and Nachman, J.: The clinical utility of preoperative therapy for sarcomas. J. Bone Joint Surg. [Am.] 68:1458–1463, 1986.

Springfield, D.S., Schmidt, R., Graham-Pole, J., et al.: Surgical treatment for osteosarcoma. J. Bone Joint Surg. [Am.] 70:1124–1130, 1988.

Sung, H.W., Kuo, D.P., Shu, W.P., Chai, Y.B., Liu, C.C., and Li, S.M.: Giant-cell tumor of bone: Analysis of 208 cases in Chinese patients. J. Bone Joint Surg. [Am.] 64:755–761, 1982.

Tepper, J., Glaubiger, D., Lichter, A., Wackenhut, J., and Glatstein, E.: Local control of Ewing's sarcoma of bone with radiotherapy and combination chemotherapy. Cancer 46:1969–1973, 1980.

Wold, L.E., McLeod, R.A., Sim, F.H., and Unni, K.K.: Atlas of Orthopedic Pathology. Philadelphia, W.B. Saunders, 1990.

Wuisman, P., and Enneking, W.F.: Prognosis for patients who have osteosarcoma with skip metastasis. J. Bone Joint Surg. [Am.] 72:60, 1990.

Yaw, K.M., and Wurtz, D.: Resection and reconstruction for bone tumors in the proximal tibia. OCNA: 22:133–148, 1991.

Zimmer, W.D., Berquist, T.H., McLeod, R.A., Sim, F.H., Pritchard, D.J., Shives, T.C., Wold, L.E., and May, G.R.: Bone tumors: Magnetic resonance imaging versus computed tomography. Radiology 155:709–718, 1985.

CHAPTER 8

Rehabilitation Gait, Amputations, Prosthetics, and Orthotics

I. Gait

A. Introduction—Human locomotion is the process of moving from one location to another. Walking involves a cyclic pattern of bodily movements integrated and controlled to minimize energy expenditure. Human walking requires one foot to be on the ground at all times, with cyclic alterations of the supporting leg and a transfer period when both feet are on the ground (double limb support). Prerequisites for normal gait include stability in stance, clearance in swing, preposition of the foot in terminal swing, adequate step length, and energy conservation. Running requires that both feet be off the ground simultaneously at one point in the cycle. Normal human gait is made up of two phases and eight periods (Fig. 8–1):

PHASE	PERIOD	ACTION	% CYCLE
Stance			60
	Heel strike	Foot on ground	—
	Foot flat	Shock absorption	15
	Midstance	Roll over foot	15
	Heel off	Roll beyond foot	25
	Toe off	Knee flexes	5
Swing			40
	Acceleration	Limb begins to advance	5
	Midswing	Limb advances further	30
	Deceleration	Limb deceleration/extension	5

B. Determinants of Gait—Classically, **six determinants of gait** are described (Inman): pelvic rotation, pelvic list, knee flexion, foot and ankle motion, knee motion, and lateral pelvic motion. All six elements contribute to decreasing excursion of the center of mass (normally just anterior to S2) and conservation of energy. The resultant gait pattern resembles a sinusoidal curve.

1. *Pelvic Rotation* (Fig. 8–2)—The pelvis rotates about a vertical axis alternately to the left and right of the line of progression. This rotation, about 4 degrees to each side of the central axis, prevents the center of mass from deviating as much in the horizontal plane, reducing impact forces and conserving energy.

2. *Pelvic List* (Fig. 8–3)—In the normal gait cycle, the pelvis drops about 5 degrees on the non–weight-bearing side (positive Trendelenburg). This allows the center of mass to not deviate as much superiorly as otherwise would be required, again conserving energy.

3. *Knee Flexion in Stance* (Fig. 8–4)—Knee flexion of the supporting limb of approximately 15 degrees dampens impact, "smoothing" the center of mass arc.

4. *Foot and Ankle Motion* (Fig. 8–5)—Sequential action of dorsiflexion and plantar flexion produces a small arc formed by the lever arm of the heel and allows a smooth and flattened pathway of the knee. The foot is pronated in the stance phase for shock absorption. During toe off, the foot serves as a rigid lever.

5. *Knee Motion* (Fig. 8–6)—Works in concert with foot and ankle motion. The knee flexes in response to heel strike and extends with foot flat, flexing again with heel rise.

6. *Lateral Pelvic Motion* (Fig. 8–7)—Aided by the fact that the femoral and tibial axes are aligned to effectively narrow the base of support, lateral motion of 5 cm over the weight-bearing leg with each step allows secure support of the center of gravity of the body.

C. Muscle Action—The hip flexors are responsible for advancing the limb in acceleration and midswing; the ankle dorsiflexors achieve clearance in midswing and deceleration and contract maximally at heel strike to modulate ankle plantar flexion. The hamstring muscles decelerate the thigh in terminal swing. Most **muscle action** in the gait cycle is ec-

213

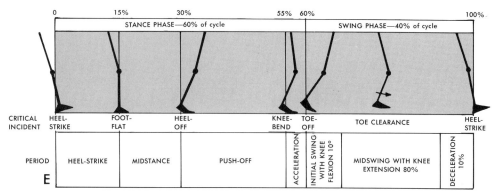

FIGURE 8–1. Gait cycle. (From Tachdjian, M.O.: Pediatric Orthopaedics, 2nd ed., p. 8. Philadelphia, W.B. Saunders, 1990; reprinted by permission.)

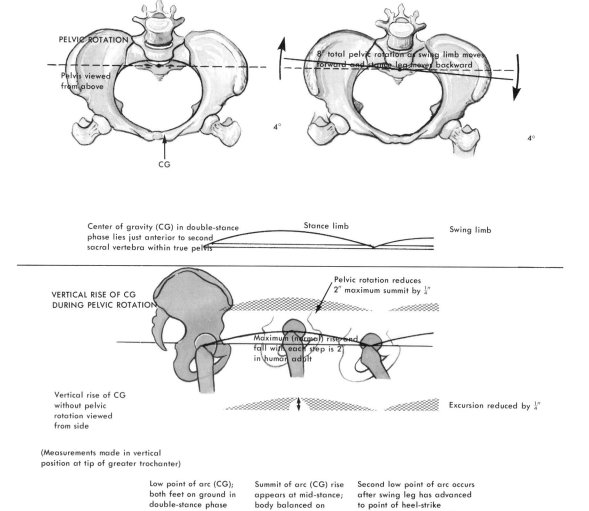

FIGURE 8–2. Pelvic rotation. (From Tachdjian, M.O.: Pediatric Orthopaedics, 2nd ed., p. 8. Philadelphia, W.B. Saunders, 1990; reprinted by permission.)

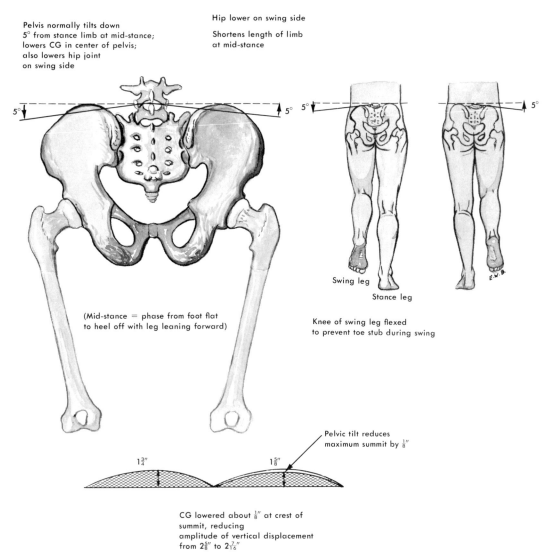

Pelvis normally tilts down
5° from stance limb at mid-stance;
lowers CG in center of pelvis;
also lowers hip joint
on swing side

Hip lower on swing side

Shortens length of limb
at mid-stance

Swing leg

Stance leg

(Mid-stance = phase from foot flat
to heel off with leg leaning forward)

Knee of swing leg flexed
to prevent toe stub during swing

Pelvic tilt reduces
maximum summit by $\frac{1}{8}$"

$1\frac{3}{4}$" $1\frac{5}{8}$"

CG lowered about $\frac{1}{8}$" at crest of
summit, reducing
amplitude of vertical displacement
from $2\frac{5}{8}$" to $2\frac{7}{16}$"

FIGURE 8–3. Pelvic list. (From Tachdjian, M.O.: Pediatric Orthopaedics, 2nd ed., p. 10. Philadelphia, W.B. Saunders, 1990; reprinted by permission.)

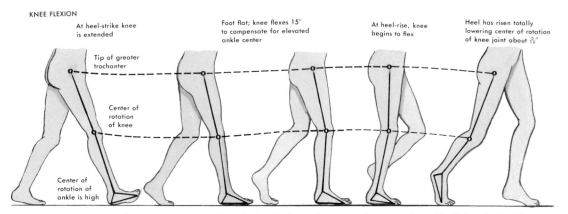

KNEE FLEXION

At heel-strike knee
is extended

Foot flat; knee flexes 15°
to compensate for elevated
ankle center

At heel-rise, knee
begins to flex

Heel has risen totally
lowering center of rotation
of knee joint about $\frac{5}{16}$"

Tip of greater
trochanter

Center of
rotation
of knee

Center of
rotation of
ankle is high

FIGURE 8–4. Knee flexion. (From Tachdjian, M.O.: Pediatric Orthopaedics, 2nd ed., p. 11. Philadelphia, W.B. Saunders, 1990; reprinted by permission.)

ANKLE ROTATION

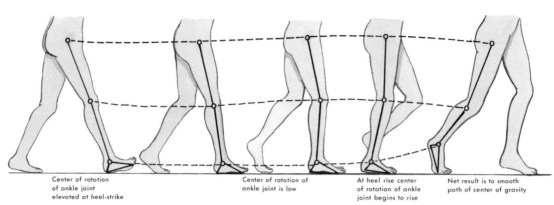

FIGURE 8–5. Foot and ankle motion. (From Tachdjian, M.O.: Pediatric Orthopaedics, 2nd ed., p. 11. Philadelphia, W.B. Saunders, 1990; reprinted by permission.)

centric, creating elongation of muscles and allowing muscles to serve as "shock absorbers," enhancing control. The following muscles are important in gait:

Muscle	Action	Function
Gluteus medius	Eccentric	Controls pelvic tilt at midstance
Gluteus maximus	Concentric	Powers hip extension
Iliopsoas	Concentric	Powers hip flexion
Hip adductors	Eccentric	Controls lateral sway (late stance)
Hip abductors	Eccentric	Controls pelvic tilt (midstance)
Quadriceps	Eccentric	Stabilizes knee at heel strike
Hamstrings	Eccentric	Controls rate of knee extension (stance)
Tibialis ant.	Concentric	Dorsiflexes ankle at swing
	Eccentric[a]	Slows plantar flexion rate (heel strike)
Gastrocnemius/soleus	Eccentric	Slows dorsiflexion rate (stance)

[a] predominate role

D. Gait Nomenclature—The **gait cycle** includes all activity between initial contact (heel strike) on one side and succeeding initial contact on the same side. The **step** or **stride** is the distance between preswing (toe off) and initial contact on the same side (mean of 1.2 m). **Velocity** (mean of 1.1 m/s) is a function of **cadence** (mean of 110 steps/minute) and stride. **Double support** is the period of cycle during which time the toe of one foot and heel of the other are both in contact with the ground. Both the vertical and horizontal oscillation of the **center of gravity** is about 5 centimeters. The line of the center of gravity (CG) changes throughout gait cycle as follows:

Phase	CG vs Hip	CG vs Knee	CG vs Ankle
Heel strike	Anterior	Through	Posterior
Foot flat	Anterior	Posterior	Posterior
Midstance	Posterior	Posterior	Anterior
Heel off	Posterior	Anterior	Anterior
Toe off	Anterior	Posterior	Anterior

E. Gait Analysis—Usually involves three different modes:

KNEE EXTENSION

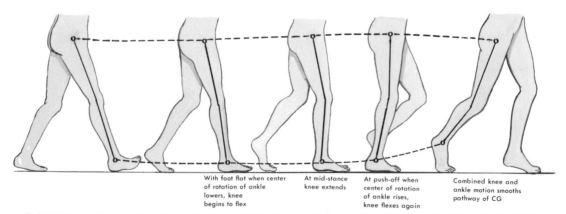

FIGURE 8–6. Knee motion. (From Tachdjian, M.O.: Pediatric Orthopaedics, 2nd ed., p. 12. Philadelphia, W.B. Saunders, 1990; reprinted by permission.)

MODE	METHOD
Motion analysis	Uses videos and computers to analyze gait
Dynamic EMGs	Determines % time of muscle activity
Floor plates	Analyzes forces imposed during foot contact

F. Pathologic Gait—Can be caused by a variety of problems.
1. Muscle Weakness—Can cause these gait abnormalities (Table 8–1).
2. Neurologic Problems—Neurologic disorders are frequently associated with gait abnormalities. Hip scissoring can be due to overactive adductors or the medial hamstrings. Knee flexion deformities can be caused by spasticity of the hamstrings, and ankle equinus can lead to a steppage gait. Neurologic conditions resulting in weakness or spasticity often cause a widened gait or an exaggerated loading response (foot slap). Degenerative disorders of the brain (spinocerebellar degeneration, Friedreich's ataxia, etc.) or spinal cord (tabes dorsalis, posterior spinal cord syndrome) may likewise have associated gait abnormalities.
3. Pain—Patients with pain in one lower extremity will usually demonstrate an **antalgic gait** pattern. In this pattern, one observes a more rapid swing phase of the contralateral (unaffected) limb with concomitant shortening of the stance phase of the ipsilateral limb. An ipsilateral abductor lurch may be present.
4. Arthrodesis—Fusion of the hip can lead to an abductor lurch. Knee fusion frequently leads to a circumduction gait. Ankle fusion often leads to exaggerated knee flexion.
5. Arthritis—Juvenile rheumatoid arthritis (JRA) patients have abnormalities with hip extension, ankle plantar flexion, and pelvic tilt. Total hip arthroplasty (THA) recipients' function is most closely associated with weight-bearing capacity and not range of motion. Upper tibial osteotomy recipients do best with low preoperative knee adduction moments. Total knee arthroplasty (TKA) recipients have a gait with decreased stride length, decreased midstance knee flexion and abnormal knee flexion/extension. Cruciate retaining TKA designs allow better stair climbing.
6. Cerebral Palsy—Gait is associated with abnormal time-distance parameters and abnormal timing of lower extremity muscle contraction, both resulting in significant increases in energy expenditure. Stance phase stability and the shortened swing phase may be mediated by hamstring lengthening where appropriate. Phasic activity of long toe flexors is not important to gait abnormalities. (See Chapter 1, Pediatric Orthopaedics, for further discussion and treatment options.)
7. Paraplegia—Functional electrical stimulation (FES) may help in supporting gait by activating

LATERAL HORIZONTAL PELVIC MOTION

CG shifts over stance
limb to prevent fall

Medial inclination of femur
and valgus vertical alignment of tibia
narrows support base

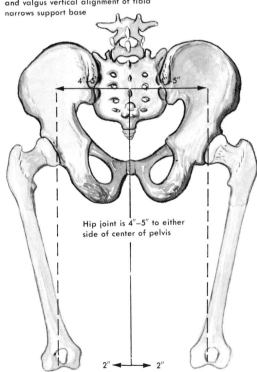

4"–5"   5"

Hip joint is 4"–5" to either
side of center of pelvis

2"   2"

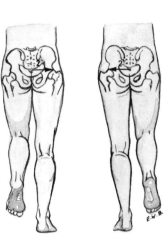

Total lateral displacement
of CG in full gait cycle
is about 2"

FIGURE 8–7. Lateral pelvic motion. (From Tachdjian, M.O.: Pediatric Orthopaedics, 2nd ed., p. 13. Philadelphia, W.B. Saunders, 1990; reprinted by permission.)

TABLE 8–1.   GAIT ABNORMALITIES CAUSED BY MUSCLE WEAKNESS

Muscle	Phase	Direction	Type of Gait	Treatment
Gluteus medius	Stance	Lateral	Abductor lurch	Cane
Gluteus maximus	Stance	Backward	Lurch (hip hyperextension)	
Quadriceps	Stance	Forward	Lurch/back knee gait	AFO
	Swing	Forward	Abnormal hip rotation	
Gastrocnemius/soleus	Stance	Forward	Flat foot (calcaneal) gait	± AFO
	Swing	Forward	Delayed heel rise	
Tibialis anterior	Stance	Forward	Foot drop/slap	AFO
	Swing	Forward	Steppage gait	

muscles that are still physiologically viable (especially in T4–T12 paraplegics). This can allow standing and even walking (with proper orthotics).

8. Hemiplegia—Prolongation of the stance and double support phases is characteristic of the disorder. Associated anomalies include ankle equinus, limitation of knee flexion, and increased hip flexion. Gait analysis may be useful in determining whether a flexor or extensor pattern exists and defining appropriate treatment modalities. Surgical correction of equinus (1 year after onset) and FES of calf muscles can be helpful. Common patterns of gait impairment in hemiplegics include excessive plantar flexion, swing phase foot varus, weakness, and impaired proprioception (balance problems).

9. Muscular Dystrophy—Responds poorly to surgical correction of equinus because it is a necessary adaptation to control forces at the knee and because of muscle weakness. The goal in surgery for this disorder is to correct deformities to make bracing more effective.

10. Crutches and Canes—The use of crutches increases stability by providing two additional points of contact for the body. The following gait patterns are described with the use of crutches:

Pattern	Sequence	Use
4-point	R crutch—L foot—L crutch—R foot	Ataxia (most stable)
2-point alt.	R crutch & L foot—L crutch & R foot	Limited weight bearing
3-point	R&L crutch & injured leg—good leg	Non–weight bearing
Tripod	Crutches advanced—body dragged	Nonfunctional limbs
Swing-to	Advance crutches, swing to them	
Swing-thru	Body is lifted and swung beyond crutches	

Canes offer less support than crutches, but do provide some support. When used in the contralateral hand, they widen the base of support and decrease stress on the affected limb by shifting the center of gravity toward the contralateral arm.

II. Amputations

A. Introduction—Historically, trauma and infection were the major causes of amputations, followed by congenital amputation and tumors. Currently, the majority of amputations performed in the United

States are a result of vascular disease. Amputation surgery has two goals: ablation (of all abnormal pathology) and reconstruction (for the optimum prosthetic substitution and restoration of function). Amputation surgery serves to remove an injured or diseased part and construct a physiologic end organ. It should not be relegated to the junior resident to be done unsupervised.

B. Amputation Level (Fig. 8–8)—Selection of amputation level is determined by pathological, anatomical, surgery, prosthetic, and biomechanical factors. In order to conserve energy expenditure, **the most distal level** that will heal and still provide a functional stump is selected. Energy expenditure depends on amputation level, etiology leading to amputation, aerobic capacity, cardiopulmonary efficiency, speed of gait, and a variety of other factors. The following are generally recognized values for a given individual:

Amputation Level	% Energy beyond Baseline
Long BKA	10
Medium BKA	25
Short BKA	40
Bilateral medium BKA	41
Average AKA	65

Note that the energy expenditure for a bilateral below-knee amputation (BKA) is less than that of a unilateral above-knee amputation (AKA)! Energy cost is also due to gait speed. Selection of amputation level is often based on experience of the surgeon and his evaluation of the tissues involved. Patient nutrition (albumin >3 g/dl), health (Hb >10 g and WBC >1500), and adequate cardiopulmonary function are also essential. Helpful clinical criteria for preoperative planning include skin temperature measurement (clinically or with thermography), and the level of dependent rubor. Doppler studies, which measure an index of ankle pressures/brachial pressures—the ankle-brachial index (**ABI**)—are the **most helpful** measurement in determining whether a **BKA** level is appropriate. **Toe pressures** are less affected by vessel calcification and are **best** for evaluation of **distal-level amputations** (especially transmetatarsal amputations). Nuclear medicine studies (xenon-133) are sometimes helpful but are often inaccurate. Transcutaneous measurement of pO_2 is one of the more sophisticated measurements for selection of amputation level, but is difficult and expensive to perform and may not be completely ac-

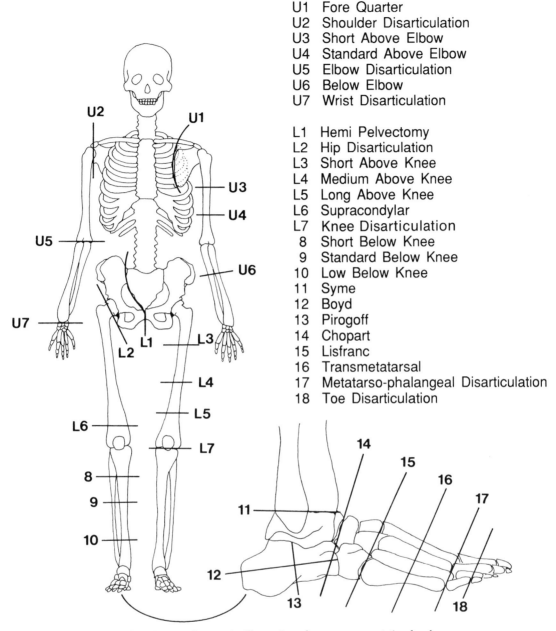

U1　Fore Quarter
U2　Shoulder Disarticulation
U3　Short Above Elbow
U4　Standard Above Elbow
U5　Elbow Disarticulation
U6　Below Elbow
U7　Wrist Disarticulation

L1　Hemi Pelvectomy
L2　Hip Disarticulation
L3　Short Above Knee
L4　Medium Above Knee
L5　Long Above Knee
L6　Supracondylar
L7　Knee Disarticulation
8　Short Below Knee
9　Standard Below Knee
10　Low Below Knee
11　Syme
12　Boyd
13　Pirogoff
14　Chopart
15　Lisfranc
16　Transmetatarsal
17　Metatarso-phalangeal Disarticulation
18　Toe Disarticulation

FIGURE 8-8.　Composite illustration of common amputation levels.

curate. A summary of these studies is presented in Table 8–2. Embolic disease usually results in higher level amputations as compared to long-standing disease, because collateral vessels have not had a chance to form. However, large vessel arteriosclerotic disease often results in lower amputations (BKA) because collateralization has usually occurred. It is helpful to consider energy expenditure and prognosis with bilateral amputees—up to 75% of bilateral BKA patients will ambulate, while only 25% of BK/AK patients will ever be functional ambulators.

C. Surgical Considerations—Modern prostheses utilize a total-contact design, making scar location and general condition of the soft tissues of the stump somewhat less important than in years past. End-bearing stumps are favored for joint disarticulations (i.e., knee disarticulation and Symes amputations), and additional care should be taken in planning incisions. Flaps should be tailored and be at least as long as the radius of the affected extremity. Muscle must be sutured to bone ends (*myodesis*—best for dysvascular cases) or into the fascia of adjoining muscles (*myoplasty*—best for nondysvascular cases) to cover the stump. Nerves should be allowed to retract into the soft tissue envelope as this confines neuromas and places them in a soft tissue cushion. Vessels must be identified and carefully ligated. Amputations performed in the face of infection are best done in stages. An open, circular (guillotine) amputation is recommended as the first stage, followed, when appropriate, by secondary revision and closure. An early rigid compressive dressing is important (pre-

TABLE 8–2. CLINICAL STUDIES FOR AMPUTATION LEVEL DETERMINATION

METHOD	VALUES NECESSARY FOR HEALING	ADVANTAGES	DISADVANTAGES
Clinical	Rubor, temperature	Easy	Inaccuracy
ABI	.35 (.45 in diabetics)	BKA healing	Vessel calcification affects results
Toe systolic BP	55 mm Hg	Distal healing	Need toes
Xenon-133	Uptake	Sometimes helpful	Time, inaccuracy
Transcutaneous pO$_2$	35	Accurate?	Time, difficulty
Thermography	Color dependent	Accurate?	Time, difficulty

vents edema, flexion contractures, and further trauma as well as helping pain control), and can sometimes be used with a pylon as a temporary prosthesis. The dressing/cast is changed every week and is maintained for 3–5 weeks. Overall rehabilitation (cardiovascular, pulmonary, psychological, etc.) is also important. Complications include infections, ischemic necrosis (from selecting too low a level), dehiscence, edema (reduced with good postop dressings), pain, and dysfunction. Pain can be from the stump itself or phantom limb pain. Stump pain is usually relieved with control of swelling and is frequently self-limited (6 weeks). Chronic pain often is difficult to manage and can be related to neuromas, psychiatric factors, or other etiologies. **Phantom limb "sensation,"** which includes an awareness of the missing portion of the limb and mild paresthesias, is common. It occurs immediately postoperatively, decays with time, rarely interferes with sleep, and is incomplete and inconsistent. **Phantom limb pain** is less common, is "stocking/glove" in distribution, is constant, may last for extended periods, and is overwhelming in severity. Management is difficult and requires a "team approach" (including psychiatric consultation).

D. Lower Extremity Amputations (Fig. 8–8)

1. Foot—Amputation of individual toes can be accomplished at any level. With the great toe, part of the proximal phalanx should be saved if possible to preserve the attachment of the short flexor and extensor tendons. Toe disarticulations are also functional. Individual metatarsal amputations (**ray**) usually do not cause excessive difficulty with the exception of the first metatarsal (affects balance and push off). Management includes fitting with a firm shoe with a metatarsal (MT) bar and/or rocker bottom. Transmetatarsal amputations (**TMAs**) are indicated for trauma, tissue loss, infection, and gangrene (limited to the toes and not the web space in diabetics [McKittrick]). TMA recipients require shoe modifications and inserts with a forefoot space replacement. This amputation can lead to a shortened stride and is often a poor choice in patients with severe peripheral vascular disease. Other foot amputations include **Lisfranc** (tarsometatarsal level), **Chopart** (midtarsal), **Boyd** (talectomy and calcaneotibial arthrodesis) and **Pirogoff** (longitudinal transcalcaneal). All of these amputations can lead to fixed equinovarus due to unopposed posterior muscles. Heel cord lengthening or tibialis anterior transfer should be considered if

these amputation levels are selected. Foot amputations are less successful in patients with ischemia and diabetes. Prosthetic fitting is difficult not only as a result of the misshapen foot but also as a result of acquired plantar flexure or equinovarus deformity of the ankle. These amputations may not have any advantage over a Symes amputation.

2. Leg—**Symes** amputation (ankle disarticulation, removal of the malleoli, and anchoring the heel pad to the weight-bearing surface) allows excellent gait with a cosmetic prosthesis. Symes-level amputations will not heal without a palpable posterior tibial artery pulse. Surgery may be performed in two stages (Hulnick), the most common indication for a two-stage procedure is the presence of infection. The ankle is disarticulated at the first stage and the amputation revised approximately 6 weeks later during the second stage. Components of the second stage include resection of the malleoli flush with the joint surface, fixation of the fat pad to residual bone, and revision of redundant skin. This amputation allows for intermittent weight bearing; however, skin breakdown may occur if a prosthesis is not used on a regular basis. Below-knee amputations (**BKAs**) are the most common level, and maximum length should be preserved. Approximately 2–3 cm of soft tissue thickness covering of bony ends is ideal. An attempt to save the knee should always be made to decrease necessary energy expenditure for gait. The goal of a BKA is to achieve a cylindrical terminal motor/sensory end organ with muscle stabilization and a nontender, nonadherent scar. Tibia-fibula synostosis (osteoplasty) can improve weight bearing in younger, active patients. **Through-knee amputations** are favored over higher level amputations because of better socket suspension and newer hydraulic knee-assist mechanisms. Through-knee amputations are end bearing, allowing direct load transfer and enhanced proprioception, and do not require intimate socket fit. However, sitting asymmetry is an important cosmetic consideration, especially in women. In this amputation, the patella and its tendon are sutured together with the hamstring tendons to the cruciate stump in the notch.

3. Thigh and Proximal—**Above-knee amputations** do better if length is preserved. Stability of the hip joint is critical and is accomplished by the adductors (keep the femur in adduction, preventing Trendelenburg gait), the quadriceps (assist the

hip flexors during forward propulsion), and the hamstrings. Muscle stabilization is an important operative consideration. Various types of prosthetic knees have been developed (hydraulic, pneumatic, mechanical, etc.). **Hip disarticulation** is occasionally necessary for trauma or malignancy. Prosthetics are only possible in young, strong individuals. **Hemipelvectomy/hemicorpectomy** may be required for pelvic malignancies, infections, and sometimes in paraplegics. Prosthetics are usually not possible except in young, motivated patients with hemipelvectomies. A supporting bucket is required.

E. Upper Extremity Amputations
   1. General Considerations—Amputations of the upper extremity are often associated with greater amounts of functional impairment. For disability ratings, loss of one upper extremity is considered 50% functional impairment, and loss of one hand is 90% of that (45% overall functional impairment). Thumb amputations are considered as 50% loss of one hand (23% overall impairment). Preservation of all viable tissue should be attempted to preserve precision handling (radial structures) and power grip (ulnar hand). Skin should be preserved anteriorly (palmar) for best prosthetic fit. Tenoplasty over amputated digits is contraindicated.
   2. Upper Extremity Amputation Levels (Fig. 8–8)— Carpometacarpal disarticulation is only occasionally indicated. **Wrist disarticulation** preserves pronation and supination and is a widely accepted level with good prosthetic use. Terminal devices for this level may require modifications. **Below-elbow amputations** again require preservation of length. Distal muscle stabilization (myodesis) is essential for myoelectric prosthetic use. Prosthesis power comes from metal or plastic cables that are activated by body movement, usually with a strap under the opposite shoulder, or utilizes external power (hydraulic, pneumatic, electric). **Elbow disarticulation** is occasionally indicated and often can be successful. Prosthesis fit is sometimes difficult, but good socket stability and a long lever arm are obtained. It may be indicated if the bicipital tuberosity of the radius is gone and can be covered with the "mobile wad" musculature. **Above-elbow amputations** require length preservation and muscle stabilization. A Marquardt supracondylar osteotomy (creates posterior bow) may facilitate suspension and provide rotational control. Two types of prosthetics are available: cosmetic (lighter) and functional (heavier and more complicated). Terminal devices and elbow joints can be controlled with body movement, electric power, or a combination of these (hybrid). **Shoulder disarticulation** and **forequarter amputation** are sometimes required for malignancy. The medial clavicle should be preserved when possible and plexus cuts should be staggered. Prosthetics are for cosmesis only. Cineplasty, which makes use of a tunnel of muscle and skin, allows better function but is technically difficult, is not durable, and has numerous associated problems.

F. Revisions—Early revisions may be required for in-

fection, trauma, gangrene, failure of wound healing, and poorly shaped stumps. Chronically, infection, stump breakdown, pressure problems, neuromas, and adherent scarring may make revisions necessary. As a general rule, do not revise for pain (unless a definite neuroma is located). Prosthetic shaping often can alleviate problems. Neuromas, especially over a bony prominence, may occasionally need moving/burying in deep soft tissues. Wedge resection adjacent to a wound breakdown with advancement of posterior tissues is recommended. Plastic surgery procedures may be useful in some cases. Verrucous hyperplasia is a skin disorder that is a result of excess keratin formation and secondary infection from nonuniform stump pressure. Treatment includes oral and topical antibiotics with a keratolytic agent, followed by prosthetic refitting. Surgery is rarely indicated.

III. Prosthetics

A. General—Prosthetics are now constructed primarily of composite plastics, graphite, and light metals. A prosthesis has three components: (1) suspension (socket) attached by straps, belts, contour, suction, friction, etc.; (2) terminal device (upper extremity) or prosthetic foot (lower extremity) that allows contact with the environment; and (3) body or shank. Energy expenditure and speed of gait are related to the weight of the prosthesis, its components, alignment of the prosthesis, and the amputation level. Fabrication is usually from a plaster mold of the residual limb and usually incorporates a check socket that can be changed in the final prosthesis.

B. Lower Extremity (LE) Prosthetics—Usually prescribed by a team composed of a surgeon, prosthetist, and therapist. Components are selected according to the patient's needs and funding available.
   1. Foot and Ankle Amputations—Distal foot amputations require only shoe fillers and rocker-bottom/stiff-soled shoes. Midfoot amputations usually call for a high shoe attached to an AFO to block dorsiflexion and improve push off. Symes amputation prostheses are designed to accommodate the bulbous end and allow proximal support. They often provide a medial (VAPC) or posterior (Canadian) opening for greater ease of insertion of the limb.
   2. Prosthetic Feet—Several varieties are available and can be generally classified into five classes based upon the design. The **single-axis** foot, which has been used since the Civil War, is based on an ankle hinge that provides dorsiflexion and plantar flexion. The disadvantages of the single-axis foot include poor durability and cosmesis. The **SACH** (solid ankle, cushioned heel) foot has been the standard for decades, and is still appropriate for general use. Its popularity is now being challenged by new prosthetic foot design. **Multiaxis** feet allow inversion/eversion and rotation of the foot and are good for work on uneven surfaces at the expense of overall utility and weight. The **energy-storing** class of foot is designed with a flexible keel and may perhaps become the new standard for general use (Fig. 8–9). These feet, also called dynamic (elastic) response feet, are designed with a cantilever spring and are best for

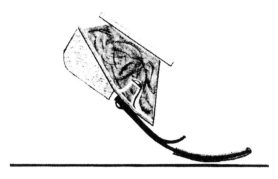

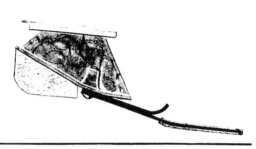

FIGURE 8–9. Dynamic response foot. Note action of dual carbon fiber deflection plates in push off. (From Michael, J.W.: Overview of prosthetic feet. Instr. Course Lect. 39:369, 1990; reprinted by permission.)

young, athletic patients. The following table summarizes these points:

CLASS	ADVANTAGES	DISADVANTAGES	USE
Single axis	Rapid foot flat	Heavy	Limited
SACH	Simple, reliable	Energy consumed	General
Multiaxis	Uneven surfaces	Lack of utility	Outdoorsman
Energy storing	Smooth rollover	Durability/cost	Active

Newer energy-storing, dynamic response feet have had significant impact on the prosthetic industry. The dynamic response feet, including the Seattle foot, Carbon Copy II/III, and the Flex Foot, allow amputees to do near-normal activities.

3. Prosthetic Shanks—Are the structural link between prosthetic components. Two varieties exist—**endoskeletal**, with a soft exterior and load-bearing tubing inside, and **exoskeletal**, with a hard load-bearing exterior shell. Rotator units are sometimes added for patients involved in twisting activities.

4. Prosthetic Knees—Used in AKA prosthetics and chosen based upon patient needs. Prosthetic knees provide controlled absorption of knee motion in the prosthesis. Alignment stability (the position of the prosthetic knee in relation to the patient's line of weight bearing) is important in design and fitting of prosthetic knees. Placing the knee center of rotation posterior to the weight line allows control in the stance phase but makes flex-

ion difficult. Alternatively, with the knee center of rotation anterior to the weight line flexion is made easier, but at the expense of control. Only the polycentric knee takes advantage of both options by having a variable center of rotation. Six basic types of knees are available.

   a. **Constant Friction** Knee—Simply a hinge that is designed to dampen knee swing via a screw or rubber pad that applies friction to the knee bolt. It is a general utility knee, and may be used on uneven terrain. It is the most common knee used in childhood prosthetics. Its major disadvantage is that it allows only single-speed walking and relies solely on alignment for stance phase stability and is therefore not recommended for older, weaker patients.

   b. **Variable Friction** (Cadence Control) Knee—Allows resistance to knee flexion to increase as the knee extends by employing a number of staggered friction pads. This knee allows walking at different speeds, but is not durable and is not available in endoskeletal systems.

   c. **Stance Phase Control** (Weight-Activated, or Safety) Knee—Functions like a constant friction knee during the swing phase but "freezes" by application of a high-friction housing when weight is applied to the limb. Its use is primarily reserved for older patients, high-level amputees, or use on uneven terrain.

   d. **Polycentric** (Four-Bar Linkage) Knees—Has a moving instant center of rotation that provides for different stability characteristics during the gait cycle and may allow increased flexion for sitting. It is favored for patients with knee disarticulations and bilateral amputees.

   e. **Manual Locking** Knee—Consists of a constant friction knee hinge with a positive lock in extension that can be unlocked to allow function similar to that of a constant friction knee. The knee is often left locked in extension for more stability. The knee has limited indications and is used primarily in weak, unstable patients, those patients just learning to use prosthetics, and blind amputees.

   f. **Fluid Control** (Hydraulic and Pneumatic) Knees—Allows adjustment of cadence response by changing resistance to knee flexion via a piston mechanism. The design prevents excessive flexion and is extended earlier in the gait cycle, allowing a more fluid gait. The knee is best used in young active patients who prefer greater utility and variability at the expense of more weight.

   g. Summary—Information on the various types of prosthetic knees is summarized in Table 8–3.

5. Suspension Systems—Suspension is provided in modern lower extremity prosthetics primarily through socket design. The use of straps and belts is usually for supplementation or redundancy. Sockets are prosthetic components that are designed to provide comfortable functional control and pressure distribution on the amputated stump. Sockets can be hard (rigid or unlined) or soft (lined with a resilient material). In general, suction (AKA) and socket contour (BKA) are the primary suspension modalities used. The suction

TABLE 8–3. CHARACTERISTICS OF VARIOUS PROSTHETIC KNEES

KNEE	ACTION	ADVANTAGES	DISADVANTAGES
Constant friction	Limits flexion	Durable, long res	Decreased stability
Variable friction	Varies with flexion	Variable cadence	Durability poor
Stance control	Friction brake	Stability during stance	Durability poor, difficult on stairs
Polycentric	Instant center moves	Stable, increased flexion	Durability poor, heavy
Manual locking	Unlock to sit	Maximum stability	Abnormal gait
Fluid control	Deceleration in swing	Variable cadence	Weight, cost

socket provides an airtight seal via a pressure differential between the socket and atmosphere. Total-contact support of the residual limb surface prevents edema formation.

a. BKA Suspension—Total-contact socket contour suspension is commonly used and can be one of two designs: patella tendon bearing (PTB) or patella tendon supporting (PTS). PTB sockets provide some weight-bearing support in the area of the patellar tendon and medial tibial flare. PTS sockets cover the condyles of the femur and have a high anterior wall enclosing the patella. PTS sockets provide more support anteriorly and add improved stability and suspension; however, they are more difficult to fit. The four important design considerations for both sockets include support (pressure distribution), control (based on the limb-socket interface), suspension (socket ± corset), and alignment (angular and linear). "Soft" PTB sockets are most commonly prescribed, especially with bony or scarred residual limbs, peripheral vascular disease, and volumetrically unstable residual limbs. Neoprene sleeves can also be used to provide additional skin protection (especially for diabetics). The addition of a supracondylar wedge of a flexible material to a PTB socket often gives more stability by providing a locking fit over the condyle. These can be designed as fixed or removable. Hard sockets are usually preferred in warm, humid climates. An above-

patella suspension strap and sometimes a pelvic belt (in obese patients) is needed. Corset-type prostheses can lead to verrucous hyperplasia and thigh atrophy, but reduce socket loads, control the direction of swing, and provide some additional weight support.

b. AKA Suspension—Quadrilateral sockets where the posterior brim abuts the ischial tuberosity have been the classic. This design made it difficult to keep the femur in adduction. Narrower medial-lateral designs (NSNA, CAT-CAM) sharing load with gluteal structures and the greater trochanteric region are now becoming popular (Fig. 8–10). The ischium and ramus are contained within the socket of these newer, more anatomic, comfortable, and functional designs. AKA suspension systems include suction (best; eliminates pistoning, better fit), Silesian belt (adds more stability), and other bands/belts (usually not necessary). **Socket design for AKA** prosthetics allows for 10 degrees of **adduction** of the femur (to stretch the gluteus medius, allowing adequate strength for midstance stability) and 5 degrees of **flexion** (to stretch the gluteus maximus and allow for greater hip extension).

6. Hip Disarticulation/Hemipelvectomy—The Canadian Hip Disarticulation prosthesis can be used for young hip disarticulation patients. Design of this prosthesis allows maximum stability in stance phase through proper alignment. The **hip should**

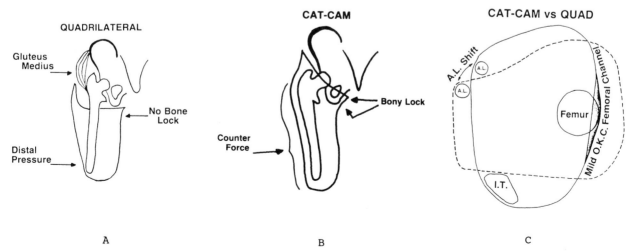

FIGURE 8–10. Comparison of AKA sockets. Note inclusion of the ischial tuberosity and narrow medial-lateral design of newer CAT-CAM socket shown as a solid line in C. (From Sabolich, J.: Contoured adducted trochanteric-controlled alignment method. Clin. Prosthet. Orthot. 9:13, 17, 1985; reprinted by permission.)

be anterior and the knee posterior to the weight-bearing line. The ischial tuberosity is important for weight bearing. Hemipelvectomy patients are much harder to fit because the ischial tuberosity is not preserved. Ambulation is difficult for these patients, and most prefer to use wheelchairs. A pelvic bucket with hydraulic or mechanical hip joint mechanisms attached to an AKA prosthesis can be used in extremely motivated patients.

C. Upper Extremity (UE) Prosthetics
    1. General Considerations—UE prosthetic selection also requires a team approach. These prostheses are rejected at a much higher rate (50%) than lower limb prostheses. They are less likely to be accepted in younger patients, nondominant arm amputations, below-elbow amputations (BEAs), with delayed fitting, and patients given conventional (vs. myoelectric) prostheses. Temporary prostheses should be used early; open wounds are not a contraindication to temporary fitting.
    2. Terminal Devices—Hand substitutes can be grouped into two general categories—the more functional hooks and the more cosmetic hands. Most devices are interchangeable and many patients own more than one terminal device. Typically, hands are passive devices, as are opposition posts and sports adaptations. Mechanical hands can be heavy. Hooks are active devices and are designed for use in one of two modes: voluntary opening (VO) or voluntary closing (VC). VO prosthetics are more popular and can be readily recognized by their rubber bands (number of rubber bands is proportional to pinch strength, with three bands [about 3 pounds of strength] needed for most activities of daily living). VO hooks are numerically classified according to the Hosmer-Dorrance system:

Number	Use
5	Adults
7	Farmer's hook—laborers
8	Ladies
9	Teenagers
10	Children
12	Infants
X	(Suffix) Neoprene fingers
A	(Suffix) Aluminum (lightweight, less rugged)
P	(Suffix) Plastic coated

VC prosthetics are held open by a spring and allow graded prehension and a powerful grip. However, patients may tire with prolonged holding of objects with VC components. They are bulkier, less durable, and more expensive. The APRL hook is a VC hook with many features, including the capability to lock in any position and a variable opening width, but its expense precludes routine use. Mechanical hands are somewhat cosmetic and are acceptable for nonprehensile activities, but they allow less precision, are heavy, and are less functional than hooks. However, they can be effective in patients with myoelectric prostheses. Mechanical hands also can be VO (most commonly) or VC and function via palmar prehension.
    3. Wrist Units—Allow attachment and positioning

of the terminal device in pronation/supination. Three types are used:

Unit	Function	Advantages	Disadvantages
Friction	Most common	Easy	Slips with heavy load
Quick change	Button disc	Adaptable	Reliability
Flexion	Incr. flexion	Can operate midline (bilat. amputees)	Reliability

    4. Elbow Hinges/Joints
       a. Elbow Hinges—Used in BEA, and can be flexible (permit pronation/supination in long BEAs) or rigid (for higher level amputees). Single-axis hinges are most commonly used, but polycentric and step-up hinges are also available. Polycentric hinges help increase elbow flexion by reducing soft tissue bunching. They are often indicated in obese patients. **Step-up hinges amplify elbow excursion** in a 2:1 ratio, but require twice the force to do so. Step-up hinges also require a split socket design.
       b. Outside Locking Hinges—Used for elbow disarticulation and transcondylar amputations where joints are not possible due to aesthetic and functional considerations. These hinges have seven locking positions.
       c. Elbow Joints—Used for above-elbow amputations (AEAs) that are at least 5 centimeters proximal to the elbow and commonly consist of an internal locking joint with 11 locking positions. The elbow is locked to operate the terminal device. A friction-held turntable is also included, permitting manual prepositioning of the prosthetic forearm.
    5. Upper Extremity Prosthetic Socket Design—Sockets cover the residual limb or stump and transmit motions normally associated with the remaining anatomy. Optimal socket design provides motion, stability, and comfort. Long BEA (with >55% of the forearm remaining) sockets are elliptically shaped in cross section and are designed to allow pronation and supination. Short BEA sockets are circular in shape and allow notching for the biceps tendon. AEA sockets are typically more oval in cross section and must snugly fit the residual stump. AEAs with more than 30% of length remaining retain a bony lever arm and musculature for effective range of motion.
    6. Suspension and Control—UE prosthetics are suspended by a system of Dacron straps (harness) and controlled by a cabling system. The following harnesses are commonly used:

Harness	Characteristics	Use
Figure 8	Most Common, cross in back	Most patients
Figure 9	No suspension, terminal device control	Self-suspended sockets
Saddle	Shoulder saddle and chest strap	Heavy lifting, intolerant patient
Strap	Chest strap, expansion controls	Short AEA, disarticulation

Bilateral AEA harnessing is composed of two figure of 8 harnesses (without axillary loops) and an across-the-back strap. BEA prostheses are controlled with a one-cable system (single control). Ipsilateral shoulder motion applies tension on a prehensile terminal to allow it to function. AEA prostheses are usually operated by two separate control cables. One cable flexes the elbow and controls the terminal device and the other cable controls prosthetic elbow locking/unlocking. Elbow flexion is made possible by split housing of the control cable. Locking/unlocking of the elbow joint is controlled by a cable running from the anterior suspension strap to the elbow that operates on an alternator principle. **The elbow is controlled by slight extension, abduction, and depression of the shoulder**. The terminal devices operates after the elbow is locked in the desired position. **Humeral flexion or biscapular abduction (protraction) opens the terminal device** using figure of 8 or 9 harnesses. Optimal mechanical efficiency of figure of 8 harnesses occurs with placement of the straps to **cross** just **below** the **spinous process** of **C7** and slightly **toward the nonamputated side**.

7. Electric Powered Prosthetics—Allow a powerful grasp, graded prehension, ease of operation, and improved cosmesis. They have the additional advantage that they **can be operated in any position** and are superior for **midline** and **overhead** activities. However, they are heavier, slower, and much more expensive than standard prosthetics. These devices are more readily accepted by patients but they are less reliable and rugged. A hybrid of body controlled and electric powered components may be the ideal solution for many patients, particularly short above-elbow amputees.

D. Common Prosthetic Problems
   1. BKA—**Pistoning** during **swing phase** of gait is usually caused by an **ineffective suspension system**. Pistoning in the **stance phase** is due to poor **socket fit** or volume changes in the stump (may require a change in stump sock thickness). Alignment problems are common and include the following:

FOOT POSITION	GAIT ABNORMALITY
Inset	Varus strain, pain (proximedial, distolateral), circumduction
Outset	Valgus strain, pain (proxilateral, distomedial), broad based gait
Forward placement	Increased knee extension (patellar pain), but stable
Posterior placement	Increased knee flexion/instability
Dorsiflexed foot	Increased patellar pressure
Plantar-flexed foot	Drop off, patellar pressure

Pressure-related pain or redness should be corrected with relief of the prosthesis in the affected area. Other problems may be related to the foot—**too soft a foot results in excessive knee extension**, while **too hard a foot causes knee flexion and lateral rotation of the** toes.

2. AKA—Excessive prosthetic length and weak hip abductors or flexors can lead to circumduction, vaulting, and lateral trunk bending. Hip flexion contractures and insufficient anterior socket support can lead to excessive lumbar lordosis (compensatory). Inadequate prosthetic knee flexion can lead to terminal knee snap. Medial whip (heel in, knee out) can be caused by a varus knee, excessive external rotation of the knee axis, or muscle weakness. Lateral whip (heel out, knee in) is caused by the opposite (valgus knee, internal rotation at knee, and weakness). The following table summarizes common AKA prosthetic gait problems:

GAIT ABNORMALITY	PROSTHETIC PROBLEM
Lateral trunk bending	Short prosthesis, weak abductors, poor fit
Abducted gait	Poor socket fit medially
Circumducted gait	Prosthetic too long, excess knee friction
Vaulted gait	Prosthetic too long, poor suspension
Foot rotation at heel strike	Heel too stiff, loose socket
Short stance phase	Painful stump, knee too loose
Knee instability	Knee too anterior, foot too stiff
Medial/lateral whip	Excessive knee rotation, tight socket
Terminal snap	Quadricep weakness, insecure patient
Foot slap, knee hyperextension	Heel too soft
Knee flexion	Heel too hard
Excessive lordosis	Hip flexion contracture, socket problems

3. Stair Climbing—In general, amputees climb stairs by leading with their normal limb and descend by leading with their prosthetic limb ("the good goes up and the bad comes down").

IV. Childhood Amputations and Prosthetics
   A. Introduction—Childhood amputations make up about 10% of amputations. Most are unilateral, and boys are more frequently affected than girls. Amputations can be congenital (most common) or acquired.
      1. Congenital Amputations—**Terminal BEA** is the **most common congenital amputation**. Risk is increased with thalidomides, maternal diabetes, hydramniosis, rubella, amniotic bands, and chromosomal abnormalities. Congenital amputations are classified based on the extent of amputation. **Amelia** connotes complete absence of a limb; **meromelia** is a partial defect. Meromelia is further subclassified based on whether it is terminal (at the end of the limb), or intercalary (in the middle), and can also be defined by the terms preaxial (radial or tibial) or postaxial (ulnar or fibular). Evaluation to rule out other anomalies (GI, respiratory, cardiovascular, GU), and scoliosis (esp. with UE involvement) is necessary. As a general rule, deformed feet should be amputated early, but a more conservative approach is favored in the upper extremity. Early use of the residual extremity should be encouraged. The use of a passive device at 3–6 months for unilateral UE amputations ("fit when they sit"), and a monolithic (unjointed) device at 6–12 months for unilateral LE

amputations is recommended, with active devices used at age 2–3.

2. Acquired Amputations—Most are the result of **trauma** (esp. motor vehicle accidents), and **involve the LE**. Prosthetic management begins preoperatively. Greater acceptance of prostheses is gained if immediate fitting is done, especially in tumor patients. Preservation of the epiphysis should be attempted. Malignancies can sometimes have surprisingly long life spans, so care and appropriate prosthetic management should not be sacrificed.

B. LE Amputations/Prosthetics—Usually should be initially fit at 9–12 months. A SACH foot with a thigh cuff often required. Syme amputations should be done before 2 years of age and should preserve the distal tibial epiphysis. Monolithic devices are favored for AKAs until 36–48 months, when the knee joint is included. A constant friction knee is favored early, followed by a hydraulic knee later. Pelvic suspension is with a Silesian belt. With phocomelia a rocker-bottom prosthesis or swivel walker at 18 months is selected, with the definitive prosthetic fitting at school age. With hip disarticulation or hemipelvectomy, a bucket prosthesis with a shoulder harness is required.

C. UE Amputations/Prosthetics—As noted, a passive device is used at 3–6 months. Later use of a terminal device with a figure of 8 harness is recommended. A hand is offered at school age. For AEA, elbow lock cables are favored at 30–36 months. With **bilateral amelia** (especially in blind children), a **Krukenberg** kineplastic operation (lobster claw) is offered early. Otherwise, the first devices are usually used at 24 months, with frequent refitting and modular components used. Myoelectric prostheses are becoming increasingly popular for use in children.

D. Complications—Include bony overgrowth (most common in the humerus in the upper extremity and the fibula in the lower extremity), painful spurs (may require revision), leg length discrepancies, neuromas, and contractures.

V. Orthotics

A. Introduction—The primary function of an orthosis is control of motion of certain body segments. An ideal orthosis controls only those motions that are abnormal or undesirable and permits motion where normal function can occur. Evaluation of the biomechanical defect that needs correcting leads to the selection of the proper orthotic. Orthotics are used for protection (e.g., in fracture management); for support (e.g., correction of flexible deformities using biomechanical principles), and to allow increased function (e.g., with spinal cord and nerve injuries). Orthotics can be static (immobilizes only), dynamic (allows controlled motion), or functional (activates a joint). **Orthotics are not indicated for correction of fixed deformities or for patients with spasticity that cannot be overpowered manually.**

B. Lower Extremity Orthotics

1. Shoes—In addition to specially designed shoewear for pediatric problems (e.g., clubfoot and metatarsus adductus), special shoewear is frequently indicated in the adult population as well. Extra depth and extra width shoes accommodate foot deformities and are required in order to use plas-

tazote liners. Wooden shoes are useful following foot operations, for treatment of certain fractures, and in the treatment of diabetic foot ulcers.

2. Shoe Modifications—Include special modifications to the heel (SACH, Thomas Heel) and sole (wedge, bars). **SACH heels** allow better shock absorption and reduce forward tibial thrust. They are useful in patients with restricted ankle motion (degenerative joint disease, fusion) and are often combined with a rocker-bottom sole. The **Thomas Heel** (medial heel wedge) tilts the heel into varus and may be helpful in the treatment of symptomatic pes planus and plantar fasciitis. Metatarsal pads transfer weight proximally and can be helpful for patients with sesamoiditis and metatarsalgia. **Rocker-bottom shoes** and Denver Bars are also used in the treatment of metatarsalgia, as well as hallux rigidus, malperferans ulcers, and partial foot amputations. Heel and sole elevations are helpful in patients with leg length discrepancies, but can add excess weight to the shoe. It is not necessary to make up the entire amount of the discrepancy with these wedges, but the appropriate amount is determined on a case-by-case basis. Other devices (wedges, etc.) alter the weight-bearing pattern of the foot.

3. Shoe Inserts—Molded shoe inserts help distribute plantar pressure, can be made from a wide variety of materials, and have many different uses. **Plastazote liners** are helpful in patients with hammer toe and claw toe deformities. The **UCBL** (University of California Biomechanics Laboratory) orthotic controls the calcaneus and helps in the correction of flexible hindfoot valgus, pes planus, and lateral ligamentous laxity. UCBL inserts may also be helpful in the treatment of plantar fasciitis and posterior tibial tendonitis. Medial inserts may be helpful in treating runners with medial knee pain and foot pronation. Other inserts commonly used include various ankle braces and stirrups for treatment of ankle sprains/instability. Rigid shoe orthotics can irritate neuromas, cause sesamoiditis, and lead to stress fractures, and it may be difficult to adjust to their wear.

4. Ankle-Foot Orthotic (**AFO**)—Controls the alignment and motions of the joints of the foot and ankle. Commonly used for patients with weak ankle dorsiflexors and medial/lateral instability and pain. AFOs can be metal (adjustable, attach to the shoe, and are heavier) or plastic. Metal AFOs usually have two (double) uprights and are connected to a shoe attachment (usually with a stirrup) or a molded shoe insert. Ankle components can be solid, limited motion (using ankle stops), or free motion, or can assist motion (with springs that aid in dorsiflexion). Varus/valgus correction straps (T-straps) can be added to the AFO (on the side opposite the instability) to provide additional ankle stability in select cases. Single upright AFOs are sometimes used for patients with mild dorsiflexion weakness. Newer thermoplastic materials are lightweight and cosmetic and offer better stability. However, they offer limited adjustability and are not good in patients with fluctuating edema. The posterior leaf spring is the most commonly used AFO. It allows ankle movement based on its narrow width proximal to the shoe insert. Extension of the trim lines an-

teriorly will result in a solid ankle AFO, and the addition of flanges will help control varus/valgus forces. Special AFOs can be made for patients with weak quadriceps (floor reaction AFO). Other AFOs include articulating AFOs, PTB AFOs (tibia fracture treatment), and spiral/hemispiral AFOs (allow some rotation).

5. Knee-Ankle-Foot Orthotic (**KAFO**)—Extend from the thigh to the foot and are often used in patients with knee instability and genu recurvatum. KAFOs are also used in patients requiring femoral and/or tibial support. KAFOs consists of two uprights that extend up the thigh, a mechanical knee joint and two thigh bands. It adds medial and lateral ankle stability as well. KAFOs attempt to balance the body weight over the feet with the CG posterior to the hip and anterior to the knee. The following knee joints are available for KAFOs:

Joint	Characteristics	Use
Free motion	Full flexion, hyperextension stop	Recurvatum
Offset	Axis posterior to uprights	Stance stability
Droplock	Ring drops to lock w/ full extension	Stance stability
Adjustable	Can lock in any degree of flexion	Protective

Supracondylar KAFOs can stabilize the knee in some cases, and may be used for treatment of recurvatum as well.

6. Hip-Knee-Ankle-Foot Orthotic (**HKAFO**)—The addition of a hip joint and pelvic band can help control selected hip motions. This orthosis provides pelvic stability and forward progression and controls uneven leg swing. Hip joints are usually a single-axis design with a ring lock. A double pelvic band or girdle is commonly used for enhanced stability. Much like prosthetics for hip disarticulation, design should ensure that the hip is **anterior** and **knee posterior to the weight-bearing line**. Thoracic-hip-knee-ankle-foot orthotics (**THKAFOs**) provide even more stability. They can be utilized for patients with osteogenesis imperfecta or other disorders. Reciprocating gait orthoses are modified THKAFO **swivel walkers** that can be used in younger patients with high lumbar myelomeningocele, other neuromuscular disorders, and spinal cord lesions. The design combines flexion of one hip with obligatory extension of the opposite hip via a cable coupling system.

7. Knee Orthotics
   a. Patellofemoral Disorders—These orthotics are designed to help control tracking of the patella throughout the range of motion of the knee. The infrapatellar strap, which is worn only during periods of activity, encircles the knee below the patella, stabilizing the patellar tendon. The Palumbo orthosis consists of an elastic sleeve with two dynamic straps that stabilize the patella.
   b. Angular Stability—The Swedish knee cage and supracondylar orthosis are designed to restrict hyperextension. Medial and lateral sta-

bility is provided by standard knee orthoses with medial and lateral bars.
   c. Axial Rotation—Various orthotics have been designed to provide both angular and rotatory stability, including the Lenox Hill, Don Joy, and Orthotech braces. However, all these braces may not withstand instantaneous forces often associated with athletic injuries.

C. Upper Extremity Orthotics
   1. Introduction—Upper extremity orthoses assist or substitute for weak or paralyzed motor power, protect parts from pain or potential deformity, or correct an existing deformity.
   2. Shoulder and Elbow Orthotics—Mostly serve a protective function. A shoulder abduction stabilizer (**airplane splint**) functions to protect the shoulder from adduction contractures and relieves tension on the superior aspect of the shoulder. It is commonly used following rotator cuff surgery when excess tension is placed on the supraspinatus tendon following repair. A shoulder harness is used for recurrent dislocations in patients who are not operative candidates. Various shoulder slings are also available (single strap, multiple strap, vertical arm, abduction, and overhead [suspension] slings are commonly used). A **Kenny Howard brace** can be used in patients with grade II or III acromioclavicular separations. This orthosis applies direct pressure on the clavicle, holding it in a reduced position with the acromion. The dorsal elbow extensor and dorsal elbow flexor orthoses are corrective orthotics that attempt to gradually elongate soft tissues to overcome contractures. Assistive and substitution orthoses for quadraplegics or severely impaired patients include orthotics with various elbow and shoulder locks and one of three principle suspension systems (hoop, shoulder cap, or harness). Various wheelchair attachments are also available, such as the balanced forearm orthoses with various attachments.
   3. Hand and Wrist Orthotics—Unlike shoulder and elbow orthoses, hand and wrist orthoses are mainly designed to augment motor power and are less commonly used for protective purposes. Several assistive or substitutive orthoses have been designed to enable patients with partial or complete paralysis to perform activities of daily living. Some of these orthotics are listed in Table 8–4. An **opponens splint** serves to maintain, assist, or provide opposition by stabilizing the thumb and fingers in a functional position. It can also be used in patients with de Quervain's syndrome. Wrist-hand orthotics (**WHOs**) include the wrist-driven flexor hinge orthosis, which can be used in C6/C7 quadraplegics who do not have active finger flexors. It allows the patient to pinch with a three-jaw chuck apparatus. A ratchet type of orthosis can be used for C5 quadraplegics. It allows some finger function. Corrective orthoses are usually used for specified periods each day. Theses devices include knuckle benders, reverse knuckle benders, adjustable WHOs (used following MCP arthroplasty), and fingernail hook devices. Protective orthoses restrict active function and protect the limb from potential deformity or damage. Orthoses include wrist-hand stabilizers (resting

TABLE 8–4. WRIST AND HAND ORTHOSES

Orthosis	Category	Function	Indication
Opponens	Positional	Stabilizes thumb	Weak thenar muscle
Lumbrical bar	Positional	Prevents MCP hyperextension	Intrinsic paralysis
Finger extension assistive	Positional	DIP/PIP extension assistance	Intrinsic paralysis
Wrist control	Positional	Dorsiflexion assistance	Weak grasp, functional finger flexors
WHO	Prehension	Stabilizes wrist & thumb	Extensive paralysis
Universal	Utensil holder	Holds small objects	Hand paralysis

splints), PIP stabilizers (swan neck splint), and thumb CMC stabilizers (thumb post). A dorsal extension outrigger is often used in radial nerve injuries. Splints are also available for median nerve injuries (opponens splint with wrist extension) and ulnar nerve injuries. Thermoplastic cock-up splints are commonly used in patients with carpal tunnel syndrome. A temporary wrist extension orthotic can be used in patients with caput ulnae syndrome.

D. Orthotics and Fracture Management—Fracture bracing, popularized originally by Dr. Vert Mooney, and later by Dr. Augusto Sarmiento, can be efficacious for follow on treatment of certain injuries. Functional bracing relies on some motion at the fracture site, leading to the formation of a stronger peripheral callus (versus the primary callus that forms following rigid fixation). Bracing is used following a period of initial immobilization in a cast or in traction. Functional bracing relies on hydrostatic forces in the affected limb to enhance physiologic healing of fractures and may also decrease the incidence of "fracture disease" (e.g., joint stiffness and osteopenia). Braces used in the treatment of diaphyseal fractures do not prevent shortening, but assist in preventing further shortening of the affected limb. Orthoses can be prefabricated or custom molded. Functional bracing is most commonly used for humerus and tibia fractures. They can also be used for protection (especially after ORIF of fractures [e.g., tibial plateau fractures]). Prefabricated orthotics (knee and ankle braces that control varus/valgus) and custom orthotics for immobilization and protection are also used.

E. Childhood Orthotics—In addition to AFOs, KAFOs, and other orthotics used in adults, there are many specialized orthotics designed for management of childhood skeletal abnormalities. Hip abduction braces are helpful in children with cerebral palsy and hip dysplasia (e.g., Lorenz brace), and Legg Calvé Perthes disease (Toronto, Tachdjian, Newington, and Atlanta **Scottish Rite Brace**). **Pavlic Harnesses**, developed for developmental dysplasia of the hip, flex and abduct affected hips. The Pavlic Harness is generally considered to be superior to the Von Rosen orthosis, Ilfeld splint, and Frejka Pillow. Specialized HKAFOs with varus molding are designed for treatment of Blount's disease. Standing frames, "A" frames, and parapodiums are useful for children with severe neuromuscular disorders. Spinal orthotics (Milwaukee Brace and TLSO) are used in management of scoliosis and kyphosis. Other orthotics (twister cables, Dennis Browne bars, etc.) have little use currently. Indications for use of various orthotics are discussed in detail in Chapter 1, Pediatric Orthopaedics.

F. Spine

1. Cervical Spine—Numerous orthotics are available for the cervical spine. Two basic designs exist: collars and post appliances. All cervical orthotics are designed to restrict motion. Most conventional orthoses limit cervical motion by about 45%. The halo vest is most stable and limits normal cervical motion by 75%. Table 8–5 lists commonly used orthoses in order of increasing stability. Torque on halo pins can safely be up to 0.90 N · m. These must be retorqued within the first 24 hours. Sizing is important in placing patients in a halo. The halo provides most stability in the upper cervical spine because "snaking" can occur at lower levels. Complications of wear include errant screw placement, loose/infected pins, osteomyelitis, and pressure sores.

2. Thoracolumbar—Most orthotics provide three effects: increased intracavity pressure, reduced trunk motion, and altered skeletal alignment. Orthotics used for back pain function as the body's abdominal support system. Control of motion in the lower lumbar segments can only be achieved by extension to the leg. Spinal alignment with three-point pressure systems may also be beneficial. Complications of orthotics include weakness/atrophy, tightness/contracture, and psychological dependence. The following orthotics are commonly used:

Orthosis	Category	Use
Sacroiliac	Soft	Pelvic pain, SI stabilization
LSO (corset)	Soft	Low back pain (decr. disc pressure)
TLSO	Soft	Mild instability/mid-low back pain
Chairback	Rigid	Reduces motion; thin patients
Taylor	Rigid	Reduces T-spine flexion-extension
Jewett	Rigid	Three-point fixation, flexion control
Knight	Rigid	Flexion-extension-lateral control
Williams	Rigid	Extension-lateral control
Cow horn	Rigid	Flexion-lateral rotation control
Plastic jacket	Rigid	Flexion-extension-lateral rotation control

G. Mobility Aids—Include walkers, crutches, canes, and wheelchairs. All assistive devices cost energy. These devices can be helpful in pain relief, balance, propulsion, and proprioception. Determining the most appropriate gait aid for a given patient is based

TABLE 8–5. CERVICAL SPINE ORTHOSES

ORTHOSIS	USE	CONTROL	COMMENTS
Soft collar	Sprain	None	Mild "whiplash"
Philadelphia collar	Trauma	Occiput–C3 (flexion)	
SOMI	Comfort	Upper flexion	
Yale	Comfort	Lower control	Lower C-spine fracture
Minerva	Comfort	Flexion/extension/rotation control	
4-poster frame	Long term	Midlevel (flexion)	
Cervicothoracic	Tracheostomy and Lower C spine Fx	Upper extension, lower flexion	
Halo vest	Unstable Fx	Lower extension and rotation	Cranial nerve VI palsy, unstable fractures

on the patient's function, amount of weight bearing desired, balance, and upper limb function. Stability is based on the number of contact points for the gait aid. Walkers are the most stable aid and often are the first aid tried after patients have learned to walk on parallel bars. Walkers should be designed to be placed at the waistline of patients. Special forearm supports can be added for patients with weak or malformed hands. Crutches can be standard axillary support (transmit up to 80% of body weight), forearm support (Canadian style, which transmit up to 50% of body weight), or newer forearm supporting versions. Canes are used in the hand opposite the involved side and widen the support base and reduce stress on the involved limb by shifting the center of gravity toward the uninvolved side. Quad canes have extra legs on their bases, allowing more stable support for elderly patients and stroke victims. Standard canes can be helpful in patients with pain or in need of minimal assistance. The height of a cane should be adjusted so that the highest point is at the level of the greater trochanter. The handle should also be fit to the patients hand. Wheelchairs are required when patients are unable to ambulate or energy expenditure for ambulation is excessive. **The location of the axle posterior to the seat is the key to wheelchair stability.** Wheelchair prescriptions must be individualized. Special cushions with air cells (ROHO) are useful in neuromuscular patients as a means of preventing pressure sores. Electric wheelchairs are required for C5 quadraplegics. Special chairs can be powered by inspiration/expiration for higher level quadraplegics.

VI. Functional Rehabilitation

A. Introduction—Special attention must be given to spinal cord injury and stroke victims because these problems can occur at a relatively young age and the effects can be devastating. With proper training, certain patients can live independent or semi-independent lives.

B. Spinal Cord Injury—Impairment and/or loss of motor and/or sensory function secondary to neurologic damage. Spinal cord injury (SCI) is frequently a result of trauma, and its incidence is increased in the summer, motor vehicle accidents, gunshot wounds, and cervical and head trauma. The **functional level** in SCI is the anatomic level where the **majority of the muscles at that level function at least at a "fair" grade.** The neurologic level is the lowest normal segment. Consideration must be given to the following factors.

1. Mobility—The level of SCI is the prime determinant of the level of function that may be achieved in a neurologically impaired patient. C4 and higher quadraplegics require high back and head support and may be mobile in a wheelchair through the addition of mouth-driven accessories. C5 levels may use an electric wheelchair and a ratchet wrist-hand orthotic (WHO) for mobilization. C6 levels and below may use a manual wheelchair and a flexor hinge WHO. C6 levels and below can usually drive specially equipped automobiles. Transfers are dependent for C4 levels and above, assisted for C5 levels, and independent for C6 levels and below.

2. Activities of Daily Living (ADL)—C6 levels can groom and dress themselves, C7 levels can cut their own meat. Bowel and bladder function can be done via daily rectal stimulation/suppositories initially and intermittent catheterization.

3. Residence—Changes such as ramps (12:1 slope), 5' × 5' platforms (for wheelchair turning), rails, etc. are helpful.

4. Psychosocial—These factors must not be overlooked, and professional assistance should be included in rehabilitation. Families of affected patients are an important component in this process. Males may be impotent but can sometimes achieve a reflex erection.

5. Education/Vocation—Occupational therapy should include activities of daily living and reintegration back into the work force when possible.

6. Other Medical Problems—Cervical level injuries often have compromised pulmonary status due to loss of abdominal musculature support. Coughing assistance and special support is required. Tracheostomies should be avoided unless there is no option. Skin breakdown must also be closely monitored. Bowel and bladder training should begin early, and problems such as kidney stones and bowel obstruction should be identified early. Autonomic dysreflexia (discussed in Chapter 6, Spine) can occur in all injuries above T5 and is usually caused by an obstructed urinary catheter or fecal impaction.

7. Cost—Management of paraplegics exceeds $100,000 annually. This can cause significant strain on patients and their families.

8. Summary—Functional levels are important in assessing orthotic treatment and rehabilitation for spinal cord injuries (Table 8–6).

C. Stroke and Head Injury—Can affect young patients (mean 56 years for CVA and mean 25 years for head

TABLE 8–6. SPINAL CORD INJURY TREATMENT BY FUNCTIONAL LEVEL

FUNCTIONAL LEVEL	WORKING	NOT WORKING	TREATMENT/MOBILITY
Above C4	—	Diaphragm, upper extremity muscles	Respirator dependent
C4	Diaphragm	Upper extremity muscles	Wheelchair chin/puff
*C5	Biceps	Below elbow	Electric wheelchair, rachet
C6	Wrist extensors	Elbow extensors	Wheelchair, flexor hinge
*C7	Triceps	Grasp	Wheelchair, independent
T1	Intrinsic muscles	Abdominals/lower extremity muscles	Wheelchair, independent
T2–T12	Upper extremity muscles, abdominals	Lower extremity muscles	Wheelchair, HKAFO (Nonfunctional ambulation)
L1	Upper extremity muscles, abdominals, quadriceps	Lower extremity muscles	KAFO, minimal ambulation
L2	Iliopsoas	Knee/ankle	KAFO, household ambulation
*L3	Quadriceps	Ankle	AFO, community ambulation
L4	Tibialis anterior	Toe, plantar flexors	AFO, community ambulation
L5	Ext. hallucis longus, ext. digitorum longus	Plantar flexors	AFO, independent
S1	Gastrocnemius/soleus	Bowel/bladder	± Metatarsal bar

* Important levels.

injuries). Early treatment is critical. The majority of neurologic return is within the first 6 months for CVAs and within the first 18 months in head injury patients. Careful assessment of neurologic function is essential. Strength, balance, and good contralateral hip flexion are required for a hemiplegic to ambulate. Treatment with AFOs is required with weak calf muscles, calf spasticity, foot drop, and mild ankle varus, and in patients with inadequate proprioception. Rarely, the use of other orthotics, including slings, resting orthotics, and wrist-hand orthotics, is required. Shoulder problems occur frequently in stroke patients and may include laxity, instability, and painful contractures.

D. Spasticity—Occurs in upper motor neuron injuries, including CVA, cervical or thoracic (not lumbar) spinal cord injuries, head injuries, and childhood disorders (e.g., CP). Spasticity is increased by noxious stimuli and can sometimes be controlled by various medications (valium, dantrolene, baclofen). Surgical control is sometimes possible with tenotomies, neurectomies, cordotomy, myelotomy, or rhizotomy, but this is still under investigation. Orthotics in spastic patients, when required, should be rigid ("no elastics for spastics"). Special problems, including pressure sores and knee malalignment, must be treated.

E. Polio—A viral infection of the anterior horn cells of the spinal cord that affects motor units preferentially (position sense and sensation are left intact). Considerations in orthotic management include atrophy and profound weakness. Spasticity is not a problem. Spring-loaded lightweight orthotics are favored. Postpolio syndrome, or development of renewed pain, fatigue, muscle weakness, and functional impairment 30–35 years after acute poliomyelitis, can cause severe problems in affected patients. The four factors associated with this syndrome include age at onset (>10), four-extremity involvement, ventilator dependence, and hospitalization during the preceding acute illness. This can occur in 20–80% of surviving patients (more than 300,000 patients in the U.S.), and must be recognized by the astute orthopaedist.

Selected Bibliography

Amputation and prosthetic management of the lower limb. Instr. Course Lect. 39:335–378, 1990.

Atlas of Prosthetics, nth ed. Chicago, American Academy of Orthopaedic Surgeons, 1900.

Bedbrook, G.M.: The Care and Management of Spinal Cord Injuries. New York, Springer-Verlag, 1981.

Brotman, S., Browner, B.D., and Cowley, R.A.: Proper timing of amputation for open fractures of the lower extremities. Am. Surg. 48:484–486, 1982.

Brown, P.W.: Sacrifice of the unsatisfactory hand. J. Hand Surg. 4:417–423, 1979.

Bunch, W.H., et al., eds.: Atlas of Orthotics, 2nd ed. St. Louis, C.V. Mosby Company, 1985.

Burgess, E.M., Matsen, F.A., Wyss, C.R., and Simmons, C.W.: Segmental transcutaneous measurements of PO_2 in patients requiring below-the-knee amputation for peripheral vascular insufficiency. J. Bone Joint Surg. [Am.] 64:378–382, 1982.

Cederberg, P.A., Pritchard, D.J., and Joyce, J.W.: Doppler-determined segmental pressures and wound-healing in amputations for vascular disease. J. Bone Joint Surg. [Am.] 65:363–365, 1983.

Cerny, K., Waters, R., Hislop, H., and Perry, J.: Walking and wheelchair energetics in persons with paraplegia. Phys. Ther. 60:1133–1139, 1980.

Dallas Orthotic and Prosthetic Course (Dallas Short Course), October 25–27, 1990. University of Texas Southwest Medical Center, Dallas, TX.

Flandry, F., Beskin, J., Chambers, R.B., et al.: The effect of the CAT-CAM above-knee prosthesis on functional rehabilitation. Clin. Orthop. 239:249–262, 1989.

Goh, J.C.H., Solomonidis, S.E., Spence, W.D., and Paul, J.P.: Biomechanical evaluation of SACH and uniaxial feet. Prosthet. Orthot. Int. 8:147–154, 1984.

Grace, R.G., Skipper, B.J., Newberry, J.C., Nelson, M.A., Sweetser, E.R., and Rothman, M.L.: Prophylactic knee braces and injury to the lower extremity. J. Bone Joint Surg. [Am.] 70:422, 1988.

Greene, W.B., and Cary, J.M.: Partial foot amputations in children: A comparison of the several types with the Syme amputation. J. Bone Joint Surg. [Am.] 64:438–443, 1982.

Hannah, R.E., Morrison, J.B., and Chapman, A.E.: Prostheses alignment: Effect on gait of persons with below-knee amputations. Arch. Phys. Med. Rehabil. 65:159–162, 1984.

Herberts, P., Almstrom, C., and Caine, K.: Clinical application study of multifunctional prosthetic hands. J. Bone Joint Surg. [Br.] 60:552–560, 1978.

Inman, V.T., Ralston, H.J., and Todd, F.: Human Walking. Baltimore, Williams & Wilkins, 1981.

Johnson, R.M., Owen, J.R., Hart, D.L., and Callahan, R.A.: Cervical orthoses: A guide to their selection and use. Clin. Orthop. 154:34–45, 1981.

Kacy, S.S., Wolma, F.J., and Flye, M.W.: Factors affecting the results of below knee amputation in patients with and without diabetes. Surg. Gynecol. Obstet. 155:513–518, 1982.

Lehmann, J.F., Esselman, P.C., Ko, M.J., Smith, J.C., deLateur, B.J., and Dralle, A.J.: Plastic ankle-foot orthoses: Evaluation of function. Arch. Phys. Med. Rehabil. 64:402–407, 1983.

Marquardt, E.: The Multiple Limb-Deficient Child: Special Surgical Procedures. St Louis, C.V. Mosby, 1981.

McCall, R.E., and Schmidt, W.T.: Clinical experience with the reciprocal gait orthosis in myelodysplasia. J. Pediatr. Orthop. 6:157–161, 1986.

McClenaghan, B.A., Krajbich, J.I., Pirone, A.M., et al.: Comparative assessment of gait after limb-salvage procedures. J. Bone Joint Surg. [Am.] 71:1178, 1989.

Mikelberg, R., and Reid, S.: Spinal cord lesions and lower extremity bracing: An overview and follow-up study. Paraplegia 19:379–385, 1981.

Moore, W.S., Henry, R.E., Malone, J.M., Daly, M.J., Patton, D., and Childers, S.J.: Prospective use of Xenon Xe 133 clearance for amputation level selection. Arch. Surg. 116:86–88, 1981.

Nickel, V.L.: Orthopedic Rehabilitation. New York, Churchill Livingstone, 1982.

Northmore-Ball, M.D., Heger, H., and Hunter, G.A.: The below-elbow myo-electric prosthesis: A comparison of the Otto Bock myo-electric prosthesis with the hook and functional hand. J. Bone Joint Surg. [Br.] 62:363–367, 1980.

Northwestern University Medical School Prosthetic and Orthotic Center. Lower and Upper Limb Prosthetics for Physicians, Surgeons and Therapists. Chicago, August 1987.

Northwestern University Medical School Prosthetic and Orthotic Center. Spinal, Lower, and Upper Limb Orthotics for Physicians and Surgeons. Chicago, February 1989.

Oishi, C.S., Fronek, A., and Golbranson, F.L.: The role of non-invasive vascular studies in determining levels of amputation. J. Bone Joint Surg. [Am.] 70:1520 1988.

Pinzur, M.S., Smith, D.G., Daluga, D.J., and Osterman, H.: Selection of patients for through-the-knee amputation. J. Bone Joint Surg. [Am.] 70:746, 1988.

Sabolich, J.: Contoured adducted trochanteric-controlled alignment method (CAT-CAM): Introduction and basic principles. Clin. Prosthet. Orthot. 9:15–26, 1985.

Shaperman, J., and Sumida, C.T.: Recent advances in research in prosthetics for children. Clin. Orthop. 148:26–33, 1980.

Shiavi, R., Bugle, H.J., and Limbird, T.: Electromyographic gait assessment. J. Rehabil. Res. Dev. 24:13–30, 1987.

Sutherland, D.H.: Gait analysis in cerebral palsy. Dev. Med. Child Neurol. 20:807–813, 1978.

Sutherland, D.H., Olshen, R., Cooper, L., and Woo, S.L.: The development of mature gait. J. Bone Joint Surg. [Am.] 62:336–353, 1980.

Tubiana, R.: Krukenberg's operation. Orthop. Clin. North Am. 12:819–826, 1981.

Wang, G.J., Moskal, J.T., Albert, T., Pritts, C., Schuch, C.M., and Stamp, W.G.: The effect of Halo-vest length on stability of the cervical spine. A study of normal subjects. J. Bone Joint Surg. [Am.] 70:357, 1988.

Wyss, C.R., Harrington, R.M., Burgess, E.M., and Matsen, F.A., III: Transcutaneous oxygen tension as a predictor of success after an amputation. J. Bone Joint Surg. [Am.] 70:203, 1988.

CHAPTER 9

Trauma

Part **1**

Adult Trauma

I. Introduction—There are many ways to describe a fracture, and a thorough understanding of the basics is necessary before addressing specific fractures. Fractures can be classified based upon location (e.g., proximal, middle and distal thirds), direction (transverse, spiral, oblique, comminuted, segmental), alignment (angulation [apex], displacement [of distal fragment], articular involvement), and associated factors (open fractures, dislocations, etc.), and classified by a variety of schemes. Many factors come into play in the description and ultimate management of fractures. Although not detailed in Table 9–2 through 9–5 (end of Part 1), the mechanism of injury provides important clues to the nature of the injury and may even be used in the classification schemes for those injuries (e.g., ankle and spine fractures). For example, traction injuries result in avulsion fractures, compression forces yield angulated or "T"-type fractures, and rotational forces cause spiral fractures.

II. Open Fractures

   A. Introduction—Open fractures, whether obvious or subtle, always communicate with the environment. Therefore, special consideration should be given to these injuries. Infection and poor healing are frequently the consequences of open fractures (although less so with hand injuries because of an excellent blood supply). Formal radical débridement and irrigation (ideally within 4–8 hours of the injury), IV antibiotics (consisting of a first- or second-generation cephalosporin and an aminoglycoside [and penicillin for barnyard or *clostridium* infections]) for 48 hours and after each subsequent procedure, appropriate immobilization and fixation, and careful wound management will reduce these risks. Early flap coverage (48 hours to 1 week after injury) has also been shown to reduce risk of chronic infections.

   B. Classification—Based on the size of the wound and amount of soft tissue injury (Gustilo):

Type	Size	Other Factors
I	<1 cm	Low energy
II	<10 cm	Moderate energy
III	>10 cm	High energy; High-velocity gunshot wounds, close range shotgun wounds, barnyard injuries, segmental fractures, neurovascular injury, open >8 hours

Type III fractures are further classified as follows:

Subclass	Description
IIIA	Adequate soft tissue coverage
IIIB	Massive soft tissue destruction, bony exposure
IIIC	Fractures associated with repairable vascular injury

   C. Gunshot Wounds (GSWs)—Often result in open fractures. Soft tissue and bony destruction is based on the velocity of the missile (KE = ½ mv^2). Low-velocity GSW's (<2000 ft/sec—most handguns) cause less soft tissue destruction, and treatment usually consists of entry wound débridement. High-velocity GSWs (>2000 ft/sec—military rifles) can cause massive soft tissue destruction and require two-stage débridement of the entire missile tract. Partially jacketed (dum-dum), unjacketed, and hollow point bullets cause greater soft tissue destruction. Shotgun wounds, especially at short range, often result in type III wounds because of extensive soft tissue injury. The wadding has a high potential for contamination of wounds and must be searched for at the time of débridement. Intra-articular missiles should be removed because of the potential for lead intoxication. Nerve injuries associated with GSWs are often temporary (neurapraxia) and are caused by the blast effect of missiles traversing the tissue. Arterial injuries may present with decreased or absent pulses, an expanding hematoma, a thrill, or massive blood loss. Arteriograms should be used liberally if there is any question of an arterial injury.

III. General Treatment Principles

A. ATLS Guidelines—Treatment of orthopaedic injuries must follow adequate stabilization of the patient (life before limb). ATLS guidelines should be rigidly followed. An adequate airway should be secured before checking for pulses and bleeding. **Nasotracheal intubation** is recommended in **breathing patients with cervical spine injuries**; **oral endotracheal intubation** with in line traction is favored **for all nonbreathing patients**. A chest x-ray should be checked for mediastinal widening and pneumo- or hemothorax, and the C-spine must be evaluated prior to proceeding to the secondary survey. ATLS principles practiced at Trauma Centers have decreased preventable death from 14% to 3%. The Trauma Score (based on respiratory, cardiovascular, and neurological parameters) is predictive of injury severity and prognosis. The most common abdominal injuries include rupture of the spleen followed by liver injuries (10–20% mortality rate). Diagnostic peritoneal lavage is favored over CT for abdominal assessment. **False positive** results can be seen in patients with **pelvic fractures** and on **expanding retropertoneal hematoma**. Pericardial tamponade should be suspected with a narrow pulse pressure and an elevated diastolic blood pressure. IVP studies are indicated for gross hematuria only. Head injuries are the most common cause of early death with trauma (Glasgow Coma Scale score <8 being severe). Hemorrhage can occur from ruptured viscera and is also commonly seen with pelvic fractures. The orthopaedist plays a key role in these latter injuries with early application of external fixation to select pelvic fractures. Once stabilized, the patient should be carefully assessed for extremity injuries, which must be reduced and stabilized. Determining the mechanism of injury, careful physical exam, and obtaining appropriate radiographs should be done in every trauma patient.

B. Reduction—Generally, less than anatomic apposition is better than angulation in reduction of fractures. Joint surface involvement demands near-anatomic reduction. Age and function of the patient is important in considering the goals in reduction. Reduction can be closed (manipulation or traction) or open (usually combined with internal fixation). Manipulative reduction usually involves exaggeration of the mechanism of injury followed by reversal of these forces. Traction, often applied to the femur or cervical spine through weights and skeletal fixation, may be temporary or prolonged. Open reduction, either primarily or after failure of other methods, should restore the fracture to as near anatomic alignment as possible.

C. Immobilization—Used to prevent displacement or angulation, to decrease movement at the fracture site, or to relieve pain. Immobilization can be through casting, splinting, orthotics, traction, external fixation, or internal fixation. Internal fixation

is indicated when closed methods have failed, when experience dictates it to be necessary (e.g., Galeazzi fractures of the forearm), for displaced intra-articular fractures, with tumors, with associated vascular injuries, and in multiply injured patients for mobilization.

D. Preservation of Function—Rehabilitation during and after fracture treatment is essential for good results. Judicious use of physical and occupational therapy will often improve eventual fracture outcome. Lower extremity intra-articular fractures should be fixed anatomically and affected patients should be kept non–weight bearing with early range of motion for best results.

E. Fracture Healing (See Chapter 2, Basic Sciences)— Optimal conditions for fracture healing are an adequate vascular supply, minimal necrosis, anatomic reduction, immobilization, the presence of physiologic stress, and the absence of infection.

IV. Radiographs

A. Introduction—Standard AP and lateral radiographs, to include the joint above and below the fracture level, are the minimal requirement for most fractures. In addition, certain special radiographic views are helpful for many fractures. The use of special imaging studies (tomograms, CT, bone scans, etc.) are also very helpful in certain instances.

B. Special Views—The radiographs listed in Table 9–1 are helpful to ascertain fracture patterns in particular areas/injuries.

C. Additional Studies—Other studies are often helpful as well. Tomograms are useful in evaluating sternoclavicular injures, tibial plateau fractures and some carpal and tarsal fractures. CT scans are vital in evaluating complex spinal, pelvic, calcaneal, sternoclavicular, and other fractures. Arthrograms are still useful in evaluating intra-articular pathology. MRI is also becoming very helpful, particularly in diagnosing soft tissue injuries. Nuclear medicine studies are useful in finding stress fractures and subtle wrist injuries.

V. Complications

A. Introduction—Complications occur commonly following trauma, and can be a direct result of the injury (intrinsic) or can be associated with other organ systems (extrinsic). General complications are discussed in this section; specific complications unique to individual fractures/dislocations are listed in Tables 9–2 through 9–5 (following Part 1).

B. Bone Healing Abnormalities—Can include delayed union, nonunion, malunion, and avascular necrosis. These problems are more common with high-energy injuries and occur more frequently in bones with limited blood supply/healing potential.

1. Delayed Union/Nonunion—Although the distinction is not always clear, fractures that still allow free movement of the bone ends at 3–4 months after injury demonstrate delayed union, and if this persists (usually for more than 6 months) then a diagnosis of nonunion can be made. Too much or too little motion at the fracture site, excessive space between fracture fragments, inadequate fixation, infection, soft tissue

TABLE 9–1. SPECIAL RADIOGRAPHIC VIEWS FOR SPECIFIC INJURIES

Injury/Location	Eponym/Description	Technique
Hand and Wrist		
Hand injuries		AP, lat., & obl., digit: dental film
4th & 5th MC	Reverse obl.	Hand placed 45 degrees tilted
MC head	Brewerton	30 degrees pronated from full supination
Gamekeeper's		Stress view (with anesthesia)
Thumb	Robert	AP hypersupinated (dorsum on cassette)
1st MC-trapezium	Burnam	Robert with 15-degree cephalic tilt
Hamate hook/CT	CT view	Tangential through carpal tunnel
Dorsal carpal chip	Dorsal tangential	Tangential of dorsal carpus
Wrist—ulnar var.	Zero rotation	AP, shoulder and elbow at 90 degrees
Carpal instability	Motion	Cineradiography
Radial wrist	Pronation oblique	AP with 45 degrees' pronation
Ulnar wrist	Bura	Sup. obl.; AP with 35 degrees' supination
Scaphoid	Series	PA/lat./obl. fist, PA in ulnar deviation
Forearm and Elbow		
Forearm	Tuberosity	AP elbow with 20-degree tilt to olecranon
Radial head		45-degree lateral of elbow, magnification
Elbow		Check fat pad, ant. humeral line, radius-capitellum
Elbow contracture	AP/lateral	AP humerus, AP forearm
Shoulder		
Shoulder	Trauma	True AP (scapula—45 degrees obl.), scapular lat. (Y)
Shoulder	Axillary lateral	Through axilla with arm abducted
Tuberosities	AP ER/IR	AP with arm in full extension & internal rotation
Impingement	Caudal tilt	AP with 30-degree caudal tilt
Impingement	Supraspinatus outlet	Scapula lat. with 10-degree caudal tilt
Hill Sachs	Stryker Notch	Supine, hand on head, 10-degree cephalic tilt
Bankart	West Point	Prone axillary lat. with 25-degree lat. & post. tilt
Bankart	Garth	Apical obl. with 45-degree caudal & AP tilt
AC injury	Stress	AP both AC (large cassette) with 10 pounds **hanging** weight
AC injury	Alexander	Scapular lat. with shoulders forward
AC arthritis	Zanca	10-degree cephalic tilt of AC
SC injury	Hobbs	PA, patient leans over cassette
SC injury	Serendipity	40-degree cephalic tilt center on manubrium
Clavicle		AP 30-degree cephalic tilt
Spine		
C-spine	Series	AP/lat./obls., open-mouth odontoid
C7	Swimmers view	Lat. through maximally abducted arm
Instability	Flex/Ext	AP with flexion & extension
L-spine	Series	AP, lat., obliques (foramina), L5/S1 spot lat.
Pelvis and Hip		
Pelvic injury	Inlet	45–50 degrees caudad (assess AP displacement)
Pelvic injury	Outlet	45 degrees cephalad (assess SI superior displacement)
Pelvic injury-Judet	Iliac obl.	Oblique on ilium (**post. column, ant. acetabulum**)
Pelvic injury-Judet	Obturator obl.	Oblique on obturator (**ant. column, post. acetabulum**)
Pelvic injury	Push-pull	Outlet view with stress (assess stability)
SI injury		Judet views centered on SI joints
Hip	Surgical lat.	Lat. from opposite side with that hip flexed
Femoral neck		AP with 15 degrees' internal rotation
Knee		
Knee AP & lat.		AP with 5 degrees' flexion, lat. with 30 degrees' flexion
Osteochondroid Fx	Notch	Prone 45 degrees from vertical
Knee DJD	Rosenberg	Weight-bearing PA with 45 degrees' flexion
Patella	Merchant	45 degrees' flexion, cassette perpendicular to tibia
Tibial plateau		AP with 10-degree caudal tilt
Foot and Ankle		
Ankle	Mortise	AP with 15 degrees' internal rotation
Ankle	Stress	AP with lat. stress, lat. with drawer
Foot	Weight bearing	AP & lat. weight bearing
Midfoot		Include obliques
Talus	Canale	AP with 75-degree cephalic tilt, pronate 15 degrees
Talar Neck		AP with 15 degrees' pronation
Subtalar	Broden	45-degree rotation lat. with varying tilts
Calcaneus	Harris	AP standing, 45-degree tilt
Sesamoid		Tangentials with dorsiflexed toes

interposition, inadequate blood supply, and many other factors can lead to delay in bone healing. Nonunions are classified as hypervascular (hypertrophic) or avascular (atrophic) based upon their capability of biologic reaction (vitality of the bone ends) and are classified as follows (Weber & Cech) (Fig. 9–1):

Nonunion	Type	Common Cause
Elephant foot	Hypervascular	Insecure fixation
Horse hoof	Hypervascular	Unstable fixation—plate & screws
Oligotrophic	Hypervascular	Displacement/distraction
Torsion wedge	Avascular	Intermediate fragment heals only on one side
Comminuted	Avascular	Necrotic intermediate fragment
Defect	Avascular	Sequestrum
Atrophic	Avascular	Intervening scar tissue

Delayed and nonunions are more common in the tibia, ulna, proximal scaphoid, fifth metatarsal metaphysis, talus, and other areas with limited soft tissue cover or blood supply. Treatment includes allowing more motion, surgical excision of intervening tissue, more secure internal fixation, electrical stimulation, bone grafting, injection of marrow or other materials with osteogenic potential, and prosthetic replacement. Three types of electrical stimulation are available:

Type	Application
Direct current	Electrode placed at fracture site, subcutaneous battery
Inductive coupling	External coil with external power source required
Capacitive coupling	External coil with portable battery source required

Contraindications to electrical stimulation include inadequate fixation, poor alignment, pseudarthrosis, and nonviability of mesenchymal cells. Many methods of bone grafting have been described. The **Phemister** technique involves bone grafts placed in a healing granulation bed. Tibia fractures can be grafted posterolaterally to avoid the actual fracture site. Bone grafting done at the time of fixation for highly comminuted fractures and forearm fractures with comminution involving more than 1/3 of the diameter of the bone may help to avoid future problems with delayed bone healing.

2. Malunion—Union in a clinically significant imperfect position. Initial fracture care is critical to help avoid this result, but it often cannot be avoided. Treatment, if necessary, is directed at correcting the anatomic abnormality. Malunion may cause shortening (with overlap), or shortening may result from bone loss or growth plate injuries (see Part 2: Pediatric Trauma). Shortening is rarely a problem in the upper extremity.

3. Avascular Necrosis—Caused by disruption of the blood supply and can lead to nonunion, osteoarthritis, collapse, and other problems. It is more common with intra-articular fractures, especially of the femoral head/neck, femoral condyles, proximal scaphoid, proximal humerus, and talar neck. It is often recognized some time after injury when relative osteodensity in the affected area is noted in comparison to disuse osteopenia of normal bone. Excision of the avascular fragment, arthroplasty, or arthrodesis is required in advanced cases. Osteonecrosis, which is the general term for all conditions causing bone death, is discussed in greater detail in Chapter 2, Basic Sciences.

C. Infection—Usually is a complication of open fractures and can lead to osteomyelitis (often chronic). Involvement of joints leads to persistent pain, stiffness, and progressive concentric joint space narrowing. Soft tissue infections may produce soft tissue air on radiographs from gangrene (*Clostridium*—a gram-positive anaerobe) and gas-producing gram-negative organisms. The most critical factor in avoiding infection in open injuries is adequate débridement. Prophylactic antibiotics for grade III open fractures should include a first-generation cephalosporin, penicillin, *and* an aminoglycoside. Tetanus (caused by *Clostridium tetani*) can lead to devastating systemic complications and requires early treatment with boosters and toxoid for susceptible injuries. Recommended treatment includes 0.5 mg tetanus toxoid for patients with current immunizations and the addition of 250 units of tetanus immune globulin (in the opposite arm) for patients with unknown immunization history or whose immunizations have lapsed. Fight bites often are not appreciated early because of inaccurate patient histories, and can cause significant infections with organisms such as *Eikenella corrodens* (an anaerobic gram-negative rod). Dog and cat bites are often infected with *Pasteurella multocida* (a gram-negative coccobacillus). Toxic shock syndrome, caused by gram-positive bacteria superinfection, can occur in an otherwise benign-appearing wound following internal fixation. Necrotizing fasciitis can cause severe, life-threatening infections following streptococci contamination of wounds. Osteomyelitis, other infections, and appropriate antibiotic coverage are discussed in Chapter 2, Basic Sciences.

D. Soft Tissue Injuries—Include direct injuries to vessels, nerves, and soft tissues as well as indirect compromise of these tissues.

1. Arterial Injury—Injuries to major arteries with fractures and dislocations are rare, but the consequences can be severe. A high index of suspicion is required, particularly with shoulder dislocations, supracondylar elbow fractures, and severe knee injuries/dislocations. Immediate diagnosis (with arteriograms if necessary) and repair (within 6 hours of injury) are essential. Although controversial, fracture fixation usually is helpful to protect vascular repairs. Fasciotomy, discussed below, is also necessary in most cases.

2. Compartment Syndrome—Increased pressure within enclosed soft tissue compartments of the

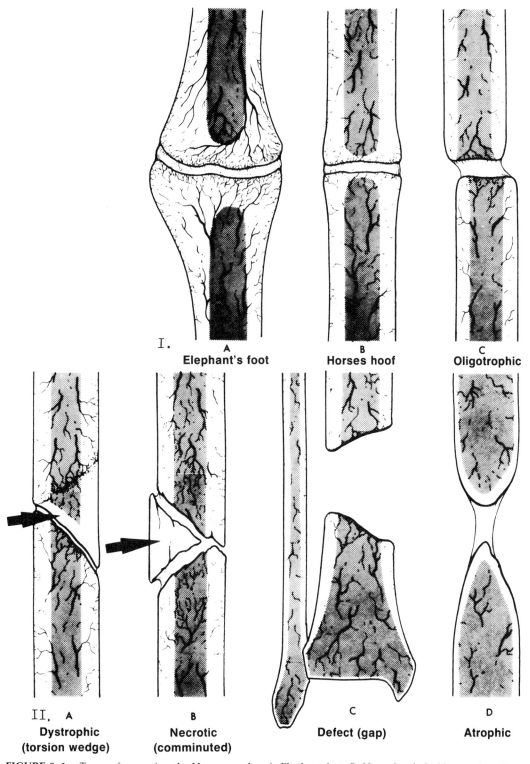

FIGURE 9–1. Types of nonunion. I—Hypervascular: *A*, Elephant foot; *B*, Horse hoof; *C*, Oligotrophic. II—Avascular: *A*, Torsion wedge; *B*, Comminuted; *C*, Defect; *D*, Atrophic. (From Weber, B.G., and Brunner, C.: The treatment of nonunions without electrical stimulation. Clin. Orthop. 161:25, 1981; reprinted by permission.)

extremities can lead to serious sequelae. Elevated compartment pressures commonly follow significant injuries to the forearm and leg and should be diagnosed early with careful patient monitoring. Risk is also increased with prolonged use of pneumatic antishock garments. **Pain** (especially with passive flexion of the digits) is the **earliest** and **most reliable** indicator, but pallor, paralysis, paresthesia, and pulselessness are also indicative of elevated pressures. Compartment pressures should be measured with a Whitesides or indwelling catheter device for any suspected compartment syndrome and for patients who are unable to adequately feel pain (paralysis, intoxication, etc.). Compartment pressures >40 mm Hg or within 10–30 mm Hg of the diastolic blood pressure are highly suggestive of the diagnosis. Fasciotomy within 4 hours of onset will usually prevent muscle necrosis (Fig. 9–2). Concomitant muscle débridement is necessary for any ischemic muscle (lacking normal color, consistency, contraction, and capacity to bleed). Irreversible nerve injury may follow in <12 hours. Thallium scans are useful for chronic exercise-induced compartment syndrome.

3. Nerve Injuries—Acute nerve injury is also relatively uncommon, but is more often associated with fractures than arterial injuries. Most injuries are neurapraxias from stretch and 70% will resolve in a few weeks. Common nervous system injuries with trauma include the spinal cord and cauda equina (spine fractures), axillary nerve (shoulder fractures and dislocations), radial nerve (humerus fractures), ulnar nerve (medial epicondyle fracture), posterior interosseous nerve (radial head and monteggia fractures), sciatic nerve (hip dislocation and acetabular fractures), and common peroneal nerve (lateral knee injuries). Nerve injury and repair are discussed in Chapter 2, Basic Sciences, and Chapter 5, Hand.

E. Pulmonary Complications
1. Adult Respiratory Distress Syndrome (ARDS)—Pulmonary edema and decreased function commonly follow severe trauma. ARDS can be a result of direct (aspiration, inhalation, etc.), or indirect (sepsis, shock, etc.) insults. It is exacerbated by prolonged hypovolemia and decreased left ventricular function. ARDS is characterized by increased intrapulmonary shunting and decreased pulmonary compliance and functional reserve capacity. ABG measurements are best for diagnosing ARDS and following therapy (ventilation with PEEP). Hypoxic changes in the hypothalamus and/or cellular humeral mediators (including complement factors) may initiate the process.
2. Fat Emboli Syndrome (FES)—A form of ARDS that follows major long bone fractures (0.5–2% of patients with multiple fractures). FES may be a result of systemic release of bone marrow fat and/or changes in chylomicron stability and conversion to free fatty acids in the lung parenchyma. It classically presents 24–72 hours after injury with tachycardia, hyperthermia, tachypnea, and hypoxia. Mental status changes, oli-

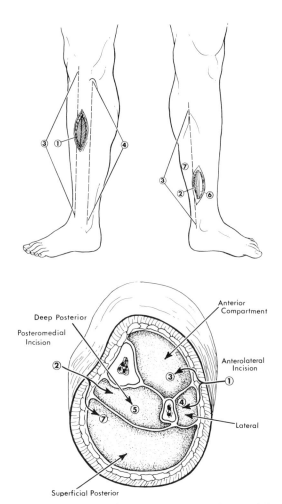

FIGURE 9–2. Fasciotomy for compartment syndrome of the leg. Note anterolateral and posteromedial incisions. (From Connolly, J.F., ed.: Depalma's The Management of Fractures and Dislocations, an Atlas, 3rd ed., p. 68. Philadelphia, W.B. Saunders 1981; reprinted by permission.)

guria, and upper torso/conjunctival petechiae are also commonly seen. Early treatment is based on stabilization of long bone fractures (within 24 hours) and pulmonary support. Steroids have been shown to have a prophylactic role only.
3. Pulmonary Embolism—Thromboembolic disease is the most common complication following surgery on the extremities. This subject is covered in detail in Chapter 2, Basic Sciences. The use of intermittent pneumatic compression is useful in trauma patients.

F. Bleeding Disorders—Excessive bleeding from injuries can cause hypovolemic shock and disseminated intravascular coagulation (DIC). Shock is a manifestation of decreased blood flow to the tissues and may present with tachycardia, oliguria, and pale, cool extremities. Treatment includes immediate whole blood, IV fluids, and sometimes dextran solutions. Albumin should be avoided. DIC is caused by microvascular thrombi that consume platelets and initiate a vicious cycle. Diagnosis involves recognition of symptoms in the appropriate setting and laboratory values showing decreased antithrombin III and fibrinogen and increased values of PT/PTT and fibrin split products. Treatment should be directed at the underlying cause, and judicious use should be made of heparin, platelets, and DDAVP. DIC or excessive anticoagulation can lead to excessive bleeding into soft tissues. Deep muscle hematomas can compress neurovascular structures (e.g., **iliacus hematoma can compress the femoral nerve**). Conservative treatment of these hematomas is usually best. Thrombotic thrombocytopenic purpura can occur in a trauma setting and is treated with IV steroids.

G. GI Complications—Can be a result of the trauma itself (the **spleen** is the **most commonly injured** organ with blunt trauma, followed by the liver), or can be a late complication. Stress ulcers are common in the ICU setting and are usually treated with appropriate antacids and H_2 blockers. **Cast syndrome** is a common orthopaedic complication and is a result of **compression of the second portion of the duodenum** by the superior mesenteric artery. It may present with postoperative small bowel obstruction with projectile vomiting. Cast syndrome can occur after placing spine fractures in plaster or children in hip spica casts. Diagnosis is usually made by an UGI series. Treatment includes removing the constrictive device and decompression (nasogotic tube).

H. Reflex Sympathetic Dystrophy (RSD)—Can follow trauma or surgery for local systemic disease and is characterized by pain, swelling, discoloration, and stiffness of the affected extremity. It is a result of vasomotor dysfunction of the sympathetic nervous system. A "vicious cycle" of pain, immobility, edema, tissue reaction, and vasospasm is influenced by noxious stimuli, abnormal sympathetic reflexes, and "personality diathesis." Three stages are defined (Lankford):

STAGE	DESCRIPTION	FEATURES
1	Acute	Pain, dusky/mottled smooth skin
2	Dystrophic	Max. pain, stiff, nail changes, edema
3	Atrophic	Atrophy, contractures, demineralization (Sudeck's atrophy)

A triple-phase bone scan showing uptake in the third phase and relief with a sympathetic block is diagnostic of this disorder. Treatment includes PT (early), NSAIDs, psychological aids, and sympathetic blockade (interrupts cycle). Sympathetic blockade is obtained with long-acting anesthetic injection of the sympathetic ganglia (UE) or epidural injection (LE). Prognosis is guarded.

I. Late Complications—Can be systemic or involve local soft tissue, bones, and joints. **Myositis ossificans** can follow injuries with large hematomas. It is common after elbow fractures and dislocations and soft tissue trauma in the thigh. Histologically, the peripheral areas are more mature than the center ("zoning phenomenon"). Conservative therapy is best, but late excision (6–9 months after the injury) of symptomatic areas is sometimes required. **Posttraumatic osteoarthritis** commonly follows intraarticular fractures that are not anatomically re-

duced. Treatment is similar to other forms of osteoarthritis discussed in Chapter 3, Adult Reconstruction and Sports Medicine. **Immobilization hypercalcemia** is an unusual disorder characterized by nausea, vomiting, abdominal pain, acute personality changes, and other symptoms. It occurs most commonly in children and patients with Paget's disease.

VI. Pathologic Fractures

A. Introduction—Pathologic fractures occur through abnormal bone. These fractures can be spontaneous or follow minor trauma. Most of these fractures involve the elderly (**osteoporosis is the most common cause**), but should be suspected in any patient when minimal trauma causes a major fracture. Repeated fractures, a history of prior malignancies, increased pain, and patients with metabolic disorders are more likely to have pathologic fractures. Work-up should include a careful history and physical exam, radiographs (often including bone scan), laboratory studies (including Ca, Phos., alk. and acid phos., total protein, ESR, BUN, and appropriate hormonal and other special studies), and a biopsy if malignancy is suspected. The different categories of pathologic fractures are discussed below.

B. Systemic Skeletal Disease—Can be correctable (renal osteodystrophy, hyperparathyroidism, osteomalacia, and disuse osteoporosis) or uncorrectable (osteogenesis imperfecta, polyostotic fibrous dysplasia, postmenopausal osteoporosis, Paget's, and osteopetrosis). Goals in treating this group are to correct abnormalities amenable to correction, and attempt to reduce risks for other groups of patients.

C. Benign Local Lesion—Generally should be removed after fracture healing if it caused a pathologic fracture (except in the hand). Intralesional excision is best for disorders such as nonossifying fibroma, bone cysts, enchondromas, and chondromyxoid fibromas. Wide excision is favored for giant cell tumors, osteoblastomas, and chondroblastomas.

D. Malignant Primary Bone Disease—Complete work-up and staging are required before starting treatment. Radiation therapy is appropriate for Ewing's, myeloma, and non-Hodgkin's lymphoma of bone. Wide surgical excision is needed to treat most sarcomas and malignant fibrous histiocytoma.

E. Metastatic Disease—The second most common cause of pathologic fractures. The most common primary tumors involved are breast, lung, thyroid, prostate, and kidney. The goal is to achieve pain-free ambulation. Internal fixation (± use of PMMA) is often required. Increased bleeding is common with renal cell, thyroid, and breast carcinomas. Patients with renal cell and follicular thyroid metastases may do well with resection of the lesions. Impending fractures with increased pain, more than 50% cortical destruction, lesions >2.5 cm, and lesions in areas of increased stress should be internally fixed prophylactically.

F. Stress Fractures—Stress fractures are the result of repetitive loading below the yield strength and are most common in the lower extremity (metatarsals > calcaneus > tibia). Stress fractures are common in elderly women (insufficiency fractures), athletes, and military recruits (fatigue fractures). They are also common with steroid use (decreases trabecular bone in the axial skeleton) and may be related to an underlying metabolic bone disease. A fracture callus is not seen until 3 weeks after the initial insult, but bone scans are positive early. Treatment is usually conservative.

G. Miscellaneous—Irradiated bone (>5000 centi-Greys) will not heal and fractures require internal fixation.

VII. Soft Tissue Trauma

A. Introduction—Many of the important concepts have been discussed elsewhere, but other injuries are discussed in this section.

B. Snake Bites—Can cause extensive soft tissue destruction and may lead to compartment syndrome. Venomous snakes are most commonly pit vipers (Crotalids—rattlesnakes, copperheads, etc.). These snakes have a triangular head and a pit below their eyes. Elapids (e.g., the coral snake) are less common, but their venom includes hemo-, cyto-, and neurotoxins. Systemic symptoms (nausea and vomiting, neurologic dysfunction, bleeding) can be severe. Local symptoms with snake bites include swelling, ecchymosis, and bullous formation. Treatment includes first aid (tourniquet, suction) and hospitalization. Monitoring, use of antibiotics, checking compartment pressures, and administration of antivenin are appropriate. At least five bottles of antivenin are required for moderate-sized bites, and this treatment can cause serum sickness (sometimes requiring systemic steroids to combat). Fasciotomies are sometimes needed for compartment syndrome.

C. Thermal Injuries—Include the following.

1. Freezing Injuries—The most common cause of bilateral upper and lower extremity amputations. Injury is direct (freezing of tissues with ice crystals in the extracellular space) and indirect (vascular damage). Treatment is based on restoring core body temperature, rapid rewarming of the extremity, débridement, PT, and sometimes anticoagulation and sympathectomy. Psychologic factors often are hard to overcome.

2. Heat Injuries—Burns require close management. Treatment is based on burn depth:

Degree	Depth	Findings	Treatment
1st	Epidermis	Edema, erythema	Symptomatic
2nd	Dermis	Blisters, blanching	Topical antibiotics, splint, ROM
3rd	Subcutaneous	Waxy, dry	Excision, split-thickness skin graft
4th	Deep	Exposed tissues	Amputation/ flap/ reconstruction

Burns can also result in compartment syndrome and sometimes require escharotomy/fasci-

otomy. Contractures are common and often require Z-plasties or releases. Infection is also common.

3. Electrical Injuries—Include ignition (burns at sites of direct contact), conductant (tunnels along neurovascular structures; the number one cause of bilateral high upper extremity amputations), and arc (high-voltage current jumps across flexor surfaces of joints, leading to late contractures). AC current is more dangerous than DC. Current density zones resulting from electrical burns are as follows:

Zone	Tissue Characteristics
Charred	Unrecognizable tissue
Gray-white	Tissue necrosis
Red	Thrombosis

Treatment involves initial débridement, fasciotomy (when indicated), second-look débridement at 2–3 days, and finally definitive flap coverage or amputation.

4. Chemical Burns—Follow exposure to noxious agents. Severity is based on concentration, duration of contact, penetrability, amount, and mechanism of action. The mainstay of treatment is copious irrigation. Hydrofluoric acid burns can be successfully treated with calcium gluconate. White phosphorus burns are treated with a 1% copper sulfate solution.

5. Chemotherapeutic Extravasation—Early débridement and secondary coverage is important to reduce the high risk of soft tissue and skin necrosis.

D. High-Pressure Injection Injuries—Occur from accidental injections by paint or grease guns. They usually involve the hand. Paint gun injuries are more common and are more severe because they lead to soft tissue necrosis (grease gun injuries cause fibrosis). A seemingly innocuous entry wound may cover an area of extensive soft tissue destruction. Treatment includes IV antibiotics, thorough I&D, and occasionally steroids.

VIII. Principles of Internal Fixation

A. Basic Principles—AO/ASIF technique should be practiced as taught in AO basic and advanced courses. The following fixation devices are commonly used (Figs. 9–3 and 9–4):

Device	Function	Use
Compression plate	Increases the stiffness of bone-implant unit; tension band	Obl. diaphyseal fractures
Dynamic compression	Compression plate with mechanical adv.	Obl. diaphyseal fractures
Neutralization plate	Artificial cortex; prevents rotation	Obl. diaphyseal fractures
Tension device	Tension band wiring	Patella, olecranon
Buttress plate	Supports/shores up intact side	Metaphysis
Strut plate	Maintains alignment/length	Bone loss
Intramedullary	Mechanical stability, soft tissue conserved	Femur/tibia
External fixation	Avoids internal hardware	Infection (III B open)

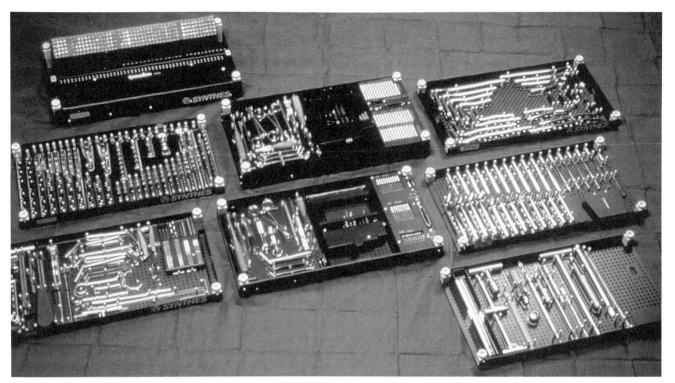

9/III

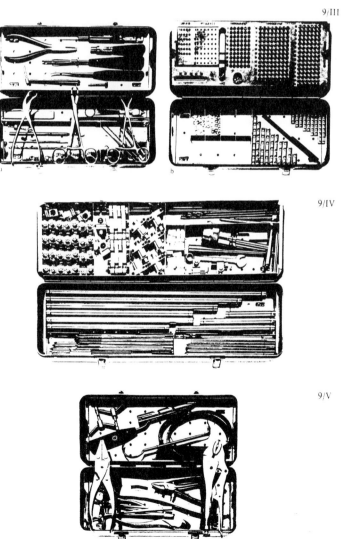

9/IV

9/V

FIGURE 9–3.   AO/ASIF instrumentation. (Courtesy of Synthes, Ltd. [USA].)

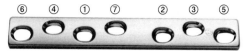

FIGURE 9–4. AO/ASIF dynamic compression plate. (Courtesy of Synthes, Ltd. [USA].)

With all devices, preoperative planning is critical, especially with complex fracture patterns.

  B. Plates and Screws

    1. Lag Screws—Allow compression of the fracture surface by overdrilling the proximal cortex or by using partially threaded screws and "drawing up" the distal cortex. Often used in conjunction with compression plating and forms the basis for AO technique. Screws are placed in a "compromise" of the best position to counteract shear forces (i.e., perpendicular to the applied load) and the optimum position for compression (i.e., perpendicular to the fracture).

    2. Compression Plates—Used on the **tension side** of transverse or short oblique fractures. They provide stability (especially vs. shear forces) and act as a **load-sharing device**. The Dynamic compression plate (DCP) is designed for self-compression by the use of offset drill guides and contoured plate holes. The sequence of screw placement is as follows (see Fig. 9–4):

      1—Neutral (green) guide used to attach plate
      2—Offset (gold) guide used to compress fracture
      3—Offset (gold) guide used to further compress fracture after screw 2 loosened
      4–6—Screws placed with neutral guide
      7—Interfragmentary screw in different plane

    A total of **six or more cortices** on each side of the fracture is required in fixation of **forearm fractures** and **at least eight cortices** are required for fixation of **lower extremity and humerus fractures**. Plates are left in place indefinitely but can be removed for contact sport participation, metal allergies, and with prominent hardware, and occasionally in patients with psychological maladaptation to hardware, usually about 1 year after insertion. Extremities must be protected after plate removal.

    3. Reconstruction Plates (Fig. 9–5)—Are more pliable and allow positioning for use as a neutralization plate not only in the pelvis, but also in distal humerus fractures and other locations.

  C. Tension Band Wiring (Fig. 9–6)—Commonly used in fixation of olecranon, patella, and sometimes ankle fractures. This method allows fixation on the tension side and relies on motion to allow union on the compression side. Parallel K-wires are placed closer to the outer cortex than the articular surface to take advantage of this design, and wire

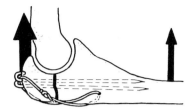

FIGURE 9–6. Tension band wiring. (From Sequin, F., and Texhammer, R.: AO/ASIF Instrumentation, p. 161. New York, Springer-Verlag, 1981; reprinted by permission.)

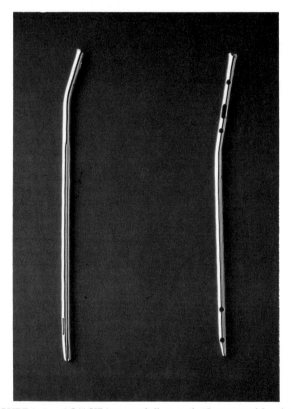

FIGURE 9–7. AO/ASIF intramedullary nail. (Courtesy of Synthes, Ltd. [USA].)

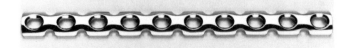

FIGURE 9–5. AO/ASIF reconstruction plate. (Courtesy of Synthes, Ltd. [USA].)

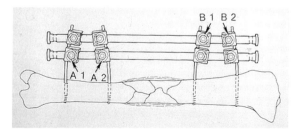

FIGURE 9–8. External fixation of an open comminuted tibial fracture. (Drawing courtesy of Synthes, Ltd. [USA].)

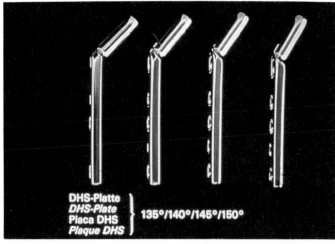

FIGURE 9–9. Side plate component of the dynamic hip screw for stabilization of intertrochanteric hip fractures. (Courtesy of Synthes, Ltd. [USA].)

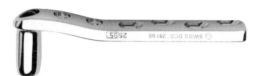

FIGURE 9–10. AO/ASIF dynamic condylar screw sideplate. (Courtesy of Synthes, Ltd. [USA].)

is placed under the K-wires, usually in figure of 8 fashion, before it is tightened.

    D. Intramedullary Fixation (Fig. 9–7)—Allows superior fixation for fractures in the diaphyses of weight bearing bones. Advantages include proper axial alignment, early weight bearing (load-sharing device), and that it can be placed in a "closed" fashion (at least it does not open the fracture site). Disadvantages include the fact that the canal diameter can limit the size of nail used, there is less rotational control (improved with interlocking nails), there is disruption of the endosteal blood supply, and it is sometimes technically difficult. Neverthe-

less, it is a popular and successful method for fixation of lower extremity diaphyseal fractures. LE intramedullary devices should be removed at 12–24 months.

    E. External Fixation (Fig. 9–8)—Useful for management of grade III open fractures with high risk of infection. Allows access to these wounds while stabilizing fractures. Other uses include stabilization of anterior disruptions of the pelvis, management of comminuted distal radius fractures, and spacing with segmental bone loss. A thorough understanding of local anatomy, injury characteristics, and mechanical demands is essential prior to placement.

    F. Special Devices—Are numerous, but include the following.

        1. Sliding Hip Screw (Fig. 9–9)—A load-sharing device that allows fixation of intertrochanteric hip fractures with screw insertion that can be placed at variable angles.

        2. Sliding Condylar Screw (Fig. 9–10)—Best used for distal femur fractures 4–9 cm proximal to the

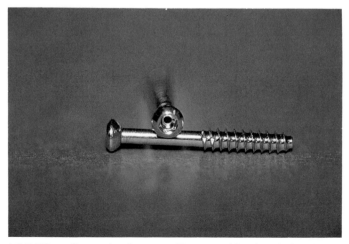

FIGURE 9–11. AO/ASIF small cannulated screws. (Courtesy of Synthes, Ltd. [USA].)

joint. Similar to the sliding hip screw, this device can achieve good compression of fracture fragments. It can also be used proximally for some unstable subtrochanteric fractures.
3. Cannulated Screws (Fig. 9–11)—Excellent for femoral neck fractures and becoming popular for fixation of a variety of fractures. Placement of small K-wires prior to insertion of large screws provides an alternative with less risk of iatrogenic neurovascular injuries.

TABLE 9–2. ADULT TRAUMATIC ORTHOPAEDIC INJURIES—UPPER EXTREMITY

INJURY	EPONYM	CLASSIFICATION	TREATMENT	COMPLICATIONS
Hand—Fractures				
Distal phalangeal Fx		Longitudinal, comminuted, transverse	Splint DIP 3–4 weeks; evacuate hematoma and repair nail bed with fine absorbable suture	Nail bed injury
EDL avulsion (Fig. 9–12)	Mallet finger	Ext. tendon stretch Ext. tendon torn Bony mallet	Volar/stack splint 6 wks + 4 wks nights Bony—splint; ORIF volar subluxation	Deformity, nail bed injury (with ORIF), subluxation
FDP avulsion (Fig. 9–13)	Jersey finger	Leddy: I—tendon to palm II—tendon to PIP	Repair within 7–10 days Repair within 3 mos	Can lead to lumbrical plus finger (late) Missed diagnosis (therapy or fuse DIP late)
		III—tendon to A4 pulley (Smith) IV—bony fragment DP base	Keep A4 pulley intact with repair Early fixation of bony fragments and tendon	
Proximal & middle phalanxes		Extra-articular stable Extra-articular unstable	Buddy tape Reduce and immobilize (PCP or ORIF if irreducible Ex fix comminuted fxs)	Decreased ROM, contractures, malunion/malrotation (may require osteotomy), lateral deviation, volar angulation (osteotomy), nonunion, tendon adherence
		Intra-articular undispaced	Buddy tape, early ROM, close on follow-up	
		Intra-articular condylar	Reduce & PCP, ORIF and restore articular surface if >2 mm displacement	
		Intra-articular PP Base	Small/nondisplaced—Buddy tape Large/displaced—ORIF	
	Boutonnière	Intra-articular MP base (D)	Splint PIP (extension) 6 wks, ORIF if large bony fragment	
		Intra-articular comminuted	Traction, Ex fix	
MC		Head	ORIF large piece, early motion comminuted fractures	Soft tissue injury, malunion (rotation); prominent MC head in palm (affects grip); loss of reduction (no volar buttress); nonunion, contractures of intrinsics
	Boxer's	Neck—4th and 5th	20–40° angulation OK, reduce/splint	
		—2nd and 3rd	Usu. requires PCP pin to adjacent MC or ORIF	
		Shaft—Transverse	Closed reduction, immobilize or PCP; Accept 50–70° angulation IV & V 20° angulation II & III, ORIF if irreducable	
		—Oblique	ORIF if >5 mm shortening or rotated—X K-wire, AO screws	
		—Comminuted	Nondisplaced splint, displaced PCP to adjacent MC or ORIF	
		Base of 5th MC	Most stable; if not, pin to adjacent MC	
1MC (Fig. 9–14) Base	Bennett's	I—Intra-articular volar lip	Attempt closed reduction and PCP MC to trapezium; ORIF if irreducable	Displaced by APL
	Rolando's	II—Intra-articular "Y" (volar & dorsal)	Large frags ORIF comminuted–Ex Fix or early motion;	DJD
		III—Extra-articular (transverse or oblique)	closed reduction spica 4 wks	
5MC	"Baby Bennett"	Base	PCP or ORIF	Displaced by ECU

(continued)

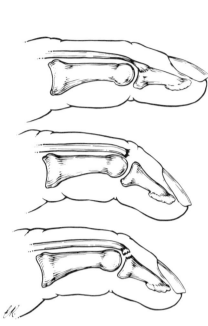

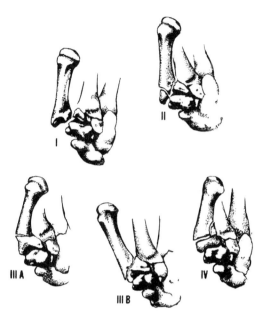

FIGURE 9–14. Classification of first metacarpal base fractures. *I,* Bennett's fracture. *II,* Rolando's fracture. *IIIA,* Transverse extra-articular fracture. *IIIB,* Oblique extra-articular fracture. *IV,* SH II epiphyseal fracture (pediatric). (From Green, D.P., and O'Brien, E.T.: Fractures of the thumb metacarpal. South. Med. J. 65:807, 1972; reprinted by permission.)

FIGURE 9–12. Mallet finger. *Top to bottom,* Extensor tendon stretch, extensor tendon rupture, bony avulsion. (From Green, D.P., and Rowland, S.A.: Fractures and dislocations in the hand. In Fractures in Adults, Rockwood, C.A., and Green, D.P., eds., 2nd ed., p. 319. Philadelphia, J.B. Lippincott, 1984; reprinted by permission.)

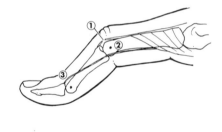

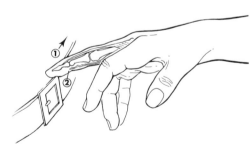

FIGURE 9–13. Avulsion of the flexor digitorum profundus. (From Connolly, J.F., ed.: Depalma's The Management of Fractures and Dislocations, an Atlas, 3rd ed., p. 1149. Philadelphia, W.B. Saunders, 1981; reprinted by permission.)

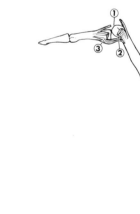

FIGURE 9–15. Boutonnière deformity, injury to central slip with volar subluxation of lateral bonds. (From Connolly, J.F., ed.: Depalma's The Management of Fractures and Dislocations, an Atlas, 3rd ed., p. 1149. Philadelphia, W.B. Saunders, 1981; reprinted by permission.)

INJURY	EPONYM	CLASSIFICATION	TREATMENT	COMPLICATIONS
Hand—Dislocations				
DIP		* Dorsal	Closed reduction, immobilize 2 weeks, late Dx or irreducable—open reduction.	
		Collateral ligament injury	Sprain—buddy tape 3–6 wks Tear—repair RCL IF, RF, MF; UCL SF (of dominant hand)	
PIP		* Dorsal (volar plate [VP] disruption):		
		I—hyperextension; VP avulsion	Buddy tape or ext. block splint	Stiffness, contractures (Rx with VP arthroplasty)
		II—dislocation major ligamentous injury	Extension block splint	
		III—proximal dislocation (middle phalanx MP Fx)	If >4 mm displacement reduce; ORIF if required	
	Boutonnière (Fig. 9–15)	Volar (central slip)	Closed reduction, splint (full extension 4–6 weeks) if congruous	Late recognition: ORIF or VP arthroplasty
		Rotatory	ORIF if irreducable or incongruous	
		Dorsal Fx-dislocation	Extension block splint if congruous, ORIF or VP arthroplasty if incongruous	
MCP		Collateral ligament injury	Splint in 50° MCP flexion 3 wks Open if >2–3 mm displacement of fragments or 20% of joint	Late recognition—injection, splinting, operate late
		* Dorsal (Fig. 9–16)—Simple	Closed reduction, 7–10 d immobilization	Failure to recognize complex dislocation
		—Complex	Soft tissue volar plate interposition (pucker, sesamoid in joint & parallelism of MC & PP on radiographs) requires open reduction volar approach	Stiffness, contractures, neurovascular injury (open)
		Volar	Rare; requires open reduction	
CMC			Closed reduction, PCP; open reduction—4CMC dislocations and open dislocations	
1MCP (Fig. 9–17)	Gamekeeper's thumb	* UCL injury	Sprain—Won't open >35–45° with stress thumb spica cast; rupture—open repair (interposition of adductor aponeurosis—Stener)	Unrecognized Stener lesion, chronic pain, instability
		RCL injury	Nonoperative: splint or PCP	
		Dorsal—Simple	Reduce and immobilize 3 wks	
		—Complex	Open after 1 attempt closed (VP ± FPL interposed)	
1CMC Dislocation (Fig. 9–18)			Hyperpronation and PCP, immobilize 6–10 weeks	
Hamatometocarpal Fx-dislocation		Cain: IA Ligamentous injury	Reduce—If stable cast; if unstable PCP	Delay in [Dx] (pronation oblique films required)
		*IB Dorsal hamate Fx	Reduce—If stable cast; if unstable ORIF	
		II Comminuted dorsal hamate Fx	ORIF, restore dorsal buttress	
		III Coronal hamate Fx	ORIF, restore congruent joint surface	
Wrist—Fractures				
Radius	Colles' (dorsal displacement)	Frykman (I–VIII; even # = ulna fx; I extra-articular, III R-C, V R-U, VII R-C & R-U) (Fig. 9–19) Melone: 4 parts (shaft, radial styloid, dorsomedial, palmar medial): I—min. displacement, II—carpus displacement, III—volar spike, IV—volar fragment rotated (Fig. 9–20)	Distract, manipulate, splint 15° palmar flexion & ulnar deviation, external fixation, &/or ORIF if comminuted/unstable; external fixation for severe comminution, ORIF large fragments with >15° DF, >1–2 mm articular displacement; bone graft comminuted fractures	Loss of reduction, nonunion, malunion, median N neuropathy, weakness, tendon adhesion, instability, EPL rupture (occurs 5–8 wks after injury), DISI (>15°DF), ulnar side pain (shortening), RSD, Volkman's ischemic contracture

246

TABLE 9–2. ADULT TRAUMATIC ORTHOPAEDIC INJURIES—UPPER EXTREMITY *(Continued)*

INJURY	EPONYM	CLASSIFICATION	TREATMENT	COMPLICATIONS
Wrist Fractures ***cont.***				
	Smith's (volar displacement)	Thomas (not used) Intra- vs. extra-articular	Distract, manipulate, splint supination, flexion; PCP often required	Missed Dx, and as for Colles' Fx
Dorsal rim	Dorsal Barton's (Fig. 9–21)		Reduce, pronation, ORIF if needed	Similar to Colles' Fx
Radial styloid (Fig. 9–22)	Chauffeur's		Reduce, PCP, immobilize in ulnar deviation	Similar to Colles' Fx, associated perilunate injury (ORIF)
Volar rim	Volar Barton's (Fig. 9–23)		Reduce, supination, PCP or ORIF common (volar buttress plate)	Similar to Colles' Fx
Distal R-U		Based on ulna displacement	Dorsal—reduce, full supination LAC 6 wks Volar—reduce (may require open reduction) LAC pronation	Osteochondral fracture, TFCC injury, ulnar nerve compression, instability
Scaphoid* (Fig. 9–24)		Based on anatomic location	Thumb spica, LAC; ORIF displacement & nonunion	Nonunion (tomographic/CT evaluation, Russe bone graft), instability, refracture, nerve injury, RSD, DJD, pain, missed Fx (bone scan helpful)
Dorsal chip		* Triquetrum	SAC 6 weeks	
Perilunate dislocation (± scaphoid Fx)		Mayfield (Fig. 9–25): I—scapholunate disassociation II—lunocapitate disruption III—lunotriquetral disruption IV—lunate dislocation	Early (6–8 wks)—open (dorsally), ligament repair and ORIF scaphoid Fx (if present) Late—triscaphe fusion, proximal row carpectomy or wrist fusion	Rotatory instability of scaphoid, median N palsy, late flexor rupture
Rotatory lunate disassociation	Terry Thomas sign	>3-mm gap on AP vs. opposite side	Closed—reduction, immobilization, ORIF if scaphoid Fx displaced; open—repair of ligaments (volar & dorsal)	Late DJD
Lunate	Kienböck's	(Osteonecrosis—Late)	Ulnar lengthening/radial shortening/resection	Disorganization, disintegration
Carpal instability		* DISI (dorsal scapholunate angle >70°) (Fig. 9–26) VISI (volar scapholunate angle <35°)	Attempt closed reduction of acute injuries; open ST reconstruction for failed reduction or late	
Hook of hamate		Based on size of fragment	Excise small fragment for chronic pain	Missed on plain films (CT view required)
Radial/ulnar Shafts Fractures/Dislocations				
R & U	Both bone	Undisplaced Displaced	LAC neutral ORIF 6 hole DCP; external fixation for type III open Fx, bone graft if >1/3 (shaft) communition	Mal/nonunion, vascular injury, PIN injury, compartment syndrome, synostosis, infection, refracture (after plate removal)
Ulna	Nightstick	Undisplaced Displaced (>10° ang, >50° disp)	LAC, ORIF if displaces ORIF—look for wrist/elbow injury	
Proximal ulna & radial head	Monteggia (Fig. 9–27)	Bado: *I—radial head ant. II—radial head post. III—radial head lat. IV—radial head ant. (& both bone Fx)	 ORIF (DCP), closed reduction head, cast 110° flexion ORIF (DCP), closed reduction head, cast 70° flexion ORIF (DCP), closed reduction head, cast 110° flexion ORIF (R + U), closed reduction head, cast 110° flexion	PIN injury (usu. spontaneously resolves), redislocation/subluxation (inadequate reduction)
Proximal radius		Undisplaced Displaced	LAC supination, close follow-up Prox 1/5 closed, 1/5–2/3 ORIF	

(continued)

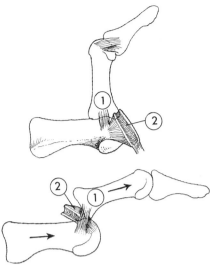

FIGURE 9–16. Thumb MCP dislocation. *Top,* Simple. *Bottom,* Complex; note interposition of volar plate. (From Connolly, J.F., ed.: Depalma's The Management of Fractures and Dislocations, an Atlas, 3rd ed., p. 1152. Philadelphia, W.B. Saunders, 1981; reprinted by permission.)

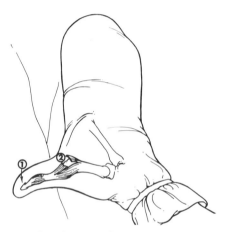

FIGURE 9–17. Gamekeeper's thumb (UCL injury). (From Connolly, J.F., ed.: Depalma's The Management of Fractures and Dislocations, an Atlas, 3rd ed., p. 1151. Philadelphia, W.B. Saunders, 1981; reprinted by permission.)

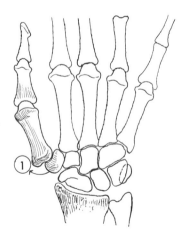

FIGURE 9–18. Subluxation/dislocation of the thumb carpometacarpal joint. (From Connolly, J.F., ed.: Depalma's The Management of Fractures and Dislocations, an Atlas, 3rd ed., p. 1165. Philadelphia, W.B. Saunders, 1981; reprinted by permission.)

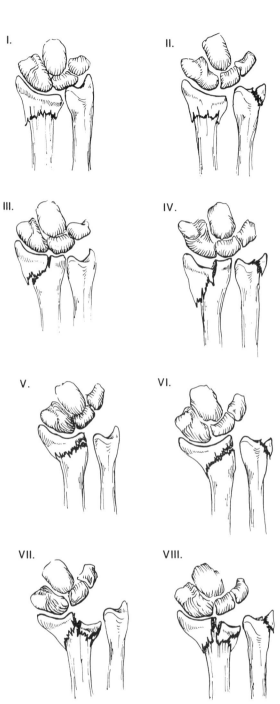

FIGURE 9–19. Frykman classification of distal radius fractures. Note even numbers with ulnar styloid involvement. (From Kozin, S.H., and Berlet, A.C.: Handbook of Common Orthopaedic Fractures, pp. 17, 19. West Chester, PA, Medical Surveillance Inc., 1989; reprinted by permission.)

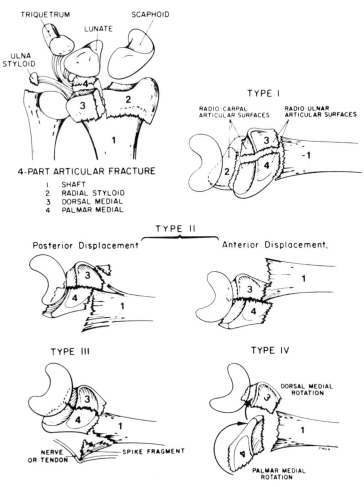

FIGURE 9–20. Melone classification of distal radius fractures. (From Melone, C.P., Jr.: Open treatment for displaced articular fractures of the distal radius. Clin. Orthop. 202:104, 1986; reprinted by permission.)

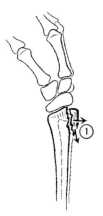

FIGURE 9–21. Dorsal Barton's fracture. (From Connolly, J.F., ed.: Depalma's The Management of Fractures and Dislocations, an Atlas, 3rd ed., p. 1032. Philadelphia, W.B. Saunders, 1981; reprinted by permission.)

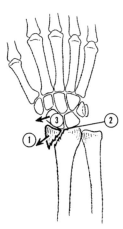

FIGURE 9–22. Radial styloid fractures. (From Connolly, J.F., ed.: Depalma's The Management of Fractures and Dislocations, an Atlas, 3rd ed., p. 1033. Philadelphia, W.B. Saunders, 1981; reprinted by permission.)

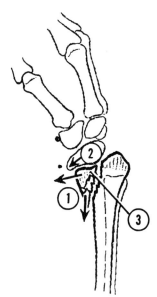

FIGURE 9–23. Volar Barton's fracture. (From Connolly, J.F., ed.: Depalma's The Management of Fractures and Dislocations, an Atlas, 3rd ed., p. 1028. Philadelphia, W.B. Saunders, 1981; reprinted by permission.)

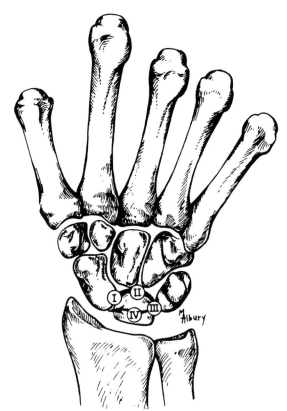

FIGURE 9–25. Perilunar instability—stages. *I*, Scapholunate. *II*, Capitolunate. *III*, Triquetrolunate. *IV*, Dorsal radiocarpal (leading to lunate dislocation). (From Mayfield, J.K.: Mechanism of carpal injuries. Clin. Orthop. 149:50, 1980; reprinted by permission.)

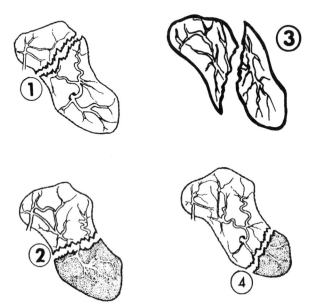

FIGURE 9–24. Classification of scaphoid fractures. *1*, Neck. *2*, Waist. *3*, Body. *4*, Proximal pole. Note progressive risk of avascular necrosis with proximal transverse fractures. (From Wiessman, B.N., and Sledge, C.B.: Orthopedic Radiology, p. 1060. Philadelphia, W.B. Saunders, 1986; reprinted by permission.)

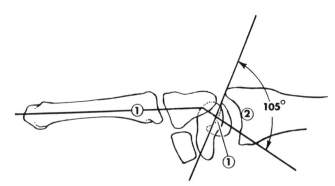

FIGURE 9–26. Dorsal intercalary segmental instability (DISI). Note scapholunate angle >70 degrees, consistent with a DISI pattern. (From Connolly, J.F., ed.: Depalma's The Management of Fractures and Dislocations, an Atlas, 3rd ed., p. 1085. Philadelphia, W.B. Saunders, 1981; reprinted by permission.)

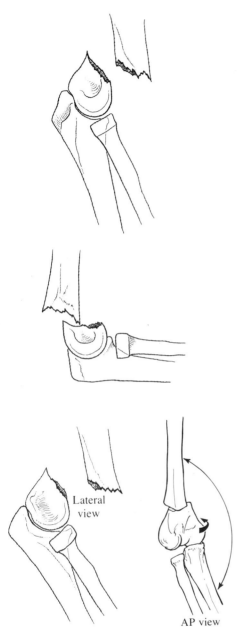

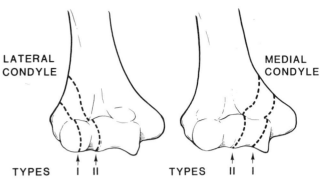

FIGURE 9–32. Humeral condyle fractures. (From Gelman, M.I.: Radiology of Orthopedic Procedures, Problems and Complications, Vol. 24, p. 56. Philadelphia, W.B. Saunders, 1984; reprinted by permission.)

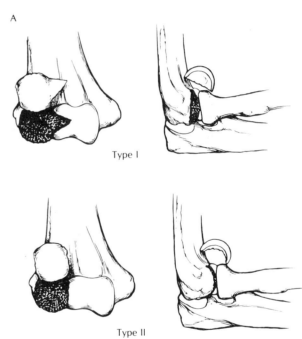

A

Type I

Type II

FIGURE 9–30. Supracondylar humerus fractures. *Top*, Extension. *Middle*, Flexion. *Bottom*, Note rotational component. (From Connolly, J.F., ed.: Depalma's The Management of Fractures and Dislocations, an Atlas, 3rd ed., p. 743. Philadelphia, W.B. Saunders, 1981; reprinted by permission.)

FIGURE 9–33. Capitellar fractures. Note presence of subchondral bone in type I fracture. (From DeLee, J.C., Green, D.P., and Wilkins, K.E.: Fractures and dislocations of the elbow. In Fractures in Adults, Rockwood, C.A., and Green, D.P., eds., 2nd ed., p. 591. Philadelphia, J.B. Lippincott, 1984; reprinted by permission.)

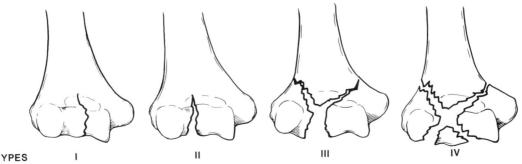

TYPES   I   II   III   IV

FIGURE 9–31. Intercondylar humerus fractures. (From Gelman, M.I.: Radiology of Orthopedic Procedures, Problems and Complications, Vol. 24, p. 55. Philadelphia, W.B. Saunders, 1984; reprinted by permission.)

INJURY	EPONYM	CLASSIFICATION	TREATMENT	COMPLICATIONS
Fractures of the Shaft of the Humerus				
Humerus shaft		Based on location/Fx pattern	Coaptation or cast brace, ORIF segmental, pathologic elbow injury, distal spiral with nerve injury (Holstein-Lewis) or with forearm Fxs (floating elbow)	Malunion (20° ant. and 30° V/V shortening and 3 cm short OK); radial N injury (5–10% incidence; observe unless follows reduction or open Fx, or persists 3–4 mos); nonunion (>4 mos ORIF); vascular injury
Shoulder Fractures				
Proximal humerus (Fig. 9–35)		Neer (parts >1 cm or 45° displacement):		Missed dislocation, adhesive capsulitis (moist heat, gentle ROM), malunion (reconstruction or TSA required), AVN (TSA required), nonunion (surgical neck, tuberosity Fxs: ORIF), disrupted rotator cuff
		*1-part	Early motion; isometrics → progressive resistance.	
		2-part	Closed reduction unless articular segment (ORIF), shaft (impacted & angulated— traction, Velpau; unimpacted— closed reduction, PCP or ORIF), greater tuberosity (rep. cuff) tuberosity with block to med. rotation (ORIF)	
		3-part	ORIF younger, prosthesis in older	
		4-part	Prosthesis, nonoperative in elderly/diabetes	
Proximal humerus	Fx-Dislocation	Ant. (greater tuberosity displacement)	If >1 cm after reduction, open repair	As above plus axillary N or plexus injury, myositis ossificans, (wait >1 yr to excise heterotopic bone)
		Post. (lesser tuberosity displacement)	Closed reduction, ORIF if 3-part	
Impression	Hill-Sach	Stable (<20% articular surface)	Closed treatment	AVN, DJD (TSA)
		Unstable (20–50%)	Transfer lesser tuberosity → defect (McLaughlin)	
		Unstable (>45%)	Prosthesis	
Head splitting			Prosthesis	
Clavicle		*Middle ⅓	Shoulder spica, sling	Vascular injury/ pneumothorax/other injury; malunion (osteotomize young active patient); nonunion (ORIF & bone graft), nerve injury (rare); muscle fatigue/weakness, DJD (if articular)
		Distal ⅓ (Neer):		
		I—min. displacement interligamentous (CC-AC)		
		II—Fx medial to CC ligaments:		
		IIA—both ligaments attached to distal fragment	ORIF	
		IIB—conoid torn, trapezoid attached to distal fragment (Fig. 9–36)	ORIF	
		III—AC joint	Closed treatment, late Mumford if required	
		Proximal ⅓	Closed treatment	
Scapula		Zdravkovic and Damholt:		Associated injuries (clavicle, rib, pneumo), axillary artery injury, plexus palsy, pressure symptoms, vascular & plexus injuries
		I—body	Most treated conservatively	
		II—coracoid & acromion	Assoc. injury common (clavicle rib, pneumo), ORIF large displaced fragments	
		III—neck & glenoid	ORIF large unstable fractures (glenoid with displaced clavicle Fx)	
Glenoid		Ideberg:		
		I—Ant avulsion Fx	>25° of surface—ORIF	
		II—Transverse/oblique Fx- inf glenoid free	Closed treatment if head is centered in glenoid—ORIF if head is subluxed with major fragment	
		III—Upper 1/3 glenoid + coracoid		
		IV—Horizontal glenoid through body		
		V—combination of II–IV		
Scapulothoracic dissociation		(Seen on scapular lateral or chest radiograph)	Closed reduction	Vascular and plexus injuries Associated clavicular fracture

TABLE 9–2. ADULT TRAUMATIC ORTHOPAEDIC INJURIES—UPPER EXTREMITY (*Continued*)

INJURY	EPONYM	CLASSIFICATION	TREATMENT	COMPLICATIONS
Shoulder Dislocations & Ligamentous Injuries				
*Ant. Dislocation (Fig. 9–37)		Subcoracoid > subglenoid (subclavicular and intrathoracic)	Reduce, immobilize (young patient 4 wks, old patient 2 wks) Passive → active rehab (Rockwood 7)	Axillary N neurapraxia, axillary A injury, cuff injury (>40 yo), recurrence (85% in <20 yo), bone injury (head, greater tuberosity, glenoid)
Ant. Subluxation		Atraumatic	Conservative (vol-psych; nonoperative)	Dead arm syndrome (nerve impingement w/ subluxation), recurrent subluxation
		Traumatic	Rehab—Rockwood 7	
Recurrent	Ant. dislocation/ subluxation		Rockwood 7 6–12 mos; if fails, consider surgery:	

Repair	Technique	Complications
Bankart	Ant. capsule → ant. rim	Late instability
Staple capsulorrhaphy	Capsule → glenoid	Late DJD, migration
Putti-Platt	Subscapularis embrication	Late DJD, decr. ER
Magnuson-Stack	Subscapularis → lesser tuberosity	Late DJD, decr. ER
Bone block	Crest graft ant.	Dec ROM, migration
Bristow	Coracoid transfer	Nonunion, decr. ER, migration
Capsular shift	Redundant capsule advanced	Min., procedure of choice with MDI

INJURY	EPONYM	CLASSIFICATION	TREATMENT	COMPLICATIONS
Post. Dislocation (Fig. 9–38)		*Subacromial (seizures & shocks)	Reduce, immobilize 4 wks; operate if recurrent (glenoid osteotomy, bone block, post. capsule shift)	Lesser tuberosity fracture Late recognition (may require advancement of lesser tuberosity into defect or TSA (place in less retroversion)
Inf. glenohumeral	Luxatio erecta (Fig. 9–39)		Reduce and immobilize	Neurovascular injury resolves after reduction; axillary A thrombosis
AC injury (Fig. 9–40)		I—AC sprain	7–10 days rest/immobilization	Joint stiffness, deformity, CC ligament and soft tissue calcification, AC DJD, associated fxs, distal clavicle osteolysis
		II—AC tear, CC sprain	Sling 2 wks, rehab, late Mumford if required	
		III—AC & CC tear	Conservative vs. ORIF (athletes, laborers)	
		IV—clavicle thru trapezius posteriorly	Closed reduction, treat like III	
		V—clavicle 100–300% elevated	ORIF	
		VI—clavicle inferior to caracoid	Closed reduction, treat like III	
SC injury (Fig. 9–41)		Anterior dislocation	Closed reduction with traction	Bump (cosmetic), DJD, mediastinal impingement, hardware migration (with operative treatment)
		Posterior dislocation	Closed reduction towel clip or open	
		Spontaneous atramatic subluxation	Nonoperative	

* Most common.

Abbreviations: PCP, percutaneous pin fixation; RCL, radial collateral ligament; LCL, lateral collateral ligament; UCL, ulnar collateral ligament; VP, volar plate; SAC, short arm cast; LAC, long arm cast; MC, metacarpal; PP, proximal phalanx; MP, middle phalanx; DP, distal phalanx; MCP, metacarpal phalangeal joint; PIP, proximal interphalangeal joint; DIP, distal interphalangeal joint; IF, index finger; RF, ring finger; MF, middle finger; SF, small finger. Fx, fractive; ORIF, open reduction and lateral fixation; ROM, range of motion; EDL, extensor digitorum longus; FDP, flexor digitorum profundus; ECU, extensor carpi ulnaris; APL, adductor pollicis longus; PIN, posterior interosseous nerve; AVN, avascular necrosis; DJD, degenerative joint disease; TSA, total shoulder arthroplasty.

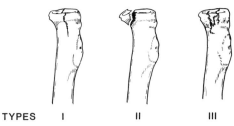

FIGURE 9–34. Classification of radial head fractures. (From Gelman, M.I.: Radiology of Orthopedic Procedures, Problems and Complications, Vol. 24, p. 59. Philadelphia, W.B. Saunders, 1984; reprinted by permission.)

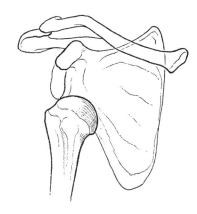

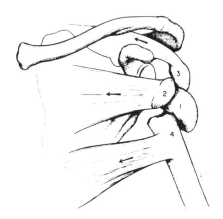

FIGURE 9–35. Proximal humeral fracture. Four parts: *1*, head; *2*, lesser tuberosity; *3*, greater tuberosity; *4*, humeral shaft. (From Neer, C.S., and Rockwood, C.A.: Fractures and dislocations of the shoulder. In Fractures in Adults, Rockwood, C.A., and Green, D.P., eds., 2nd ed., p. 696. Philadelphia, J.B. Lippincott, 1984; reprinted by permission.)

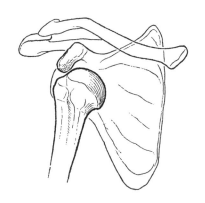

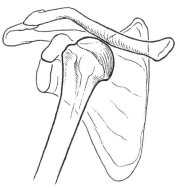

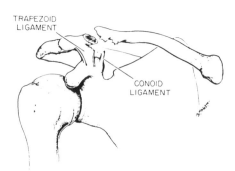

FIGURE 9–36. Neer type IIB fracture of the distal clavicle. (From Neer, C.S., II: Fracture of the distal clavicle with detachment of the coracoclavicular ligaments in adults. J. Trauma 3:101, 1963; reprinted by permission. Copyright © 1968 by Williams & Wilkins.)

FIGURE 9–37. Anterior shoulder dislocation. *Top*, Subglenoid. *Middle*, Subcoracoid. *Bottom*, Subclavicular. (From Connolly, J.F., ed.: Depalma's The Management of Fractures and Dislocations, an Atlas, 3rd ed., p. 617. Philadelphia, W.B. Saunders, 1981; reprinted by permission.)

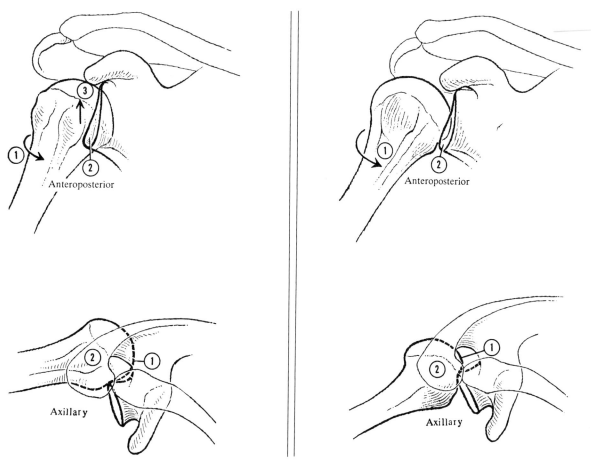

FIGURE 9–38. Posterior shoulder dislocation. *Left*, Subacromial. *Right*, Subcoracoid. (From Connolly, J.F., ed.: Depalma's The Management of Fractures and Dislocations, an Atlas, 3rd ed., p. 633. Philadelphia, W.B. Saunders, 1981; reprinted by permission.)

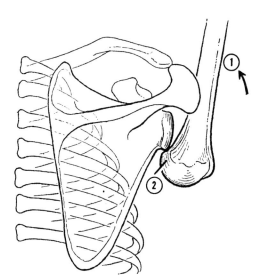

FIGURE 9–39. Luxatio erecta. (From Connolly, J.F., ed.: Depalma's The Management of Fractures and Dislocations, an Atlas, 3rd ed., p. 622. Philadelphia, W.B. Saunders, 1981; reprinted by permission.)

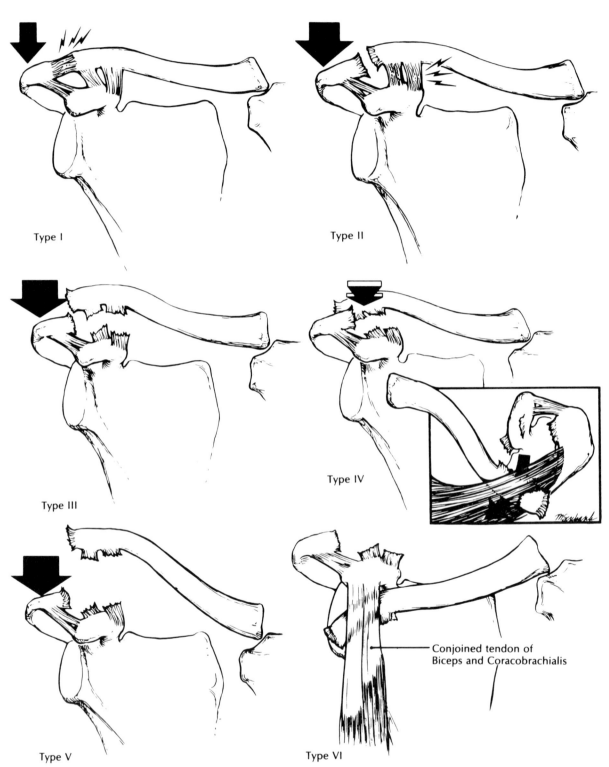

FIGURE 9–40. Classification of acromioclavicular injuries. (From Neer, C.S., and Rockwood, C.A.: Fractures and dislocations of the shoulder. In Fractures in Adults, Rockwood, C.A., and Green, D.P., eds., 2nd ed., p. 871. Philadelphia, J.B. Lippincott, 1984; reprinted by permission.)

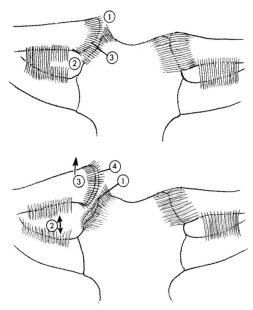

FIGURE 9–41. Sternoclavicular dislocations. *Top*, Partial injury. *Bottom*, Complete sternoclavicular dislocation. (From Connolly, J.F., ed.: Depalma's The Management of Fractures and Dislocations, an Atlas, 3rd ed., p. 560. Philadelphia, W.B. Saunders, 1981; reprinted by permission.)

TABLE 9–3. ADULT TRAUMATIC ORTHOPAEDIC INJURIES—CERVICAL SPINE

INJURY	EPONYM	MOI	CLASSIFICATION	TREATMENT	NEURO INJURY	COMPLICATIONS/OTHER
Occiput–C1 Dislocation		Distraction or translation	Anterior or posterior	Halo + Occiput–C2 fusion	Usually fatal!	Overdistration (avoid traction)
C1 Fx		Axial; + extension	Posterior	Usu. stable—orthosis (50% w/ other C-spine injuries)	Rare	Vertebral A injury (unilateral = Wallenberg's; Rx w/ heparin), CN VIII injury; diastasis of lat. masses (may require fusion late)
	Jefferson (Fg. 9–42)	Axial + flexion Axial load	Anterior Poster & anterior	Halo Halo traction, C1–C2 fusion for mal/nonunion or instabiity (>7-mm splaying)		
			Lateral mass compression Fx	Orthosis		
C1–C2 subluxation		Transverse ligament rupture	Increased atalanto-dens interval	C1–C2 fusion		
C1–C2 dislocation (Fig. 9–43)	"Cock robin"		Ant. ± Fx Post. ± Fx	Reduction (traction)—orthosis Usu. requires post. fusion (recurrence)	Ant. common	AP x-ray—"wink" sign (overlap fo C1–C2 lat. masses)
			Rotatory	Requires traction → halo or fusion (C₁C₂)		
C2 Fx odontoid (Fig. 9–44)		Flexion, extension, rotation	Anderson & D'Alonzo: I—upper tip II—at junction of odontoid & C2 body III—thru C2 body	Orthosis PSF C1–C2 if >5 mm, post. displacement, imperfect reduction Halo × 12 wks	Rare	Nonunion
C2 isthmus Fx	Hangman's (Fig. 9–45)	Hyperextension + axial	Spondylolisthesis (odontoid, ant. body, superior facet)	Halo vest reduction and immobilization; operative traction rarely; ant.—C2–C3 fusion; post.—C1–C2 fusion	Uncommon	Follow for loss of reduction, often assoc. w/ other lower C-spine injuries
C3–C7 facet dislocation	"Jumped facet (Fig. 9–46)	Flexion-distraction/rotation	Unilateral (<25% body) Bilateral (25–50% body)	Traction—sequential weight addition (10 lb. + 5 lb./level; open reduction post. fusion if fails or unstable	Common (incr. risk w/ greater displacements)	Neuro injury at offset, disc herniation with traction → paralysis if unreducable MRI before open reduction
C3–C7 Fx			Translation Angular displacement	>3.5 mm vs. other levels → fusion >11° vs. other levels → fusion		
C3–C7 compression (Fig. 9–47)	Burst/crush		Canal compression (post. elements)	Stable—halo; unstable or neuro injury—ant. strut w/ postop orthosis; post. elements—ant. + post. fusion; AS—laminectomy (only indication)	Common	Post-traumatic kyphosis
C3–C7 spinous processes	Clay shoveler's		Spinous process avulsion	Symptomatic		

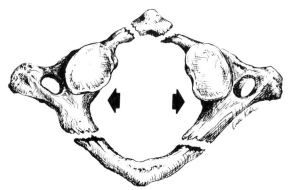

FIGURE 9–42. Jefferson fracture. (From Urbaniak, J.R.: Fractures of the spine. In Davis-Christopher Textbook of Surgery, Sabiston, D.C., Jr., ed., p. 1528. Philadelphia, W.B. Saunders, 1977; reprinted by permission.)

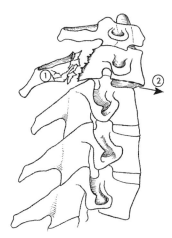

FIGURE 9–45. Hangman's fracture. (From Connolly, J.F., ed.: Depalma's The Management of Fractures and Dislocations, an Atlas, 3rd ed., p. 312. Philadelphia, W.B. Saunders, 1981; reprinted by permission.)

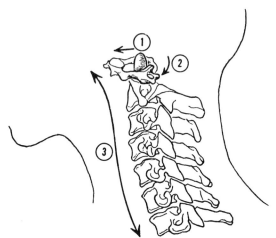

FIGURE 9–43. Rotatory subluxation of C1–C2. (From Connolly, J.F., ed.: Depalma's The Management of Fractures and Dislocations, an Atlas, 3rd ed., p. 287. Philadelphia, W.B. Saunders, 1981; reprinted by permission.)

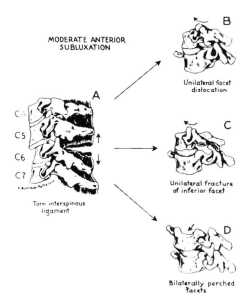

FIGURE 9–46. Jumped facet. Note 25% displacement with unilateral dislocation and 50% displacement with bilateral dislocation. (From Bohlman, H.H.: Fractures and dislocations of the cervical spine. J. Bone Joint Surg. [Am.] 61:1136, 1979; reprinted by permission.)

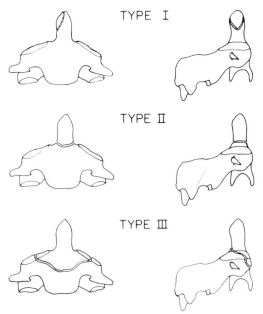

FIGURE 9–44. Odontoid fracture classification. (From Anderson, L.D., and D'Alonzono, R.T.: Fractures of the odontoid process of the axis. J. Bone Joint Surg. [Am.] 56:1664, 1974; reprinted by permission.)

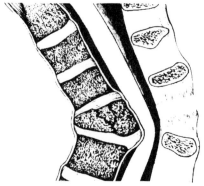

FIGURE 9–47. Crush fracture. (From Bohlman, H.H.: Fractures and dislocations of the cervical spine. J. Bone Joint Surg. [Am.] 61:1131, 1979; reprinted by permission.)

TABLE 9–4. ADULT TRAUMATIC ORTHOPAEDIC INJURIES—THORACIC AND LUMBAR SPINE
(Ferguson-Allen)

INJURY	EPONYM	COMMON FORCES			CLASSIFICATION	TREATMENT[a]	NEURO INJURIES	COMPLICATIONS/OTHER
		Ant.	Mid.	Post.				
Compression-flexion	Wedge	C+	D	D	Stage I—<50% decrease ant. height	Bed rest acute, orthosis	Rare	Progression (rare for type I but incr. for type III > II if not stabilized)
(flexion-distraction)	(Fig. 9–48)	C+	D+	D	Stage II—SP separated ± facet Fx/dislocation	Posterior fusion (compression)	Occasional	
	Blowout	C+	D+	D+	Stage III—canal impingement (superior vertebral body)	Posterior fusion (compression) ± decompression for neuro injury	More common	
Flexion-distraction	Chance (seat belt) (Fig. 9–49)	D+	D+	D	Bony Ligamentous Bony & ligamentous	Bed rest/orthosis (hyper ext) Posterior fusion (compression) Posterior fusion (compression)	Occasional (based on trans)	
Lateral flexion		C+	C+	C±	Ipsilateral compression ± contralateral facet Fx-dislocation	Based on middle & post. column disruption (fuse concave—distraction convex—compression)	Occasional (ipsilateral)	
Translational	Shear (Fig. 9–50)	T+	T+	T+	Based on position of displacement (ant., post., lat.)	If >25%, segmental instrumentation (Luque rods)	Very common	
Flexion-rotation	Slice (Fig. 9–51)	DC+	D±	DT+	Facet Fx-dislocation, superior vertebral body → ant.	Most unstable! Segmental fixation favored	Very common	Usu. in lower T-spine
Vertical compression	Burst (Fig. 9–52)	C+	C+	C±	Based on canal compromise (CT)	Post. ± ant. decompression/ fusion if increased canal compression (>50% or neuro injury), otherwise extended bed rest, then orthosis	Occasional	Progression? Dural tear, herniated roots (w/ lamina Fx)
Extension-distraction	Teardrop (Fig. 9–53)	D+		C+	Often spontaneously reduces	Nonoperative	Rare	

[a] C, compression; D, distraction; T, translation; R, rotation; +, likely disrupted; ±, may or may not be disrupted.
[b] As a general rule the axiom "rod long and fuse short" applies. Conventional Harrington rods are usually removed at 1 yr postop. Newer instrumentation (pedicle screws/plates) may allow instrumentation of fewer levels and do not require later removal. Tomograms are helpful in the evaluation of posterior element fractures.

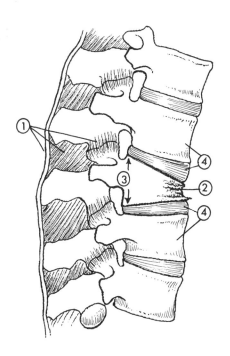

FIGURE 9–48. Wedge fracture. (From Connolly, J.F., ed.: Depalma's The Management of Fractures and Dislocations, an Atlas, 3rd ed., p. 407. Philadelphia, W.B. Saunders, 1981; reprinted by permission.)

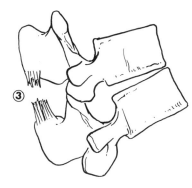

FIGURE 9–49. Chance fracture (ligamentous). (From Connolly, J.F., ed.: Depalma's The Management of Fractures and Dislocations, an Atlas, 3rd ed., p. 413. Philadelphia, W.B. Saunders, 1981; reprinted by permission.)

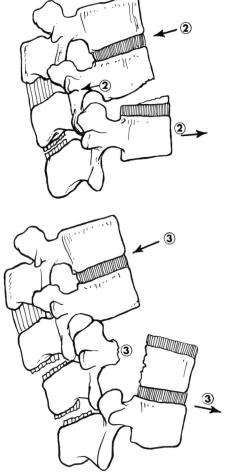

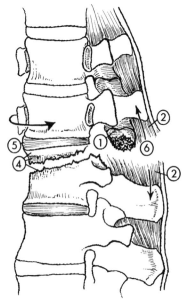

FIGURE 9–50. Shear fracture. *Top*, Stable. *Bottom*, Unstable. (From Connolly, J.F., ed.: Depalma's The Management of Fractures and Dislocations, an Atlas, 3rd ed., p. 412. Philadelphia, W.B. Saunders, 1981; reprinted by permission.)

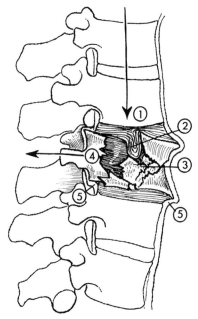

FIGURE 9–52. Burst fracture. Note retropulsion of bony fragments into spinal canal. (From Connolly, J.F., ed.: Depalma's The Management of Fractures and Dislocations, an Atlas, 3rd ed., p. 409. Philadelphia, W.B. Saunders, 1981; reprinted by permission.)

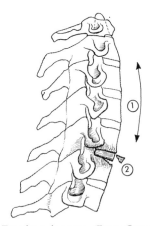

FIGURE 9–53. Teardrop fracture. (From Connolly, J.F., ed.: Depalma's The Management of Fractures and Dislocations, an Atlas, 3rd ed., p. 363. Philadelphia, W.B. Saunders, 1981; reprinted by permission.)

FIGURE 9–51. Slice fracture. (From Connolly, J.F., ed.: Depalma's The Management of Fractures and Dislocations, an Atlas, 3rd ed., p. 410. Philadelphia, W.B. Saunders, 1981; reprinted by permission.)

TABLE 9–5. ADULT TRAUMATIC ORTHOPAEDIC INJURIES—LOWER EXTREMITY

INJURY	EPONYM	CLASSIFICATION	TREATMENT	COMPLICATIONS
Pelvic Fractures				
Pelvis (Fig. 9–54)		Young:		Life-threatening hemorrhage, GI injury, GU injury (bladder, urethra, impotency), neuro injury, nonunion, DJD, pain, loss of reduction, sepsis, thrombophlebitis, malunion (leg length discrepancy, sitting problems), heterotopic bone, vascular injuries (incl. aortic rupture). APC III highest rate of associated injury.
		Lateral compression (LC):		
		*I—I/L or C/L ramii & I/L sacral compression	Bed rest	
		II—I/L or C/L ramii & I/L post. iliac	Bed rest or delayed ORIF	
		III—I/L or C/L ramii & LC I/II & C/L APC	Based on C/L injury	
		Anteroposterior compression (APC):		
		I—symphysis (<2 cm) or ramii & ant. SI ligament stretched	Bed rest	
		II—symphysis or ramii & ant. SI ligament torn	Acute external fixation/ant. ORIF if concurrent laparotomy	
		III—symphysis or ramii & ant. & post. SI ligament torn	Acute external fixation/ant. ORIF if concurrent laparotomy, post. SI ORIF	
	Malgaigne	*Vertical shear* (VS): ant. & post. vertical displacement	Acute external fixation/ant. ORIF if concurrent laparotomy, post. SI ORIF	
		Combined mechanical (CM): combination of other injuries	Based on injuries, ORIF if posterior SI displaced	
Acetabulum (Fig. 9–55)		Tile:		Nerve injury (sciatic 16–33%, femoral, sup. gluteal), vascular injury (supgluteal A) hetrotopic ossification (3–69%—consider XRT or indocin), avascular necrosis (with posterior injury), chondrolysis DJD
		Undisplaced	Nonoperative: Less than 2–5 mm displacement in the acetabular dome, low ant. column Fxs, low transverse Fxs, associated both column Fxs with secondary congruence. Operative: incongruous or unstable joint; (Posterior column/wall: Kocher-Langenbach approach; Anterior column/wall: ilioinguinal approach; both columns: extended iliofemoral combined or triradiate transtrochanteric approach)	
		Displaced		
		I—posterior ± posterior dislocation		
		A—posterior column		
		B—posterior wall		
		1—associated w/ post. column		
		2—associated with transverse Fx		
		II—anterior ± anterior dislocation		
		A—anterior column		
		B—anterior wall		
		C—associated ant. & transverse Fx		
		III—anterior ± central dislocation		
		A—pure transverse		
		B—"T" fractures		
		C—assoc. transverse & acetabular wall Fxs		
		D—double-column fractures		
Hip Fractures				
Femoral neck		Garden (Fig. 9–56):	CRIF with 3 screws or sliding compression hip screw with derotation screw; prosthesis for elderly (>70 yo physio), sick, pathologic Fx, Parkinson's, RA, dilantin Tx with displaced fractures (Garden III or IV); bipolar prosthesis for more active patients, THA for acetabular DJD (cement often indicated)	Malunion (accept <15° valgus and 10°AP displacement); AVN (25% at 12 h, 30% at 24 h, 40% at 24–48 h, 100% at 1 wk); nonunion (incr. with sliding screws); infection; PE; mortality (35% at 1 yr; incr. with advanced age, medical problems, & in males)
		I—incomplete/valgus impaction		
		II—complete, undisplaced		
		III—complete, partially displaced		
		IV—complete, totally displaced		
Neck stress		Devas:		
		Compression or transverse (distraction)	Distraction type increased propensity to displace	
		Blickenstaff & Morris:		
		I—callus	Bed rest → progressive weight bearing	Completed fracture, as above
		II—nondisplaced	SPICA or lateral fixation	
		III—displaced	CRIF ± bonegraft, followed by SPICA for 6 weeks	
Intertrochanteric (Fig. 9–57)		Boyd & Griffin:	CRIF with sliding compression hip screw most reliable; unstable fx (B&G III, or posteriomedial comminution) may require a fixation of posteromedial buttress before internal fixation in younger patients. Calcar replacing arthroplasty for patients with osteopenia and metastatic disease	Varus deformity (esp. w/ nonrigid fixation [Ender's nails]); pin migration; nail cutout; loss of fixation (incr. with superiolateral screws); joint penetration (screw ideally placed centrally) mortality, infection
		I—nondisplaced		
		*II—displaced		
		III—reverse obliquity		
		IV—subtrochlear spike		
		Evans (stable, unstable)		
Greater trochanter		Separation	>1 cm sep ORIF in younger patient	
Lesser trochanter		Separation	>2 cm sep ORIF in young athlete	
Subtrochanteric		Seinsheimer (I–V) (Fig. 9–58)		Refracture (at another site distal after Zickel nail removal) other complications similar to other hip fractures
		I—non/min. displaced	Locked intramedullary nail	
		II—2-part	Locked intramedullary nail	
		III—3-part	Recon nail or condylar plate/screw	
		IV—comminuted	Recon nail or condylar plate/screw	
		V—subtrochanteric-intertrochanteric	Sliding compression hip screw with long side plate (old patient), condylar blade plate (young patient)	
Hip Dislocations				
Hip Dislocation		*Ant.* (Epstein) (Fig. 9–59):	In general, treatment of ant. hip dislocations includes closed reduction, with open reduction if needed (irreducible or interspersed fragments, or with instability [unstable exam/<⅓ post. rim intact]) and ORIF of fractures or prosthetic replacement as indicated	Associated w/ increased energy trauma & often associated with other injuries; femoral A/N injuries (ant. dislocation), sciatic N (peroneal division) injuries; osteonecrosis (esp. with post. dislocation in elderly patients, delayed reduction; can present up to 5 yr after injury); posttraumatic DJD (esp. w/ retained fragments [CT required w/ type I dislocation to rule out fragments]); instability (with 30–40% of post. wall Fxs); incr. complications w/ instability after closed reduction
		I—superior		
		A—no Fx		
		B—head Fx		
		C—acetabular Fx		
		II—inferior		
		A—no Fx		
		B—head Fx		
		C—Acetabular Fx		

(continued)

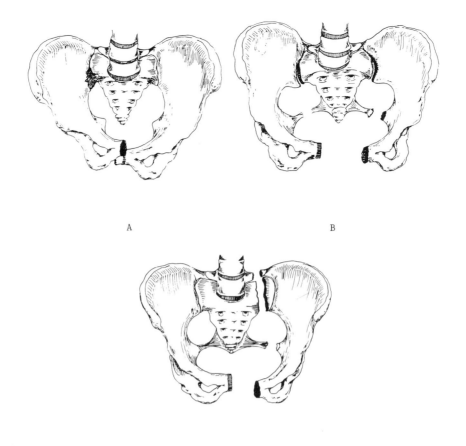

FIGURE 9–54. Young classification of pelvic fractures. *A,* Lateral compression. *B,* Anteroposterior compression. *C,* Vertical shear. (From Kozin, S.H., and Berlet, A.C.: Handbook of Common Orthopaedic Fractures, pp. 79, 83. West Chester, PA, Medical Surveillance Inc., 1989; reprinted with permission.)

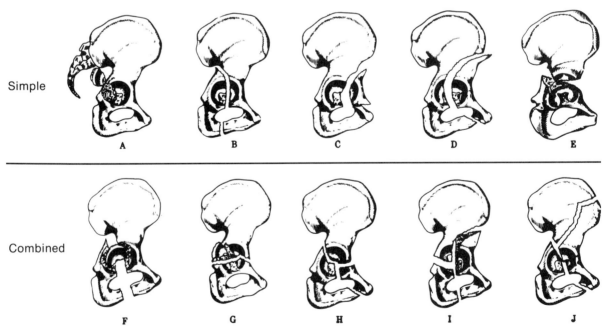

FIGURE 9–55. Letournel classification of acetabular fractures. *A,* Posterior wall. *B,* Posterior column. *C,* Anterior wall. *D,* Anterior column. *E,* Transverse. *F,* Posterior column and posterior wall. *G,* Transverse and posterior wall. *H,* "T" fracture. *I,* Anterior column and posterior hemitransverse. *J,* Both columns. (From Matta, J.M.: Trauma: Pelvis and acetabulum. In Orthopaedic Knowledge Update II, p. 348. Chicago, American Academy of Orthopaedic Surgeons, 1987; reprinted by permission.)

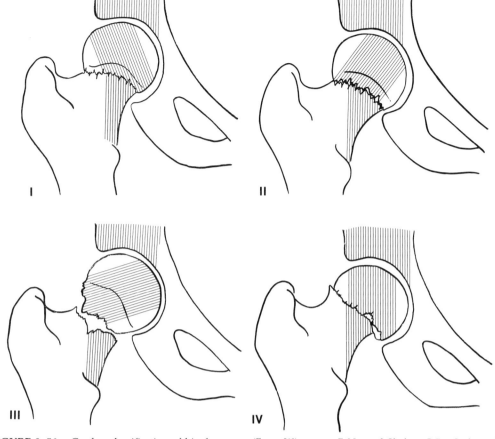

FIGURE 9–56. Garden classification of hip fractures. (From Wiessman, B.N., and Sledge, C.B.: Orthopedic Radiology, p. 408. Philadelphia, W.B. Saunders, 1986; reprinted by permission.)

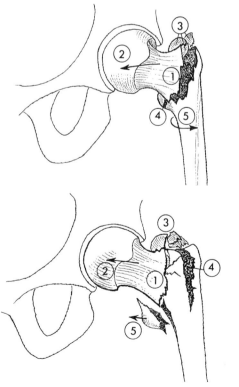

FIGURE 9–57. Intertrochanteric hip fracture classification. *Top*, Stable. *Bottom*, Unstable. (From Connolly, J.F., ed.: Depalma's The Management of Fractures and Dislocations, an Atlas, 3rd ed., p. 1372, 1373. Philadelphia, W.B. Saunders, 1981; reprinted by permission.)

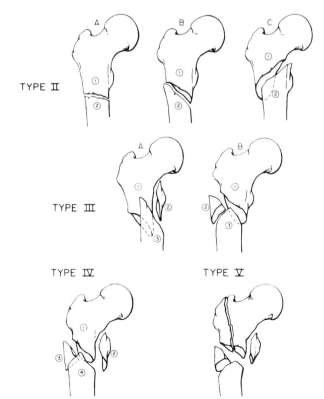

FIGURE 9–58. Classification of subtrochanteric femur fractures. (From Seinsheimer, F., III: Subtrochanteric fractures of the femur. J. Bone Joint Surg. [Am.] 60:302, 1978; reprinted by permission.)

TABLE 9–5. ADULT TRAUMATIC ORTHOPAEDIC INJURIES—LOWER EXTREMITY (*Continued*)

INJURY	EPONYM	CLASSIFICATION	TREATMENT	COMPLICATIONS
Hip Dislocations *cont.*				
		Post. (Thompson & Epstein) (Fig. 9–60)		
		I—no/min. Fx	Closed reduction, skin traction	
		II—post. acetabular rim	Primary open reduction	
		III—comminuted rim	ORIF (if possible), closed reduction (if not)	
		IV—acetabular floor	Closed reduction, open if necessary	
		V—Femoral head Fx		
		Pipkin subdivided these into:		
		I—head caudad	Closed reduction, skeletal traction	
		II—head cephalad	Closed reduction, skeletal traction	
		III—femoral head & neck Fx	ORIF (young pt) hemiarthroplasty/THA (older pt)	
		IV—associated acetabular Fx	ORIF (incongruous joint in young pt), THA (incongruous joint in older pt)	
		Central (Rowe & Lowell) (Fig. 9–61):		
		1—Undisplaced	Bed rest → crutches (nonweightbearing)	
		2—Inner wall		
		A—Femoral head beneath dome	Bedrest ± traction, early ROM	
		B—Not beneath dome	Closed reduction + traction	
		3—Superior dome		
		A—Congruent	Skeletal traction, early ROM	
		B—Incongruent	ORIF if large piece	
		4—Bursting		
		A—Congruent	Skeletal traction	
		B—Incongruent	Closed reduction ± traction, ORIF if irreducable (or late THA)	
Femoral Shaft Fractures				
Femur (2.5 cm below lesser trochanter → 8 cm from joint)		Winquist & Hansen (Fig. 9–62): I—transverse/<25% butterfly II—transverse 25–50% butterfly III—>50% comminution—unstable IV—extensive comminution no cortal abbutment—unstable V—segmental bone loss—unstable	Most Fxs are treated initially with traction followed by closed IM rodding; other options include traction, cast brace, external fixation (open IIIB); interlocking rods favored for comminuted and prox. & distal Fxs (<1.5 cm of isthmus for stability, types III & IV); dynamization usu. not indicated; I&D with immediate fixation grade I & II open Fxs, I&D with external fixation or delayed internal fixation for grade III open Fxs	Nonunion (remove rod over ream and replace with larger rod), infection (early: I&D, late: remove & re-ream intramedullary nail), missed knee ligament injury, other Fxs, neurovascular injury (peroneal N neurapraxia, femoral A), malunion (shortening & rotatory malalignment), knee stiffness (esp. with distal external fixation), refracture, failure of fixation
Femoral neck & shafts		Garden/Winquist (2.5–5% of femoral shaft fractures)	Treat neck Fx first, then the shaft (screws in neck & IM rod or plate for femur Fx or recon nail after provisional fixation of femoral neck)	Infection, delayed union, plate failure
Femoral & tibial shafts	"Floating knee"		IM rod femur, cast or IM rod tibia	Multiple other injuries, fat emboli syndrome
Knee Fractures and Dislocations				
Supracondylar		AO (Fig. 9–63)		Knee stiffness, DJD, nonunion, popliteal A injury (arteriogram required), varus angulation with buttress plate, malunion, unstable fixation, DVT
		A—extra-articular	>8 cm above joint IM locking nail, <8 cm condylar blade plate/screw	
		B—unicondylar	ORIF condylar blade plate/screw	
		C—bicondylar	Condylar blade plate/screw; buttress plate for comminuted Fx	
Patella (Fig. 9–64)		Undisplaced, transverse, lower pole, upper pole, comminuted, vertical	Undisplaced—cylinder cast ORIF if can't actively extend knee or >2 mm separation, or incongruent articular surface (tension band); excise fragments that are extremely comminuted	Separation of fragments, infection, AVN, DJD
Tibial plateau		Hohl's revised classification (Fig. 9–65): Minimally displaced (<4 mm dep/diplacement)		DJD, stiffness, loss of reduction, AVN, infection, medial plateau fractures almost always require ORIF
			Stable (<5° V/V instability)—closed treatment; unstable (>5° V/V instability)—closed reduction ± PC screw fixation	
		Displaced (>4 mm dep/displacement): *Local compression	Closed treatment if <6 mm displaced, arthroscopic assisted reduction/fixation if 6–12 mm displaced, ORIF >12 mm displaced	
		Split compression	ORIF with buttress plate (arthroscopic assisted if ≤10 mm)	
		Total depression	CRIF + PC screws or ORIF if >5 mm displaced	
		Split	Closed treatment if stable, min. fixation/collateral ligament repair if unstable	
		Rim	Elevation and fixation with collateral ligament repair	
		Bicondylar	Skeletal traction ± PC screw fixation; rarely ORIF	
Tibial spine (Fig. 9–66)		I—anterior tilt II—complete anterior tilt III—no contact A—no rotation B—rotated	I & II & IIIA closed reduction LLC 6 wks if knee can be brought into full extension; IIIB and all irreducable types require open reduction	Block to motion (arthroscopic loose body removal), ACL laxity
Tibial tubercle			ORIF with screw or staple.	Loss of fixation, quad weakness
Subcondylar tibia		Stable Displaced	Cast immobilization ORIF with buttress plate	Arterial injury (arteriography suggested), decreased ROM
Prox. fibula			Open if unstable (peroneal N, biceps)	

(continued)

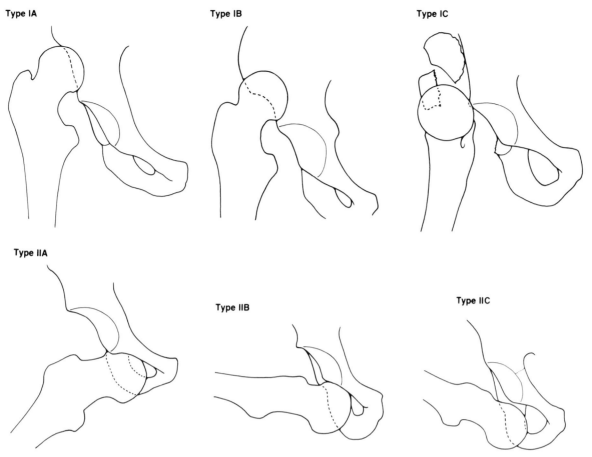

FIGURE 9–59. Classification of anterior dislocations of the femoral head. Type I: superior; type II: inferior; A: no fracture; B: femoral head fracture; C: acetabular fracture. (From DeLee, J.C.: Dislocations and fracture-dislocations of the hip. In Fractures in Adults, Rockwood, C.A., and Green, D.P., eds., 2nd ed., pp. 1288–1292. Philadelphia, J.B. Lippincott, 1984; reprinted by permission.)

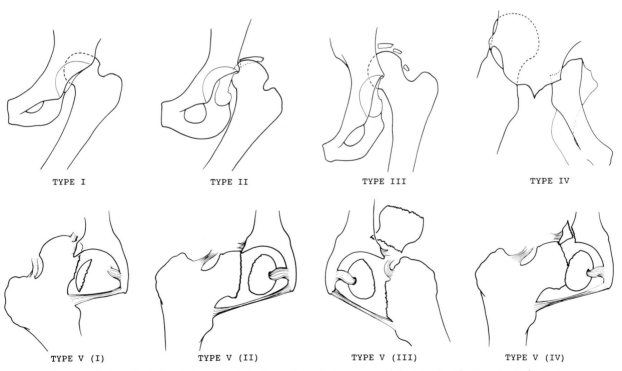

FIGURE 9–60. Posterior dislocation of the femoral head—Thomas and Epstein classification. *I*, No fracture. *II*, Posterior acetabular fracture. *III*, Comminuted rim fracture. *IV*, Acetabular floor fracture. *V*, Femoral head fracture. (From DeLee, J.C.: Dislocations and fracture-dislocations of the hip. In Fractures in Adults, Rockwood, C.A., and Green, D.P., eds., 2nd ed., pp. 1293–1297. Philadelphia, J.B. Lippincott, 1984; reprinted by permission.)

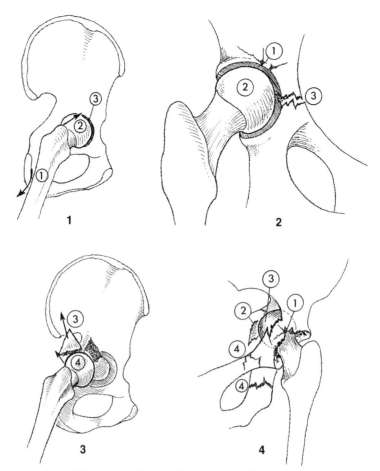

FIGURE 9-61. Central hip dislocations—Rowe and Lowell classification. *1*, Undisplaced. *2*, Inner wall. *3*, Superior dome. *4*, Bursting. (From Connolly, J.F., ed.: Depalma's The Management of Fractures and Dislocations, an Atlas, 3rd ed., p. 1348, 1349. Philadelphia, W.B. Saunders, 1981; reprinted by permission.)

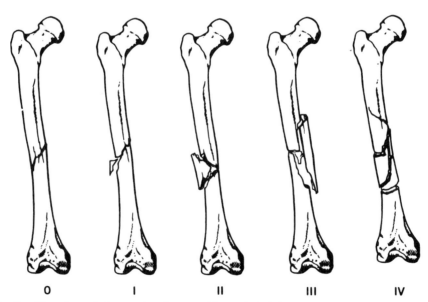

O   I   II   III   IV

FIGURE 9-62. Winquist and Hanson classification of femoral shaft fractures. (*Note:* Type V [not shown] has segmental bone loss.) (From Johnson, K.D.: Femur: Trauma. In Orthopaedic Knowledge Update III, p. 514. Chicago, American Academy of Orthopaedic Surgeons, 1990; reprinted by permission.)

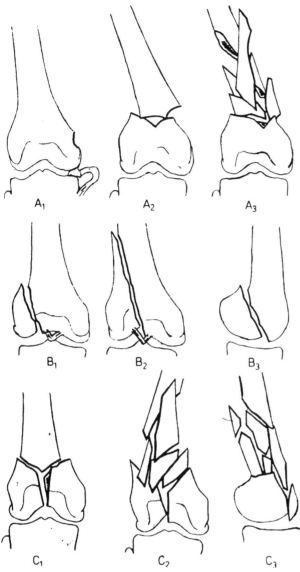

FIGURE 9–63. AO/ASIF classification of supracondylar fractures. *A*, Extra-articular. *B*, Unicondylar. *C*, Bicondylar. (From Johnson, K.D.: Femur: Trauma. In Orthopaedic Knowledge Update III, p. 521. Chicago, American Academy of Orthopaedic Surgeons, 1990; reprinted by permission.)

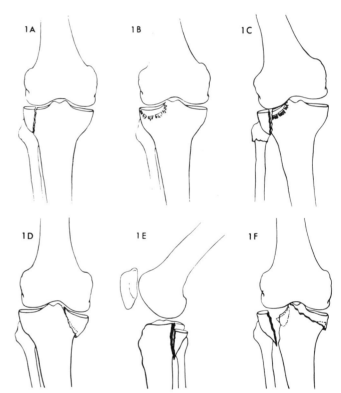

FIGURE 9–65. Classification of tibial plateau fractures. *1A*, Minimally displaced. *1B*, Local compression. *1C*, Split compression. *1D*, Total depression. *1E*, Split. *1F*. Bicondylar. (From Hohl, M.: Tibial condylar fractures. J. Bone Joint Surg. [Am.] 49:1455, 1967; reprinted by permission.)

Undisplaced **Transverse** **Lower or Upper Pole** **Comminuted** **Vertical**

FIGURE 9–64. Types of patellar fractures. (From Wiessman, B.N.W., and Sledge, C.B.: Orthopedic Radiology, p. 553. Philadelphia, W.B. Saunders, 1986; reprinted by permission.)

TABLE 9–5.   ADULT TRAUMATIC ORTHOPAEDIC INJURIES—LOWER EXTREMITY (*Continued*)

INJURY	EPONYM	CLASSIFICATION	TREATMENT	COMPLICATIONS
Knee Fracture *cont.*				
Quadriceps rupture			Repair acutely, cylinder cast	
Patella tendon rupture			Repair with tension reducing device	Missed Dx (high riding patella seen on radiographs)
Patella dislocation		Acute, recurrent, subluxation, habitual	Cylinder cast & quadriceps strengthening if congruent; arthroscopy for displaced or osteochondral Fxs; recurrent—lat. rel, med. plication, bony transplant if abnormal Q angle. Avoid surgery in habitual dislocators.	Recurrence
Knee dislocation (Fig. 9–67)		*Ant., post., lat., med., rotatory (AM, AL, PM, PL)	Reduce emergently, immobilize 6 wks; open reduction if needed (PL rotation); repair vascular injuries; ligament repair 2ndary	Popliteal A injury (arteriogram mandatory); tibial/peroneal N injuries, ACL tear (most common)
Prox. tibia-fibula dislocation		*Ant.(lat.), post.(med.), sup. (usu. w/ lat. malleolus injury)	Reduce (90° flexion) ORIF if fails or recurrent	
Chondral/ Osteochondral		Endogenous vs. exogenous	Arthroscopic evaluation of locked, acute condylar defects and remove small fragments (pin large fragments)	DJD
Tibia-Fibula Fractures				
Tibia (Fig. 9–68)		Chapman A—Transverse/short/oblique—closed reduction LLC B—Small butterfly—closed reduction LLC C—Large butterfly—IM fixation (if <50 cortical contact) D—Segmental—IM fixation E—Spiral—closed reduction LLC F—Proximal ¼—closed treatment, ORIF if unstable G—Distal ¼—closed treatment, ORIF if unstable	Most will respond to closed traction LLC, wedge as needed, PTB at 6–8 wks; IM nail for transverse oblique Fx of mid ⅓ or segmental; IM nail also vascular injury, bilateral injury, pathologic Fxs, severe knee ligamentous injuries; external fixation with large open wounds (grade III); Open Fxs: early flap coverage, delayed bone grafting. Consider early amputation in Grade IIIC injuries, posterior tibial nerve injury, warm ischemia time >6 hours, severe ipsilateral foot injury; etc.	Delayed union (>20 wks; incr. with greater initial displacement & middle third Fxs; treatment includes fibulectomy and P/L bone graft), nonunion (P/L bone graft or reamed IM nail), infection (flap/graft or amputation), malunion (V/V, shortening [accept <5° V/V, <10° AP angulation]), vascular injuries (upper ¼—ant. tibial A), compartment syndrome, peroneal N injury, RSD
Tibia stress		Upper ⅓ (recruits)	Modify activity 6–10 wks	Progression to complete Fx
Fibula shaft		Mid-lower ⅓ (athletes)	Cast only if needed for pain relief	
Tibial plafond	Pilon (Fig. 9–69)	Ruedi & Allgower: I—minimally displaced II—incongruous III—comminuted	LLC & non-weight bearing ORIF if displaced & ankle involved (fibula 1st); os calis pin if severely comminuted	DJD (may require late fusion), infection, V/V angulation
Ankle Fractures and Dislocations				

Ankle fracture (Figs. 9–70 and 9–71)		Lauge-Hansen (position of foot—direction of force):
		S-Add: 1—LM transverse (or LCL)
		    2—MM Fx
		S-ER: 1—AITFL
		    2—LM spiral Fx
		    3—PM Fx or PITFL injury
		    4—MM Fx/deltoid
		P-Abd: 1—MM Fx/deltoid
		    2—A&P ITFL/PM
		    3—LM oblique supramalleolar
		P-ER: 1—MM Fx/deltoid
		    2—AITFL/IOL
		    3—High fibular
		    4—PM Fx
		Danis Weber (AO) (position of fibular Fx):
		A—at or below joint
		B—Obliquely up from joint
		C—High fibular fx
			Treatment of ankle Fx based on position of mortise (nondisplaced fractures can be treated in a LLC >1 mm displacement after reduction requires ORIF; syndesmosis screw if interosseous ligament/membrane is disrupted); usually not necessary to reduce posteromedial fragment (not in weight-bearing area unless >⅓); use of an antiglide plate posteriolaterally on the fibula is helpful with oblique Fxs; for open Fxs grades I & II injuries can be acutely fixed with DPC, grade III injuries may require Ex Fix
			
			In general, treatment of AO type A fractures is closed and treatment of AO types B and C is with ORIF
				Nonunion, malunion, infection (esp. w/ ORIF and may present with symmetric tibiotalar joint space narrowing), DJD, vascular injury, RSD, synostisis; 1 mm of lat. talar displacement from the med. malleolus is associated with 42% decr. in tibiotalar articulation (Ramsey)

Foot Fractures and Dislocations				
Stress	March	*2MT & calcaneus	Symptomatic, SLWC if late	
Talar neck	Aviator's astragalus	Hawkins & Canale (Fig. 9–72) I—nondisplaced vertical II—displaced & subtalar dislocation/subluxation III—displaced & talar body dislocation IV—With talar head dislocation	SLC 8–12 wks (NWB 4–6 wks) Reduce dislocation, cast eq, open reduction if nonanatomic closed reduction ORIF—anatomic reduction required ORIF required	AVN (esp. type III & IV [Hawkin's sign indicates a good prognosis]; weight bearing is important in treating this complication), delayed/nonunion, malunion, DJD, skin necrosis
Talar body		Rare	Usu. requires ORIF	AVN, malunion, DJD
Talar head		Rare	Nondisplaced—splint/ice/elevation Displaced—ORIF or excision of comminuted fragments	Talonavicular DJD
Talar process		Lateral process	SLC × 6 wks, excise if comminuted	Med. malleolus fracture (26%), rule out os trigonum (50%)
	Shepherd's	Posterior process	SLC × 6 wks, excise nonunions	
Subtalar dislocation	Basketball foot	*Calcaneus medial displacement	Reduce, immobilization 4 wks, open reduction if irreducable	Posterior tibialis tendon entrapment

(continued)

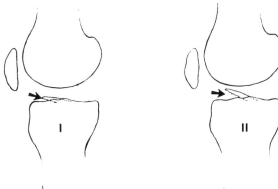

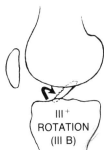

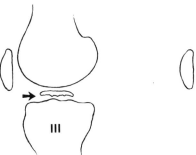

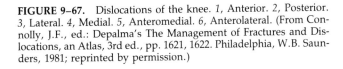

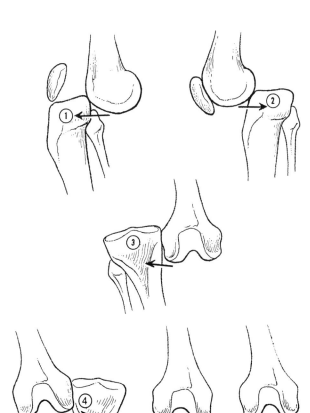

FIGURE 9–66. Classification of tibial spine fractures. (From Myers, M.H., and McKeever, F.M.: Fractures of the intercondylar eminence of the tibia. J. Bone Joint Surg. [Am.] 52:1677, 1974; reprinted by permission.)

FIGURE 9–67. Dislocations of the knee. *1,* Anterior. *2,* Posterior. *3,* Lateral. *4,* Medial. *5,* Anteromedial. *6,* Anterolateral. (From Connolly, J.F., ed.: Depalma's The Management of Fractures and Dislocations, an Atlas, 3rd ed., pp. 1621, 1622. Philadelphia, W.B. Saunders, 1981; reprinted by permission.)

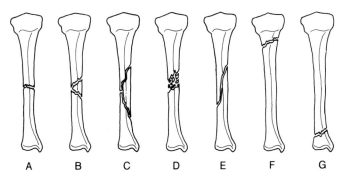

FIGURE 9–68. Classification of tibial fractures. *A,* Transverse/short oblique. *B,* Small butterfly. *C,* Large butterfly. *D,* Segmental. *E,* Spiral. *F,* Proximal. *G,* Distal. (From Chapman, M.W.: Fractures of the tibia and fibula. In Operative Orthopaedics, Chapman, M.W., ed., p. 437. Philadelphia, J.B. Lippincott, 1988; reprinted by permission.)

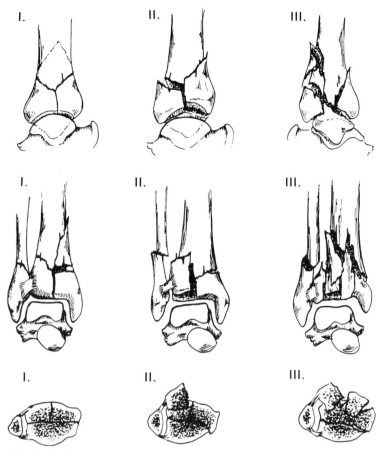

FIGURE 9–69. Tibial pilon fractures. *I*, Minimally displaced. *II*, Incongruous. *III*, Comminuted. (From Kozin, S.H., and Berlet, A.C.: Handbook of Common Orthopaedic Fractures, p. 131. West Chester, PA, Medical Surveillance Inc., 1989; reprinted by permission.)

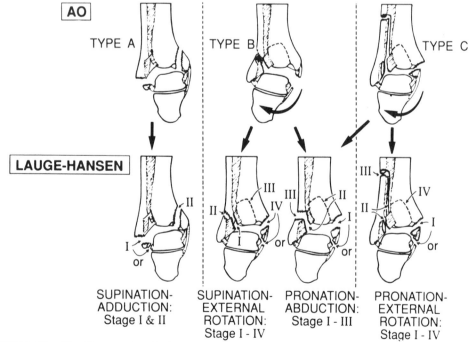

FIGURE 9–70. Classification of ankle fractures—AO (Danis-Weber) and Lauge-Hansen. (From Sangeorzan, B.J., and Hansen, S.T.: Ankle and foot: Trauma. In Orthopaedic Knowledge Update III, p. 615, Chicago, American Academy of Orthopaedic Surgeons, 1990; reprinted by permission.)

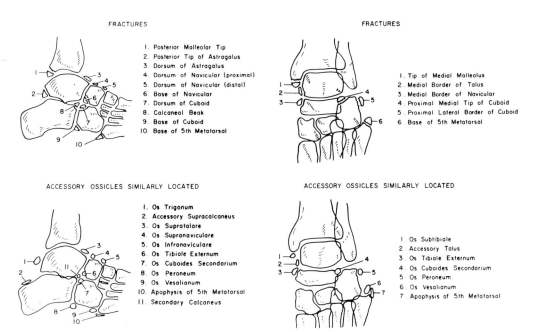

FRACTURES

1. Posterior Malleolar Tip
2. Posterior Tip of Astragalus
3. Dorsum of Astragalus
4. Dorsum of Navicular (proximal)
5. Dorsum of Navicular (distal)
6. Base of Navicular
7. Dorsum of Cuboid
8. Calcaneal Beak
9. Base of Cuboid
10. Base of 5th Metatarsal

FRACTURES

1. Tip of Medial Malleolus
2. Medial Border of Talus
3. Medial Border of Navicular
4. Proximal Medial Tip of Cuboid
5. Proximal Lateral Border of Cuboid
6. Base of 5th Metatarsal

ACCESSORY OSSICLES SIMILARLY LOCATED

1. Os Trigonum
2. Accessory Supracalcaneus
3. Os Supratalare
4. Os Supranaviculare
5. Os Infranaviculare
6. Os Tibiale Externum
7. Os Cuboides Secondarium
8. Os Peroneum
9. Os Vesalianum
10. Apophysis of 5th Metatarsal
11. Secondary Calcaneus

ACCESSORY OSSICLES SIMILARLY LOCATED

1. Os Subtibiale
2. Accessory Talus
3. Os Tibiale Externum
4. Os Cuboides Secondarium
5. Os Peroneum
6. Os Vesalianum
7. Apophysis of 5th Metatarsal

FIGURE 9–71. Avulsion fractures of the ankle. (After Zatkin, H.R. Semin. Roentgenol. 5:419, 1970. From Jahss, M.H.: Disorders of the Foot, p. 1488. Philadelphia, W.B. Saunders, 1982; reprinted by permission.)

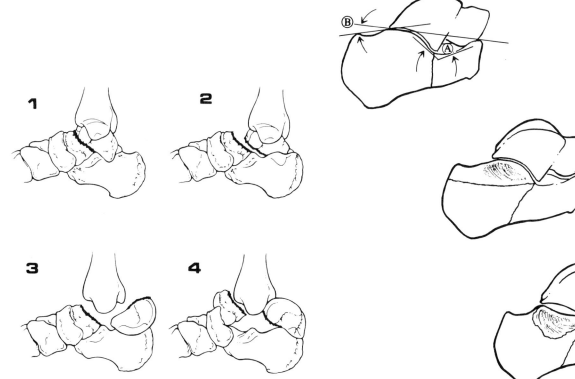

FIGURE 9–72. Hawkins (and Canale) classification of talar neck fractures. *1*, Nondisplaced. *2*, Subtalar dislocation. *3*, Talar body dislocation. *4*, Talar head dislocation. (From Sangeorzan, B.J., and Hansen, S.T.: Ankle and foot: Trauma. In Orthopaedic Knowledge Update III, p. 616, Chicago, American Academy of Orthopaedic Surgeons, 1990; reprinted by permission.)

FIGURE 9–73. Intra-articular calcaneus fractures. *1*, Nondisplaced. *2*, Tongue. *3*, Joint depression. Note: *A*, crucial angle of Gusiane; *B*, Bohler's angle. (From Connolly, J.F., ed.: Depalma's The Management of Fractures and Dislocations, an Atlas, 3rd ed., p. 2013. Philadelphia, W.B. Saunders, 1981; reprinted by permission.)

TABLE 9–5. ADULT TRAUMATIC ORTHOPAEDIC INJURIES—LOWER EXTREMITY (*Continued*)

INJURY	EPONYM	CLASSIFICATION	TREATMENT	COMPLICATIONS
Foot Fractures and Dislocations *cont.*				
Total talar dislocation		Subtalar + Chopart injury	Open reduction, late fusion	AVN
*Calcaneus	Essex-Lopresti	Extra-articular (ant. process, tuberosity, med. process, sustentaculum talus, *body). *Intra-articular (nondisplaced, tongue, joint depression comminuted) (Fig. 9–73) (Bohlers angle & Gissane angle)	Principles of treatment: CT scan helpful, reduce joint incongruity, ORIF younger active patients if possible (medial ± lateral approach); bone graft defects; late excision of symptomatic anterior process fractures; extra-articular—SLC, ORIF if displaced	Chronic pain (heel widening, nerve entrapment), peroneal tendonitis, DJD, malunion, associated Fxs (spine, LE), heel skin slough
Midtarsal injury		*Med. stress, longitudinal stress, lat. stress, plantar stress, crush	Prompt reconstruction of anatomy, ORIF often	
Navicular		Cortical avulsion Tuberosity Fx (PT avulsion) Body Fx Stress Fx	Reduce, pin large fragments (>25%) ORIF w/ screw and washer ORIF if displaced NWB cast 6–8 wks	Osteonecrosis (ORIF nonunion), associated with midfoot fractures
Cuboid compound Fx	Nutcracker	Compressed calcaneus & MT	ORIF with bone graft	
TMT Fx/ dislocation	Lisfranc (Fig. 9–74)	Homolatel. (all 5 same direction), isolated (1 or 2MT displaced), divergent (displacement in sagittal and coronal planes)	Closed reduction ± PCP required; open reduction if severe displacement, or foreign body entrapment; ORIF of MT-tarsal disruptions with screws is successful	Chronic pain (arthrodesis preferred) Delay in Dx (at neck if medial border of 2MT base aligned with medial border of middle cuneiform)
Metatarsal		Shaft Head	Reduce, pin if needed, SLWC 4 wks Reduce (traction and manipulation), cast	Posttraumatic DJD
	Pseudo-Jones (Fig. 9–75)	Base avulsion (5MT)	2–3 wks SLWC, late removal of fragments if needed	
	Jones (Fig. 9–75)	5MT base transverse Fx	4–6 wks NWB SLC, late ORIF if required	Nonunion (screw/bone graft)
MTP dislocation			Reduce promptly, immobilize	
Digits			ORIF displaced intra-articular Fx	

* Most common.

Abbreviations: I/L, ipsilateral; C/L, contralateral; CRIF, closed reduction internal fixation; ORIF, open reduction internal fixation; PC, percutaneous; PCP, percutaneous pin; V/V, varus/valgus; SLC, short leg cast; SLWC, short leg walking cast; NWB, nonweight bearing; MT, metatarsal; TMT, tarsometatarsal; MTP, metatarsal phalangeal; THA, total hip arthroplasty.

FIGURE 9–74. Lisfranc fractures—usually involve second metatarsal base ± third and fourth metatarsals (rarely involve first or fifth metatarsal). (From Connolly, J.F., ed.: Depalma's The Management of Fractures and Dislocations, an Atlas, 3rd ed., p. 2053. Philadelphia, W.B. Saunders, 1981; reprinted by permission.)

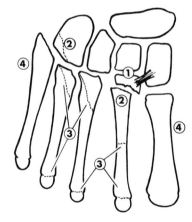

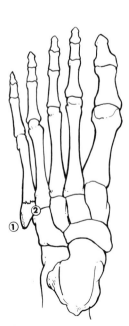

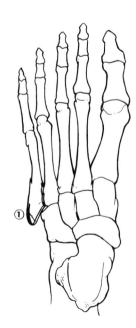

FIGURE 9–75. Jones and "pseudo-Jones" fractures. *Left,* Metaphyseal fracture (true Jones). *Right,* Avulsion fracture (pseudo-Jones). (From Connolly, J.F., ed.: Depalma's The Management of Fractures and Dislocations, an Atlas, 3rd ed., pp. 2065, 2066. Philadelphia, W.B. Saunders, 1981; reprinted by permission.)

PART 2

Pediatric Trauma

I. Introduction—Because fractures and dislocations in children are often unique, several features of these injuries are not found in adults (see Table 9–6, at the end of Part 2). Children's bones are more ductile than adult bones, and bowing (especially in the fibula and ulna), "greenstick," and "torus" fractures are unique to children. The periosteum in children is much thicker, and often remains intact on the concave (compression) side, allowing less displacement and better reduction of fractures. Children's fractures heal much quicker, and less immobilization time is required. Children are also less likely to develop contractures from immobilization and therefore this is less of a concern. However, because bones are actively growing in pediatric patients, malunion and growth plate injuries are an important concern. Remodeling is more thorough, especially in younger children, so displacement and angulation that would not be tolerated in an adult are often acceptable in the management of children's fractures (except intra-articular fractures, where the same axioms apply).

II. Child Abuse—The "Battered Child" Syndrome

    A. Introduction—Unfortunately, child abuse does occur in this population and one must always be wary of the "battered child." This is especially true when fractures are encountered in the infant. All states now obligate physicians to report suspected child abuse. Suspicions should be raised with fractures in children less than 3 years old with multiple healing bruises, skin marks, burns, unreasonable histories, signs of neglect, etc.

    B. Fracture Locations—The most common locations of fractures in children are the humerus, tibia, and femur, in that order. **Skeletal surveys** are appropriate if a "battered child" is encountered, in children with delayed development, in some metaphyseal and metaphyseal-epiphyseal fractures, and in spiral fractures. Diaphyseal fractures, generally considered less suspicious of child abuse, are in fact four times more common. The skeletal survey consists of skull, T-L–spine AP and lateral views, and AP views of ribs and extremities. Skeletal surveys are rarely helpful in children over the age of 5. Bone scans can identify fractures earlier and can be a helpful adjunct, especially in children less than 2 years old. Other nonorthopaedic injuries commonly encountered in child abuse include head injuries ("shaken baby" leading to avulsion of the cerebral bridging veins), burns, and blunt abdominal visceral injuries.

    C. Treatment—In addition to normal fracture care, early involvement of social workers and pediatricians is essential. If child abuse is missed, there is a greater than 1/3 chance of further abuse, and a 5–10% chance of death in affected children.

III. Physeal Fractures

    A. Introduction—The physis, or growth plate, is more susceptible to fracture than injury to attached ligaments, and therefore, if there is any question, one must assume that there is a fracture of the physis until proven otherwise.

    B. Characteristics—Most physeal injuries (except about the elbow) occur toward the end of skeletal maturity, and are therefore most common in adolescents. Although physeal fractures are classically thought to be through the zone of provisional calcification (within the zone of hypertrophy) of the growth plate, the fracture can actually involve several of the layers. Failure is usually from torsion and not tension at the growth plate. The blood supply of the epiphysis is tenuous, and injuries can disrupt small epiphyseal vessels supplying the growth center. This can lead to the many complications associated with these injuries (limb length discrepancies, malunion, bony bars, etc.). Physeal fractures are most common in the distal radius, followed by the distal tibia.

    C. Classification—The Salter-Harris (SH) classification, modified by Rang, is used to classify physeal fractures (Fig. 9–76):

TYPE	DESCRIPTION	CHARACTERISTICS
I	Transverse fractures through physis	Younger children
II	Fractures through physis with metaphyseal fragment	Children >10 yo
III	Fractures through physis and epiphysis	Intra-articular
IV	Fractures through epiphysis, physis, and metaphysis	Migration/growth arrest
V	Crush injury of physis	Growth arrest late
VI	Injury to perichondrial ring	Bridging/angular deformity

    D. Treatment—A few general guidelines regarding treatment of these fractures is in order. Gentle reduction should be attempted initially for SH I and II fractures, often requiring general anesthesia. With appropriate reduction and immobilization, these fractures will usually do well without a significant amount of growth arrest (except in the distal femur, where SH II fractures can result in malalignment and arrest, and proximal tibia fractures, which can develop a valgus deformity). SH III and IV injuries are intra-articular and will usually require open reduction to correctly align the growth plate. Fixation, if used, should not cross the physis if at all possible. SH V and VI fractures are usually not identified early, and have a high complication rate. The cartilaginous growth plate will usually heal in about half the time required for the adjacent bone to heal. Follow-up radiographs are required for all physeal fractures. Minor injuries can often be appreciated on late radiographs by the presence of transversely oriented Harris-Park growth arrest lines. With severe injuries where limb salvage is

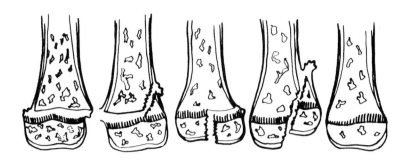

FIGURE 9–76. Salter-Harris classification of injuries to the physis. (From Bora, F.W.: The Pediatric Upper Extremity, p. 154. Philadelphia, W.B. Saunders, 1986; reprinted by permission.)

not possible, disarticulation is often favored over amputation in children in order to retain the proximal growth plate.

E. Partial Growth Arrest—Physeal bars or bridges result from growth plate injuries that arrest growth of part of the physis, and the uninjured portion of the physis continues to grow normally. Three types of physeal arrest have been characterized (Bright):

Type	Location	Common Etiology
I	Peripheral	SH II fractures
II	Central	Infection
III	Combined	SH IV fractures

Physeal bridge resection with interposition of fat graft or other materials like Silastic and Cranioplast (which must be removed at maturity) is reserved for patients with >2 cm of growth remaining, and <50% physeal involvement. Smaller, peripheral bars in younger patients do the best, and the procedure is contraindicated with active infection (resection should be delayed 6–12 months following infection) and inadequate skin coverage. Hypocycloidal tomograms or CT is useful in planning the resection, and intact physeal cartilage must be preserved. Arrest involving >50% of the physis should be treated with ipsilateral completion of the arrest and contralateral epiphysiodesis, or ipsilateral limb lengthening.

TABLE 9–6. PEDIATRIC TRAUMATIC ORTHOPAEDIC INJURIES

Injury	Eponym	Classification	Treatment	Complications
Wrist and Hand Fractures				
Phalanx fractures (Figs. 9–77 and 9–78)		Based on phalanx and SH classification	Closed reduction for most, PCP if unstable; condylar & SH III/IV Fxs may require ORIF	Residual deformities, tendon imbalance, nail deformities
MC fractures		Based on location	Reduce, ORIF if unreducible	
Thumb MC Fxs (Fig. 9–79)		A—metaphyseal B—SH II (medial) C—SH II (lateral)	Closed reduction Closed reduction Closed reduction	
	Bennett equivalent	D—SH III	ORIF	
IP dislocation			Closed reduction and splint; open if irreducible, incongruous on x-ray, or redisplaces with ROM	
MCP dislocation*			Attempt closed reduction, open if irreducible	
CMC dislocation			Reduce with finger traps, PCP K-wire to carpus and adjacent MC	
Distal radius (Fig. 9–80)	SH fractures	I–V	PCP types III & IV (transepiphyseal)	Deformity, loss of reduction, infection (open fracture), Volkmann's contracture, growth arrest, malunion, refracture
	Torus	Tension side intact	SAC for 3 wks	
	Greenstick	Tension side plastic deformation	Reduce if angulation > 10°, LAC in supination	
	Complete	Both cortices disrupted	Reduce and place in LAC in supination	

(continued)

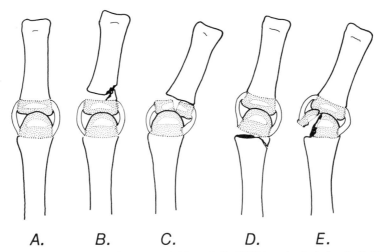

FIGURE 9–77. Pediatric finger MCP fractures. *A*, Normal. *B*, SH II (proximal phalanx). *C*, SH III (proximal phalanx). *D*, SH II (metacarpal). *E*, SH III (metacarpal). (From Ogden, J.A.: Skeletal Injury in the Child, 2nd ed., p. 531. Philadelphia, W.B. Saunders, 1990; reprinted by permission.)

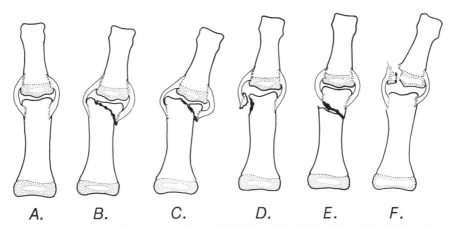

FIGURE 9–78. Pediatric finger IP fractures. *A*, Normal. *B*, Unicondylar. *C*, Partial condylar. *D*, Lateral avulsion. *E*, Bicondylar. *F*, SH III. (From Ogden, J.A.: Skeletal Injury in the Child, 2nd ed., p. 530. Philadelphia, W.B. Saunders, 1990; reprinted by permission.)

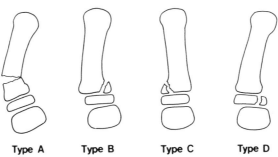

FIGURE 9–79. Classification of pediatric thumb metacarpal fractures. *A*, Metaphyseal. *B*, SH II (medial). *C*, SH II (lateral). *D*, SH III. (From O'Brien, E.T.: Fractures of the hand and wrist region. In Fractures in Children, Rockwood, C.A., Jr., Wilkins, K.E., and King, RE., eds., 2nd ed., p. 257. Philadelphia, J.B. Lippincott, 1984; reprinted by permission.)

TABLE 9–6. PEDIATRIC TRAUMATIC ORTHOPAEDIC INJURIES (*Continued*)

INJURY	EPONYM	CLASSIFICATION	TREATMENT	COMPLICATIONS
Radial and Ulnar Shafts				
Radius & ulna	Both bone	Greenstick (incomplete) Compression (buckle or torus) Complete	Correct rotation w/ pronation/ supination, and w/ pressure with <10° angulation: SAC 3–4 wks in <10 yo (even w/ bayonet opposition); match rotation of distal fragment with proximal (bicep tuberosity [points opposite of thumb])	Refracture, limb ischemia, malunion (esp. in <10 yo w/ inadequate reduction), nerve injury, synostosis
Plastic Deformation		Based on bones involved (Ulna > Radius)	Great pressure with fulcrum (reduce most deformed bone first)	Persistance of deformity
Ulna Fx & radial head dislocation	Monteggia (Fig. 9–81)	I—*ulna angulation & radial head ant. (extension) II—ulna angulation & rad head post. (flexion) III—ulna ant. angulation, radial head lat. (adduction) IV—ulna and proximal 1/3 radius Fx (both angulated ant.)	Reduce (traction, flexion), LAC 100° flexion, supination Reduce (traction, extension), LAC in some extension Reduce (extension & pressure), LAC 90° flexion, supination Reduce (supinate), may require ORIF	Late diagnosis (reconstruct annular ligament—Bell Tawse), decreased ROM, missed wrist injury, nonunion, persistent radial head dislocation (Bell Tawse & ulnar osteotomy if ulna healed), para-articular ossification
Radial head dislocation (ant.)	Monteggia equivalent		Supination & pressure on radial head, LAC 100° flexion, supination	Synostosis, nerve injury (PIN), loss of reduction (Bell Tawse)
Ulna Fx & radial neck Fx	Check for Monteggia equivalent	Min. displaced radial head Completely displaced radial head	Reduce (traction, pressure on radial head, varus stress), ORIF	LAC
Ulna Fx & prox. radius Fx	Check for Monteggia equivalent		Reduce (traction, supination), LAC 90° flexion, supination	
Ulna Fx, radial neck Fx & radial shaft dislocation	Check for Monteggia equivalent		Reduce (traction, reduce shaft), LAC (extension & supination)	
Radius Fx & dist radioulnar dislocation	Galeazzi		Reduce (traction, supination), LAC (90° flexion, supination); ORIF if >12 yo and closed reduction fails	Malunion, nerve injury (ulnar, ant. IO), RU subluxation, loss of radial bow
Elbow				
Supracondylar (6–8 yo) (Fig. 9–82)		*Extension: I—undisplaced II—displaced (post. cortex intact) III—displaced (A—PM*; B—PL)	Immobilize 3 weeks Reduce ± PCP (or hold in flexion >90°) CR PCP; open reduction or closed traction if fails	Nerve injury (radial > median), vascular (acute or Volkmann's), decr. ROM, myositis ossificans, C. varus (osteotomy cosmetic), ipsilateral Fxs (forearm, wrist 10%)
		Flexion (distal fragment ant.)	Reduce in extension, Cast in extension or PCT pin (best) ORIF often required if completely displaced	Nerve injury (ulnar), malunion, decr. ROM
Lat. condyle (6 yo) (Fig. 9–83)		Milch: I—SH IV, II—SH II into trochlea Displacement: I—undisplaced, II—min. displaced, III—rotated	Min. displaced (<2 mm): splint; displaced: ORIF	Overgrowth/spur, delayed/ nonunion, C. valgus, tardy ulnar N palsy, physeal arrest, AVN
Med. condyle (10 yo) (Fig. 9–84)		Milch: I—to trochlear apex, II—to C-T groove Displacement: I—undisplaced, II—min. displaced, III—rotated	Min. Displaced: splint; displaced: ORIF	Missed Dx, C. varus, AVN
Entire distal humumeral physis (<7 yo) (Fig. 9–85)		A—infant (SH I) B—7 mo–3 yo (SH I) C—3–7 yo (SH II)	Closed reduction LAC	Child abuse commonly associated, Late Dx (osteotomy), cubitus varus

(*continued*)

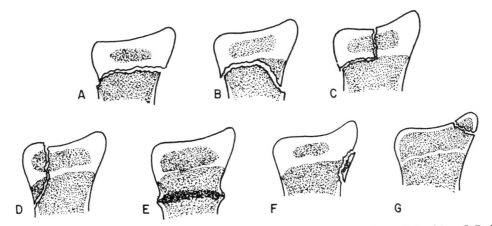

FIGURE 9–80. Pediatric wrist fractures. *A*, SH I. *B*, SH II. *C*, SH III. *D*, SH IV. *E*, Torus. *F*, Avulsion. *G*, Radial styloid. (From Ogden, J.A.: Skeletal Injury in the Child, 2nd ed., p. 513. Philadelphia, W.B. Saunders, 1990; reprinted by permission.)

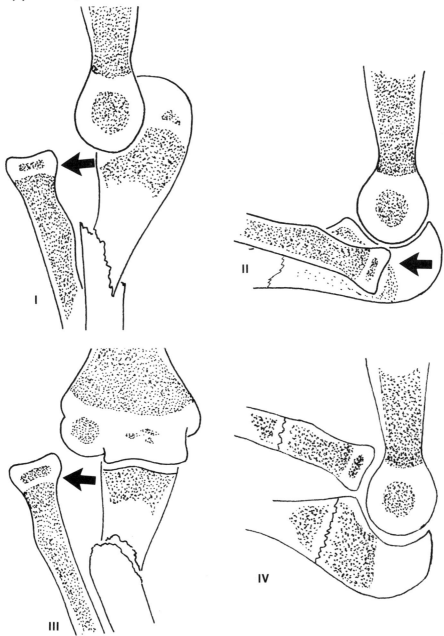

FIGURE 9–81. Pediatric Monteggia fractures. *I*, Anterior, *II*, Posterior. *III*, Lateral. *IV*, BB fracture. (Figs. I–III from Ogden, J.A.: Skeletal Injury in the Child, 2nd ed., pp. 480, 481. Philadelphia, W.B. Saunders, 1990; reprinted by permission.)

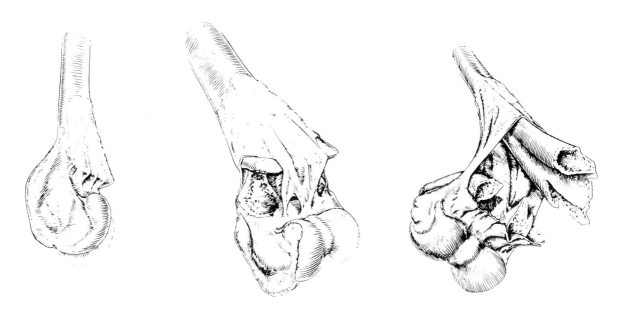

TYPE I

TYPE II

TYPE III

FIGURE 9–82. Supracondylar fractures. (From Abraham, E., Powers, T., Witt, P., and Ray, R.D.: Experimental hyperextension supracondylar fractures in monkeys. Clin. Orthop. 171:313, 314, 1982; reprinted by permission.)

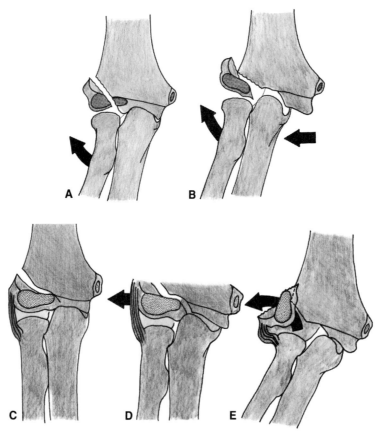

FIGURE 9–83. Lateral condyle fractures. *A*, Milch I. *B*, Milch II. *C*, Undisplaced. *D*, Displaced. *E*, Rotated. (From Tachdjian, M.O.: Pediatric Orthopaedics, 2nd ed., pp. 3109, 3110. Philadelphia, W.B. Saunders, 1990; reprinted by permission.)

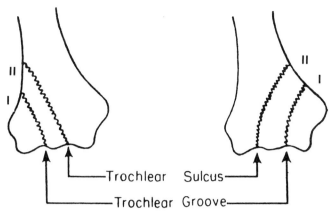

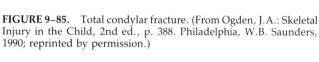

Trochlear Sulcus

Trochlear Groove

FIGURE 9–84. Milch classification of humeral condyle fractures. (Modified from Milch, H.: Fracture and fracture dislocations of the humeral condyles. J. Trauma 4:601, 1964; reprinted by permission. Copyright © 1964 by Williams & Wilkins.)

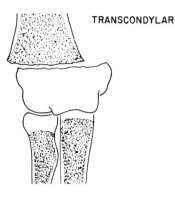

TRANSCONDYLAR

FIGURE 9–85. Total condylar fracture. (From Ogden, J.A.: Skeletal Injury in the Child, 2nd ed., p. 388. Philadelphia, W.B. Saunders, 1990; reprinted by permission.)

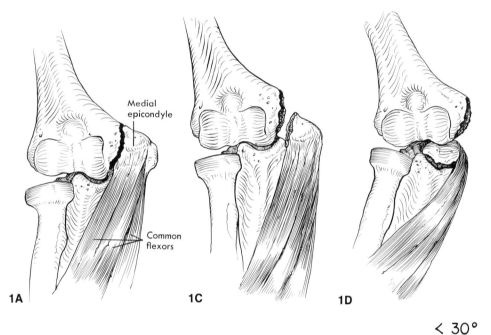

Medial epicondyle

Common flexors

1A   1C   1D

FIGURE 9–86. Medial epicondyle fractures. *IA*, Undisplaced. *IC*, Displaced. *ID*, Entrapped. (From Tachdjian, M.O.: Pediatric Orthopaedics, 2nd ed., p. 3122. Philadelphia, W.B. Saunders, 1990; reprinted by permission.)

< 30°   30°– 60°   > 60°

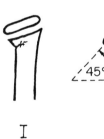

45°

I   II   III

FIGURE 9–87. Radial head fractures; type III requires primary ORIF. (From Tachdjian, M.O.: Pediatric Orthopaedics, 2nd ed., p. 3140. Philadelphia, W.B. Saunders, 1990; reprinted by permission.)

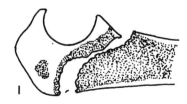

I

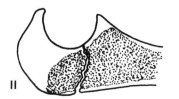

II

FIGURE 9–88. Proximal ulna fractures. (From Ogden, J.A.: Skeletal Injury in the Child, 2nd ed., p. 463. Philadelphia, W.B. Saunders, 1990; reprinted by permission.)

TABLE 9–6. PEDIATRIC TRAUMATIC ORTHOPAEDIC INJURIES (*Continued*)

INJURY	EPONYM	CLASSIFICATION	TREATMENT	COMPLICATIONS
Elbow *cont.*				
Trochlea AVN	"Fishtail"	A—lateral trochlea	Involves only internal ossification center	Early DJD, some decreased ROM
		B—entire trochlea	Involves medial and lateral centers	Cubitus varus, decreased ROM
Med. epicondylar apophysis (11 yo) (Fig. 9–86)		I—Acute injury A—undisplaced	Immobilize 1 week	Highly associated with elbow dislocation, reduce dislocation and treat Fx accordingly; ulnar N dysfunction (ORIF), valgus instability, loss of full extension (mild)
		B—minimally displaced	Immobilize 1 week	
		C—significantly displaced (± dislocation)	ORIF for valgus instability in athlete, otherwise early ROM	
		D—entrapment of fragment in joint	Manipulative extraction, ORIF (esp w/ ulnar nerve entrapment or fragment remains)	
		E—Fracture thru epicondylar apophysis	Immobilize or ORIF or excision if unstable in athlete	
	Little League elbow	II—Chronic tension stress injury	Change in throwing activities	
Lat. epicondylar apophysis (rare)			Immobilize for comfort, open reduction & excision if fragment incarcerated	
"T" condylar Fx (rare)		Based on fracture	Hanging arm cast or ORIF	Dec ROM, neurovascular complications
Radial head/neck (9–10 yo) (Fig. 9–87)		A—SH I or II physeal fracture B—SH IV fracture C—Transmetaphyseal fracture D—with elbow dislocation—reduction injury E—with elbow dislocation—dislocation injury	Immobilize if <30° angulation or <45° angulation after reduction (or 70° of pro/supination) or Fx >4 days old with angulation up to 90°; ORIF translocated, >60° primarily; ORIF if markedly displaced	Decr. ROM, radial head overgrowth, neck notching, premature physeal closure, nonunion, AVN, proximal synostosis (esp. with late treatment)
Prox. olecranon physis (rare) (Fig. 9–88)		I—physeal-metaphyseal border (younger children) II—physis with large metaphyseal fragment (older children)	ORIF if significantly displaced	Epiphyseal overgrowth, spurs (may require excision)
Olecranon metaphysis (rare)		A—flexion	If undisplaced, immobilize 3 wks; ORIF if defect	Rare: delay/nonunion, Volkmann's, ulnar N irritation
		B—extension (1—valgus, 2—varus)	Reduce (forceful manipulation in extension)	
		C—shear	Immobilize in hyperflexion, ORIF periosteal tear	
Coronoid process (rare)			Immobilize in flexion	Assoc. with elbow dislocation
Elbow dislocation (10–19 yo)		I—prox. RU intact: A—posterior (1—postmed., 2—postlat.) B—anterior C—medial D—lateral II—prox. RU divergent: A—anteroposterior B—medial-lateral (transverse)	Reduction (push off younger, pull off older patients)	Assoc. Fxs (med. epicondylar apophysis, prox. radius, coronoid), nerve injuries (ulnar > median) (median N entrapment: 1 in joint, 2 between epicondyle and condyle, 3 kinked anteriorly [Fig. 9–89]), myositis ossificans, recurrent dislocation, prox. RU translocation, OC Fx
Radial head subluxation	Nursemaid's elbow	(Stretching of annular/orbicular ligaments)	Reduce (supination, flex, snap)	Unreduced subluxations, recurrence, irreducible (rare)
Shoulder				
Humerus shaft (Fig. 9–90)		Neonate (birth injury) 0–3 yo 3–12 yo >12 yo	Small splint or splint to side Collar and cuff Velpeau Sugar tong splints	Compartment syndrome, radial N injury, rotational deformity (Ok if <12°), growth disturbance (<15 mm not noticeable)
Prox. humeral physis (Fig. 9–91)		Salter-Harris (I most common in <5 yo, II most common in older children) Neer-Horowitz (based on	Velpeau if min. displaced, gentle manipulation for displaced fractures with immobilization to side in	Growth disorders

TABLE 9–6. PEDIATRIC TRAUMATIC ORTHOPAEDIC INJURIES (*Continued*)

INJURY	EPONYM	CLASSIFICATION	TREATMENT	COMPLICATIONS
Shoulder *cont.*				
		displacement): I—<5 mm, II—<⅓ shaft, III—<⅔, IV—>⅔	younger patients, and "salute" position in older children ± PCP; ORIF <50% opposition, >45° angulation	
Prox. physis stress Fx	LL shoulder	Stress fracture	Activity modification	
Prox. humeral metaphysis		(Common), based on location	Sling and swathe/Velpeau	
Midshaft clavicle		0–2 yo	Supportive, bind to side if symptomatic	Rare: neurovascular injury, mal/nonunion
		>2 yo	Figure of 8 dressing for 3 wks	
Med. clavicle (rare)		Usually SH I or II physeal separations	Sling for 1 wk	Rare
Lat. clavicle		I—nondisplaced, intact AC and CC ligaments IIA—clavicle displaced sup., Fx med. to CC ligament IIB—clavicle displaced sup., conoid ligament tear III—fracture into AC joint	Figure of 8 dressing; some recommend ORIF of Type II injuries	
AC joint (Fig. 9–92)		I—Sprain II—Partial tear dorsal periosteal tube III—Large tear of dorsal tube, sup. displacement IV—Clavicle displaced posteriorly V—Clavicle displaced significantly sup. VI—Inferior dislocation of clavicle	Types I, II, & III, closed treatment Closed reduction, open if required Open reduction, repair and reconstruction Open reduction may be required	Coracoid fracture (treated nonoperatively)
SC joint		Anterior Posterior	Sling/reassurance Acute—reduce, chronic/leave alone	
Clavicle dislocation (rare)			Open reduction with repair of periosteal tube	
Scapula fractures		Based on location	Treatment similar to adult fractures	
Glenohumeral dislocation		Traumatic vs. atraumatic	Rehabilitation; reconstruction for unstable posttraumatic shoulders after 6 mos of rehab	
Spine Fractures				
C2–C3 laxity	Pseudosubluxation	<4 mm translation in child <7 yo	None—normal variant	
Occiput–C1 lesions			Reduced with traction, craniovertebral fusion later	Often fatal injuries
C1–C2 lesions		Traumatic ligament disruption	Reduce in extension, immobilize (Minerva or halo) 8–12 wks	Vertebral A—risk with surgery
	Grisel's syndrome	Ligament laxity from local inflammation Rotatory (I—w/o C1 shift, II—<5 mm C1 ant. shift, III—>5 mm C1 ant. shift, IV—post. shift (Fig. 9–93) Odontoid—physeal or os odontoideum	Traction, immobilize (Minerva) 6–8 wks I—soft collar, II, III & IV—Traction + immobilization 6 wks C1–C2 fusion ant. esp. w/ recurrence/neuro Sx Reduce (hyperextension), immobilize (Minerva) 12 wks	Vertebral A—risk with surgery
C2–C3 dislocation		True vs. pseudo more likely with trauma history, PLL ossification, chip Fxs, and failure to correct with extension		

(*continued*)

Type 1   Type 2   Type 3

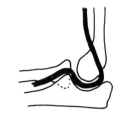
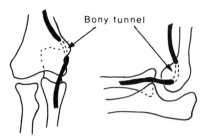
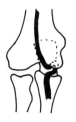
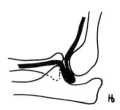

Bony tunnel

FIGURE 9–89. Median nerve entrapment. (From Hallett, J.: Entrapment of the median nerve after dislocation of the elbow. J. Bone Joint Surg. [Br.] 63:410, 1981; reprinted by permission.)

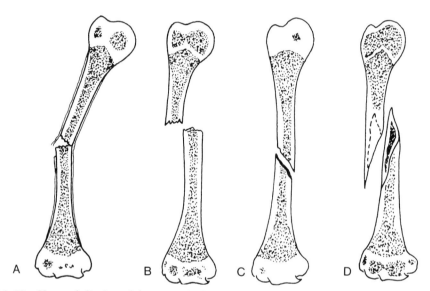

A   B   C   D

FIGURE 9–90. Humeral diaphyseal fractures. *A*, Transverse, periosteum intact. *B*, Transverse, periosteum ruptured. *C*, Oblique. *D*, Spiral. (From Ogden, J.A.: Skeletal Injury in the Child, 2nd ed., p. 367. Philadelphia, W.B. Saunders, 1990; reprinted by permission.)

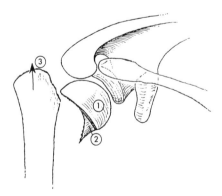

FIGURE 9–91. Proximal humeral epicondylar fracture (SH II); note superior displacement of humeral shaft. (From Connolly, J.F., ed.: Depalma's The Management of Fractures and Dislocations, an Atlas, 3rd ed., p. 458. Philadelphia, W.B. Saunders, 1981; reprinted by permission.)

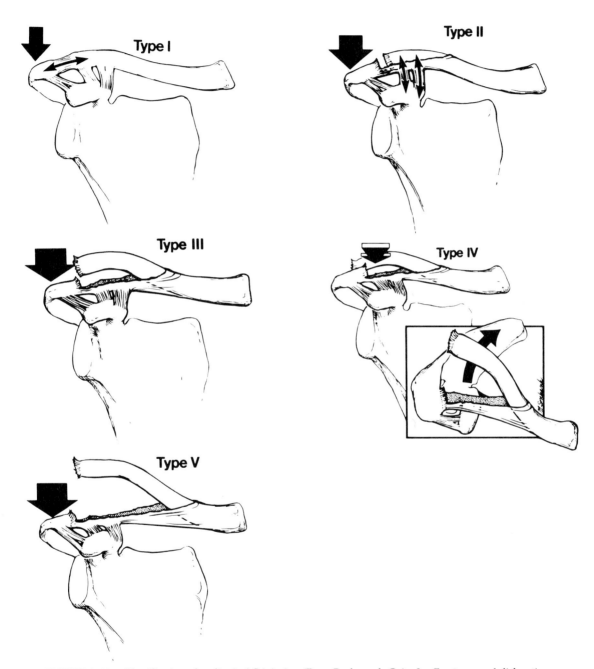

FIGURE 9–92. Classification of pediatric AC injuries. (From Rockwood, C.A., Jr.: Fractures and dislocations of the ends of the clavicle, scapula, and glenohumeral joint. In Fractures in Children, Rockwood, C.A., Jr., Wilkins, K.E., and King, R.E., eds., 2nd ed., p. 636. Philadelphia, J.B. Lippincott, 1984; reprinted by permission.)

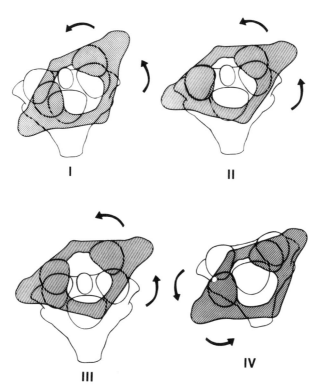

FIGURE 9–93. Atlantoaxial rotatory displacement. *I*, No shift. *II*, Shift <5 mm. *III*, Shift >5 mm. *IV*, Post shift. (From Bailey, D.K.: Normal cervical spine in infants and children. Radiology 59:37, 1952; reprinted by permission.)

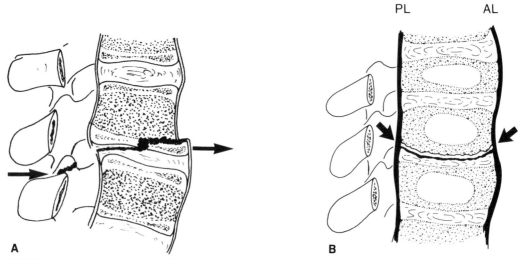

FIGURE 9–94. Classification of pediatric spine fractures. *Left*, Unstable SH III. *Right*, Stable SH I. (From Ogden, J.A.: Skeletal Injury in the Child, 2nd ed., p. 599. Philadelphia, W.B. Saunders, 1990; reprinted by permission.)

TABLE 9–6. PEDIATRIC TRAUMATIC ORTHOPAEDIC INJURIES (*Continued*)

INJURY	EPONYM	CLASSIFICATION	TREATMENT	COMPLICATIONS
Spine Fractures *cont.*				
T&L fractures (Fig. 9–94)		Compression fractures Unstable fractures	Bed rest/symptomatic Treated like adults	Neurologic injuries
Kyphosis	Scheurmann's disease	3 adjacent vertebrae with >5° wedging	Milwakee bracing occasionally indicated	
Spondolysis		Stress Fx of pars (L5–S1)	Acute—immobilize, conservative otherwise, L4–S1 fusion in refractory cases	
SCIWORA		(Spinal cord injury without radiographic abnormality)	Evaluation with MRI and appropriate treatment	Scoliosis (esp. <8 yo)
Pelvic Fractures				
Pelvic Fxs (Figs. 9–95, 9–96, and 9–97)		Key & Conwell: I—ring Intact: Avulsion (ASIS—sartorius; AIIS—rectus; IT—hamstring)	BR flexed hip 2 wks, guarded WB 4 wks	In general less than adults, includes loss of reduction, delayed/non-union, DJD, malunion, problems with organ injury (vs adult)
	Duverney	*Pubis/ischium	BR 3–7 days, limited WB 4 wks	Asymmetric ossification is not a Fx
		Iliac wing	BR leg abducted, progress to graudal WB	
		Sacrum/coccyx II—single break in ring: *Ipsilateral ramii	BR 3–6 Wks if severe (sacral) BR 2–4 wks, non–weight bearing	Sacral N injury
		Symphysis pubis SI joint (rare) III—double break in ring:	BR with sling or spica cast BR, progress to guarded WB	Often unstable with associated injuries
	Straddle Malgaigne	Bilateral pubic fractures Ant. & post. ring with migration Severe multiple fractures	BR flexed hip 4–6 wks Skeletal traction, pelvic sling 3–6 wks, avoid compression Treatment on a case-by-case basis	LLD with vertical shear
		IV—acetabular fractures: Small fragment w/ dis-location (post. ≥ ant.)	BR, progress to guarded ambulation	
		Linear—nondisplaced Linear—hip unstable	Treat associated pelvic fracture Skeletal traction, ORIF if incongruous	
		Central	Lateral traction, ORIF severe	Heterotopic ossification especially w/ ORIF
Hip Fractures				
Hip Fxs (Fig. 9–98)		Delbet: IA—transepiphyseal w/ dislocation IB—transepiphyseal w/o dislocation II—*transcervical IIIA—cervical trochanteric, displaced IIIB—cervical trochanteric, nondisplaced IV—intertrochanteric	Closed reduction or ORIF and pin Closed reduction and pin Closed reduction and pin Closed reduction and pin Abduction spica cast Traction and abduction spica, ORIF unstable	AVN in up to 40% (higher in more proximal Fxs, related to displacement, 100% in IA) Ratliff classification of AVN: I—complete, II—physeal, III—neck only (Fig. 9–99); Coxa vara (25%—osteotomy if severe); nonunion (6%, treat w/ subtrochanteric valgus osteotomy); growth arrest
Femoral neck stress Fx		Devas: Superior transverse Inferior (compressive)	Pin (displaces otherwise) NWB	Displacement causes incr. complications; varus deformities
Traumatic dislocation (Fig. 9–100)		*Posterior Anterior	Closed reduction (Stimson), open if incongrus after two attempts at closed reduction, greater trochenteric Fxs common	AVN (10%), recurrent dislocation, myositis ossificans, DJD
Femoral Shaft Fractures				
Femur Fx		0–2 years old 2–10 years old	Spica cast Spica cast if <2 cm override; split Russel >2 cm	*LLD, angular deformity (avoid >10° frontal and >30° sagittal malalignment,

(*continued*)

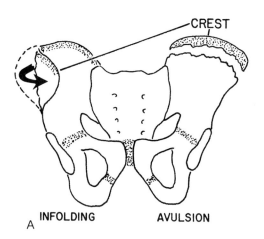

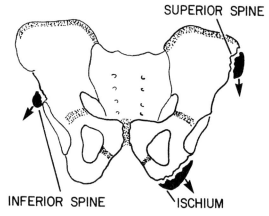

FIGURE 9–95. Avulsion fractures of the pelvis. Superior spine, sartorius avulsion; inferior spine, rectus avulsion; ischium, hamstring avulsion. (From Ogden, J.A.: Skeletal Injury in the Child, 2nd ed., p. 635. Philadelphia, W.B. Saunders, 1990; reprinted by permission.)

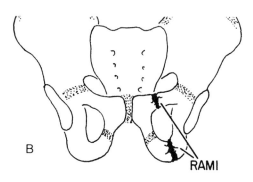

FIGURE 9–96. Stable pelvic fractures. (From Ogden, J.A.: Skeletal Injury in the Child, 2nd ed., p. 634. Philadelphia, W.B. Saunders, 1990; reprinted by permission.)

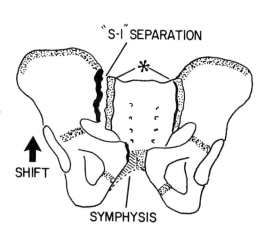

FIGURE 9–97. Unstable pelvic fracture. (From Ogden, J.A.: Skeletal Injury in the Child, 2nd ed., p. 634. Philadelphia, W.B. Saunders, 1990; reprinted by permission.)

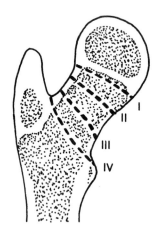

FIGURE 9–98. Femoral neck fractures in children. *I,* Transepiphyseal. *II,* Transcervical. *III,* Cervical-trochanteric. *IV,* Intertrochanteric. (From Ogden, J.A.: Skeletal Injury in the Child, 2nd ed., p. 689. Philadelphia, W.B. Saunders, 1990; reprinted by permission.)

FIGURE 9–99. Patterns of avascular necrosis in children following hip fractures (Ratliff). *I,* Complete. *II,* Physeal. *III,* Neck. (From Ogden, J.A.: Skeletal Injury in the Child, 2nd ed., p. 701. Philadelphia, W.B. Saunders, 1990; reprinted by permission.)

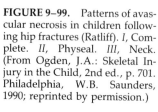
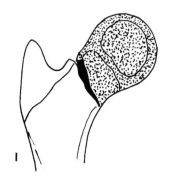
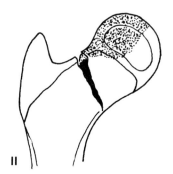
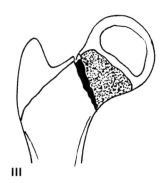

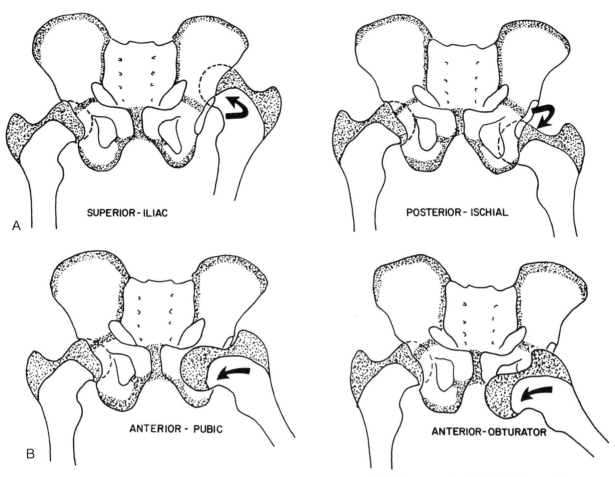

FIGURE 9–100. Hip dislocations in children. (From Ogden, J.A.: Skeletal Injury in the Child, 2nd ed., p. 663. Philadelphia, W.B. Saunders, 1990; reprinted by permission.)

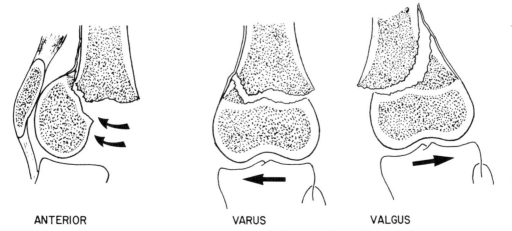

FIGURE 9–101. Distal femoral physeal fractures. (From Ogden, J.A.: Skeletal Injury in the Child, 2nd ed., p. 725. Philadelphia, W.B. Saunders, 1990; reprinted by permission.)

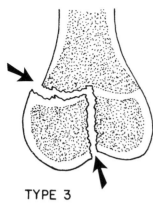

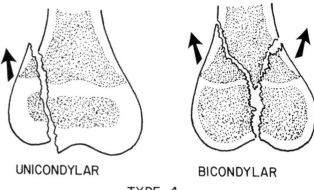

FIGURE 9–102. Distal femoral Salter-Harris III fracture. (From Ogden, J.A.: Skeletal Injury in the Child, 2nd ed., p. 727. Philadelphia, W.B. Saunders, 1990; reprinted by permission.)

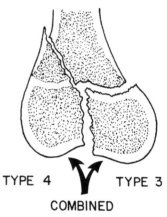

FIGURE 9–104. Salter-Harris III and IV fractures of the distal femur. (From Ogden, J.A.: Skeletal Injury in the Child, 2nd ed., p. 729. Philadelphia, W.B. Saunders, 1990; reprinted by permission.)

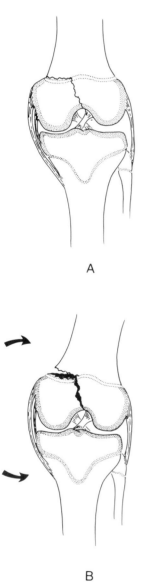

FIGURE 9–103. Stress test used to diagnose subtle fractures about the knee. (From Ogden, J.A.: Skeletal Injury in the Child, 2nd ed., p. 728. Philadelphia, W.B. Saunders, 1990; reprinted by permission.)

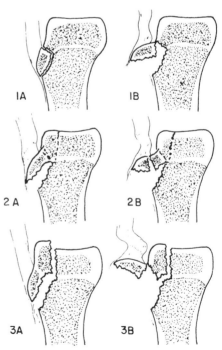

FIGURE 9–105. Fractures of the tibial tuberosity. (From Ogden, J.A.: Skeletal Injury in the Child, 2nd ed., p. 808. Philadelphia, W.B. Saunders, 1990; reprinted by permission.)

TABLE 9–6. PEDIATRIC TRAUMATIC ORTHOPAEDIC INJURIES (*Continued*)

INJURY	EPONYM	CLASSIFICATION	TREATMENT	COMPLICATIONS
Femoral Shaft Fractures *cont.*				
		10–15 years old >15 years old	90–90 skeletal traction IM rod Consider IM rod or external fixatioin in younger children with CHI	rotational deformity (>10°), ischemia, SMA syndrome (with casting)
Subtrochlear		Based on anatomic location	90–90 traction ORIF w/head injury (can't control)	LLD
Knee Injuries				
Distal femoral epiphysis separation (Figs. 9–101, 9–102, 9–103, 9–104)	"Wagon Wheel"	SH I–IV (*II) or based on displacement or based on child's age	Closed reduction → LLC, PCP in SH III or IV; Open only for soft tissue interposition	Popliteal A or Peroneal N injury, recurrent displacement, growth plate injuries (angulation and shortening)
Proximal tibial epiphysis fracture		SH I–IV (*II)	Nondisplaced: LLC in 30° flexion; displaced: closed reduction, PCP	Popliteal A injury, growth plate injuries
Floating knee		Letts: A—both fractures diaphyseal	ORIF 1, closed reduction other	Infection, nonunion, malunion, growth arrest
		B—1 fracture diaphyseal, 1 metaphyseal	ORIF diaphyseal, closed reduction metaphyseal	
		C—1 fracture diaphyseal, 1 epiphyseal	Closed reduction & pin epiphyseal, closed traction diaphyseal	
		D—1 fracture open, 1 fracture closed	Débride/external fixation open, closed treatment closed Fx	
		E—both fractures open	Débride/external fixation or traction for both	

Tibial tubercle avulsion		Ogden (Fig. 9–105):
		   1—Small distal piece fractured
		   2—Fx junction of 1° and 2° oss centers
		   3—Fx thru 1 epiphysis (SH III)
			Small fragment, min. displaced with full extension—cast; ORIF all other fractures	Genu recurvatum, decr. ROM, prominence, patella alta

Osteochondral Fxs		Kennedy & Smillie:
		   Med. femoral condyle exogenous or endogenous
		   Lat. femoral condyle exogenous or endogenous
		   Patella (med.) endogenous (dislocation)
			Operative—remove small fragments, attempt ORIF large fragments (Steiman pin in condyles, small screws in patella [remove at 3 mos]).	Recurrent patella dislocation, DJD

Intercondylar eminence tibia (Fig. 9–106)		Meyers & McKeever:
		   I—incomplete/nondisplaced
		   II—hinged (posterior rim intact)
		   III—completely displaced (supinated & rotated)
			Attempt closed reduction in all (with extension); ORIF for soft tissue interposition	Decr. extension (if not completely reduced), MCL or meniscal injury, postop complications

Patella		Undisplaced	Aspiration, cylinder cast (<5° flexion)	Patella alta, extensor lag, quadriceps atrophy, infection
		Displaced transverse "Sleeve" Fx (avulsion of distal Pole & articular cartilage) (Fig. 9–107)	ORIF tension band ORIF tension band	
Marginal fractures			Excision, ORIF if involves articular surface	
Knee Dislocations and Ligamentous Injuries				
Ligament injuries		Based on ligament and location	Stress radiographs, primary repair	Instability; heterotopic bone & other complications with open repair
Patella osteochondrosis	Sinding-Larsen-Johansson	Acute	Cylinder cast in extension 3–4 wks	Patella alta, distal pole prominence
		Chronic	Activity limitation, quadriceps/hamstring stent	

(*continued*)

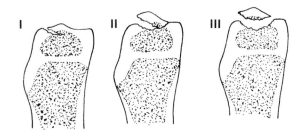

FIGURE 9–106. Tibial spine fractures. (From Ogden, J.A.: Skeletal Injury in the Child, 2nd ed., p. 796. Philadelphia, W.B. Saunders, 1990; reprinted by permission.)

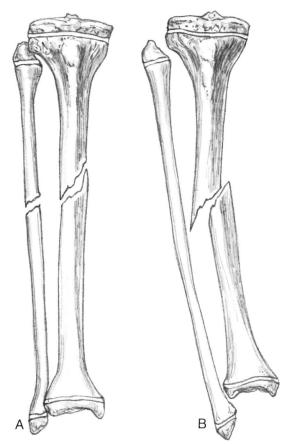

FIGURE 9–108. Spiral fracture of the tibia. Note deforming influence of intact fibula (B). (From Tachdjian, M.O.: Pediatric Orthopaedics, 2nd ed., p. 3296. Philadelphia, W.B. Saunders, 1990; reprinted by permission.)

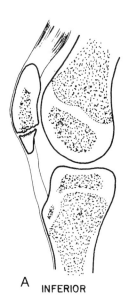

A INFERIOR

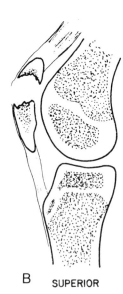

B SUPERIOR

FIGURE 9–107. Patellar sleeve fractures. (From Ogden, J.A.: Skeletal Injury in the Child, 2nd ed., p. 762. Philadelphia, W.B. Saunders, 1990; reprinted by permission.)

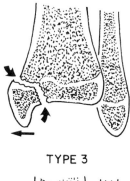

TYPE 3

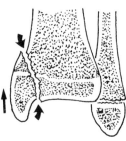

TYPE 4

SUPINATION-INVERSION

FIGURE 9–109. Supination-inversion ankle fracture. (From Ogden, J.A.: Skeletal Injury in the Child, 2nd ed., p. 837. Philadelphia, W.B. Saunders, 1990; reprinted by permission.)

292

TABLE 9–6. PEDIATRIC TRAUMATIC ORTHOPAEDIC INJURIES (*Continued*)

INJURY	EPONYM	CLASSIFICATION	TREATMENT	COMPLICATIONS
Knee Dislocations *cont.*				
Tibial tuberosity osteochondrosis	Osgood-Schlatter	Woolfry & Chandler radiographic changes: I—irregular, II—irregular & small ossicle, III—normal tubercle with free ossicle	Activity limitation or immobilization Excision of ununited ossicles at maturity	
Meniscal injury		Based on injury	Arthroscopic examination & repair	DJD
Discoid meniscus		Intact or torn	Most favor leaving intact; resect only if torn	
Femorotibial dislocations		Femorotibial (rare)	Like adult, arteriogram	Popliteal A injury
Patella dislocations		Patella-intra-articular dislocation	Closed reduction, cast 3–6 wks, open if fragment	Predisposition: Down's, MD, arthrogryposis, neurologic disorders
Tibiofibular dislocations		Prox. tibiofibular joint dislocation	Intra-articular	Clicking, instability, peroneal neuropathy
Tibia-Fibula				
Tibia-Fibula	Greenstick	Incomplete	LLC slight flexion—8–10 wks	Angular deformity G. valgus (don't accept >10° AP or >5° V/V)
		Complete	Closed reduction and cast	LLD, malrotation, delayed/nonunion, vascular injury
Tibial Spiral (Fig. 9–108)	Toddler's	Spiral tibial Fx in child <6 yo	LLC 3–4 wks	
Bike spoke injury		Soft tissue disruption	Admit, observe, débride	
Stress Fx		Usually involves upper ⅓ of tibia	Bone scan helpful, activity restriction	
Prox. tibial metaphysis	Cozen's	Greenstick in 3–6-yo, complete older	LLC in varus 6 wks	Arterial injury, valgus deformity (usually self-correcting, varus osteotomy if >10 yo), physeal injury
Distal tibial metaphysis		Usually greenstick	Closed reduction, LLC	
Ankle and Foot Injuries				
Ankle fractures		Dias & Tachdijian: *SI I—Fx of distal fibular physis (Fig. 9–109)	Reduce with foot eversion—SLWC	Angular deformity, bony bridge, LLD, DJD, rotational deformity, AVN
		SI II—SI I + SH III or IV of Tib Physis	ORIF, transepiphyseal	
		PEER—SH II w/ lat. metaphyseal fragment + high fibular Fx (Fig. 9–110)		
		SER I—SH II with ant. metaphyseal fragment (Fig. 9–111)	Closed reduction, LLC 3 wks, SLC 3 wks	
		SER II—SER I + spiral Fx fibula	Open reduction if not acceptable	
		SPF—SH II ant. metaphyseal fragment (Fig. 9–112)		
	Axial compression	SH V of distal tibia	Seen late	Growth arrest, AVN of epiphysis
	Juvenile Tillaux (Fig. 9–113)	SH III of lat. tibial physis	Closed reduction, cast (S, IR), open if required	Missed triplane Fx
	Wagstaff	SH III of distal fibular physis	Closed reduction cast (S, IR), open if required	
	Triplane (Fig. 9–114)	SH III tibia ant.-lat. + SH IV post.-med. + SH I	ORIF fixing all 3 fragments (internally rotate to reduce, fix metaphysis then epiphysis)	

(continued)

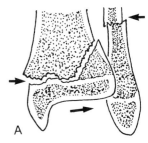

FIGURE 9–110. Pronation-eversion–external rotation ankle fracture. (From Ogden, J.A.: Skeletal Injury in the Child, 2nd ed., p. 836. Philadelphia, W.B. Saunders, 1990; reprinted by permission.)

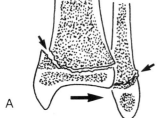

FIGURE 9–111. Supination–external rotation ankle fracture. (From Ogden, J.A.: Skeletal Injury in the Child, 2nd ed., p. 835. Philadelphia, W.B. Saunders, 1990; reprinted by permission.)

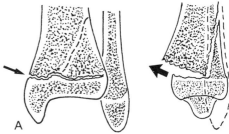
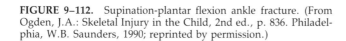

FIGURE 9–112. Supination-plantar flexion ankle fracture. (From Ogden, J.A.: Skeletal Injury in the Child, 2nd ed., p. 836. Philadelphia, W.B. Saunders, 1990; reprinted by permission.)

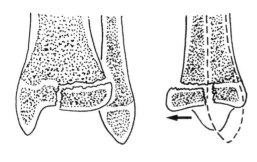
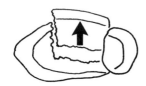

FIGURE 9–113. Juvenile Tillaux fracture. (From Ogden, J.A.: Skeletal Injury in the Child, 2nd ed., p. 838. Philadelphia, W.B. Saunders, 1990; reprinted by permission.)

TYPE 3 - FRACTURE OF TILLAUX

TABLE 9–6. PEDIATRIC TRAUMATIC ORTHOPAEDIC INJURIES (*Continued*)

INJURY	EPONYM	CLASSIFICATION	TREATMENT	COMPLICATIONS
Knee Dislocations *cont.*				
Tibial tuberosity osteochondrosis	Osgood-Schlatter	Woolfry & Chandler radiographic changes: I—irregular, II—irregular & small ossicle, III—normal tubercle with free ossicle	Activity limitation or immobilization Excision of ununited ossicles at maturity	
Meniscal injury		Based on injury	Arthroscopic examination & repair	DJD
Discoid meniscus		Intact or torn	Most favor leaving intact; resect only if torn	
Femorotibial dislocations		Femorotibial (rare)	Like adult, arteriogram	Popliteal A injury
Patella dislocations		Patella-intra-articular dislocation	Closed reduction, cast 3–6 wks, open if fragment	Predisposition: Down's, MD, arthrogryposis, neurologic disorders
Tibiofibular dislocations		Prox. tibiofibular joint dislocation	Intra-articular	Clicking, instability, peroneal neuropathy
Tibia-Fibula				
Tibia-Fibula	Greenstick	Incomplete	LLC slight flexion—8–10 wks	Angular deformity G. valgus (don't accept >10° AP or >5° V/V)
		Complete	Closed reduction and cast	LLD, malrotation, delayed/nonunion, vascular injury
Tibial Spiral (Fig. 9–108)	Toddler's	Spiral tibial Fx in child <6 yo	LLC 3–4 wks	
Bike spoke injury		Soft tissue disruption	Admit, observe, débride	
Stress Fx		Usually involves upper ⅓ of tibia	Bone scan helpful, activity restriction	
Prox. tibial metaphysis	Cozen's	Greenstick in 3–6-yo, complete older	LLC in varus 6 wks	Arterial injury, valgus deformity (usually self-correcting, varus osteotomy if >10 yo), physeal injury
Distal tibial metaphysis		Usually greenstick	Closed reduction, LLC	
Ankle and Foot Injuries				
Ankle fractures		Dias & Tachdijian: *SI I—Fx of distal fibular physis (Fig. 9–109)	Reduce with foot eversion—SLWC	Angular deformity, bony bridge, LLD, DJD, rotational deformity, AVN
		SI II—SI I + SH III or IV of Tib Physis PEER—SH II w/ lat. metaphyseal fragment + high fibular Fx (Fig. 9–110)	ORIF, transepiphyseal	
		SER I—SH II with ant. metaphyseal fragment (Fig. 9–111)	Closed reduction, LLC 3 wks, SLC 3 wks	
		SER II—SER I + spiral Fx fibula SPF—SH II ant. metaphyseal fragment (Fig. 9–112)	Open reduction if not acceptable	
	Axial compression	SH V of distal tibia	Seen late	Growth arrest, AVN of epiphysis
	Juvenile Tillaux (Fig. 9–113)	SH III of lat. tibial physis	Closed reduction, cast (S, IR), open if required	Missed triplane Fx
	Wagstaff	SH III of distal fibular physis	Closed reduction cast (S, IR), open if required	
	Triplane (Fig. 9–114)	SH III tibia ant.-lat. + SH IV post.-med. + SH I	ORIF fixing all 3 fragments (internally rotate to reduce, fix metaphysis then epiphysis)	

(*continued*)

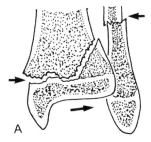

FIGURE 9–110. Pronation-eversion–external rotation ankle fracture. (From Ogden, J.A.: Skeletal Injury in the Child, 2nd ed., p. 836. Philadelphia, W.B. Saunders, 1990; reprinted by permission.)

TYPE 2
PRONATION – EVERSION

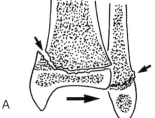

FIGURE 9–111. Supination–external rotation ankle fracture. (From Ogden, J.A.: Skeletal Injury in the Child, 2nd ed., p. 835. Philadelphia, W.B. Saunders, 1990; reprinted by permission.)

TYPE 2
SUPINATION-EXTERNAL ROTATION

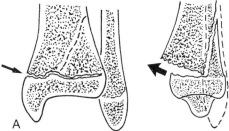

FIGURE 9–112. Supination-plantar flexion ankle fracture. (From Ogden, J.A.: Skeletal Injury in the Child, 2nd ed., p. 836. Philadelphia, W.B. Saunders, 1990; reprinted by permission.)

TYPE 2
SUPINATION – PLANTAR FLEXION

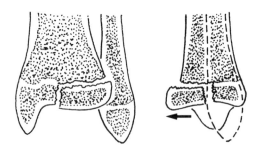

FIGURE 9–113. Juvenile Tillaux fracture. (From Ogden, J.A.: Skeletal Injury in the Child, 2nd ed., p. 838. Philadelphia, W.B. Saunders, 1990; reprinted by permission.)

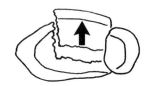

TYPE 3 - FRACTURE OF TILLAUX

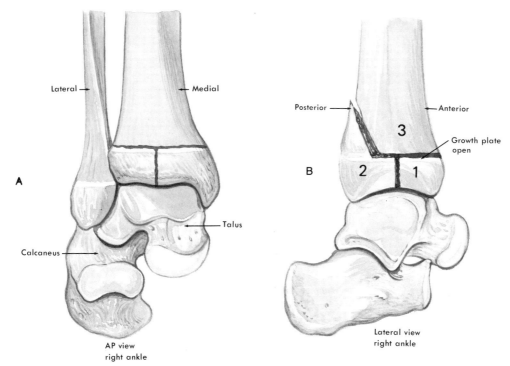

FIGURE 9–114. Triplane fracture. (From Tachdjian, M.O.: Pediatric Orthopaedics, 2nd ed., p. 3324. Philadelphia, W.B. Saunders, 1990; reprinted by permission.)

TABLE 9–6. PEDIATRIC TRAUMATIC ORTHOPAEDIC INJURIES (*Continued*)

INJURY	EPONYM	CLASSIFICATION	TREATMENT	COMPLICATIONS
Ankle & Foot *cont.*				
Isolated distal fibula		SH	Anatomic reduction, axial screw	Failure to recognize, DJD
Talar Fxs		Talar neck	Closed reduction, cast in PF, open >5 mm or 5° displacement	AVN (Hawkins sign = good prognosis)
		Talar dome—osteochondral Fx	Open esp. if lat.; excise small, ORIF large fragments	
Calcaneus	Essex-Lopresti	Intra-articular (tongue or joint dep)	NWB, nonoperative traction	
		Extra-articular	Nonoperative	
Tarsometatarsal		Fx at base of 2MT + cuboid Fx	Closed reduction, PCT if unstable	
MT Fxs		Location	Most treated closed	
Base of 5MT	Jones Pseudo-Jones	Metaphyseal Avulsion of PB	SLC, ORIF ± bone graft nonunion SLC or postop shoe	Increased incidence of nonunion
Navicular ostchondrosis	Kohler's	Navicular	Symptomatic	

* Most common
Abbreviations: SCIWORA, spinal cord injury without radiologic abnormality; BR, bed rest; LLD, leg length discrepancy.

Selected Bibliography

Akbarnia, B., Torg, J.S., Kirkpatrick, J., and Sussman, S.: Manifestations of the battered-child syndrome. J. Bone Joint Surg. [Am.] 56:1159–1166, 1974.

Allen, B.L., Jr., Ferguson, R.L., Lehmann, T.R., and O'Brien, R.P.: A mechanistic classification of closed, indirect fractures and dislocations of the lower cervical spine. Spine 7:1–27, 1982.

Amato, J.J., Rhinelander, H.F., and Cleveland, R.J.: Post-traumatic adult respiratory distress syndrome. Orthop. Clin. North Am. 9:693–713, 1978.

AO Course, Principles of Internal Fixation of Fractures. Monterey, California, 1989.

Arneson, T.J., Melton, L.J., III, Lewallen, D.G., et al.: Epidemiology of diaphyseal and distal femoral fractures in Rochester, Minnesota, 1965–1984. Clin. Orthop. 234:188–194, 1988.

Berquist, T.H., ed.: Imaging of Orthopedic Trauma and Surgery. Philadelphia, W.B. Saunders Company, 1986.

Blick, S.S., Brumback, R.J., Poka, A., et al.: Compartment syndrome in open tibia fractures. J. Bone Joint Surg. [Am.] 68:1348–1353, 1986.

Bohler, J.: Anterior stabilization for acute fractures and non-unions of the dens. J. Bone Joint Surg. [Am.] 64:18–27, 1982.

Bohlman, H.H.: Acute fractures and dislocations of the cervical spine: An analysis of three hundred hospitalized patients and review of the literature. J. Bone Joint Surg. [Am.] 61:1119–1142, 1979.

Bohlman, H.H.: Treatment of fractures and dislocations of the thoracic and lumbar spine. J. Bone Joint Surg. [Am.] 67:165–169, 1985.

Bone, L., and Bucholz, R.: The management of fractures in the patient with multiple trauma. J. Bone Joint Surg. [Am.] 68:945–949, 1986.

Bone, L.B., Johnson, K.D., Weigelt, J., et al.: Early versus delayed stabilization of femoral fractures. A prospective randomized study. J. Bone Joint Surg. [Am.] 71:336, 1989.

Bosse, M.J., Poka, A., Reinert, C.M., et al.: Heterotopic ossification as a complication of acetabular fracture: Prophylaxis with low-dose irradiation. J. Bone Joint Surg. [Am.] 70:1231–1237, 1988.

Bradford, D.S., and McBride, G.G.: Surgical management of thoracolumbar spine fractures in incomplete neurologic deficits. Clin. Orthop. 218:201–216, 1987.

Bradway, J.K., Amadio, P.C., and Cooney, W.P.: Open reduction and internal fixation of displaced, comminuted intra-articular fractures of the distal end of the radius. J. Bone Joint Surg. [Am.] 71:839, 1989.

Bright, R.W.: Partial growth arrest: Identification, classification, and results of treatment. Orthop. Trans. 6:65–66, 1982.

Brighton, C.T.: Current concepts review. The treatment of nonunions with electricity. J. Bone Joint Surg. [Am.] 63:847–851, 1981.

Broberg, M.A., and Morrey, B.F.: Results of delayed excision of the radial head after fracture. J. Bone Joint Surg. [Am.] 68:669–674, 1986.

Bryan, W.J., and Tullos, H.S.: Pediatric pelvic fractures: Review of 52 patients. J. Trauma 19:799–805, 1979.

Bucholz, R.W.: The pathologic anatomy of Malgaigne fracture-dislocations of the pelvis. J. Bone Joint Surg. [Am.] 63:400–404, 1981.

Cain, J.E., Jr., Shepler, T.R., and Nelson, M.R.: Hematometacarpal fracture–dislocation classification and treatment. J. Hand Surg. 12A:762–767, 1987.

Canale, S.T.: Traumatic dislocation and fracture-dislocation of the hips in children. In The Hip—Proceedings of the Ninth Open Scientific Meeting of the Hip Society, pp. 219–245. St. Louis, C.V. Mosby, 1981.

Canale, S.T., and Kelly, F.B.: Fractures of the neck of the talus. J. Bone Joint Surg. [Am.] 60:143–156, 1978.

Chapman, M.W., ed.: Operative Orthopaedics. Philadelphia, J.B. Lippincott, 1988.

Chapman, M.W., Gordon, J.E., and Zissimos, A.G.: Compression-plate fixation of acute fractures of the diaphyses of the radius and ulna. J. Bone Joint Surg. [Am.] 71:159, 1989.

Cierny, G., III, Byrd, H.S., and Jones, R.E.: Primary versus delayed soft tissue coverage for severe open tibial fractures: A comparison of results. Clin. Orthop. 178:54–63, 1983.

Connolly, J.F., ed.: Depalma's The Management of Fractures and Dislocations, An Atlas, 3rd ed. Philadelphia, W.B. Saunders, 1981.

DeLee, J.C., and Curtis, R.: Subtalar dislocation of the foot. J. Bone Joint Surg. [Am.] 64:433–437, 1982.

DeLee, J.C., and Stiehl, J.B.: Open tibia fracture with compartment syndrome. Clin. Orthop. 160:175–184, 1981.

DeLuca, P.A., Lindsey, R.W., and Ruwe, P.A.: Refracture of bones in the forearm after removal of compression plates. J. Bone Joint Surg. [Am.] 70:1372–1376, 1988.

Denis, F.: The three column spine and its significance in the classification of acute thoracolumbar spinal injuries. Spine 8:817–831, 1983.

Denis, F.: Updated classification of thoracolumbar fractures. Orthop. Trans. 6:8, 1982.

Denis, F., Davis, S., and Comfort, T.: Sacral fractures: An important problem. Retrospective analysis of 236 cases. Clin. Orthop. 227:67–81, 1988.

Drummond, D., Guadagni, J., Keene, J.S., Breed, A., and Narechania, R.: Interspinous process segmental spinal instrumentation. J. Pediatr. Orthop. 4:397–404, 1984.

Epstein, H.C.: Traumatic Dislocation of the Hip. Baltimore, Williams & Wilkins, 1980.

Epstein, H.C., Wiss, D.A., and Cozen, L.: Posterior fracture dislocation of the hip with fractures of the femoral head. Clin. Orthop. 201:9–17, 1985.

Ertl, J.P., Barrack, R.L., Alexander, A.H., and VanBuecken, K.: Triplane fracture of the distal tibial epiphysis. Long term follow-up. J. Bone Joint Surg. [Am.] 70:967, 1988.

Faciszewski, T., Burks, R.T., and Manaster, B.J.: Subtle injuries of the Lisfranc joint. J. Bone Joint Surg. [Am.] 72:1519, 1990.

Fernandez, D.L.: Anterior approach to the knee with osteotomy of the tibial tubercle for bicondylar tibial fractures. J. Bone Joint Surg. [Am.] 70:208–219, 1988.

Fielding, J.W., and Hawkins, R.J.: Atlanto-axial rotatory fixation (fixed rotatory subluxation of the atlanto-axial joint). J. Bone Joint Surg. [Am.] 59:37–44, 1977.

Foster, D.E., Sullivan, J.A., and Gross, R.H.: Lateral humeral condylar fractures in children. J. Pediatr. Orthop. 5:16–22, 1985.

Fowles, J.V., and Kassab, M.T.: Displaced fractures of the medial humeral condyle in children. J. Bone Joint Surg. [Am.] 62:1159–1163, 1980.

Fowles, J.V., Sliman, N., and Kassab, M.T.: The Monteggia lesion in children: Fracture of the ulna and dislocation of the radial head. J. Bone Joint Surg. [Am.] 65:1276–1283, 1983.

Galleno, H., and Oppenheim, W.L.: The battered child syndrome revisited. Clin. Orthop. 162:11–19, 1982.

Gelberman, R.H., Garfin, S.R., Hergenroeder, P.T., Mubarak, S.J., and Menon, J.: Compartment syndromes of the forearm: Diagnosis and treatment. Clin. Orthop. 161:252–261, 1981.

Gelman, M.I.: Radiology of Orthopedic Procedures, Problems and Complications, Vol. 24. Philadelphia, W.B. Saunders, 1984.

Giachino, A.A., and Uhthoff, H.K.: Current concepts review. Intra-articular fractures of the calcaneus. J. Bone Joint Surg. [Am.] 71:784, 1989.

Godina, M.: Early microsurgical reconstruction of complex trauma of the extremities. Plast. Reconstr. Surg. 78:285–292, 1986.

Goossens, M., and De Stoop, N.: Lisfranc's fracture-dislocations: Etiology, radiology, and results of treatment; A review of 20 cases. Clin. Orthop. 176:154–162, 1983.

Gossling, H.R., and Pellegrini, V.D., Jr.: Fat embolism syndrome: A review of the pathophysiology and physiological basis of treatment. Clin. Orthop. 165:68–82, 1982.

Grace, T.G., and Eversmann, W.W.: Forearm fractures. J. Bone Joint Surg. [Am.] 62:433–438, 1980.

Gustilo, R.B., Mendoza, R.M., and Williams, D.N.: Problems in the management of type III (severe) open fractures: A new classification of type III open fractures. J. Trauma 24:742–746, 1984.

Gustilo, R.B., Merkow, R.L., and Templeman, D.: Current concepts review. The management of open fractures. J. Bone Joint Surg. [Am.] 72:299, 1990.

Hansen, S.T., and Winquist, R.A.: Closed intramedullary nailing of the femur, Kuntscher technique with reaming. Clin. Orthop. 138:56–61, 1979.

Harper, M.C., and Hardin, G.: Posterior malleolar fractures of the ankle associated with external rotation-abduction injuries: Results with and without internal fixation. J. Bone Joint Surg. [Am.] 70:1348–1356, 1988.

Helfer, R.E., and Kempe, R.S., eds.: The Battered Child, 4th ed. Chicago, University of Chicago Press, 1987.

Herbert, T.J., and Fisher, W.E.: Management of the fractured scaphoid using a new bone screw. J. Bone Joint Surg. [Br.] 66:114–123, 1984.

Holbrook, J.L., Swiontkowski, M.F., and Sanders, R.: Treatment of open fractures of the tibial shaft: Ender nailing versus external fixation. A randomized, prospective comparison. J. Bone Joint Surg. [Am.] 71:1231, 1989.

Horne, G.: Supracondylar fractures of the humerus in adults. J. Trauma 20:71–74, 1980.

Jacobs, R.R., and Casey, M.P.: Surgical management of thoracolumbar injuries. General principles and controversial considerations. Clin. Orthop. 189:22–35, 1984.

Johnson, K.D., Cadambi, A., and Seibert, G.B.: Incidence of adult respiratory distress syndrome in patients with multiple musculoskeletal injuries: Effect of early operative stabilization of fractures. J. Trauma 25:375–383, 1985.

Judet, R., Judet, J., and Letournel, E.: Fractures of the acetabulum: Classification and surgical approaches for open reduction. J. Bone Joint Surg. [Am.] 46:1615–1646, 1964.

Jupiter, J.B., Neff, U., Holzach, P., et al.: Intercondylar fractures of the humerus: An operative approach. J. Bone Joint Surg. [Am.] 67:226–239, 1985.

King, J., Diefendorf, D., Apthorp, J., et al.: Analysis of 429 fractures in 189 battered children. J. Pediatr. Orthop. 8:585–589, 1988.

Klassen, R.A., and Peterson, H.A.: Excision of physeal bars: The Mayo Clinic experience, 1968–1978. Orthop. Trans. 6:65, 1982.

Kozin, S.H., and Berlet, A.C.: Handbook of Common Orthopaedic Fractures. West Chester, PA, Medical Surveillance Inc., 1990.

Kramer, K.M., and Levine, A.M.: Unilateral facet dislocation of the lumbosacral junction. A case report and review of the literature. J. Bone Joint Surg. [Am.] 71:1258, 1989.

Kyle, R.F., Wright, T.M., and Burstein, A.H.: Biomechanical analysis of the sliding characteristics of compression hip screw. J. Bone Joint Surg. [Am.] 62:1308–1314, 1980.

Lange, R.H., and Hansen, S.T., Jr.: Pelvic ring disruptions with symphysis pubis diastasis: Indications, technique, and limitations of anterior internal fixation. Clin. Orthop. 201:130–137, 1985.

Letournel, E., and Judet, R.: Fractures of the Acetabulum (Transl. and edited by R.A. Elson). New York, Springer-Verlag, 1981.

Matsen, F.A., III, Winquist, R.A., and Krugmire, R.B., Jr.: Diagnosis and management of compartmental syndromes. J. Bone Joint Surg. [Am.] 62:286–291, 1980.

Matta, J., Anderson, L., Epstein, H., and Henricks, P.: Fractures of the acetabulum: A retrospective analysis. Clin. Orthop. 205:230–240, 1986.

Matta, J.M., Mehne, D.K., and Roffi, R.: Fractures of the acetabulum: Early results of a prospective study. Clin. Orthop. 205:241–250, 1986.

Matta, J.M., and Saucedo, T.: Internal fixation of pelvic ring fractures. Clin. Orthop. 242:83–97, 1989.

May, J.W., Jr., Jupiter, J.B., Weiland, A.J., et al.: Current concepts review. Clinical classification of post-traumatic osteomyelitis. J. Bone Joint Surg. [Am.] 71:1422, 1989.

McDonald, G.A.: Pelvic disruptions in children. Clin. Orthop. 151:130–134, 1980.

McMurtry, R., Walton, D., Dickinson, D., Kellam, J., and Tile, M.: Pelvic disruption in the polytraumatized patient: A management protocol. Clin. Orthop. 151:22–30, 1980.

McReynolds, I.S.: The Case for Operative Treatment of Fractures of the Os Calcis. Philadelphia, W.B. Saunders, 1982.

Mears, D.C., Capito, C.P., and Deleeuw, H.: Posterior pelvic disruptions managed by the use of the Double Cobra plate. Instr. Course Lect. 37:143–150, 1988.

Mears, D.C., and Rubash, H.: Pelvic and Acetabular Fractures. Thorofare, N.J., Slack, 1986.

Mehlhoff, T.L., Noble, P.C., Bennett, J.B., and Tullos, H.S.: Simple dislocation of the elbow in the adult. Results after closed treatment. J. Bone Joint Surg. [Am.] 70:244, 1988.

Melone, C.P., Jr.: Open treatment for displaced articular fractures of the distal radius. Clin. Orthop. 202:103–111, 1986.

Miller, M.E., Allgower, M., Schneider, R., et al.: Manual of Internal Fixation. Berlin, Springer-Verlag, 1979.

Millis, M.B., Singer, I.J., and Hall, J.E.: Supracondylar fracture of the humerus in children: Further experience with a study in orthopaedic decision-making. Clin. Orthop. 188:90–97, 1984.

Morrissey, R.T.: Fractured Hip in Childhood. St. Louis, C.V. Mosby, 1984.

Naam, N.H., Brown, W.M., Hurd, R., Burdge, R.E., and Kaminski, D.L.: Major pelvic fractures. Arch. Surg. 118:610–616, 1983.

Ogden, J.A.: Skeletal Injury in the Child, 2nd ed. Philadelphia, W.B. Saunders, 1990.

Odgen, J.A., Tross, R.B., and Murphy, M.J.: Fractures of the tibial tuberosity in adolescents. J. Bone Joint Surg. [Am.] 62:205–215, 1980.

Orthopaedic Knowledge Update Home Study Syllabus I, II, and III. Chicago, American Academy of Orthopaedic Surgeons, 1984, 1987, 1990.

Ovadia, D.N., and Beals, R.K.: Fractures of the tibial plafond. J. Bone Joint Surg. [Am.] 68:543–551, 1986.

Phillips, T.F., and Contreras, D.M.: Current concepts review. Timing of operative treatment of fractures in patients who have multiple injuries. J. Bone Joint Surg. [Am.] 72:784, 1990.

Phillips, W.A., and Hensinger, R.N.: The management of rotatory atlanto-axial subluxation in children. J. Bone Joint Surg. [Am.] 71:664, 1989.

Pirone, A.M., Graham, H.K., and Krajbich, J.I.: Management of displaced extension-type supracondylar fractures of the humerus in children. J. Bone Joint Surg. [Am.] 70:641–650, 1988.

Pollak, R., and Myers, R.A.M.: Early diagnosis of the fat embolism syndrome. J. Trauma 18:121–123, 1978.

Pollock, F.H., Drake, D., Bovill, E.G., Day, L., and Trafton, P.G.: Treatment of radial neuropathy associated with fractures of the humerus. J. Bone Joint Surg. [Am.] 63:239–243, 1981.

Prietto, C.A.: Supracondylar fractures of the humerus. J. Bone Joint Surg. [Am.] 61:425–428, 1979.

Pritchett, J.W.: Supracondylar fractures of the femur. Clin. Orthop. 184:173–177, 1984.

Rang, M.: Children's Fractures. Philadelphia, J.B. Lippincott Company, 1974.

Regan, W., and Morrey, B.: Fractures of the coronoid process of the ulna. J. Bone Joint Surg. [Am.] 71:1348, 1989.

Rockwood, C.A., Jr., and Green, D.P., eds.: Fractures in Adults. 3rd ed. Philadelphia, J.B. Lippincott, 1991.

Rockwood, C.A., Jr., Wilkins, K.E., and King, R.E., eds.: Fractures in Children. 3rd ed. Philadelphia, J.B. Lippincott, 1991.

Routt, M.L.C., Jr., and Swiontkowski, M.F.: Operative treatment of complex acetabular fractures. Combined anterior and posterior exposures during the same procedure. J. Bone Joint Surg. [Am.] 72:897, 1990.

Saltzman, C.L., Goulet, J.A., McClellan, R.T., et al.: Results of treatment of displaced patellar fractures by partial patellectomy. J. Bone Joint Surg. [Am.] 72:1279, 1990.

Sangeorzan, B.J., Benirschke, S.K., Mosca, V., et al.: Displaced intra-articular fractures of the tarsal navicular. J. Bone Joint Surg. [Am.] 71:1504, 1989.

Schatzker, J., and Lambert, D.C.: Supracondylar fractures of the femur. Clin. Orthop. 138:77–83, 1979.

Schatzker, J., McBroom, R., and Bruce, D.: The tibial plateau fracture: The Toronto experience, 1968–1975. Clin. Orthop. 138:94–104, 1979.

Schatzker, J., Rorabeck, C.H., and Waddell, J.P.: Fractures of the dens (odontoid process): An analysis of thirty-seven cases. J. Bone Joint Surg. [Br.] 53:392–405, 1971.

Segal, D.: Displaced Ankle Fractures Treated Surgically and Postoperative Management. St. Louis, C.V. Mosby, 1979.

Silberstein, M.J., Brodeur, A.E., and Graviss, E.R.: Some vagaries of the lateral epicondyle. J. Bone Joint Surg. [Am.] 64:444–448, 1982.

Southwick, W.O.: Current concepts review. Management of fractures of the dens (odontoid process). J. Bone Joint Surg. [Am.] 62:482–486, 1980.

Staeheli, J.W., Frassica, F.J., and Sim, F.H.: Prosthetic replacement of the femoral head for fracture of the femoral neck in patients who have Parkinson disease. J. Bone Joint Surg. [Am.] 70:565–568, 1988.

Steinberg, E.L., Golomb, D., Salama, R., et al.: Radial head and neck fractures in children. J. Pediatr. Orthop. 8:35–40, 1988.

Stephenson, J.R.: Treatment of displaced intra-articular fractures of the calcaneus using medial and lateral approaches, internal fixation, and early motion. J. Bone Joint Surg. [Am.] 69:115–130, 1987.

Strickland, J.W., and Steichen, J.B., eds.: Difficult Problems in Hand Surgery. St Louis, C.V. Mosby, 1982.

Swiontkowski, M.F., Hansen, S.T., Jr., and Kellam, J.: Ipsilateral fractures of the femoral neck and shaft: A treatment protocol. J. Bone Joint Surg. [Am.] 66:260–268, 1984.

Talucci, R.C., Manning, J., Lampard, S., Bach, A., and Carrico, C.J.: Early intramedullary nailing of femoral shaft fractures: A cause of fat embolism syndrome. Am. J. Surg. 146:107–110, 1983.

Tanner, M.W., and Cofield, R.H.: Prosthetic arthroplasty for fractures and fracture-dislocations of the proximal humerus. Clin. Orthop. 179:116–128, 1983.

Tibone, J.E., and Stoltz, M.: Fractures of the radial head and neck in children. J. Bone Joint Surg. [Am.] 63:100–106, 1981.

Tile, M.: Pelvic ring fractures: Should they be fixed? J. Bone Joint Surg. [Br.] 70:1–12, 1988.

Tile, M.: Fractures of the Pelvis and Acetabulum. Baltimore, Williams & Wilkins, 1984.

Weber, B.G. and Cech, O.: Pseuanthrosen. Bern, Stuttgart-Wien, Huber, 1973.

Weber, M.J., Janecki, C.J., McLeod, P., Nelson, C.L., and Thompson, J.A.: Efficacy of various forms of fixation of transverse fractures of the patella. J. Bone Joint Surg. [Am.] 62:215–220, 1980.

White, A.A., Southwick, W.O., and Panjabi, M.M.: Clinical instability in the lower cervical spine: A review of past and current concepts. Spine 1:15–27, 1976.

Wiley, J.J., and Galey, J.P.: Monteggia injuries in children. J. Bone Joint Surg. [Br.] 67:728–731, 1985.

Wilkins, R.M., and Johnston, R.M.: Ununited fractures of the clavicle. J. Bone Joint Surg. [Am.] 65:773–778, 1983.

Winquist, R.R., Waddell, J.P., Sullivan, T.R., Ashworth, M.A., and Rorabeck, C.H.: Infra-isthmal fractures of the femur: A review of 82 cases. J. Trauma 24:735–741, 1984.

Young, J.W.R., and Burgess A.R.: Radiographic management of pelvic ring fractures: Systematic Radiographic Diagnosis. Baltimore: Urban & Schwarzenberg, 1987.

Zdrovkovic, D. and Damholt, V.V. Comminuted and severely displaced fractures of the sepula. Acta Orthop. Scand. 45:60–65, 1974.

Zickel, R.E.: Subtrochanteric femoral fractures. Orthop. Clin. North Am. 11:555–568, 1980.

CHAPTER 10

Anatomy

I. Introduction

  A. Osteology—The study of bones. Eighty bones make up the axial skeleton and 126 bones are in the appendicular skeleton, for a total of 206 bones in the human skeleton. There are four general types of bones: long (e.g., femur), short (e.g., phalanges), flat (e.g., scapulae), and irregular (e.g., vertebrae). Ossification, or the formation of bone, can be intramembranous (without a cartilage model, as in the skull) or enchondral (with a cartilage model; most bones). Enchondral growth begins in the diaphyses of long bones at a primary ossification center, most of which are present at birth. Secondary ossification centers usually develop in the periphery of bone, and are important in growth and in treatment of childhood fractures. Anatomic landmarks of the skeleton and their related structures are listed in Table 10–1.

  B. Arthrology—The study of joints, specialized structures that allow articulation of various bones. Joints are reinforced by ligaments, capsules, and other structures that may restrict movement and add stability. Joints are commonly classified into three types based on their freedom of movement: (1) Synarthroses, (2) Amphiarthroses, (3) Diarthroses. Although **synarthroses**, such as the sutures in the skull, may have motion in early childhood, they usually have no motion at maturity and simply serve to join two bony elements. **Amphiarthrodial** joints, such as the symphysis pubis, have hyaline cartilage and intervening discs. Limited motion is possible. In true **diarthrodial** joints, motion is enhanced and is characterized by hyaline cartilage, synovial membranes, capsules, and ligaments. Diarthrodial joints are further classified based upon their degrees of freedom of motion and their shape. Uniaxial joints (ginglymus [e.g., hinge] and trochoid [e.g., pivot]) allow movement in one plane. Biaxial joints (e.g., condyloid, ellipsoid, and saddle joints) allow movement in two planes. Polyaxial (spheroidal [e.g., ball and socket]) allow movement in any direction. Finally, plane (gliding) joints allow only slight sliding of one joint surface over another.

  C. Myology—The study of muscles, structures that are capable of contraction and power movement. Fascia (dense connective tissue) surrounds muscle groups, divides them into compartments, and serves as attachments for muscles. Several different arrangements of fibers allows classification of muscles into the following categories: parallel (e.g., rhomboids), fusiform (e.g., biceps brachii), oblique (with tendinous interdigitation—further subclassified as pennate, bipennate, and multipennate), triangular (e.g., pectoralis minor), and spiral (e.g., latissimus dorsi). Knowledge of origins and insertions of skeletal muscle is critical in understanding their functions.

  D. Nerves—Most peripheral nerves originate from the ventral rami of spinal nerves and are distributed via several plexii (cervical, brachial, and lumbosacral). Efferent, or motor, fibers carry impulses from the CNS to muscles; afferent, or sensory, fibers carry information toward the CNS. The autonomic nervous system controls visceral structures and consists of the parasympathetic

TABLE 10–1. SKELETAL GROOVES, NOTCHES, AND POINTS

REGION	GROOVE OR NOTCH	IMPORTANT RELATED STRUCTURES
Hand	Hook of Hamate	Ulnar nerve
	Trapezial groove	FCR tendon
Wrist	Distal ulna	ECU
	Radial styloid	EPL
Elbow	Medial Supracondylar process	Median nerve, brachial artery
Shoulder	Scapular notch	Suprascapular nerve
	Supraglenoid tubercle	Long head biceps brachii
	Infraglenoid tubercule	Long head triceps brachii
Hip	ASIS	Sartorius
	AIIS	Dir. head of rectus femoris
	Ischial spine	Coccygeus, levator ani
	Lesser sciatic foramen	Pudendal nerve
	Piriformis fossa	Obturator externus
	Tip of greater trochanter	Piriformis
	Quadrate tubercle	Quadratus femoris
	Lesser trochanter	Psoas minor
Knee	Hunter's canal	Femoral → popliteal artery
	Adductor tubercle	Adductor magnus
	Gerdy's tubercle	IT band
	Fibular neck	Common peroneal nerve
Foot	Henry's knot	FDL & FHL intersection
	Sustentaculum tali	Spring ligament (FHL inferior)
	Base of fifth metatarsal	Peroneus brevis/Plantar aponeurosis
	Tuberosity of navicular	Tibialis posterior
	Cuboid groove	Peroneus longus
	Sinus tarsi	Ligamentum cervis tali & EDB

(craniosacral) and the sympathetic (thoracolumbar) divisions. Preganglionic neurons of parasympathetic nerves arise in the nuclei of CNs III, VII, IX, and X and in the S2, S3, and S4 segments of the spinal cord and synapse in peripheral ganglia. Preganglionic neurons in the sympathetic system are located in the spinal cord (T1–L3) and synapse in chain ganglia adjacent to the spine and collateral ganglia along major abdominal blood vessels.

  E. Vessels—Consist of arteries, veins, and lymphatics. Of primary concern to the orthopaedist is avoiding major injury to these structures. Their courses and relationships are important.

  F. Surgical Approaches (Table 10–2)—Usually are based on entering an internervous interval and are planned for as little disruption to other structures as possible.

II. Shoulder

  A. Osteology—The shoulder girdle is composed of the scapula and the clavicle, and serves to attach the upper limb to the trunk. The shoulder (gle-

nohumeral) joint is the attachment of the upper humerus (discussed in Section III: Upper Arm) to the shoulder girdle.

  1. Scapula–spans the second through seventh ribs and serves as an attachment for 17 separate muscles and four ligaments. It has two surfaces, costal and dorsal, and has three processes: the spine, the acromion, and the coracoid. It also has three borders (superior, lateral, and medial) and three angles (inferior, superior, and lateral). The scapula has one primary and six secondary ossification centers:

OSSIFICATION CENTER	AGE APPEARS	ORDER FUSES
Body (primary)	8 wks (fetal)	1
Coracoid (tip)	1 year	2
Coracoid	15 years	3
Acromion	15 years	4
Acromion	16 years	5
Inferior angle	16 years	6
Medial border	16 years	7

TABLE 10–2. SUMMARY OF POPULAR ORTHOPAEDIC SURGICAL APPROACHES

REGION	APPROACH	EPONYM	MUSCULAR INTERVAL 1 (NERVE)	MUSCULAR INTERVAL 2 (NERVE)	DANGERS
			Upper Extremity		
Shoulder	Anterior	Henry	Deltoid (Axillary)	Pec. major (Med./Lat. pectoral)	MC N/Cephalic V
	Lateral		Deltoid (splitting) (Axillary)	Deltoid (splitting) (Axillary)	Axillary N
	Posterior		Infraspinatus (Suprascapular)	Teres minor (Axillary)	Ax. N/Post. cir. hum. A
Prox. humerus	Anterolateral		Deltoid (Axillary)	Pec. major (Med./Lat. pectoral)	Radial & Axillary N/Ant circ. hum. A
Distal humerus	Anterolateral		Brachialis (Musculocutaneous)	Brachioradialis (Radial)	Radial N
	Lateral		Triceps (Radial)	Brachioradialis (Radial)	Radial N
Humerus	Posterior		Lat. triceps (Radial)	Long triceps (Radial)	Radial N/Brachial A
Elbow	Anterolateral	Henry	Brachialis/Pron. teres (Musculocut./Median)	Brachioradialis (Radial)	Lat. ABC N/Radial N
	Posterolateral	Kocher	Anconeus (Radial)	Ext. carpi ulnaris (PIN)	PIN (diss. to ann. lig.)
	Medial		Brachialis (Musculocutaneous)	Triceps/Pron. teres (Radial/Median)	Ulnar N
Forearm	Anterior	Henry	Brachioradialis (Radial)	Pronator teres/FCR (Median)	PIN
	Dorsal	Thompson	ECRB (Radial)	EDC/EPL (PIN)	PIN
	Ulnar		ECU (PIN)	FCU (Ulnar)	Ulnar N & A
Wrist	Dorsal		Third compartment (PIN)	Fourth compartment (PIN)	
Scaphoid	Volar	Russe	FCR or thru sheath (Median)	Radial A	Radial A
	Dorsolateral	Matti	First compartment (PIN)	Third compartment (PIN)	Sup. rad. N/Radial A

N, nerve; A, artery; V, vein; PIN, posterior intervosseous nerve; ABC, antebrachial cutaneous.

(continued)

TABLE 10–2. SUMMARY OF POPULAR ORTHOPAEDIC SURGICAL APPROACHES (*Continued*)

REGION	APPROACH	EPONYM	MUSCULAR INTERVAL 1 (NERVE)	MUSCULAR INTERVAL 2 (NERVE)	DANGERS
			Lower Extremity		
Iliac crest	Posterior		Gluteus maximus (Inferior gluteal)	Latissimus dorsi (Long thoracic)	Clunial N, SGA, Sciatic N
	Anterior		TFL/Glut. med. & min. (Superior gluteal)	Ext. abd. oblique (Segmental)	ASIS/LFCN
Hip	Anterior	Smith-Peterson	Sartorius/Rectus fem. (Femoral)	TFL/Gluteus medius (Superior gluteal)	LFCN, Fem. N, Asc. br. LFCA
	Anterolateral	Watson-Jones	Tensor fasciae latae (Sup. gluteal)	Gluteus medius (Sup. gluteal)	Fem. NAV/Profunda A
	Lateral	Hardinge	Splits glut. med. (Sup. gluteal)	Splits vastus lat. (Femoral)	Femoral NAV/LFCA (transverse br.)
	Posterior	Moore-Southern	Splits glut. max. (Inf. gluteal)	N/A	Sciatic, inf. glut. A
	Medial	Ludloff	Add. longus/Add. brevis (Ant. div. obt.)	Gracilis/Add. magnus (Obt./Tibial)	Ant. div. obt. N/MFCA
Thigh	Lateral		Vastus lateralis (Femoral)	Vastus lateralis (Femoral)	Perf. br. profundus
	Posterolateral		Vastus lateralis (Femoral)	Hamstrings (Sciatic)	Perf. br. profundus
	Anteromedial		Rectus femoris (Femoral)	Vastus medialis (Femoral)	Med. sup. geniculate A
	Posterior		Biceps femoris (Sciatic)	Vastus lateralis (Femoral)	Sciatic/N PFCN
Knee	Med. parapatellar		Vastus medialis (Femoral)	Rectus femoris (Femoral)	Infrapatellar br. saphenous N
	Medial		Vastus medialis (Femoral)	Sartorius (Femoral)	Infrapatellar br. saphenous N
	Lateral		Iliotibial band (Superior gluteal)	Biceps femoris (Sciatic)	Peroneal N/Popliteus Ten.
	Posterior		Semimem./Lat. Gastroc. (Tibial)	Biceps/Lat. gastroc. (Tib.)/(Tib.)	Med. sural cut. N/Tib. N/ Peroneal N
Distal femur	Lateral		Vastus lateralis (Femoral)	Biceps femoris (Sciatic)	Peroneal N/Lat. sup. gen. A
Tibia	Posterolateral		GS & Soleus & FHL (Tibial)	Peroneus L&B (Sup. peroneal)	Sm saph. V/Post. tib. A
	Anterior		Tibialis anterior (Peroneal)	Periosteum	Long saph. V
Ankle	Anterior		EHL (Deep peroneal)	EDL (Deep peroneal)	S&D peroneal N/Ant. tib. A
Med. malleolus	Posterior		Tibialis posterior	FDL	Saphenous N & V
Ankle	Posterolateral		Peroneus brevis (Sup. peroneal)	FHL (Tibial)	Sural N/Sm saph. V
Distal fibula	Lateral		Peroneus tertius (Deep peroneal)	Peroneus brevis (Sup. peroneal)	Sural N
Ankle	Anterolateral		Peroneal muscles (Sup. peroneal)	EDC and Per. tertius (Deep peroneal)	Deep per. N/Ant. tib. A
	Posteromedial		TP or FDL	FDL or FHL	Post. tib. A/Tib. N

A, artery; V, vein; N, nerve; S, superficial; D, decr; LFCA, lateral femoral circumflex artery; MFCA, medial femoral circumflex artery; SGA, superior gluteal artery; PFCN, posterior femoral cutaneous nerve; LFCN, lateral femoral cutaneous nerve.

2. Clavicle—Acts as a fulcrum for lateral movement of the arm. It has a double curvature (sternal–ventral, acromial–dorsal), and serves as an attachment for the upper extremity. The clavicle is the **first bone in the body to ossify, and the last to fuse**. It has two primary and one secondary ossification centers:

OSSIFICATION CENTER	AGE APPEARS	AGE FUSES
Medial (primary)	5 wks (fetal)	
Lateral (primary)	5 wks (fetal)	
Sternal	19 years	25 years

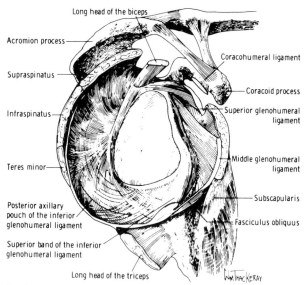

FIGURE 10–1. Glenohumeral ligaments and rotator cuff muscles. (From Turkel, S.J., et al.: Stabilizing mechanisms preventing anterior dislocation of the gleno-humeral joint. J. Bone Joint Surg. [Am.] 63:1209; reprinted by permission.)

B. Arthrology—The shoulder area has one major (glenohumeral) and several minor (sternoclavicular, acromioclavicular, and scapulothoracic) articulations. Additionally, there are numerous ligaments associated with each articulation.

1. Glenohumeral Joint—The articulation between the glenoid fossa and the proximal humerus. It is classified as a spheroidal, or ball-and-socket, joint. The articular surface of the glenoid is thickest at the periphery. This joint has the greatest ROM of any joint, but has very limited inherent stability, and relies on the rotator cuff tendons and the following ligaments for support (Fig. 10–1):

Ligament	Function
Capsule	Support/boundary layer
Coracohumeral	Anterior support; tightens with flexion
Glenohumeral	Sup., mid., and inferior (inferior strongest)
Glenoid labrum	Increases surface area, stability
Transverse humeral	Maintains biceps (long head) in groove

2. Sternoclavicular (SC) Joint—Is a double gliding joint and has a articular disc. Its ligaments include the capsule, anterior and posterior sternoclavicular ligaments, an interclavicular

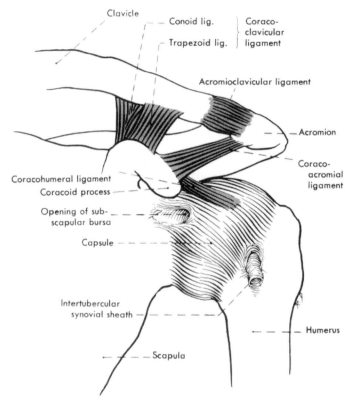

FIGURE 10–2. Ligaments about the shoulder. (From Jenkins, D.B.: Hollinshead's Functional Anatomy of the Limbs and Back, 6th ed., p. 71. Philadelphia, W.B. Saunders, 1991; reprinted by permission.)

FIGURE 10–3. Origins ▨ and insertions ▧ of muscles about the shoulder girdle. (From Jenkins, D.B.: Hollinshead's Functional Anatomy of the Limbs and Back, 6th ed., fig. 5–3. Philadelphia, W.B. Saunders, 1991; reprinted by permission.)

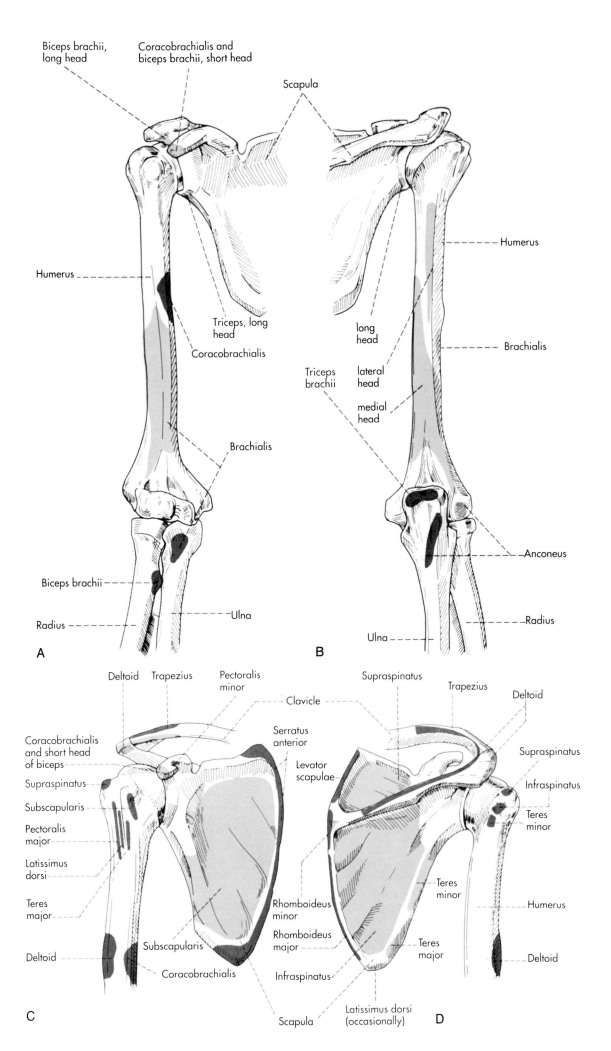

Biceps brachii, long head

Coracobrachialis and biceps brachii, short head

Scapula

Humerus

Triceps, long head

Coracobrachialis

Brachialis

Biceps brachii

Radius

Ulna

A

Humerus

long head

Triceps brachii

lateral head

medial head

Brachialis

Anconeus

Ulna

Radius

B

Deltoid

Trapezius

Pectoralis minor

Clavicle

Serratus anterior

Levator scapulae

Coracobrachialis and short head of biceps

Supraspinatus

Subscapularis

Pectoralis major

Latissimus dorsi

Teres major

Deltoid

Subscapularis

Coracobrachialis

Rhomboideus minor

Rhomboideus major

Infraspinatus

Scapula

C

Supraspinatus

Trapezius

Deltoid

Supraspinatus

Infraspinatus

Teres minor

Teres minor

Teres major

Humerus

Deltoid

Latissimus dorsi (occasionally)

D

ligament, and a costoclavicular ligament (strongest). The SC joint rotates 30 degrees with shoulder motion.

3. Acromioclavicular (AC) Joint—A plane/gliding joint that also possesses a disc. Its ligaments (Fig. 10–2) include the capsule, acromioclavicular ligament, and coracoclavicular (CC) ligament (with trapezoid [anterolateral] and conoid [posteromedial and stronger] component ligaments). The AC ligament prevents anteroposterior displacement of the distal clavicle. The CC ligament prevents superior displacement of the distal clavicle.

4. Scapulothoracic Joint—Although not a true joint, this attachment allows scapular movement against the posterior rib cage. It is fixed primarily by the scapular muscle attachments.

5. Intrinsic Ligaments of the Scapula—Include the superior transverse scapular ligament (which separates the suprascapular nerve and vessels), and the coracoacromial ligament (which is a frequent cause of impingement).

C. Muscles of the Shoulder (Fig. 10–3)—Serve a variety of functions. Five muscles help connect the upper limb to the vertebral column (trapezius, latissimus, both rhomboids, and the levator scapulae). Four muscles connect the upper limb to the thoracic wall (both pectoralis muscles, subclavius, and serratus anterior). Finally, six muscles act on the shoulder joint itself (deltoid, teres major, and the four rotator cuff muscles [supraspinatus, infraspinatus, teres minor, and subscapularis]). The rotator cuff muscles serve to depress and stabilize the humeral head against the glenoid. Table 10–3 presents specifics on these muscles.

D. Nerves—Peripheral nerves that innervate muscles about the upper extremity derive from the brachial plexus. This plexus is formed from the ventral primary ramii of C5–T1, and lies under the clavicle, extending from the scalenus anterior to the axilla. The brachial plexus is organized into five components: **r**oots, **t**runks, **d**ivisions, **c**ords, and **b**ranches (remember the mnemonic **R**ob **T**aylor **d**rinks **c**old **b**eer). There are five roots (C5–T1—although C4 and T2 can have small contributions), three trunks (upper, middle, and lower), six divi-

sions (two from each trunk), three cords (posterior, lateral, and medial), and multiple branches, as illustrated in Figure 10–4. Note that there are four preclavicular branches (from roots and upper trunk): dorsal scapular nerve, long thoracic nerve, suprascapular nerve, and nerve to subclavius.

E. Vessels (Fig. 10–5)—The subclavian artery arises either directly from the aorta (left subclavian) or from the brachiocephalic trunk (right subclavian). It then emerges between the scalenus anterior and medius muscles and becomes the axillary artery at the outer border of the first rib. The axillary artery is divided into three portions, based on its relationship to the pectoralis minor (the first is medial to it, the second is under it, and the third is lateral to it). Each part of the artery has as many branches as the number of that portion (e.g., the second part has two branches):

Part	Branch	Course
1	Supreme thoracic	Medial—to serratus ant and pecs
2	Thoracoacromial	4 branches (deltoid, anterior, pectoralis, clavicular)
	Lateral thoracic	Descends to serratus ant.
3	Subscapular	2 branches (thoracodorsal and circumflex scapular → triangular space)
	Ant. circumflex humeral	Circles humerus anteriorly, blood supply to humeral head
	Post. circumflex humeral	Post. humerus → quadrangular space

F. Surgical Approaches to the Shoulder—Include the anterior approach (reconstructions and arthroplasties), the lateral approach (acromioplasty and cuff repair), and the posterior approach (posterior reconstruction).

1. Anterior Approach (Henry) (Fig. 10–6)—Explores the interval between the deltoid (axillary N) and the pectoralis major (medial and lateral pectoral N). The cephalic vein is dissected and retracted laterally with the deltoid, and the underlying subscapularis is exposed. This is then

TABLE 10–3. MUSCLES OF THE SHOULDER

Muscle	Origin	Insertion	Action	Innervation
Trapezius	Spin. proc. C7–T12	Clavicle, scapula (AC, SP)	Rotate scapula	CN XI
Lat. dorsii	Spin. proc. T6–S5, Ilm	Humerus (ITG)	Ex., add., IR humerus	Thoracodorsal
Rhomboid maj.	Spin. proc. T2–T5	Scapula (med. border)	Adduct scapula	Dorsal scapular
Rhomboid min.	Spin. proc. C7–T1	Scapula (med. spine)	Adduct scapula	Dorsal scapular
Lev. scapulae	T. proc. C1–C4	Scapula (sup. med.)	Elevate, rotate scapula	C3, C4
Pectoralis maj.	Sternum, ribs, clavicle	Humerus (L-ITG)	Add., IR arm	M & L PN
Pectoralis min.	Ribs 3–5	Scapula (coracoid)	Protract scapula	MPN
Subclavius	Rib 1	Inf. clavicle	Depress clavicle	U trunk
Serratus ant.	Ribs 1–9	Scapula (vent. med.)	Prevent winging	Long thoracic
Deltoid	L. clavicle, scapula	Humerus (deltoid tub.)	Abduct arm (2)	Axillary
Teres major	Inf. scapula	Humerus (M-ITG)	Add., IR, ext.	L subscapular
Subscapularis	Ventral scapula	Humerus (LT)	IR arm, ant. stability	U & L subscapular
Supraspinatus	Sup. scapula	Humerus (GT)	Abd. (1), ER arm stability	Suprascapular
Infraspinatus	Dorsal scapula	Humerus (GT)	Stability, ER arm	Suprascapular
Teres minor	Scapula (dorsolateral)	Humerus (GT)	Stability, ER arm	Axillary

ITG, intertubercular groove; AC, acromion; SP, spinous process; LT, lesser tuberosity; GT, greater tuberosity.

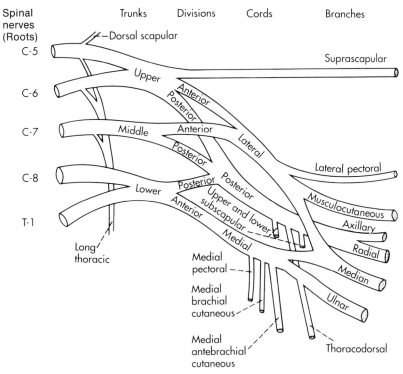

FIGURE 10–4. Brachial plexus. (From Jenkins, D.B.: Hollinshead's Functional Anatomy of the Limbs and Back, 6th ed., fig. 5–7. Philadelphia, W.B. Saunders, 1991; reprinted by permission.)

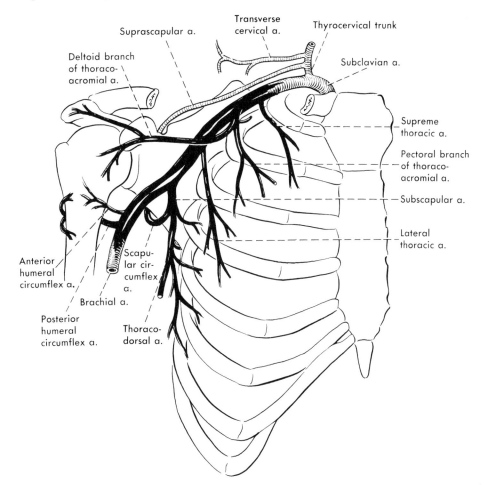

FIGURE 10–5. Branches of the axillary artery. (From Jenkins, D.B.: Hollinshead's Functional Anatomy of the Limbs and Back, 6th ed., p. 77. Philadelphia, W.B. Saunders, 1991; reprinted by permission.)

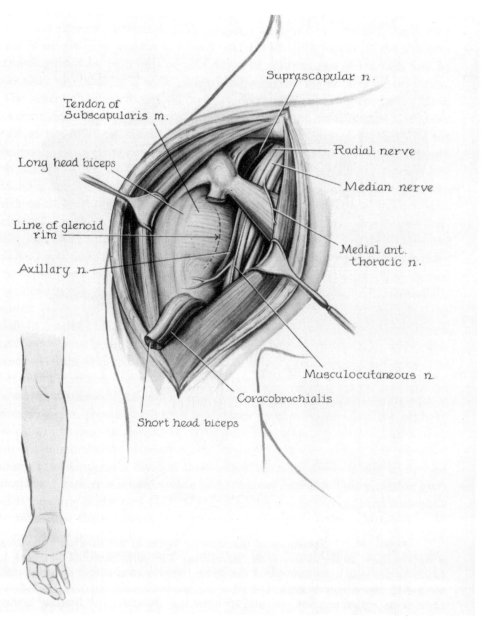

Tendon of
Subscapularis m.

Long head biceps

Line of glenoid
rim

Axillary n.

Short head biceps

Coracobrachialis

Suprascapular n.

Radial nerve

Median nerve

Medial ant.
thoracic n.

Musculocutaneous n.

FIGURE 10–6. Anterior approach to the shoulder through the deltopectoral interval. (From Kaplan, E.B.: Surgical Approaches to the Neck, Cervical Spine, and Upper Extremity, p. 57. Philadelphia, W.B. Saunders, 1966; reprinted by permission.)

divided (preserving the most inferior fibers to protect the axillary N), and the shoulder capsule is encountered. The **musculocutaneous nerve** should be protected by avoiding dissection medial to the coracobrachialis. This nerve usually penetrates the biceps/coracobrachialis 5–8 cm below the coracoid, but it enters these muscles proximal to this **5-cm "safe zone"** almost 30% of the time. The **axillary nerve**, which is **just inferior** to the shoulder **capsule** must be protected during procedures in this area.

2. Lateral Approach—Involves splitting the deltoid muscle or subperiosteal dissection of the muscle from the acromion. This exposes the supraspinatus tendon well, and allows for repairs of the rotator cuff. The deltoid should not be split more than **5 cm below the acromion** to avoid injury to the **axillary nerve**.

3. Posterior Approach (Fig. 10–7)—Uses the internervous plane between the infraspinatus (suprascapular nerve) and teres minor (axillary nerve). This plane can be approached by detaching the deltoid from the scapular spine or by splitting the deltoid (Rockwood). After finding this interval, the posterior capsule lies immediately below it. The axillary nerve and the posterior circumflex humeral artery both run in the **quadrangular space** below the teres minor, so it is important to stay above this muscle. Excessive medial retraction of the infraspinatus can injure the suprascapular nerve.

III. The Arm

A. Osteology—The humerus is the only bone of the arm, and the largest and longest bone of the upper

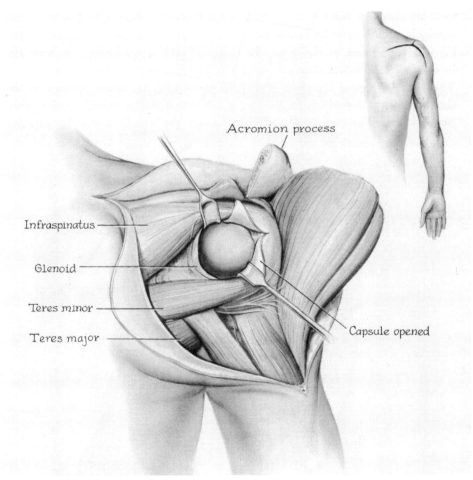

FIGURE 10–7. Posterior approach to the shoulder through the infraspinatus–teres minor interval. (From Kaplan, E.B.: Surgical Approaches to the Neck, Cervical Spine, and Upper Extremity, p. 61. Philadelphia, W.B. Saunders, 1966; reprinted by permission.)

extremity. The humerus is composed of a shaft and two articular extremities. The hemispherical head, directed superiorly, medially, and slightly dorsally, articulates with the much smaller scapular glenoid cavity. The *anatomical* neck, directly below the head, serves as an attachment for the shoulder capsule. The *surgical neck* is lower, and is more often involved in fractures. The greater tuberosity, lateral to the head, serves as the attachment for the supraspinatus, infraspinatus, and teres minor (SIT) muscles (anterior to posterior, respectively). The lesser tuberosity, located anteriorly, has only one muscular insertion: the last rotator cuff muscle, the subscapularis. The bicipital groove (for the tendon of the long head of the biceps) is situated between the two tuberosities. The shaft of the humerus has a notable groove for the radial nerve posteriorly in its midportion, adjacent to the deltoid tuberosity. Distally, the humerus flares into medial and lateral epicondyles, and forms half of the elbow joint with a medial spool-shaped trochlea (articulates with the olecranon of the ulna), and a globular capitulum (which opposes the radial head). The humerus has one primary and seven secondary ossification centers:

Ossification Center	Age Appears	Age Fuses
Body (primary)	8 weeks (fetal)	Blend at 6 years, unite at 20 years
Head	1 year	
Greater tuberosity	3 years	
Lesser tuberosity	5 years	
Capitulum	2 years	Blend and unite with body at 16–18 years
Medial epicondyle	5 years	
Trochlea	9 years	
Lateral epicondyle	13 years	

B. Arthrology—The humerus articulates with the scapula on its upper end, forming the glenohumeral joint (discussed above), and with the radius and ulna on its lower end, forming the elbow joint. The elbow is composed of a compound ginglymus (hinge) joint (humeroulnar) and a trochoid (pivot) joint (humeroradial):

Articulation	Components
Humeroulnar	Trochlea & Trochlear notch
Humeroradial	Capitulum & Radial head
Proximal R-U	Radial notch & Radial head

The ligaments of the elbow joint include a relatively weak capsule and the following ligaments (Fig. 10–8):

Ligament	Components	Comments
Ulnar Collateral	Anterior & Posterior	Ant. fibers key
Radial collateral	Triangular	Weaker, less distinct
Annular	Osseofibrous ring	Rotatory movements
Quadrate	Annular lig. → Radial neck	
Oblique cord	Coronoid base → Radius	

C. Muscles of the Arm—There are four muscles of the arm (Table 10–4). The triceps muscle helps form borders for two important spaces (Fig. 10–9). The **triangular space** is bordered by the teres minor (superiorly), teres major (inferiorly), and long head of the triceps (laterally) and contains the circumflex scapular vessels. The **quadrangular space** is also bordered by the teres minor (superiorly) and the teres major (inferiorly), with the long head of the triceps forming its medial border and the humerus forming the lateral border. The quadrangular space transmits the posterior humeral circumflex vessels and the axillary nerve. The **triangular interval** is immediately inferior to the quadrangular space and is bordered by the teres major (superiorly), long head of the triceps (medially), and lateral head of the triceps or the humerus (laterally). Through this interval, the profunda brachii artery and radial nerve can be seen.

D. Nerves—Four major nerves traverse the arm, two giving off branches to arm musculature, and two that innervate distal musculature (Fig. 10–10). Most of the cutaneous innervation of the arm arises directly from the brachial plexus.

1. Musculocutaneous Nerve—Formed from the lateral cord of the brachial plexus, this nerve pierces the coracobrachialis 5–8 cm distal to the coracoid, and then branches to supply this muscle, the biceps, and the brachialis. It also gives off a branch to the elbow joint before it becomes the lateral antebrachial cutaneous nerve of the forearm.
2. Radial Nerve—Formed from the posterior cord of the brachial plexus, this nerve spirals around the humerus (medial → lateral), supplying the triceps muscles. It emerges on the lateral side·

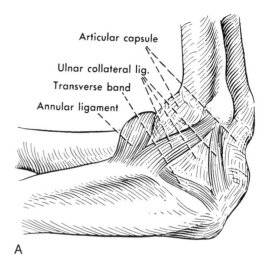

A

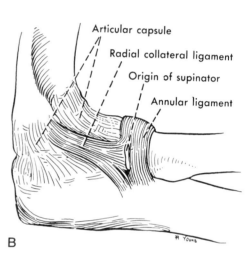

B

FIGURE 10–8. Elbow ligaments. *A*, Medial view. *B*, Lateral view. (From Jenkins, D.B.: Hollinshead's Functional Anatomy of the Limbs and Back, 6th ed., p. 108. Philadelphia, W.B. Saunders, 1991; reprinted by permission.)

of the arm between the brachialis and brachioradialis anterior to the lateral epicondyle.

3. Median Nerve—From the medial and lateral cords of the brachial plexus, this nerve accompanies the brachial artery along the arm, crossing it in its course (lateral → medial). It supplies some branches to the elbow joint, but has no branches in the arm itself.

TABLE 10–4. MUSCLES OF THE ARM

Muscle	Origin	Insertion	Action	Innervation
Coracobrachialis	Coracoid	Mid. humerus medial	Flexion, Adduction	Musculocutaneous
Biceps	Coracoid (SH) Supraglenoid (LH)	Radial tuberosity	Supination, Flexion	Musculocutaneous
Brachialis	Ant. humerus	Ulnar tuberosity (ant.)	Flexes forearm	Musculocut. & Radial
Triceps	Infraglenoid (LH) Post. humerus (lat H) Post. humerus (MH)	Olecranon	Extends forearm	Radial

SH, short head; LH, long head; lat H, lateral head; MH, medial head.

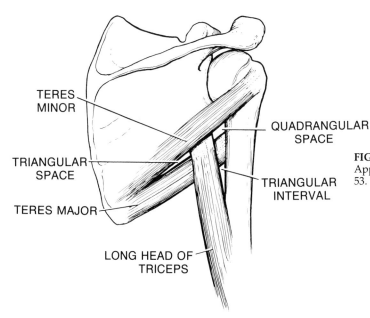

FIGURE 10–9. Quadrangular space. (From Kaplan, E.B.: Surgical Approaches to the Neck, Cervical Spine, and Upper Extremity, p. 53. Philadelphia, W.B. Saunders, 1966; reprinted by permission.)

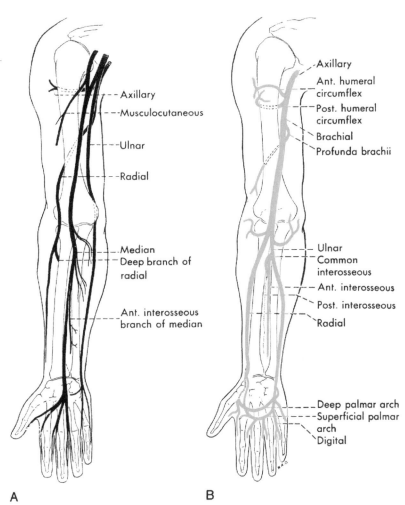

A   B

FIGURE 10–10. Nerves and vessels of the upper extremity. *A*, Principal nerves. *B*, Chief arteries. (From Jenkins, D.B.: Hollinshead's Functional Anatomy of the Limbs and Back, 6th ed., p. 62. Philadelphia, W.B. Saunders, 1991; reprinted by permission.)

4. Ulnar Nerve—The continuation of the medial cord of the brachial plexus, this nerve remains medial to the brachial artery in the arm, and then runs behind the medial epicondyle of the humerus, where it is quite superficial. It also has branches to the elbow but no arm branches.

5. Cutaneous Nerves—The supraclavicular nerve (C3, C4) supplies the upper shoulder. The axillary nerve supplies the shoulder joint and the overlying skin (in accordance with Hilton's Law). The medial, lateral, and dorsal brachial cutaneous nerves supply the balance of the cutaneous innervation of the arm.

E. Vessels—The brachial artery originates at the lower border of the tendon of the teres major and continues to the elbow, where it bifurcates into the radial and ulnar arteries (Fig. 10–10). Lying medial in the arm, the brachial artery curves laterally to enter the cubital fossa (formed by the distal humerus proximally, the brachioradialis laterally, and the pronator teres medially). Its principal branches include the deep brachial, the superior and inferior ulnar collaterals, and nutrient and muscular branches. Anastomoses around the elbow (medial→lateral) are as follows:

SUPERIOR BRANCH	INFERIOR BRANCH
Superior ulnar collateral	Posterior ulnar recurrent
Inferior ulnar collateral	Anterior ulnar recurrent
Mid. collateral branch of deep brachial	Interosseous recurrent
Rad. collateral branch of deep brachial	Radial recurrent

F. Surgical Approaches to the Arm and Elbow—Proximally include the anterior and posterior approaches, and distally include anterolateral and lateral approaches to the humerus and numerous approaches to the elbow.

1. Anterorolateral Approach to the Humerus (Fig. 10–11)—Depends on the internervous plane between the deltoid (axillary nerve) and the pectoralis major (med. & lat. pectoral nerves) proximally, and between the fibers of the brachialis (radial nerve and musculocutaneous nerve) distally. The radial and axillary nerves are at risk mainly with forceful retraction. The anterior circumflex humeral vessels may need to be ligated with a proximal approach.

2. Posterior Approach to the Humerus (Fig. 10–12)—Utilizes the interval between the lateral and long heads of the triceps superficially, and a muscle-splitting approach for the medial (deep) head. The radial nerve and deep brachial artery must be identified and protected, and the ulnar nerve is jeopardized unless subperiosteal dissection of the humerus is meticulous.

3. Anterolateral Approach to the Distal Humerus (Fig. 10–13)—Uses the interval between the brachialis (musculocutaneous and radial nerves) and the brachioradialis (radial nerve). The radial nerve again must be identified and protected.

4. Lateral Approach to the Distal Humerus—Exploits the interval between the triceps and the brachioradialis by elevating a portion of the common extensor origin from the lateral epicondyle. Proximal extension jeopardizes the radial nerve.

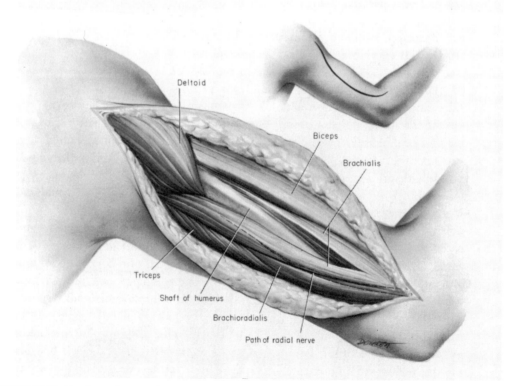

FIGURE 10–11. Lateral approach to the arm. (From Kaplan, E.B.: Surgical Approaches to the Neck, Cervical Spine, and Upper Extremity, p. 74. Philadelphia, W.B. Saunders, 1966; reprinted by permission.)

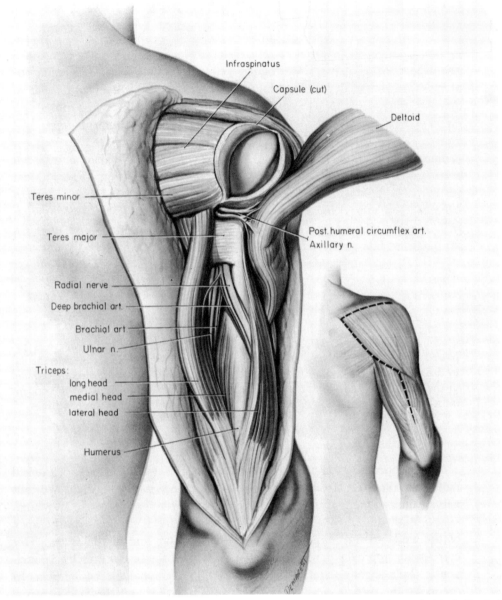

Infraspinatus

Capsule (cut)

Deltoid

Teres minor

Teres major

Post. humeral circumflex art.
Axillary n.

Radial nerve

Deep brachial art.

Brachial art.

Ulnar n.

Triceps:
  long head
  medial head
  lateral head

Humerus

FIGURE 10–12. Posterior approach to the arm. (From Kaplan, E.B.: Surgical Approaches to the Neck, Cervical Spine, and Upper Extremity, p. 73. Philadelphia, W.B. Saunders, 1966; reprinted by permission.)

5. Posterior Approach to the Elbow (Fig. 10–14)—Detachment of the extensor mechanism of the elbow gives excellent exposure for many elbow fractures. The olecranon osteotomy (best done with a chevron cut 2 cm distal to the tip) should be predrilled, and the ulnar nerve protected.
6. Medial Approach to the Elbow—Exploits the interval between the brachialis (musculocutaneous nerve) and the triceps (radial nerve) proximally, and the brachialis and pronator teres (median nerve) distally. The ulnar and medial antebrachial cutaneous nerves are in the field and must be protected.
7. Anterolateral Approach to the Elbow (Henry)—An extension of the same approach to the distal humerus, this approach is a brachialis (musculocutaneous nerve) splitting approach proximally and is between the pronator teres (me-

dian nerve), and the brachioradialis distally. The lateral antebrachial cutaneous nerve must be protected superficially, and the radial nerve (and its branches) deep (supinate the forearm).
8. (Postero)Lateral (Kocher) Approach to the Elbow (Fig. 10–15)—Uses the interval between the anconeus (radial nerve) and the main extensor origin (ECU—posterior interosseous branch of the radial nerve [PIN]). Pronation of the arm moves the PIN radially, and the radial head is approached through the proximal supinator fibers. Extending this approach distal to the annular ligament increases the risk to the posterior interosseous nerve.

IV. The Forearm

  A. Osteology—The forearm includes two long bones—the ulna and radius, which articulate with

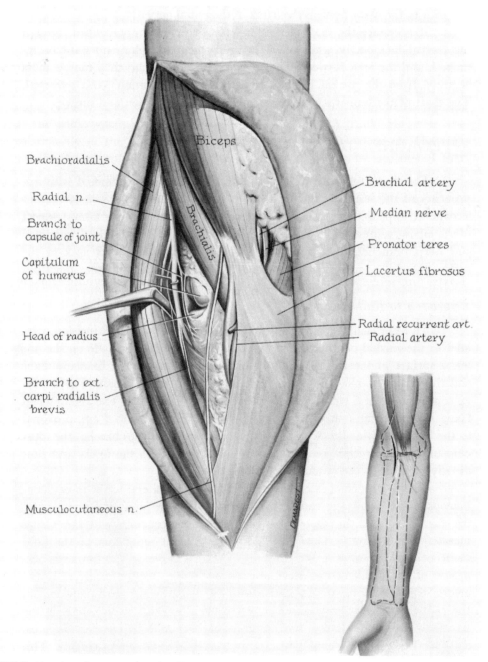

FIGURE 10–13. Anterior approach to the elbow. (From Kaplan, E.B.: Surgical Approaches to the Neck, Cervical Spine, and Upper Extremity, p. 77. Philadelphia, W.B. Saunders, 1966; reprinted by permission.)

the humerus (principally the ulna)—and the carpii (articulate principally with the radius).

1. Ulna—A long prismatic bone occupying the medial forearm and consisting of a body and two extremities. Proximally, the ulna is composed of two curved processes, the olecranon and the coronoid processes, with an intervening trochlear notch. Distally, the ulna tapers and ends in a lateral head and a medial styloid process. The ulna has one primary and two secondary ossification centers:

OSSIFICATION CENTER	AGE APPEARS	AGE FUSES
Body (primary)	8 weeks (fetal)	
Distal ulna	5 years	20 years
Olecranon	10 years	16 years

2. Radius—Like the ulna, the radius has a body and two extremities. The proximal radius is composed of a head with a central fovea, a neck, and a proximal medial radial tuberosity (for the

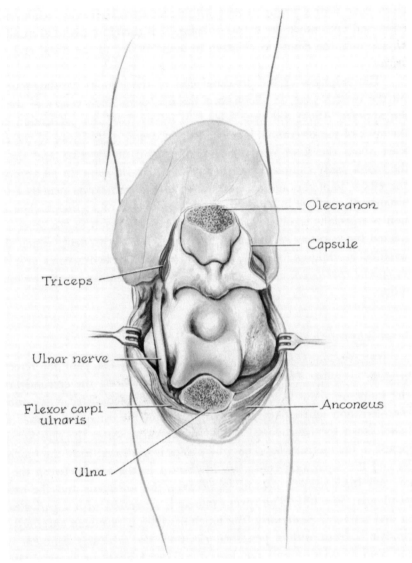

FIGURE 10–14. Posterior approach to the elbow. (From Kaplan, E.B.: Surgical Approaches to the Neck, Cervical Spine, and Upper Extremity, p. 82. Philadelphia, W.B. Saunders, 1966; reprinted by permission.)

insertion of the biceps tendon). The radius has a gradual bend (convex laterally), and gradually increases in size distally. The distal extremity of the radius is composed of the carpal articular surface, an ulnar notch, a dorsal tubercle, and a lateral styloid process. The radius is also ossified via three centers:

Ossification Center	Age Appears	Age Fuses
Body (primary)	8 weeks (fetal)	
Distal radius	2 years	17–20 years
Proximal radius	5 years	15–18 years

B. Arthrology—The radius and ulna articulate proximally at the elbow joint (discussed above) and distally at the wrist. The wrist consists primarily of the radiocarpal joint, but also includes the distal radioulnar articulation with its triangular fibrocartilage complex (TFCC).

1. Radiocarpal Joint—An ellipsoid joint involving the distal radius and the scaphoid, lunate, and triquetrum. Covered by a loose capsule, the wrist relies heavily on ligaments, especially volar ligaments, for stability. These include the volar and dorsal radiocarpal ligaments and the ulnar and radial collateral ligaments.
2. The TFCC (Fig. 10–16)—Originates from the most ulnar portion of the radius and extends into the caput ulna and the ulnar wrist to the base of the fifth metacarpal, and includes the following components:

Component	Origin	Insertion
Dorsal & volar radioulnar ligament (RUL)	Ulnar radius	Caput ulna
Articular disc	Radius/ulna	Triquetrum
Prestyloid recess	Disc	Meniscus homologue
Meniscus homologue	Ulna/disc	Triquetrum/UCL
Ulnar collateral ligament	Ulna	5th metacarpal

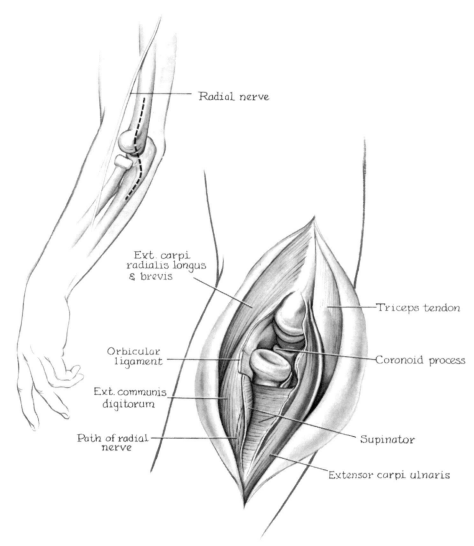

FIGURE 10–15. Lateral approach to the elbow. (From Kaplan, E.B.: Surgical Approaches to the Neck, Cervical Spine, and Upper Extremity, p. 83. Philadelphia, W.B. Saunders, 1966; reprinted by permission.)

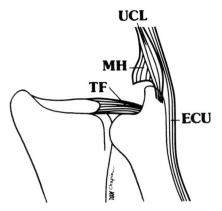

FIGURE 10–16. The triangular fibrocartilage complex (TFCC). *UCL*, ulnar collateral ligament; *MH*, meniscal homologue; *TF*, transverse fibers (radioulnar ligament); *ECU*, extensor carpi ulnaris. (From Wiessman, B.N., and Sledge, C.B.: Orthopedic Radiology, p. 115. Philadelphia, W.B. Saunders, 1986; reprinted by permission.)

C. Muscles of the Forearm (Fig. 10–17)—Are arranged based upon both location and function into volar flexors (superficial and deep) and dorsal extensors (superficial and deep) (Table 10–5).

D. Nerves—The nerves of the upper arm continue into the forearm (Fig. 10–18).

1. Radial Nerve—Anterior to the lateral epicondyle, the radial nerve runs between the brachialis and brachioradialis and divides into anterior and deep (posterior interosseous nerve [PIN]) branches. The PIN splits the supinator and supplies all of the extensor muscles (except the mobile wad [brachioradialis, ECRB, ECRL]). The superficial branch of the radial nerve passes to the dorsal radial surface of the hand in the distal third of the forearm by passing between the brachioradialis and ECRL.

2. Median Nerve—Lies medial to the brachial artery at the elbow, superficial to the brachialis muscle. In the forearm, the median nerve **splits** the two heads of the **pronator teres** and then **runs between the FDS and FDP**, becoming more superficial at the flexor retinaculum, where it continues into the hand. It has

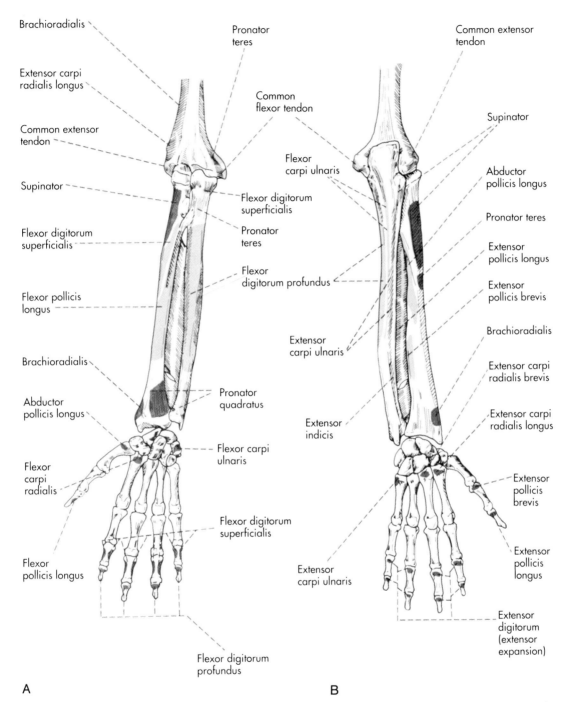

Brachioradialis

Extensor carpi radialis longus

Common extensor tendon

Supinator

Flexor digitorum superficialis

Flexor pollicis longus

Brachioradialis

Abductor pollicis longus

Flexor carpi radialis

Flexor pollicis longus

Pronator teres

Common flexor tendon

Flexor carpi ulnaris

Flexor digitorum superficialis

Pronator teres

Flexor digitorum profundus

Pronator quadratus

Flexor carpi ulnaris

Flexor digitorum superficialis

Flexor digitorum profundus

Common extensor tendon

Supinator

Abductor pollicis longus

Pronator teres

Extensor pollicis longus

Extensor pollicis brevis

Brachioradialis

Extensor carpi radialis brevis

Extensor carpi radialis longus

Extensor pollicis brevis

Extensor pollicis longus

Extensor digitorum (extensor expansion)

Extensor carpi ulnaris

Extensor indicis

Extensor carpi ulnaris

A

B

FIGURE 10–17. Origins and insertions of muscles of the forearm. (From Jenkins, D.B.: Hollinshead's Functional Anatomy of the Limbs and Back, 6th ed., fig. 8–4. Philadelphia, W.B. Saunders, 1991; reprinted by permission.)

branches to all the superficial flexor muscles of the forearm except the FCU. Its anterior interosseous branch, which runs between the FPL and FDP, supplies all the deep flexors except the ulnar half of the FDP.
3. Ulnar Nerve—Enters the forearm between the two heads of the FCU, which it supplies, and then **runs between the FCU and FDP** (and innervates the ulnar half of this muscle). It lies more superficial at the wrist and enters the hand through Guyon's canal.

4. Cutaneous Nerves—In the forearm, include the lateral antebrachial cutaneous nerve (the continuation of the musculocutaneous nerve), the medial antebrachial cutaneous nerve (which is a branch from the medial cord of the brachial plexus), and the posterior antebrachial cutaneous nerve (which is a branch of the radial nerve given off in the arm).

E. Vessels (Fig. 10–18)—At the elbow, the brachial artery enters the cubital fossa (bordered by the two

TABLE 10–5. MUSCLES OF THE FOREARM

Muscle	Origin	Insertion	Action	Innervation
Superficial Flexors				
Pronator teres (PT)	Med. epicondyle & coronoid	Mid. lat. radius	Pronate, flex forearm	Median
Flexor carpi radialis (FCR)	Med. epicondyle	2nd & 3rd metacarpal bases	Flex wrist	Median
Palmaris longus (PL)	Med. epicondyle	Palmar aponeurosis	Flex wrist	Median
Flexor carpi ulnaris (FCU)	Med. epicondyle & post. ulna	Pisiform	Flex wrist	**Ulnar**
Flexor digitorum superficialis (FDS)	Med. epicondyle & ant. radius	Base of middle phalanges	Flex PIP	Median
Deep Flexors				
Flexor digitorum profundus (FDP)	Ant. & med. ulna	Base of distal phalanges	Flex DIP	**Median-ant. interosseous/ and Ulnar**
Flexor pollicis longus (FPL)	Ant. & lat. radius	Base of distal phalanges	Flex IP, thumb	Median-ant. interosseous
Pronator quadratus (PQ)	Distal ulna	Volar radius	Pronate hand	Median-ant. interosseous
Superficial Extensors				
Brachioradialis (BR)	Lat. supracondylar humerus	Lat. distal radius	Flex forearm	Radial
Ext. carpi radialis longus (ECRL)	Lat. supracondylar humerus	2nd metacarpal base	Extend wrist	Radial
Ext. carpi radialis brevis (ECRB)	Lat. epicondyle of humerus	3rd metacarpal base	Extend wrist	Radial
Anconeus	Lat. epicondyle of humerus	Proximal dorsal ulna	Extend forearm	Radial
Extensor digitorum (ED)	Lat. epicondyle of humerus	Extensor aponeurosis	Extend digits	Radial-post. interosseous
Extensor ditigi minimi (EDM)	Common extensor tendon	Small finger extensor carpi ulnaris	Extend small finger	Radial-post. interosseous
Ext. carpi ulnaris (ECU)	Lat. epicondyle of humerus	5th metacarpal base	Extend/Adduct hand	Radial-post. interosseous
Deep Extensors				
Supinator	Lat. epicondyle of humerus, ulna	Dorsolateral radius	Supinate forearm	Radial-post. interosseous
Abductor pollicis longus (APL)	Dorsal ulna/Radius	1st metacarpal base	Abduct thumb, extend	Radial-post. interosseous
Extensor pollicis brevis (EPB)	Dorsal radius	Thumb proximal phalanx base	Extend thumb MCP	Radial-post. interosseous
Extensor pollicis longus (EPL)	Dorsolateral ulna	Thumb dorsal phalanx base	Extend thumb IP	Radial-post. interosseous
Extensor indicis proprius (EIP)	Dorsolateral ulna	Index finger extensor apparatus (ulnarly)	Extend index finger	Radial-post. interosseous

epicondyles, the brachioradialis, and the pronator teres and overlying the brachialis and supinator). It then divides at the level of the radial neck into the radial and ulnar arteries.

1. Radial Artery—Runs initally on the pronator teres, deep to the brachioradialis, and continues to the wrist between this muscle and the FCR. Forearm branches include the radial recurrent (see above), and muscular branches.
2. Ulnar Artery—The larger of the two branches, it is covered by the superficial flexors proximally (between the FDS and FDP). Distally, the artery lies on the FDP, between the tendons of the FCU and FDS. Forearm branches include the anterior and posterior ulnar recurrent (discussed above), the common interosseous (with anterior and posterior branches), and several muscular and nutrient arteries.

F. Surgical Approaches to the Forearm
1. Anterior Approach (Henry) (Fig. 10–19)—Utilizes the interval between the brachioradialis (radial N) and the pronator teres (or FCR distally) (median N). Proximally, it is necessary to isolate and ligate the **leash of Henry** (radial artery branches), and subperiosteally strip the supinator from its insertion. Distally, it is necessary to dissect off the FPL and PQ. Supination of the forearm displaces the PIN ulnarly.
2. Dorsal Approach (Thompson) (Fig. 10–20)—Utilizes the interval between the ECRB (radial N) and EDC (or EPL distally) (posterior interosseous N). The posterior interosseous nerve must be identified and protected with this surgical approach.
3. Exposure of the Ulna—Is via the interval between the ECU (posterior interosseous N) and the FCU (ulnar N).

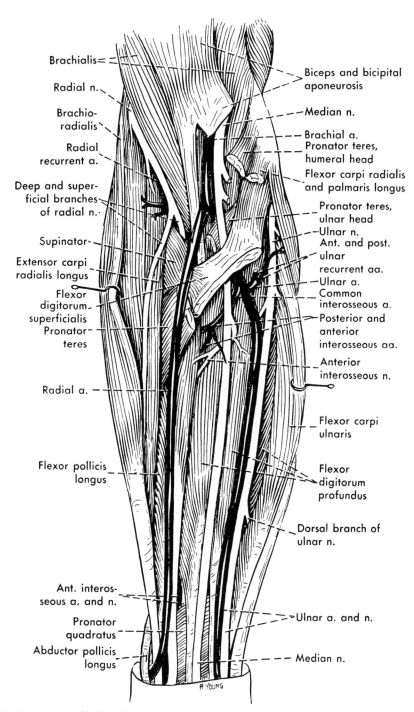

FIGURE 10–18. Arteries (*black*) and nerves (white) of the forearm. (From Jenkins, D.B.: Hollinshead's Functional Anatomy of the Limbs and Back, 6th ed., p. 131. Philadelphia, W.B. Saunders, 1991; reprinted by permission.)

V. Wrist and Hand

A. Osteology

1. Carpal Bones—Each carpal bone has six surfaces, with proximal, distal, medial, and lateral surfaces for articulation and palmar and dorsal surfaces for ligamentous insertion. Ossification begins at the capitate (usually present at 1 year of age), and proceeds in a counterclockwise direction. Therefore the hamate is the second carpus to ossify (1–2 yo), followed by the triquetrum (3 yo), lunate (4–5 yo), scaphoid (5 yo), trapezium (6 yo), and trapezoid (7 yo). The pisiform, which is actually a large sesamoid bone, is the last to ossify (9 yo). Several key features are important to recognize in the individual carpal bones:

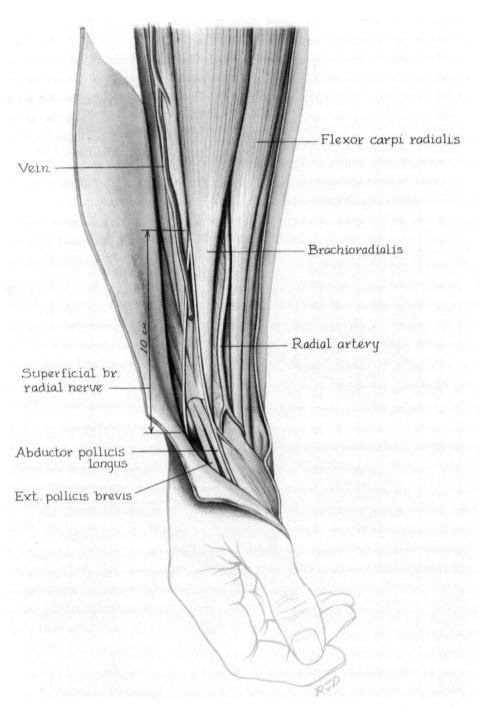

FIGURE 10–19. Anterior (Henry) approach to the forearm. (From Kaplan, E.B.: Surgical Approaches to the Neck, Cervical Spine, and Upper Extremity, p. 92. Philadelphia, W.B. Saunders, 1966; reprinted by permission.)

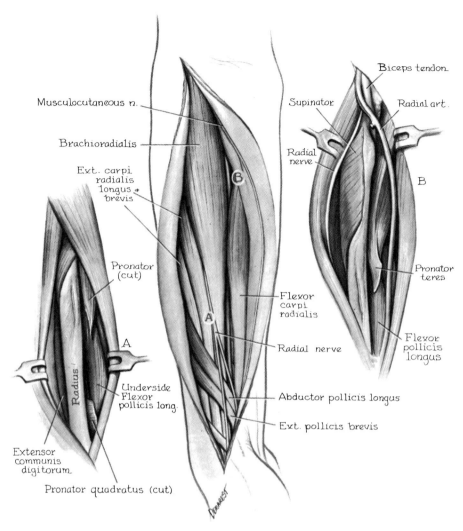

FIGURE 10–20. Dorsal (Thompson) approach to the forearm. (From Kaplan, E.B.: Surgical Approaches to the Neck, Cervical Spine, and Upper Extremity, p. 90. Philadelphia, W.B. Saunders, 1966; reprinted by permission.)

Bone	Important Features	# Articulations
Scaphoid	Tubercle (TCL, APB), distal vascular supply	5
Lunate	Lunar shape	5
Triquetrum	Pyramid shape	3
Pisiform	Spheroidal (TCL, FCR)	1
Trapezium	FCR groove, tubercle (opponens, APB, FPB, TCL)	4
Trapezoid	Wedge shape	4
Capitate	Largest bone, central location	7
Hamate	Hook (TCL)	5

TCL, transverse carpal ligament.

2. Metacarpals—Have two ossification centers: one for the body (primary center of ossification), which ossifies at 8 weeks of fetal life (like most long bones); and one at the neck that usually appears before the age of 3. The first metacarpal is a primordial phalanx, and has its secondary ossification center located at the base (like the

phalanges). Several characteristics allow identification of the individual metacarpals:

Metacarpal	Distinctive Features
I (Thumb)	Short, stout, base is saddle shaped
II (Index)	Longest, largest base, medial at base
III (Middle)	Styloid process
IV (Ring)	Small quadrilateral base, narrow shaft
V (Small)	Tubercle at base (ECU)

3. Phalanges—The 14 phalanges (three for each finger and two for the thumb) are all similar. They all have secondary ossification centers at their bases that appear at ages 3 (proximal), 4 (middle), and 5 (distal). The bases of the proximal phalanges are oval and concave, with smaller heads ending in two condyles. The middle phalanges have two concave facets at their bases and pulley-shaped heads. The distal pha-

langes are smaller and have palmar ungual tuberosities distally.

B. Arthrology

  1. Radiocarpal (Wrist) Joint—An ellipsoid joint made up of the distal radius, scaphoid, lunate, triquetrum and the following ligamentous structures (Fig. 10–21):

STRUCTURE	ATTACHMENTS	DISTINCTIVE FEATURES
Articular capsule	Surrounds joint	Reinforced by volar & dorsal RCL
Volar radiocarpal ligament (RCL)	Radius, ulna, scaphoid, lunate, triquetrum, capitate	Oblique ulnar, strong
Dorsal radiocarpal ligament	Radius, scaphoid, lunate, triquetrum	Oblique radial, weak
Ulnar collateral ligament	Ulna, triquetrum, pisiform, transverse carpal ligament	Fan shaped, two fascicles
Radial collateral ligament	Radius, scaphoid, trapezium, transverse carpal ligament	Radial artery adjacent

The palmar radiocarpal ligament is the strongest supporting structure, although it has a weak area on the radial side (the space of Poirier) that lends less support to the scaphoid, lunate, and trapezoid, and may be related to wrist instability with injury.

  2. Intercarpal Joints

    a. Proximal Row—Scaphoid, lunate, and triquetral are gliding joints. Two dorsal intercarpal ligaments connect the scaphoid and lunate and lunate and triquetral bones. Two palmar intercarpal ligaments connect the scaphoid and lunate and lunate and triquetral bones. The dorsal intercarpal ligaments are stronger. Interosseous ligaments are narrow bundles connecting the lunate and scaphoid and the lunate and triquetral bones.

    b. Pisiform Articulation—The pisotriquetral joint has a thin articular capsule. The pisiform is also connected proximally by the ulnar collateral and palmar radiocarpal ligaments. The pisohamate ligament and pisometacarpal ligaments help extend the pull of the FCU.

    c. Distal Row—Trapezium, trapezoid, capitate, and hamate gliding joints. The dorsal intercarpal ligaments connect the trapezium with the trapezoid, the trapezoid with the capitate, and the capitate with the hamate. The palmar ligaments do the same. The interosseous ligaments are much thicker in the distal row, connecting the capitate and hamate (strongest), the capitate and trapezoid, and the trapezium and trapezoid (weakest).

    d. Midcarpal joint—Transverse articulations between the proximal and distal rows are reinforced by palmar and dorsal intercarpal ligaments and carpal collateral ligaments (radial is stronger).

  3. Carpometacarpal (CMC) Joints

    a. Thumb CMC Joint—A highly mobile saddle joint. It is supported by a capsule and radial, palmar, and dorsal carpometacarpal ligaments.

    b. Finger CMC Joints—Gliding joints with capsules, dorsal CMC ligaments (strongest), palmar CMC ligaments, and interosseous CMC ligaments.

  4. Metacarpophalangeal Joints—Ellipsoid joints covered by palmar (volar plate), collateral, and deep transverse metacarpal ligaments.

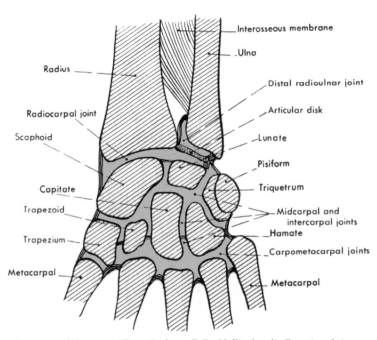

FIGURE 10–21. Anatomy of the wrist. (From Jenkins, D.B.: Hollinshead's Functional Anatomy of the Limbs and Back, 6th ed., p. 158. Philadelphia, W.B. Saunders, 1991; reprinted by permission.)

5. Interphalangeal Joints—Hinge joints with capsules and obliquely oriented collateral ligaments.
6. Other Important Structures
   a. Extensor Retinaculum—Covers the dorsum of the wrist and contains six separate synovial sheaths (Fig. 10–22):

Compartment	Contents	Pathologic Condition Involving Tendons
1	APL, EPB	de Quervain's tenosynovitis
2	ECRL, ECRB	Tennis elbow/extensor tendonitis
3	EPL	Rupture at lister's tubercle (following wrist fractures)
4	EDC, EIP	Extensor tenosynovitis
5	EDM	Rupture (rheumatoid)
6	ECU	Snapping at ulnar styloid

   b. Transverse Carpal Ligament (TCL; Flexor Retinaculum)—Forms the roof of the carpal tunnel, which contains the long flexor tendons and the median nerve (Fig. 10–23). It is attached medially to the pisiform and the hook of the hamate, and laterally to the tuberosity of the scaphoid and the ridge of the trapezium. It also forms the floor of Guyon's canal, which is also bordered by the hook of the hamate and the pisiform and is covered by the volar carpal ligament. Entrapment of the ulnar nerve in this canal is possible.
   c. Triangular Fibrocartilage Complex—Formed by the triangular fibrocartilage, ulnocarpal ligaments (volar ulnolunate and ulnotriquetral ligaments), and a meniscal homologue. Injuries to this structure are a common cause of ulnar wrist pain.
   d. Intrinsic Apparatus—A complex arrangement of structures that surrounds the digits (Fig. 10–24). The following structures are important:

Structure	Attachments	Significance
Sagittal bands	Covers MCP	Allows MCP extension
Transverse (sagittal) fibers	Volar plate	Allows MCP flexion (interosseoi)
Lateral bands	Covers PIP	Allows PIP extension (lumbricals)
Oblique retinacolor ligament (landsmeer's ligament)	A4 pully, terminal tendon	Allows DIP extension (passive)

   e. Flexor Sheath (Fig. 10–25)—Covers the flexor tendons in the finger, protecting and nourishing the tendons (vincula). Also forms five pulleys (A1–A5) with three intervening cruciate attachments (C1–C3). **The**

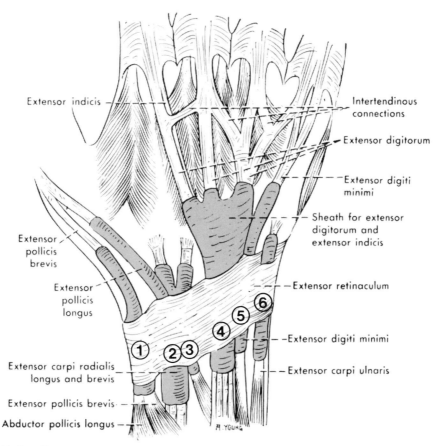

FIGURE 10–22. Extensor compartments of the wrist (1 → 6). (From Jenkins, D.B.: Hollinshead's Functional Anatomy of the Limbs and Back, 6th ed., p. 174. Philadelphia, W.B. Saunders, 1991; reprinted by permission.)

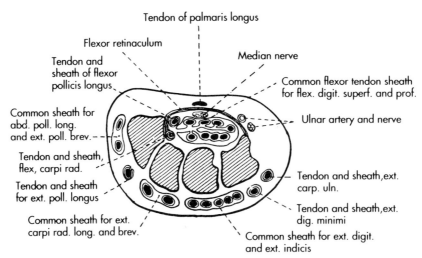

FIGURE 10–23. Components of the carpal tunnel. (From Jenkins, D.B.: Hollinshead's Functional Anatomy of the Limbs and Back, 6th ed., p. 162. Philadelphia, W.B. Saunders, 1991; reprinted by permission.)

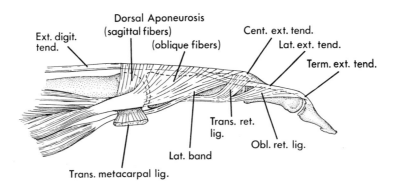

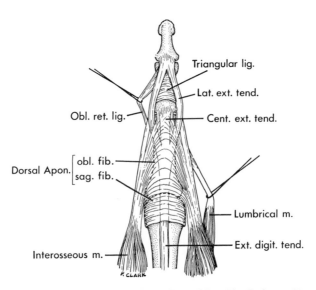

FIGURE 10–24. Dorsal extensor apparatus. (From Bora, F.W.: The Pediatric Upper Extremity, p. 93, Philadelphia, W.B. Saunders, 1986; reprinted by permission.)

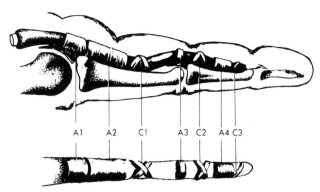

FIGURE 10–25. Flexor pulleys. (From Tubiana, R.: The Hand, Vol. 3, p. 173. Philadelphia, W.B. Saunders, 1985; reprinted by permission.)

A2 pulley, overlying the proximal phalanx, is the most important one, followed by A4, which covers the middle phalanx.

C. Muscles (Table 10–6, Fig. 10–26)

D. Nerves (Fig. 10–27)

1. Median Nerve—Enters the wrist just under the transverse carpal ligament between the FDS and the FCR. The palmar branch supplies the thenar skin. The deep (muscular) branch runs radially and supplies thenar muscles. Digital nerves supply the lumbricals and the radial 3½ digits.

2. Ulnar Nerve—Enters the wrist through Guyon's canal and divides into a superficial branch (palmaris brevis and skin) and a deep branch that passes between the ADM and FDMB, giving off motor branches to the deep musculature and terminating in digital nerves for the ulnar

1½ digits. The dorsal cutaneous branch swings dorsally at the wrist and can be injured with either arthroscopic portal placement or surgical incisions.

3. Sensation to the Thumb—Can be comprised of five different branches: lateral antebrachial cutaneous nerve, superficial and dorsal digital branches of the radial nerve, and digital and palmar branches of the median nerve.

E. Vessels (Fig. 10–27)

1. Radial Artery—At the wrist, the radial artery reaches the dorsum of the carpus by passing between the RCL and the APL and EPB tendons (snuffbox). Prior to this, it gives off a superficial palmar branch that communicates with the superficial arch (ulnar artery). In the hand, it forms the deep palmar arch.

2. Ulnar Artery—At the wrist, the ulnar artery lies on the TCL, gives off a deep palmar branch (which anastomoses with the deep arch), and then forms the superficial palmar arch, which is distal to the deep arch.

F. Surgical Approaches

1. Dorsal Approach to the Wrist (Fig. 10–28)—Through the third and fourth extensor compartment (EPL and EDC). Protecting and retracting these tendons allows access to the distal radius and the dorsal radiocarpal joint.

2. Volar Approach to the Wrist (Fig. 10–29)—Used most commonly for carpal tunnel release, the incision is usually made in line with the fourth ray to avoid the palmar cutaneous branch of the median nerve. Careful dissection through the transverse carpal ligament is necessary to avoid injury to the median nerve or its motor branch. The median nerve and flexor tendons can be

TABLE 10–6. MUSCLES OF THE HAND AND WRIST

MUSCLE	ORIGIN	INSERTION	ACTION	INNERVATION
Thenar Muscles				
Abductor pollicis brevis (APB)	Scaphoid, Trapezoid	Base of proximal phalanx—radial side	Abduct thumb	Median
Opponens pollicis	Trapezium	Thumb metacarpal	Abduct, flex, med. rotation	Median
Flexor pollicis brevis (FPB)	Trapezium, capitate	Base of proximal phalanx—radial side	Flex MCP	Median & Ulnar
Adductor pollicis (AP)	Capitate, 2nd & 3rd metacarpals	Base of proximal phalanx—ulnar side	Adduct thumb	Ulnar
Hypothenar Muscles				
Palmaris brevis (PB)	TCL, Palmar aponeurosis	Ulnar palm	Retract skin	Ulnar
Abductor digiti minimi (ADM)	Pisiform	Base of proximal phalanx—ulnar side	Abduct small finger	Ulnar
Flexor digiti minimi brevis (FDMB)	Hamate, TCL	Base of proximal phalanx—ulnar side	Flex MCP	Ulnar
Opponens digiti minimi (ODM)	Hamate, TCL	Small finger metacarpal	Abduct, flex, lat. rotation	Ulnar
Intrinsic Muscles				
Lumbricals	Flexor digitorum profundus (FDP)	Lateral bands (radial)	Extend PIP	Median & Ulnar
Dorsal interosseous (DIO)	Adjacent metacarpals	Proximal phalanx base/Extensor apparatus	Abduct, flex MCP	Ulnar
Volar interosseous (VIO)	Adjacent metacarpals	Proximal phalanx base/Extensor apparatus	Adduct, flex MCP	Ulnar

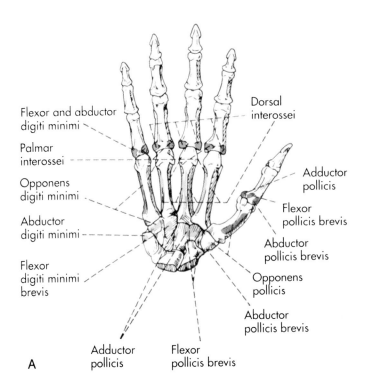

Flexor and abductor
digiti minimi

Palmar
interossei

Opponens
digiti minimi

Abductor
digiti minimi

Flexor
digiti minimi
brevis

Dorsal
interossei

Adductor
pollicis

Flexor
pollicis brevis

Abductor
pollicis brevis

Opponens
pollicis

Abductor
pollicis brevis

A

Adductor
pollicis

Flexor
pollicis brevis

FIGURE 10–26. Origins and insertions of muscles of the wrist and hand. (From Jenkins, D.B.: Hollinshead's Functional Anatomy of the Limbs and Back, 6th ed., fig. 11–9. Philadelphia, W.B. Saunders, 1991; reprinted by permission.)

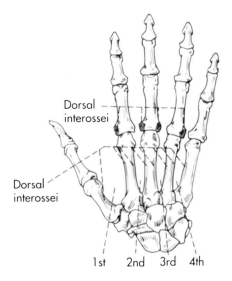

Dorsal
interossei

Dorsal
interossei

1st   2nd   3rd   4th

B

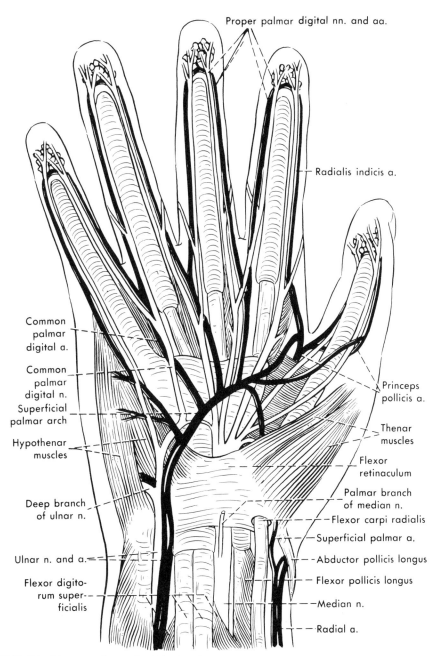

FIGURE 10–27. Nerves and vessels of the hand. (From Jenkins, D.B.: Hollinshead's Functional Anatomy of the Limbs and Back, 6th ed., fig. 11–11. Philadelphia, W.B. Saunders, 1991; reprinted by permission.)

retracted to allow access to the distal radius and carpus.

3. Volar Approach to the Scaphoid (Russe) (Fig. 10–30)—Uses the interval between the FCR and the radial artery. An approach through the radial aspect of the FCR sheath is often easier, and protects the radial artery.

4. Dorsloateral Approach to the Scaphoid (Fig. 10–31)—Utilizes an incision within the anatomic snuffbox (first and third dorsal wrist compartment) protecting the superficial radial nerve and radial artery (deep).

5. Volar Approach to the Flexor Tendons (Bunnell)—Zig-zag incisions across the flexor creases help in exposure of the flexor sheaths. The digital sheaths should be avoided.

6. Midlateral Approach to the Digits—Good for stabilization of fractures and neurovascular exposure, this approach uses a laterally placed incision at the dorsal extent of the IP creases. Exposure of the digital neurovascular bundle is carried out volar to the incision.

VI. Spine

A. Osteology

1. Introduction—The spine contains 33 vertebrae. There are 7 cervical, 12 thoracic, 5 lumbar, 5 sacral, and 4 coccygeal vertebrae. The total length of the spine averages about 71 cm. Normal curves include cervical lordosis, thoracic kyphosis, and lumbosacral lordosis. The vertebral bodies generally increase in width craniocau-

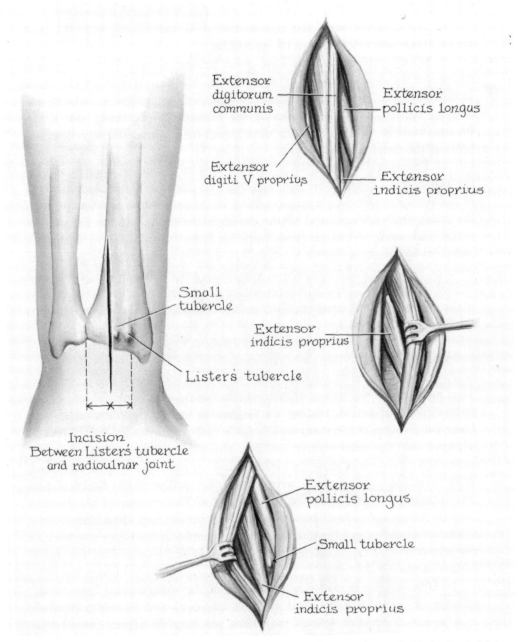

FIGURE 10–28. Dorsal wrist approach. (From Kaplan, E.B.: Surgical Approaches to the Neck, Cervical Spine, and Upper Extremity, p. 112. Philadelphia, W.B. Saunders, 1966; reprinted by permission.)

dally with the exception of T1–T3. Important topographic landmarks include the mandible (C2–C3), hyoid cartilage (C3), thyroid cartilage (C4/C5), cricoid cartilage (C6), vertebra prominens (C7), spine of scapula (T3), tip of scapula (T7), and iliac crest (L4–L5).

2. Cervical Spine—Unique features include foramina in each transverse process. The spinous processes are bifid and the vertebral foramina are triangularly shaped. The atlas (C1) is unique in that it contains no vertebral body and no spinous process. It does contain two lateral masses. The axis (C2) has a vertical projection called the dens or odontoid process that articulates with the atlas. It also possesses superior and inferior facets. The seventh cervical verte-

bra is unique because it has a prominent non-bifid posterior spinous process and no anterior tubercle.

3. Thoracic Spine—Unique features include costal facets (present on all 12 vertebral bodies and the transverse processes of T1–T9) and a rounded vertebral foramen. The first thoracic vertebra contains a large and prominent spinous process.

4. Lumbar Spine—These vertebrae are the largest. They contain short laminae and pedicles and massive vertebral bodies. They also have mammillary processes that project posteriorly from the superior articular facet. The transverse processes are thin and long (with the exception of the fifth lumbar vertebra).

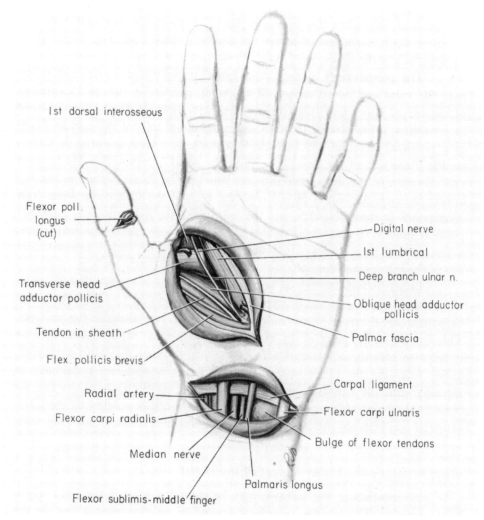

1st dorsal interosseous

Flexor poll. longus (cut)

Transverse head adductor pollicis

Tendon in sheath

Flex. pollicis brevis

Radial artery

Flexor carpi radialis

Median nerve

Flexor sublimis-middle finger

Palmaris longus

Digital nerve

1st lumbrical

Deep branch ulnar n.

Oblique head adductor pollicis

Palmar fascia

Carpal ligament

Flexor carpi ulnaris

Bulge of flexor tendons

FIGURE 10–29. Approach to the carpal tunnel and thenar muscles. (From Kaplan, E.B.: Surgical Approaches to the Neck, Cervical Spine, and Upper Extremity, p. 97. Philadelphia, W.B. Saunders, 1966; reprinted by permission.)

5. Sacrum—This is a fusion of five spinal elements. The promontory is the anterosuperior portion that projects into the pelvis. There are usually four pairs of pelvic sacral foramina located both anteriorly and posteriorly that transmit respective branches of the upper four sacral nerves. There is also a sacral canal, which opens caudally into the sacral hiatus.

6. Coccyx—This is a fusion of the lowest four spinal elements and attaches dorsally to the gluteus maximus, the external anal sphincter, and the coccygeal muscles.

7. Ossification—There are three primary ossification centers for each vertebra: two ossification centers in the centrum and one cartilaginous center for each arch. The arches unite dorsally at the third month of fetal life. Five secondary ossification centers (two transverse processes, one spinous process, and two body end plates) do not appear until after puberty. Ossification of the atlas, axis, sacral, and coccygeal vertebrae are unique. The axis (C2) ossifies from five primary and two secondary centers. Of note, the dens is formed from two primary growth cen-

ters that originate from the "centrum", or body of the atlas (C1). Mamillary processes arise from additional ossification centers in the lumbar vertebrae. The arches fuse with the centrum in the seventh year in the following order: thoracic, cervical, lumbar, and finally sacral. Failure of arch formation results in spina bifida.

B. Arthrology
   1. Ligaments
      a. General Arrangement—The vertebral bodies are bound together by the stronger anterior longitudinal ligament (**ALL**) and the weaker posterior longitudinal ligament (**PLL**). The ALL is usually thickest at the center of the vertebral body and thins at the periphery. Separate fibers extend from one to five levels. The PLL extends from the occiput to the posterior sacrum. It is separated from the center of the vertebral body by a space that allows passage of the dorsal branches of the spinal artery. The PLL is hourglass shaped, with the wider (yet thinner) sections located over the discs. Ruptured discs tend

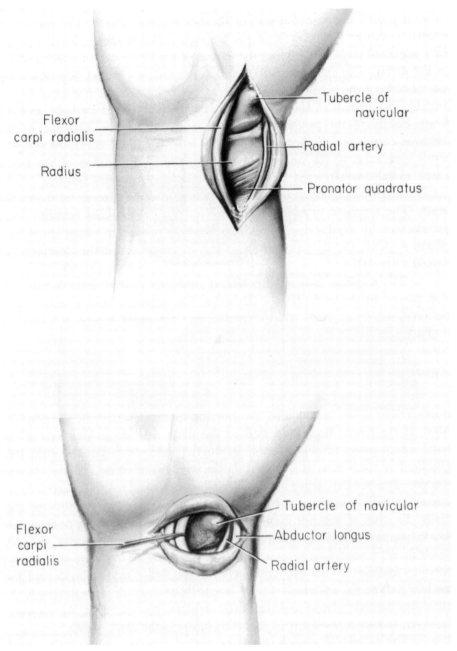

FIGURE 10–30. Russe approach to the scaphoid. (From Kaplan, E.B.: Surgical Approaches to the Neck, Cervical Spine, and Upper Extremity, p. 101. Philadelphia, W.B. Saunders, 1966; reprinted by permission.)

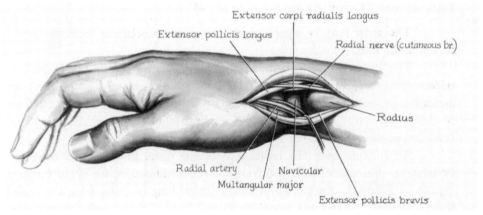

FIGURE 10–31. Dorsal approaches to the scaphoid. (From Kaplan, E.B.: Surgical Approaches to the Neck, Cervical Spine, and Upper Extremity, p. 107. Philadelphia, W.B. Saunders, 1966; reprinted by permission.)

to occur lateral to these expansions. Ligamentous capsules over lying the zygapophyseal joints and the intertransverse ligaments contribute little to interspinous stability. The **ligamentum flavum** is a strong, yellow, elastic ligament connecting the laminae. It runs from the anterior surface of the superior lamina to the posterior surface of the inferior lamina and is constantly in tension. Hypertrophy of the ligamentum flavum is said to contribute to nerve root compression. The **supraspinous** and **interspinous** ligaments lie dorsal to or in between the spinous processes, respectively. The supraspinous ligament begins at C7 and is in continuity with the ligamentum nuchae (which runs from C7 to the occiput). Their relative contribution to interspinous stability is unknown.

   b. Specialized Ligaments

      (1) Atlanto-occipital Joint-Consists of two articular capsules (anterior and posterior) and the **tectoral membrane** (a cephalad extension of the PLL), and is further stabilized by the ligamentous attachments to the dens.

      (2) Atlantoaxial Joint—The **transverse** ligament is the major stabilizer of the median atlantoaxial joint. This articulation is further stabilized by the apical ligament (longitudinal) that, together with the transverse ligament, comprises the **cruciate** ligament. Additionally, a pair of **alar**, or "check," ligaments run obliquely from the the tip of the dens to the occiput.

      (3) Iliolumbar Ligament—This stout ligament connects the transverse process of L5 with the ilium. Tension on this ligament in patients with unstable vertical shear pelvic fractures can lead to avulsion fractures of the transverse process.

2. Facet (Apophyseal) Joints—The orientation of the facets of the spine dictates the plane of motion at each relative level. The facet orientation varies with spinal level. In the sagittal plane, the orientation is 45 degrees in the cervical spine, 60 degrees in the thoracic spine, and 90 degrees in the lumbar spine. In the coronal plane, the orientation is 0 degrees (neutral) in the cervical spine, 20 degrees posterior in the thoracic spine, and 45 degrees anterior in the lumbar spine. In the cervical spine the superior articular facet is anterior and inferior to the inferior articular process of the vertebra above. In the lumbar spine the superior articular facet is anterior and lateral to the inferior articular facet.

3. Discs—The intervertebral discs are fibrocartilaginous, with obliquely oriented **annulus** fibrosis comprised of **type I collagen** and a softer central **nucleus pulposus** made of **type II collagen**. The discs account for 25% of the total spinal columnar height. They are attached to the vertebral bodies by hyaline cartilage, which is responsible for vertical growth of the column. The distinction between the nucleus and annulus becomes less apparent as one ages.

C. Spinal Musculature

1. Neck—The neck is divided, for functional purposes into the anterior and posterior regions.

   a. Anterior—The anterior neck muscles include the superficial platysma muscle (CN VII innervated), the stylohyoid and digastric muscles (CN XII) above the hyoid, and the "strap" muscles below the hyoid. Important strap muscles include the sternohyoid and omohyoid in the superficial layer, and the thyrohyoid and sternothyroid in the deep layer, all are innervated by the ansa cervicalis. Laterally the sternocleidomastoid (CN XI and ansa) runs obliquely across the neck and inserts into the mastoid process. It bends the neck to the ipsilateral side and rotates the head to the contralateral side.

   b. Posterior—The posterior neck muscles form the border of the **suboccipital triangle**. This triangle is formed by the superior and inferior heads of the obliquus capitis muscle and the rectus capitis posterior major muscle. The vertebral artery and the first cervical nerve are within this triangle and the greater occipital nerve is superficial.

2. Back—The back is blanketed by the trapezius (superiorly) and the latissimus dorsi (inferiorly). The rhomboids and levator scapulae are deep to this layer. Refer to table 10–3 for specifics on these muscles. The deep muscles of the back are arranged into two groups: the erector spinae and the transversospinalis group. The erector spinae run from the transverse and spinous processes of inferior vertebrae to the spinous processes of the superior vertebrae. They stabilize and extend the back. All of the deep back musculature is innervated by dorsal primary rami of spinal nerves.

D. Nerves

1. Spinal Cord—The cord extends from the brainstem to L1, where it terminates as the conus medularis. It is enclosed within the bony spinal canal with variable amounts of space (greatest in the upper cervical spine). The cord also varies in diameter (widest at the origin of plexi). In cross section, the cord has both geographic and functional boundaries (Fig. 10–32). It is divided in the midline anteriorly by a fissure and posteriorly by the sulcus. The posterior funiculi (**dorsal columns**) are located dorsally and receive ascending fibers, which deliver deep touch, proprioception, and vibratory sensation. The **lateral spinothalamic tract** transmits pain and temperature (this is the site for chordotomy for intractable pain). Descending in the **lateral corticospinal tract** are fibers transmitting instructions for voluntary muscle contraction. The **ventral spinothalamic tract** transmits light touch sensation while the ventral corticospinal tract delivers cortical messages of voluntary contraction. Pathways to the hand and upper extremity are usually localized centrally within this area (hence clinical findings of anterior cord syndrome). The spinal cord tapers at L1–L2 (conus medularis), and a small filum terminale continues with surrounding nerve roots contained within a common dural sac (cauda equina) to its termination in the coccyx.

POSTERIOR FUNUCULI
[Dorsal Columns]
(Sensory - Deep touch, Prop, Vib)

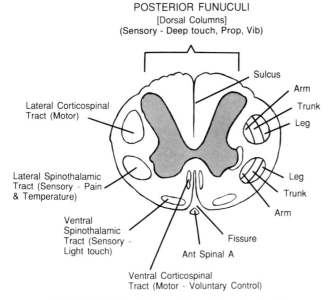

FIGURE 10–32. Cross section of the spinal cord.

2. Nerve Roots (Fig. 10–33)—Within the subarachnoid space, the dorsal root (and ganglia) and ventral roots converge to form the spinal nerve. The nerve becomes "extradural" as it approaches the intervertebral foramen (dura becomes epineurium) at all levels above L1. Below this level, the nerves are contained within the cauda equina. In the cervical spine the numbered nerve exists at a level *above* the corresponding vertebral level (e.g., C_2 exists at C_1C_2). In the lumbar spine the nerve root traverses the respective disc space above the named vertebral body and exits the respective foramen under the pedicle (Fig. 10–34). Herniated discs will usually impinge upon the traversing nerve root and the facet joint. After exiting the foramen, the spinal nerve delivers dorsal primary rami that supply the muscles and skin of the neck and back regions. The ventral rami supply the anteromedial trunk and the limbs. With exception of the thoracic nerves, ventral rami are grouped in plexuses before delivering sensorimotor functions to a general region.

3. Sympathetic Chain—The cervical sympathetic chain is a deep structure closely associated with the longus capitus and colli muscles, posterior to the carotid sheath. The sympathetic chain has three ganglia—superior, middle and inferior.

GANGLIA	LOCATION	OTHER
Superior	C_2–C_3	Largest
Middle	C_6	Variable
Inferior	C_7–T_1	"Stellate"

E. Vascular Supply to the Spine—Spinal blood supply is usually derived from the segmental arteries via the aorta. The primary supply to the dura and posterior elements is from the dorsal branches. The ventral branches supply the vertebral bodies via ascending and descending branches, which are delivered beneath the posterior longitudinal ligament in four separate ostia. The vertebral artery (a branch of the subclavian) ascends through the transverse foramina of C1–C6 (anterior to and not through C7), then posterior to the lateral masses, along the cephalad surface of the posterior arch of C_1 (atlas), then through the foramen magnum before uniting at the midline basilar artery. The **artery of Adamkiewicz** (great anterior medullary artery) enters through the left intervertebral foramen in the lower thoracic spine. It should be preserved in dissections at this level. Arterial supply to the spinal cord is from anterior and posterior spinal arteries and segmental branches of the vertebral artery and dorsal arteries, which travel via the dorsal and ventral rootlets to the respective dorsal and anterolateral portions of the cord. The venous

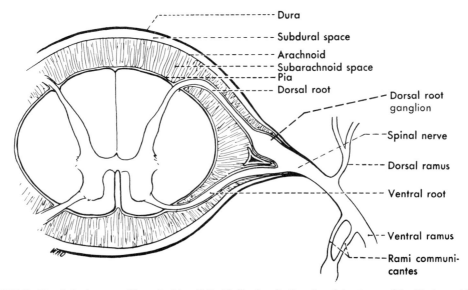

FIGURE 10–33. Spinal nerves. (From Jenkins, D.B.: Hollinshead's Functional Anatomy of the Limbs and Back, 6th ed., p. 205. Philadelphia, W.B. Saunders, 1991; reprinted by permission.)

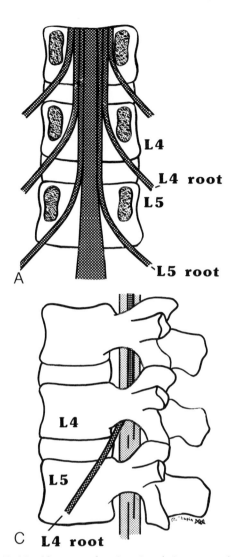

FIGURE 10–34. Nerve root locations in relation to vertebral landmarks. (From Wiessman, B.N., and Sledge, C.B.: Orthopedic Radiology, p. 283. Philadelphia, W.B. Saunders, 1986; reprinted by permission.)

drainage of the vertebral bodies is primarily via the central sinusoid located on the dorsum of each vertebral body.

F. Surgical Approaches to the Spine

1. Anterior Approach to the Cervical Spine (Fig. 10–35)—A transverse incision is based on the desired level (e.g., for C5 one should enter the carotid triangle). The platysma is retracted with the skin. The pretracheal fascia is exposed to explore the interval between the carotid sheath and the trachea. The prevertebral fascia is sharply incised and the longus colli muscle gently retracted (protecting the recurrent laryngeal nerve) to expose the vertebral body. The right recurrent laryngeal nerve can lie outside the carotid sheath and must be identified. By dissecting the longus muscles subperiosteally, one also will protect the stellate ganglion (avoiding Horner's syndrome). Occasionally it is necessary to split the fibers of the omohyoid.

2. Posterior Approach to the Cervical Spine—

After a midline approach through the ligamentum nuchae, the superficial layer (trapezius) and intermediate layer (splenius, semispinalis, and longissimus capitis) are reflected laterally and the vertebrae are exposed. The vertebral artery is especially vulnerable as it leaves the foramen transversarium and travels above and medially to pierce the atlanto-occipital membrane at its lateral angle. The greater occipital nerve (C2) and the third occipital nerve (C3) should also be protected in the suboccipital region. Access to the spinal canal is via laminectomy or facetectomy (Fig. 10–36).

3. Anterior Approach to the Thoracic Spine—A transverse incision is made approximately two ribs above the level of interest. Dissection over the top of the rib is carried out to avoid injuring the intercostal neurovascular bundle. The rib is further dissected and removed from the field. The right-sided approach is favored to avoid the aorta, segmental arteries, artery of Adamkiewicz, as well as the thoracic duct. The esophagus, aorta, vena cava, and pleura of the lungs should be identified and protected.

4. Posterior Approach to the Thoracolumbar Spine—A straight midline incision is made over the spinous processes and carried down through the thoracolumbar fascia. Paraspinal musculature is subperiosteally dissected from the attached spinous processes, exposing the posterior elements. Structures at risk include the posterior primary rami (near facet joints) and segmental vessels (anterior to the plane connecting the transverse processes). Partial laminectomy allows greater exposure of the cord and discs. Pedicle screw placement is at the junction of the lateral border of the superior facet and the middle of the transverse process. These screws should be angled 15 degrees medially and in line with the slope of the vertebra as seen on lateral radiographs.

5. Anterior Approach to the Thoracolumbar Spine—An oblique incision is centered over the 10th rib, which is exposed and removed. The diaphragm is incised near its periphery and dissection is carried into the retroperitoneum. The peritoneum is swept away from the psoas and vertebral bodies. Segmental arteries are ligated. Dangers include the ureter, internal iliac vessels, and lumbar plexus nerves.

VII. Pelvis and Hip

A. Osteology— The pelvic girdle is composed of two innominate (coxal) bones that articulate with the sacrum. Each innominate bone, in turn, is composed of three united bones: the ilium, ischium, and pubis. Distinctive parts of each innominate bone include the acetabulum (vinegar cup) and the obturator foramen. The acetabulum is anteverted and obliquely oriented. The posterior superior articular surface is thickened to accommodate weight bearing. The inferior surface is deficient and contains the acetabular or cotyloid notch. This notch is bound by the transverse acetabular ligament. The greater sciatic notch is located posterior and superior to the acetabulum, between the posterior inferior iliac spine (PIIS) and the ischial spine. The anterior superior iliac spine (ASIS) is prominent and palpable at the lateral edge of the inguinal lig-

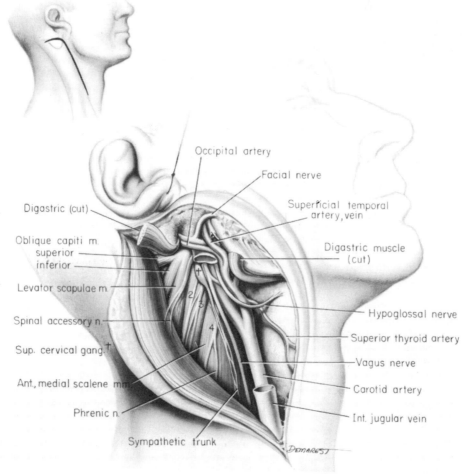

Occipital artery

Facial nerve

Superficial temporal artery, vein

Digastric muscle (cut)

Digastric (cut)

Oblique capiti m.
superior
inferior

Levator scapulae m.

Spinal accessory n.

Sup. cervical gang.

Ant., medial scalene mm.

Phrenic n.

Sympathetic trunk

Hypoglossal nerve

Superior thyroid artery

Vagus nerve

Carotid artery

Int. jugular vein

DEMAREST

FIGURE 10–35. Approach to the anterior neck. (From Kaplan, E.B.: Surgical Approaches to the Neck, Cervical Spine, and Upper Extremity, p. 23. Philadelphia, W.B. Saunders, 1966; reprinted by permission.)

ament. It is the origin for the sartorious muscle and the transverse and internal abdominal muscles. The posterior superior iliac spine (PSIS) is usually located 4–5 cm lateral to the S2 spinous process. It may be marked topographically by a dimple and is an excellent source for bone graft. The anterior inferior iliac spine (AIIS) is less prominent and provides the origin of the direct head of the rectus

femoris. The arcuate line delineates a thick column of bone that extends from the auricular process of the ilium to the pectineal line and represents the weight-bearing column. The outer surface of the iliac wing contains the anterior, posterior, and inferior gluteal lines, which form borders for the origins of the gluteal muscles. The iliopectineal eminence is a raised region anteriorly that represents the union of the ilium and pubis. The iliopsoas muscle traverses a groove between this eminence and the anterior inferior iliac spine. Ossification centers of the pelvis are as follows:

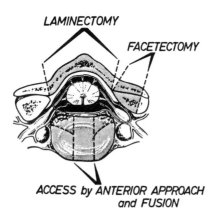

LAMINECTOMY

FACETECTOMY

ACCESS by ANTERIOR APPROACH and FUSION

FIGURE 10–36. Approach to the cervical spine. (From Rothman, R.H., and Simeon, F.A.: The Spine, 2nd ed., p. 484. Philadelphia, W.B. Saunders, 1982; reprinted by permission.)

CENTER	TYPE	AGE APPEARS	AGE FUSES
Ilium	Primary	2 mo	15 yr
Ischium	Primary	4 mo	15 yr
Pubis	Primary	6 mo	15 yr
Acetabulum	Secondary	12 yr	15 yr
Iliac crest	Secondary	16 yr	25 yr
Ant. inf. iliac spine	Secondary	16 yr	25 yr
Ischial tuberosity	Secondary	16 yr	25 yr
Pubis	Secondary	16 yr	30 yr

The proximal femur is composed of the femoral head (articulates with the acetabulum), neck, and greater and lesser trochanters. The inner architecture of the proximal femur includes an intricate ar-

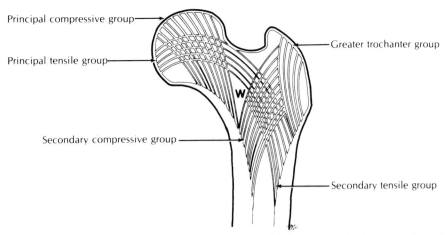

FIGURE 10–37. Hip trabeculae. (From DeLee, J.C.: Fractures and dislocations of the hip. In Rockwood, C.A., Jr., Green D.P., and Buchholz, R.W., eds., Fractures in Adults, 3rd ed., p. 1488. Philadelphia, J.B. Lippincott, 1991; reprinted by permission.)

rangement of primary and secondary trabeculae (Fig. 10–37).

B. Arthrology

1. Hip—The hip joint is a spheroid, or ball-and-socket, type of diarthrodial joint. Its stability is based primarily on the bony architecture, which also allows good motion. The acetabulum is deepened by the fibrocartilaginous rim, called the labrum. The joint capsule extends anteriorly across the femoral neck to the trochanteric crest; however, posteriorly it extends only partially across the femoral neck (Fig. 10–38). The fibrous capsule that encloses the joint contains circular fibers that can be recognized better posteriorly as the zona orbicularis. A series of three ligaments comprise the capsule anteriorly. The *iliofemoral* or Y ligament of Bigelow is the strongest ligament in the body and attaches the anterior inferior iliac spine (AIIS) to the intertrochanteric line in an inverted Y fashion. The remaining anterior ligaments, the *ischiofemoral* and *pubofemoral* ligaments, are weaker but lend additional stability. Inside the joint, the ligament on teres

arises from the apex of the cotyloid notch and attaches to the fovea of the femoral head. It transmits an arterial branch of the posterior division of the **obturator artery** to the femoral head (less significant in adults).

2. Sacroiliac (SI) Joint—A true diarthrodial gliding joint that is supported by three groups of ligaments. They include the posterior SI ligaments, the anterior SI ligaments, and the interosseous ligaments. Of these, the posterior ligaments, which have been compared to the trusses of a suspension bridge (Tile), provide the most stability and strength to the joint.

3. Symphysis Pubis—Connects the two hemipelvii anteriorly, and is united with a fibrocartilaginous disc and supported by the superior pubic ligament and the arcuate pubic ligament.

4. Other ligaments include the sacrospinous and sacrotuberous ligaments, which outline the boundaries for the greater and lesser sciatic foramina. **The sacrospinous ligament** (anterior sacrum → ischial spine) is the inferior border of the **greater** sciatic foramen and the superior border of the **lesser** sciatic foramen. The lesser

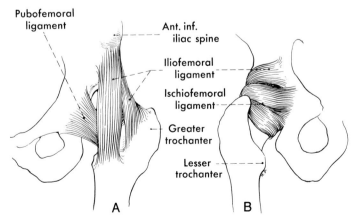

FIGURE 10–38. Hip capsule. *A*, Anterior view. *B*, Posterior view. (From Jenkins, D.B.: Hollinshead's Functional Anatomy of the Limbs and Back, 6th ed., p. 230. Philadelphia, W.B. Saunders, 1991; reprinted by permission.)

sciatic foramen is bordered inferiorly by the **sacrotuberous ligament** (anterior sacrum → ischial tuberosity). The piriformis, sciatic nerve, and other important structures exit the greater sciatic foramen. The short external rotators of the hip exit the lesser sciatic foramen.

C. Muscles of the Pelvis and Hip (Table 10–7; Fig. 10–39)

D. Nerves

    1. Lumbosacral Plexus (Fig. 10–40)

        a. Lumbar Plexus—The lumbar plexus involves the ventral primary rami for T12 to L4 but may display the usual prefixed (T11–L3) and postfixed (L1–L5) variations.

Nerves	Level	Innervation
Anterior Division		
Subcostal	T12	Sensory: subxiphoid region
Iliohypogastric	L1	Sensory: posterolat. buttock/above pubis
		Motor: transversus abdominis/Int. oblique
Ilioinguinal	L1	Sensory: inguinal area
Genitofemoral	L1–L2	Sensory: Proximal anteromed thigh, scrotum/mons
		Motor: cremaster
Obturator	L2–L4	Motor: Ext. oblique/adductor longus/adductor magnus (ant.)/gracilis
Posterior Division		
Lateral femoral cutaneous (LFCN)	L2–L3	Sensory: Lateral thigh
Femoral	L2–L4	Motor: Psoas/iliacus/quadratus/sartorius/pectineus/articularis genu
Accessory obturator	L2–L4	Motor: Psoas

        b. Sacral Plexus—The sacral plexus typically involves the ventral primary rami of L4 to S3. It is formed in the pelvis both anterior and lateral to the sacrum. It provides a significant amount of innervation to the limb.

Nerves	Level	Innervation
Anterior Division		
Tibial	L4–S3	Semimembranosus/semitendinosus/Biceps (long head)/Adductor magnus/Sup. gemellus/Soleus/Plantaris/Popliteus/Tibialis posterior/Flexor digitorum longus/Flexor hallucis longus
Quadratus femoris	L4–S1	Quadratus femoris/Inf. gemellus
Obturator internus	L5–S2	Obturatorius internus/Sup. gemellus
Pudendal	S2–S4	Sensory: Perineal
		Motor: bulbocavernosus/urethra/urogenital diaphragm
Coccygeus	S4	Coccygeus
Levator ani	S3–S4	Levator ani

Table continues at top of next column

Nerves	Level	Innervation
Posterior Division		
Peroneal	L4–S2	Biceps (short head)/Tibialis anterior/Extensor digitorum longus/Peroneus tertius/Extensor hallucis longus
		Peroneus longus & brevis/Extensor hallucis brevis/Extensor digitorum brevis
Sup. gluteal	L4–S1	Gluteus medius & minimus/TFL
Inf. gluteal	L5–S2	Gluteus maximus
Piriformis	S2	Piriformis
Post. femoral cutaneous (PFCN)	S1–S3	Sensory: posterior thigh

2. Relationships—The lumbar plexus is found on the surface of the quadratus lumborum under (and within) the substance of the psoas major muscle. The genitofemoral nerve pierces the psoas and then lies on the anteromedial surface of the psoas. The femoral nerve lies between the iliacus and the psoas. The lateral femoral cutaneous nerve lies on the surface of the iliacus muscle and exits the pelvis under the lateral attachment of the inguinal ligament. Virtually all important nerves about the hip leave the pelvis by way of the sciatic foramen. The major reference point for the greater sciatic nerve and related structures in the hip is the piriformis muscle ("key" to the sciatic foramen). The **superior gluteal nerve and artery lie above the piriformis** and virtually everything else leaves below the muscle (remember POP'S IQ [lateral to medial]: **P**udendal, **O**bturator internus, **P**ost femoral cutaneous, **S**ciatic, **I**nferior gluteal, **Q**uadratus femoris). Two nerves will leave the greater sciatic foramen and re-enter the pelvis via the lesser foramen (pudendal and nerve to obturator internus). In addition to the peripheral nerves, a plexus of parasympathetic nerves cover the lower aorta and the anterior sacrum. These nerves should be protected to prevent sexual dysfunction. Anteriorly, the great nerves and vessels enter the thigh (and into the **femoral triangle**) under the inguinal ligament (Fig. 10–41). The borders of this triangle include the sartorius laterally, the pectineus medially, and the inguinal ligament superiorly. Within the triangle, from lateral to medial are the femoral nerve, artery, and vein and lymphatic vessels (remember NAVAL). The femoral nerve descends between the iliacus and psoas and delivers numerous branches to muscle, overlying skin, and the hip joint (in accordance with Hilton's Law). A spontaneous iliacus hematoma may irritate the femoral nerve due to its proximity. At the apex of the triangle, the saphenous nerve branches off and travels under the sartorius muscle. The obturator nerve exits the pelvis via the obturator canal. It splits into anterior and posterior divisions within the canal. The anterior division proceeds anterior to the obturator externus and posterior to the pectineus and supplies the adductor longus and brevis and the gracilis; then it delivers cutaneous branches to the medial thigh. The posterior di-

TABLE 10–7. MUSCLES OF THE PELVIS AND HIP

Muscle	Origin	Insertion	Nerve	Segment
Flexors				
Iliacus	Iliac fossa	Lesser trochanter	Femoral	L234 (P)
Psoas	Transverse processes of L1–L5	Lesser trochanter	Femoral	L234 (P)
Pectineus	Pectineal line of pubis	Pectineal line of femur	Femoral	L234 (P)
Rectus femoris	AIIS, Acetabular rim	Patella → Tibial tubercle	Femoral	L234 (P)
Sartorius	ASIS	Proximal medial tibia	Femoral	L234 (P)
Adductors				
Post Adductor magnus	Inferior pubic ramus/ Ischial tuberosity	Linea aspera/Adductor tubercle	Obturator (P) & Sciatic (Tibial)	L234 (A)
Adductor brevis	Inferior pubic ramus	Linea aspera/Pectineal line	Obturator (P)	L234 (A)
Adductor longus	Anterior pubic ramus	Linea aspera	Obturator (A)	L234 (A)
Gracilis	Inf. symphysis/Pubic arch	Proximal medial tibia	Obturator (A)	L234 (A)
External Rotators				
Gluteus maximus	Ilium post to posterior gluteal line	Iliotibial band/Gluteal sling (femur)	Inf. gluteal	L5-S2 (P)
Piriformis	Ant. sacrum/Sciatic notch	Proximal greater trochanter	Piriformis	S12 (P)
Obturator externus	Ischiopubic rami/ Obturator membrane	Trochlear fossa	Obturator (P)	L234 (A)
Obturator internus	Ischiopubic rami/ Obturator membrane	Medial greater trochanter (MGT)	Obturator internus	L5-S2 (A)
Superior gemellus	Outer ischial spine	MGT	Obturator internus	L5-S2 (A)
Inferior gemellus	Ischial tuberosity	MGT	Quadratus femoris	L4-S1 (A)
Quadratus femoris	Ischial tuberosity	Quadrate line of femur	Quadratus femoris	L4-S1 (A)
Abductors				
Gluteus medius	Ilium/between post. and ant. gluteal lines	Greater trochanter	Superior gluteal	L4-S1 (P)
Gluteus minimus	Ilium between ant. & inf. gluteal lines	Ant. border of greater trochanter	Superior gluteal	L4-S1 (P)
Tensor fasciae latae (TFL) (tensor fascia femoris [TFF])	Anterior iliac crest	Iliotibial band	Superior gluteal	L4-S1 (P)

vision supplies the obturator externus, the adductor brevis, and the upper part of the adductor magnus and delivers other branches to the knee joint. The obturator nerve can be injured by retractors placed behind the transverse acetabular ligament.

E. Vessels (Fig. 10–42)—The aorta branches into the common iliacs arteries anterior to the L4 vertebral body. The common iliac vessels, in turn, divide into the internal (or *hypogastric*; medial) and external (lateral) iliacs at the S1 level. Important internal iliac branches include the obturator, superior gluteal (can be injured in the sciatic notch), and inferior gluteal (supplies the gluteus maximus and the short external rotators) (Fig. 10–43). The external iliac artery continues under the inguinal ligament to become the femoral artery. The external iliac vein lies inferior to the artery. It can be injured by anterosuperior quadrant acetabular screw placement in total hip arthroplasty, while the obturator artery and vein are jeopardized by anteroinferior screws. The femoral artery enters the femoral triangle and delivers the profunda femoris, which supplies to the anteromedial portion of the thigh as well as the perforators. The profunda has two other important branches, the medial and lateral femoral circumflex arteries. The lateral femoral circumflex travels obliquely and deep to the sartorius and rectus femoris. It delivers an ascending branch (at risk during anterolateral approaches) that proceeds to the greater trochanteric region, and a descending branch that travels laterally under the rectus femoris. The **medial femoral circumflex**, which supplies the majority of the blood to the **femoral head**, runs between the pectineus and the iliopsoas and then in the interval between the obturator externus and adductor brevis muscles. The cruciate anastomosis is the confluence of the ascending branch of the first perforating artery, the descending branch of the inferior gluteal artery, and the transverse branches of the medial and lateral femoral circumflex arteries. It lies at the inferior margin of the quatratus femoris muscle. The superficial femoral artery continues on the medial side of the thigh (between the vastus medialis and adductor longus) toward the adductor [Hunter's] canal. In the posteromedial thigh, it becomes the popliteal artery in the popliteal fossa.

F. Approaches to the Pelvis and Hip

1. Posterior Approach to the Iliac Crest—A curvilinear incision is made just inferior to the crest beginning at the PSIS. After identifying the iliac crest, the gluteus maximus fibers are subperiosteally dissected from the outer table. Risks of this approach include the greater sciatic notch

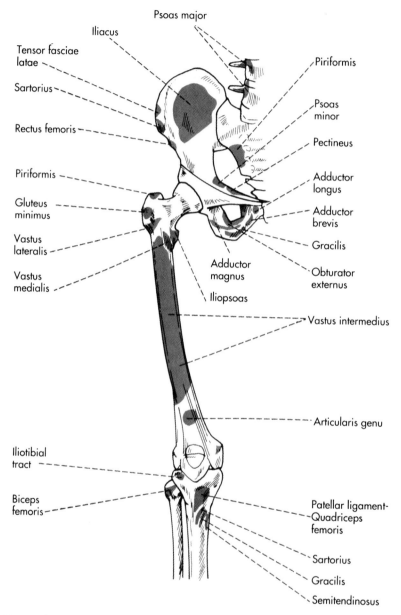

FIGURE 10–39. Origins and insertions of muscles of the hip and leg. (From Jenkins, D.B.: Hollinshead's Functional Anatomy of the Limbs and Back, 6th ed., fig. 16–7 and 17–3. Philadelphia, W.B. Saunders, 1991; reprinted by permission.)

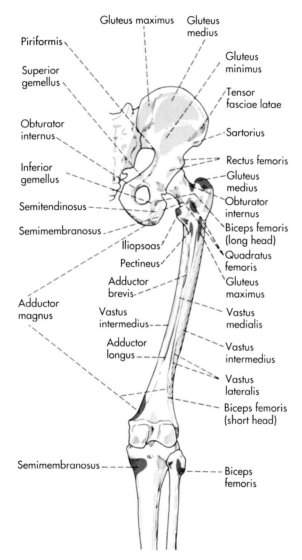

Piriformis

Superior
gemellus

Obturator
internus

Inferior
gemellus

Semitendinosus

Semimembranosus

Adductor
magnus

Gluteus maximus   Gluteus
medius

Gluteus
minimus

Tensor
fasciae latae

Sartorius

Rectus femoris

Gluteus
medius

Obturator
internus

Biceps femoris
(long head)

Quadratus
femoris

Gluteus
maximus

Vastus
medialis

Vastus
intermedius

Vastus
lateralis

Biceps femoris
(short head)

Iliopsoas

Pectineus

Adductor
brevis

Vastus
intermedius

Adductor
longus

Semimembranosus

Biceps
femoris

FIGURE 10–39. *(Continued)*

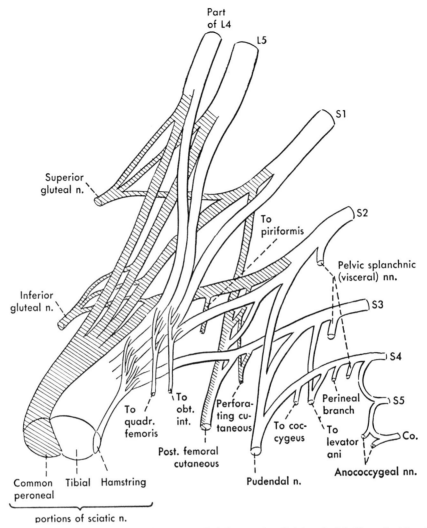

FIGURE 10–40. Sacral plexus. Anterior division *unshaded*, posterior division *shaded*. (From Jenkins, D.B.: Hollinshead's Functional Anatomy of the Limbs and Back, 6th ed., p. 256. Philadelphia, W.B. Saunders, 1991; reprinted by permission.)

(superior gluteal artery and sciatic nerve) and the clunial nerves (8 cm anterolateral to the PSIS).

2. Anterior Approach to the Iliac Crest—An oblique incision is made lateral to the ASIS and the crest is exposed through the interval between the external oblique and the gluteus medius. Risks include the greater sciatic notch, the inguinal ligament, and the lateral femoral cutaneous nerve.

3. Anterior (Smith-Peterson) Approach to the Hip (Fig. 10–44)—Takes advantage of the internervous plane between the sartorious (femoral nerve) and the tensor fascia femoris (superior gluteal nerve). It is useful for hemiarthroplasty and open reduction of the congenitally dislocated hip. Retract the lateral femoral cutaneous nerve anteriorly and ligate the ascending branch of lateral femoral circumflex artery. For deeper dissection, approach the interval between the gluteus medius and rectus femoris. Detach the origin of both heads of the rectus femoris. Retract the rectus medially and the gluteus medius laterally. Dissect any attachments of the iliop-

soas to the inferior capsule and perform a capsulotomy. Dangers include the lateral femoral cutaneous nerve, which is located anterior or medial to the sartorius about 6–8 cm below the ASIS. The femoral nerve and vessels can sometimes be injured with aggressive medial retraction of the sartorius.

4. Anterolateral (Watson-Jones) Approach to the Hip (Fig. 10–45)—This approach can be used for total hip arthroplasty (THA) as popularized by Watson-Jones. There is no true internervous plane, but it utilizes the intermuscular plane between the tensor fascia femoris and gluteus medius. After the incision and superficial dissection, the fascia lata is split to expose the vastus lateralis. Detach the anterior ⅓ of the gluteus medius from the greater trochanter and the entire gluteus minimus. Dissect the reflected head of the rectus femoris (and capsular attachment of the iliopsoas if necessary) and retract medially. Perform a capsulotomy. Dangers of this approach include damage to the femoral nerve by excessive medial retraction and denervation of the tensor fascia femoris if the in-

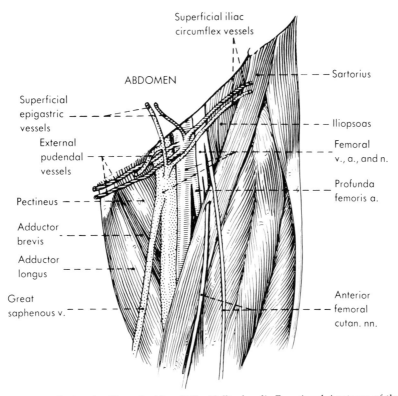

FIGURE 10–41. Femoral triangle. (From Jenkins, D.B.: Hollinshead's Functional Anatomy of the Limbs and Back, 6th ed., p. 243. Philadelphia, W.B. Saunders, 1991; reprinted by permission.)

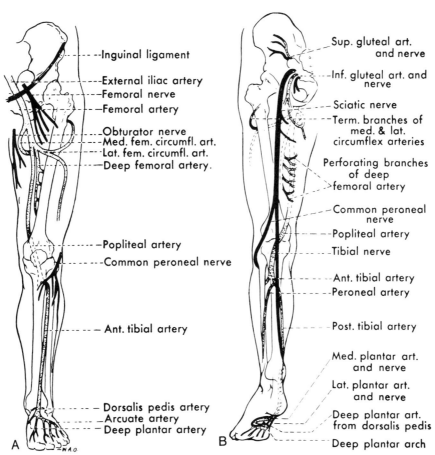

FIGURE 10–42. Nerves and vessels of the lower extremity. *A*, Anterior view. *B*, Posterior view. (From Jenkins, D.B.: Hollinshead's Functional Anatomy of the Limbs and Back, 6th ed., p. 221. Philadelphia, W.B. Saunders, 1991; reprinted by permission.)

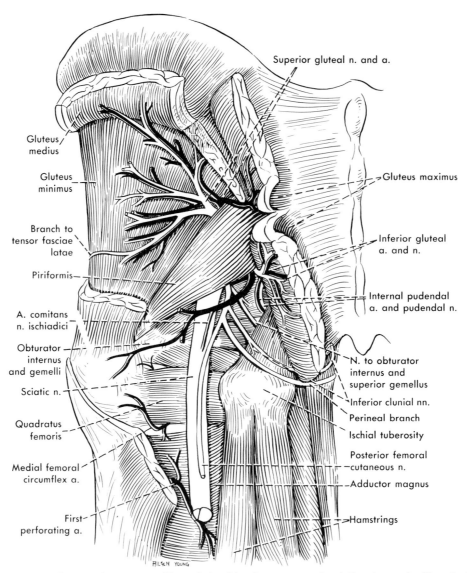

Superior gluteal n. and a.

Gluteus medius

Gluteus minimus

Branch to tensor fasciae latae

Piriformis

A. comitans n. ischiadici

Obturator internus and gemelli

Sciatic n.

Quadratus femoris

Medial femoral circumflex a.

First perforating a.

Gluteus maximus

Inferior gluteal a. and n.

Internal pudendal a. and pudendal n.

N. to obturator internus and superior gemellus

Inferior clunial nn.

Perineal branch

Ischial tuberosity

Posterior femoral cutaneous n.

Adductor magnus

Hamstrings

FIGURE 10–43. Posterior hip anatomy. Note relationship of structures to the pisiformis muscle. (From Jenkins, D.B.: Hollinshead's Functional Anatomy of the Limbs and Back, 6th ed., p. 260. Philadelphia, W.B. Saunders, 1991; reprinted by permission.)

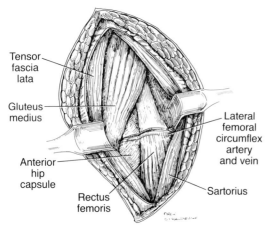

Tensor fascia lata

Gluteus medius

Anterior hip capsule

Rectus femoris

Lateral femoral circumflex artery and vein

Sartorius

FIGURE 10–44. Anterior approach to the hip. (From Steinberg, M.E.: The Hip and Its Disorders, p. 92. Philadelphia, W.B. Saunders, 1991; reprinted by permission.)

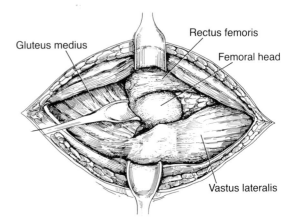

Gluteus medius

Rectus femoris

Femoral head

Vastus lateralis

FIGURE 10–45. Anterolateral approach to the hip. (From Steinberg, M.E.: The Hip and Its Disorders, p. 93. Philadelphia, W.B. Saunders, 1991; reprinted by permission.)

termuscular interval is exploited too superiorly (the superior gluteal nerve lies about 5 cm above the acetabular rim), and the lateral femoral circumflex artery (anterior and inferior).

5. Lateral (Hardinge) Approach to the Hip (Fig. 10–46)—Useful for THA bipolar hemiarthroplasty, and revision work, this approach utilizes an incision that splits both the gluteus medius and vastus lateralis in tandem. Incise the skin and the fascia lata to expose the gluteus medius and the vastus. Incise the gluteus medius from the greater trochanter, leaving a cuff of tissue and the posterior ½ to ⅔ attached. Extend this incision to split the gluteus medius proximally. Distally, split the vastus along its anterior ¼ down to the femoral shaft. Detach the gluteus minimus from its insertion. The hip capsule is exposed for further dissection. Dangers include the femoral nerve as well as possible denervation of the gluteus medius (superior gluteal nerve) if the split is generous.

6. Posterior (Moore or Southern) Approach to the Hip (Fig. 10–47)—The internervous plane in one version is between the gluteus maximus (inferior gluteal nerve) and the gluteus medius and the tensor fascia femoris (superior gluteal nerve). Most surgeons, however, approach the hip by splitting the fibers of the gluteus maximus. Incise the skin and the fascia lata along the posterior border of the femur. Then split the fibers of the gluteus maximus bluntly. Next expose the short external rotators. With the leg internally rotated, divide the tendons of the short external rotators close to their insertion into the greater trochanter. Reflect them laterally to protect the sciatic nerve and expose the posterior hip capsule. A portion of the quadratus femoris may be taken down with the short external rotators, but one must be aware of the significant bleeding that can come from the inferior portion of this muscle (ascending branches of medial femoral circumflex artery). Dangers include sciatic neurapraxia if the sciatic nerve is not properly protected by the short external rotators. Additional trouble can be encountered if the inferior gluteal artery is damaged during the splitting of the gluteus maximus.

7. Medial (Ludloff) Approach to the Hip (Fig. 10–48)—Used occasionally for pediatric adductor releases and open reductions, this approach uses the interval between the adductor longus and gracilis. Deep, the interval is between the adductor brevis and magnus. Structures at risk include the anterior division of the obturator nerve and medial femoral circumflex artery (between adductor brevis and adductor magnus/pectineus).

8. Acetabular Approaches—Used primarily for ORIF of pelvic fractures, these approaches are basically extensions of incisions for exposure of the hip discussed above. The Kocher-Langenbeck incision is a posterolateral approach that provides access to the posterior column/acetabulum (Fig. 10–49). The ilioinguinal incision relies on mobilization of the rectus abdominis and iliacus and exposes the anterior column (Fig. 10–50). The extended iliofemoral incision

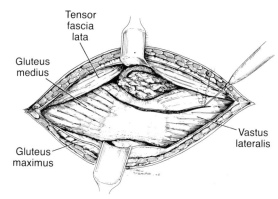

FIGURE 10–46. Lateral approach to the hip. (From Steinberg, M.E.: The Hip and Its Disorders, p. 95. Philadelphia, W.B. Saunders, 1991; reprinted by permission.)

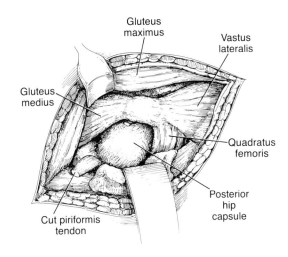

FIGURE 10–47. Posterior approach to the hip. (From Steinberg, M.E.: The Hip and Its Disorders, p. 98. Philadelphia, W.B. Saunders, 1991; reprinted by permission.)

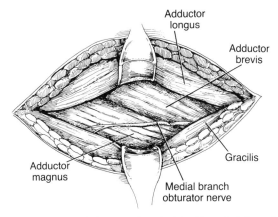

FIGURE 10–48. Medial approach to the hip. (From Steinberg, M.E.: The Hip and Its Disorders, p. 99. Philadelphia, W.B. Saunders, 1991; reprinted by permission.)

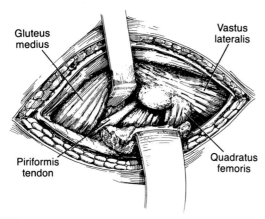

FIGURE 10–49. Posterolateral approach to the hip. (From Steinberg, M.E.: The Hip and Its Disorders, p. 96. Philadelphia, W.B. Saunders, 1991; reprinted by permission.)

allows access to both columns by reflecting the gluteal muscles and tensor posteriorly and dividing the obturator internus and piriformis.

VIII. Thigh

    A. Osteology of the Femur

        1. Introduction—The femur is the largest bone of the body. The upper portion contains a head, neck, and two trochanters connected posteriorly by a crest. The neck-shaft angle averages about 127 degrees, although it begins at 141 degrees in the fetus. The anteversion varies from 1 to 40 degrees but averages 14 degrees. Below the lesser trochanter is a ridge known as the pectineal line. This continues as the linea aspera with medial and lateral ridges that diverge at the lower end to meet the medial and lateral supracondylar ridges. There are two femoral condyles. The medial condyle is larger. The more prominent medial epicondyle supports the adductor tubercle.

        2. Ossification—The ossification center of the body of the femur appears at the seventh fetal

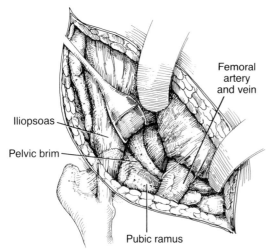

FIGURE 10–50. Ilioinguinal approach to the hip. (From Steinberg, M.E.: The Hip and Its Disorders, p. 103. Philadelphia, W.B. Saunders, 1991; reprinted by permission.)

week. The femoral head is usually not present at birth, but appears as one large physis that includes both trochanters at about 11 months and fuse at 18 years. The greater trochanter becomes distinct at 5 years and the lesser at 9 years, and both will fuse at 16 years. The distal femoral physis will appear at birth and fuse at 19 years.

    B. Muscles of the Thigh

        1. Anterior Thigh (Table 10–8)—See Table 10–7 for rectus femoris, sartorius)

        2. Medial Thigh—See Adductors in Table 10–7

        3. Posterior Thigh (Table 10–9)

    C. Nerves and Vessels (See Also Section VII: Thigh and Hip, and Section IX: Leg)—The sciatic nerve emerges from its foramen below the piriformis muscle and lies posterior to the other short external rotators. It descends below the gluteus maximus and proceeds posterior to the adductor magnus and between the long head of the biceps and the semimembranosus. Before it emerges from the popliteal fossa, it divides into the common peroneal nerve and the tibial nerve. The common peroneal nerve diverges laterally and traverses the lateral knee region under cover of the biceps femoris. The tibial nerve emerges into the popliteal fossa lateral, then posterior, to the vessel, then it descends between the heads of the gastrocnemius. After supplying the profundus (described above) the superficial femoral artery descends under cover of the sartorius muscle and proceeds between the adductor group and the vastus medialis into the adductor canal. At the level above the medial epicondyle, the artery supplies a supreme geniculate branch, then passes through a defect in the adductor magnus (adductor hiatus) and emerges into the popliteal fossa. The vein is usually posterior to the artery.

    D. Approaches to the Thigh

        1. Lateral Approach to the Thigh—The lateral approach is used for open reduction and internal fixation of intertrochanteric and femoral neck fractures. This approach can be extended for access to shaft and supracondylar fractures. There is no true internervous plane. Split the fascia lata in line with the femoral shaft. Include part of the tensor fascia femoris if necessary. Then bluntly dissect the vastus lateralis in line with its fibers or dissect the fibers of the intermus-

TABLE 10–8. MUSCLES OF THE ANTERIOR THIGH

MUSCLE	ORIGIN	INSERTION	INNERVATION
Vastus lateralis	Iliotibial line/ Greater trochanter/ Lateral linea aspera	Lateral patella	Femoral
Vastus medialis	Iliotibial line/ Medial linea aspera/ Supracondylar line	Medial patella	Femoral
Vastus intermedius	Proximal anterior femoral shaft	Patella	Femoral

TABLE 10–9. MUSCLES OF THE POSTERIOR THIGH

Muscle	Origin	Insertion	Innervation
Biceps (long head)	Medial ischial tuberosity	Fibular head/Lateral tibia	Tibial
Biceps (short head)	Lat. linea aspera/Lat. intermuscular septum	Lateral tibial condyle	Peroneal
Semitendinosus	Distal med. ischial tuberosity	Anterior tibial crest	Tibial
Semimembranosus	Proximal lat. ischial tuberosity	1. Oblique popliteal ligament 2. Posterior capsule 3. Posterior/Medial tibia 4. Popliteus 5. Medial meniscus	Tibial

cular septum. Identify and coagulate the various perforators from the profunda femoris.

2. Posterolateral Approach to the Thigh—This may be used for exposure of the entire length of the femur through an internervous plane. It exploits the interval between the vastus lateralis (femoral nerve) and the hamstrings (sciatic nerve). Incise the fascia under the iliotibial band and retract the vastus superiorly. Continue anterior to the lateral intermuscular septum with blunt dissection until the periosteum over the linea aspira is reached. The danger in this dissection is the series of perforating vessels from the profundus that pierce the lateral intermuscular septum to reach the vastus. If approached without care, these vessels will retract and bleed underneath the septum.

3. Anteromedial Approach to the Distal Femur—This approach may be used for open reduction and internal fixation of distal femoral and femoral shaft fractures. Explore the interval between the rectus femoris and the vastus medialis and extended to a point medial to the patella. Retract the rectus laterally. Explore the interval to reveal the vastus intermedius. It may be necessary to open the knee joint. If this is the case, then incise the medial patellar retinaculum and split a portion of the quadriceps tendon just lateral to the medial border. After identifying the vastus intermedius, split this along its fibers to expose the femur. Dangers include the medial superior geniculate artery and the infrapatellar branch of the saphenous nerve, as both will cross the site of exposure. Additionally, one must leave an adequate cuff of tissue for a strong patellar retinacular repair or risk lateral subluxation of the patella.

4. Posterior Approach to the Thigh—This rare approach may be used for exploration of the sciatic nerve. It makes use of the internervous interval between the sciatic nerve (biceps femoris) and the femoral nerve (vastus lateralis). Identify and protect the posterior femoral cutaneous nerve (between the biceps and the semitendinosus). Next, explore the interval between the biceps and the lateral intermuscular septum. Detach the origin of the short head of the biceps from the linea aspera. This will allow exposure of the femur at the midshaft level. In the lower thigh, retract the long head of the biceps laterally to expose the sciatic nerve. It lies on the surface of the adductor magnus and may be retracted laterally for exposure of this portion of the femur.

IX. Leg

A. Osteology

1. Patella—Commonly known as the kneecap, the patella is the largest sesamoid bone (about 5 cm in diameter). It serves three functions: It is a fulcrum for the quadriceps, it protects the knee joint, and it enhances lubrication and nutrition of the knee. The patella is said to have the thickest articular surface in the body, probably because of the loads it must transmit. Although sometimes subdivided, the articular surface of the patella has two facets, medial and lateral, separated by a vertical ridge. The lateral facet is broader and deeper than the medial facet. Somewhat triangular in shape, the apex of the patella gives rise to the patella tendon, which attaches to the tibial tubercle. Several ossification centers make up the patella and they fuse sometime between the second and sixth year. An accessory or "bipartite" patella may represent failure of fusion of the superiolateral corner of the patella and is commonly confused with patellar fractures.

2. Tibia—This is the second longest bone in the body (behind the femur). It consists of a proximal extremity with medial (oval and concave) and lateral (circular and convex) facets. The intercondylar eminence separates the medial and lateral facets and the anterior and posterior cruciate ligaments. The tibial tubercle is an oblong elevation on the anterior surface of the tibia where the patella tendon inserts. Gerdy's tubercle lies on the lateral side of the proximal tibia and is the insertion of the iliotibial tract. The tibial shaft is triangular in cross section and tapers to its thinnest point at the junction of the middle and distal third and again widens to form the tibial plafond. Distally, the tibia forms an inferior quadrilateral surface for articulation with the talus and the pyramid-shaped medial malleolus. Laterally, the fibular notch forms an articulation with the fibula. The tibia is formed from three ossification centers:

Ossification Center	Age Appears	Age Fuses
Body (primary)	7 wks (fetal)	
Proximal (secondary)	Birth	20 years
Distal (secondary)	Second year	18 years

3. Fibula—This long slender bone is composed of a head, a shaft, and a distal lateral malleolus.

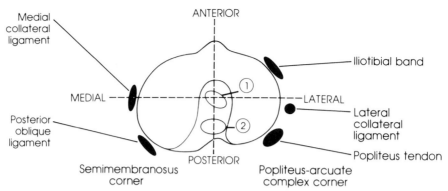

FIGURE 10–51. Ligaments of the knee. *1*, Anterior cruciate ligament. *2*, Posterior cruciate ligament. (From Magee, D.J.: Orthopedic Physical Assessment, p. 285. Philadelphia, W.B. Saunders, 1987; reprinted by permission.)

The styloid process of the head serves as the attachment for the fibular collateral ligament and the biceps tendon. Lying just below the head, the neck of the fibula is grooved by the common peroneal nerve. The expanded distal fibula is known as the lateral malleolus and extends beyond the distal margin of the medial malleolus. Together with the inferior distal surface of the tibia, these structures make up the ankle mortise. Like the tibia, the fibula is also formed from three ossification centers:

Ossification Center	Age Appears	Age Fuses
Body (primary)	8 wks (fetal)	
Proximal (secondary)	Third year	25 years
Distal (secondary)	Second year	20 years

B. Arthrology
 1. Knee (Fig. 10–51)—Much more than a simple ginglymus or hinge-type of joint, the knee is a compound joint consisting of two condyloid joints and one sellar joint (patellofemoral articulation). The medial and lateral femoral condyles articulate with the corresponding tibial facets. Intervening menisci serve to deepen the concavity of the facets, help protect the articular surface, and assist in rotation of the knee. The peripheral ⅓ of the menisci are vascular (and can be repaired), the inner ⅔ are nourished by synovial fluid. Stability of the knee is enhanced by a complex arrangement of ligaments (Table 10–10; Fig. 10–52). In addition, several muscles and tendons traverse the knee, giving it dynamic stability:

Location	Muscles
Anterior	Quadriceps
Lateral	Biceps and popliteus
Medial	Pes anserinus (sartorius, gracilis, semitendinosis), semimembranosus (with five attachments)
Posterior	Medial and lateral heads of the gastrocnemius, plantaris

 2. Superior Tibiofibular Joint—A plane or gliding joint that is strengthened by the anterior and posterior ligaments of the head of the fibula.
C. Muscles of the Leg—Commonly divided into groups based upon compartments (anterior, lateral, superficial posterior, and deep posterior) (Table 10–11; Fig. 10–53).

TABLE 10–10. LIGAMENTS OF THE KNEE

Ligament	Origin	Insertion	Function
Retinacular	Vastus medialis & lateralis	Tibial condyles	Forms anterior capsule
Posterior fibers	Femoral condyles	Tibial condyles	Forms posterior capsule
Oblique popliteal	Semimembranosus tendon	Lateral femoral condyle/Posterior capsule	Strengthens capsule
Deep medial collateral (MCL)	Medial epicondyle	Medial meniscus	Holds med. meniscus to femur
Superficial MCL	Medial epicondyle	Medial condyle of tibia	Resists valgus force
Arcuate	Lat. femoral condyle, over popliteus	Post. tibia/Fibular head	Posterior support
Lateral collateral (LCL)	Lateral epicondyle	Lateral fibular head	Resists varus force
Anterior cruciate (ACL)	Anterior intercondylar tibia	Posteromed. lat. femoral condyle	Limits hyperextension/Slide
Posterior cruciate (PCL)	Posterior intercondylar tibia	Anteromed. femoral condyle	Prevents hyperflexion/Sliding
Coronary	Meniscus	Tibial periphery	Meniscal attachment
Wrisberg	Posterolateral meniscus	Med. femoral condyle (behind PCL)	Stabilizes lat. meniscus
Humphrey	Posterolateral meniscus	Med. femoral condyle (in front)	Stabilizes lat. meniscus
Transverse meniscal	Anterolateral meniscus	Anteromedial meniscus	Stabilizes menisci

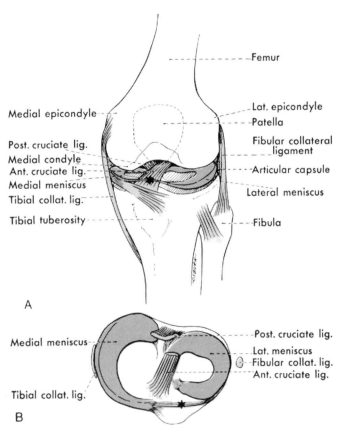

A

B

FIGURE 10–52. Ligaments of the knee. (From Jenkins, D.B.: Hollinshead's Functional Anatomy of the Limbs and Back, 6th ed., fig. 16–1. Philadelphia, W.B. Saunders, 1991; reprinted by permission.)

TABLE 10–11.   MUSCLES OF THE LEG

MUSCLE	ORIGIN	INSERTION	ACTION	INNERVATION
Anterior Compartment				
Tibialis anterior	Lateral tibia	Med. cuneiform, 1st metatarsal	Dorsiflex, invert foot	Deep peroneal (L_4)
Extensor hallucis longus (EHL)	Mid. fibula	Great toe distal phalanx	Dorsiflex, extend toe	Deep peroneal (L_5)
Extensor digitorum longus (EDL)	Tibial condyle/Fibula	Toe middle and distal phalanges	Dorsiflex, extend toes	Deep peroneal (L_5)
Peroneus tertius	Fibula & EDL tendon	5th metatarsal	Evert, plantar flex, abduct foot	Deep peroneal (S_1)
Lateral Compartment				
Peroneus longus	Proximal fibula	Med. cuneiform, 1st metatarsal	Evert, plantar flex, abduct foot	Superficial peroneal (S_1)
Peroneus brevis	Distal fibula	Tuberosity of 5th metatarsal	Evert foot	Superficial peroneal (S_1)
Superficial Posterior Compartment				
Gastrocnemius	Post. med. & lat. femoral condyles	Calcaneus	Plantar flex foot	Tibial (S_1)
Soleus	Fibula/Tibia	Calcaneus	Plantar flex foot	Tibial (S_1)
Plantaris	Lat. femoral condyle	Calcaneus	Plantar flex foot	Tibial (S_1)
Deep Posterior Compartment				
Popliteus	Lat. femoral condyle, fibular head	Proximal tibia	Flex, IR knee	Tibial (L_5S_1)
Flexor hallucis longus (FHL)	Fibula	Great toe distal phalanx	Plantar flex great toe	Tibial (S_1)
Flexor digitorum longus (FDL)	Tibia	2nd–5th toe distal phalanges	Plantar flex toes, foot	Tibial (S_1S_2)
Tibialis posterior	Tibia, fibula, interosseous membrane	Navicular, med. cuneiform	Invert/Plantar flex foot	Tibial (L_4L_5)

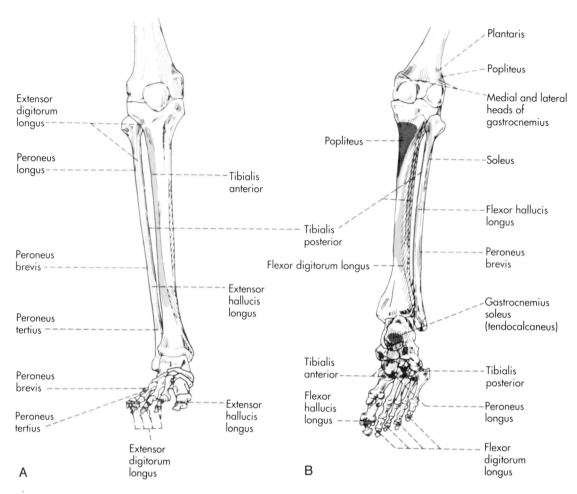

Extensor digitorum longus

Peroneus longus

Peroneus brevis

Peroneus tertius

Peroneus brevis

Peroneus tertius

Tibialis anterior

Extensor hallucis longus

Extensor hallucis longus

Extensor digitorum longus

A

Plantaris

Popliteus

Medial and lateral heads of gastrocnemius

Popliteus

Soleus

Flexor hallucis longus

Tibialis posterior

Peroneus brevis

Flexor digitorum longus

Gastrocnemius soleus (tendocalcaneus)

Tibialis anterior

Flexor hallucis longus

Tibialis posterior

Peroneus longus

Flexor digitorum longus

B

FIGURE 10–53. Origins and insertions of leg and foot muscles. (From Jenkins, D.B.: Hollinshead's Functional Anatomy of the Limbs and Back, 6th ed., fig. 19–3. Philadelphia, W.B. Saunders, 1991; reprinted by permission.)

D. Nerves (Fig. 10–54)—Motor branches to the muscles of the leg are from terminal divisions of the sciatic nerve (in the distal thigh) and the tibial and common peroneal nerves and their branches.
  1. Tibial Nerve—Continues in the thigh deep to the long head of the biceps and enters the popliteal fossa. It then crosses over the popliteus muscle and splits the two heads of the gastrocnemius, passing deep to the soleus on its course to the posterior aspect of the medial malleolus. It terminates as the medial and lateral plantar nerves. Muscular branches supply the posterior leg along its course.
  2. Common Peroneal Nerve—The smaller terminal division of the sciatic, this nerve runs laterally in the popliteal fossa in the interval between the medial border of the biceps and the lateral head of the gastrocnemius. Then it winds around the neck of the fibula, deep to the peroneus longus, where it divides into superficial and deep branches.
    a. Superficial Peroneal Nerve—Runs along the border between the lateral and anterior compartments in the leg, supplying muscular branches to the peroneus longus and brevis. It terminates in two cutaneous branches supplying the dorsal foot.

    b. Deep Peroneal Nerve—Sometimes known as the anterior tibial nerve, this nerve runs along the anterior surface of the interosseous membrane, supplying the musculature of the anterior compartment.
  3. Cutaneous Nerves—Important cutaneous nerves include the saphenous nerve and the sural nerve. The saphenous nerve is the continuation of the femoral nerve of the thigh, and it becomes subcutaneous on the medial aspect of the knee between the sartorius and gracilis (where it is sometimes injured during procedures about the knee—e.g., meniscoresis). The saphenous nerve supplies sensation to the medial aspect of the leg and foot. The sural nerve, which is often used in nerve grafting, and which can cause painful neuromas when inadvertently cut, is formed by cutaneous branches of both the tibial (medial sural cutaneous) and common peroneal (lateral sural cutaneous) nerves. It lies on the lateral aspect of the leg and foot.
E. Vessels (Fig. 10–54)—Branches of the popliteal artery, the continuation of the femoral artery, supply the leg. The artery enters the popliteal fossa between the biceps and semimembranosus and descends beneath the tibial nerve and terminates between the medial and lateral heads of the

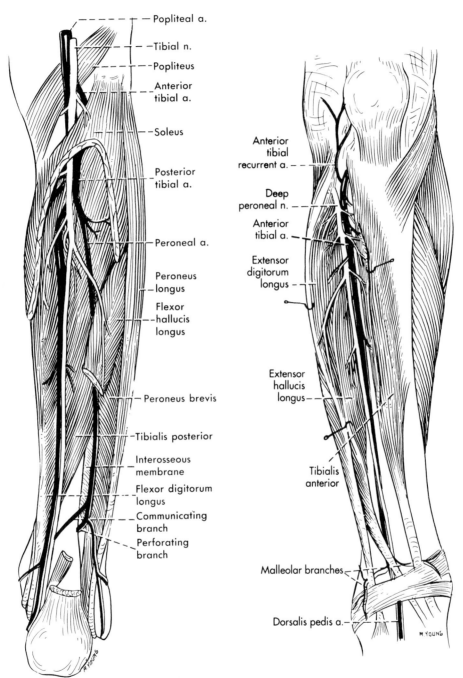

Popliteal a.

Tibial n.

Popliteus

Anterior
tibial a.

Soleus

Posterior
tibial a.

Peroneal a.

Peroneus
longus

Flexor
hallucis
longus

Peroneus brevis

Tibialis posterior

Interosseous
membrane

Flexor digitorum
longus

Communicating
branch

Perforating
branch

Anterior
tibial
recurrent a.

Deep
peroneal n.

Anterior
tibial a.

Extensor
digitorum
longus

Extensor
hallucis
longus

Tibialis
anterior

Malleolar branches

Dorsalis pedis a.

FIGURE 10–54. Nerves and vessels of the leg (left-posterior, right anterior). (From Jenkins, D.B.: Hollinshead's Functional Anatomy of the Limbs and Back, 6th ed., pp. 292, 296. Philadelphia, W.B. Saunders, 1991; reprinted by permission.)

gastrocnemius, dividing into the anterior and posterior tibial arteries. Several genicular branches are given off in the popliteal fossa, including the medial and lateral geniculates, which supply the menisci, and the middle geniculate, which supplies the cruciate ligaments.

1. Anterior Tibial Artery—The first branch of the popliteal artery, this vessel passes between the two heads of the tibialis posterior and the interosseous membrane to lie on the anterior surface of that membrane between the tibialis anterior and extensor hallicus longus until it terminates as the dorsalis pedis artery.

2. Posterior Tibial Artery—Continues in the deep posterior compartment of the leg, coursing obliquely to pass behind the medial malleolus, where it terminates by dividing into medial and lateral plantar arteries. Its main branch, the peroneal artery, is given off 2.5 cm distal to the popliteal fossa and continues in the deep posterior compartment, lateral to its parent artery, between the tibialis posterior and flexor hallicus longus, eventually terminating in calcaneal branches.

F. Surgical Approaches to the Knee and Leg

1. Medial Parapatellar Approach to the Knee—Used most commonly for total knee arthroplasty, this approach utilizes a midline incision and a medial parapatellar capsular incision. The infrapatellar branch of the saphenous nerve can sometimes be cut with incisions that stray too far medially, leading to a painful neuroma.

2. Medial Approach to the Knee (Fig. 10–55)—Used for repair of the MCL and capsule, this approach is in the interval between the sartorius and medial patellar retinaculum. Three layers are commonly recognized (from superficial to deep):

Layer	Components
1	Pes anserinus tendons
2	Superficial MCL
3	Deep MCL, capsule, POL

The saphenous nerve and vein must be identified and protected.

3. Lateral Approach to the Knee (Fig. 10–56)—Used primarily for exploring and repairing damaged ligaments, this approach utilizes the plane between the iliotibial band (superior gluteal nerve) and the biceps (sciatic nerve). The common peroneal nerve, located near the posterior border of the biceps, must be isolated and retracted. The popliteus tendon is also at risk and should be identified.

4. Posterior Approach to the Knee—Occasionally required to address posterior capsular pathology, this approach uses an S-shaped incision beginning laterally and ending medially (distally). The popliteal fossa is exposed using the small saphenous vein and medial sural cutaneous nerves as landmarks. The two heads of the gastrocnemius can be detached if greater exposure is necessary.

5. Anterior Approach to the Tibia—May be used for ORIF of fractures, bone grafting, etc., and relies on subperiosteal elevation of the tibialis anterior.

6. Posterolateral Approach to the Tibia—Used typically for bone grafting of tibial nonunions, this approach utilizes the internervous plane between the soleus and FHL (tibial nerve) and the peroneal muscles (superficial peroneal nerve). The FHL is detached from its origin on the fibula and the tibialis posterior is detached from its origin along the interosseous membrane to reach the tibia. Neurovascular structures in the posterior compartment are protected by the muscle bellies of the FHL and tibialis posterior.

7. Approach to the Fibula—Through the same interval as the posterolateral approach to the tibia, but stays more anterior, and relies on isolation and protection of the common peroneal nerve in the proximal dissection.

X. Ankle and Foot

A. Osteology—The 26 bones of the foot include seven tarsal bones, five metatarsals, and 14 phalanges.

1. Tarsus—Includes the talus, calcaneus, cuboid, navicular and three cuneiforms.

a. Talus—Articulates with the tibia and fibula in the ankle mortise, and with the calcaneus and navicular distally. It is made up of a body with three articular surfaces (the trochlea, including surfaces for the malleoli articulations, and the posterior and middle calcaneal facets) and a posterior process (for the posterior talofibular ligament). The neck of the talus connects with the head, which in turn articulates with the navicular distally and the calcaneus inferiorly.

b. Calcaneus—The largest and strongest bone in the foot. It has three surfaces that articulate with the talus: a large posterior surface, an anterior surface, and a middle surface. Distally, there is an articular surface that receives the cuboid bone. The sustentaculum tali is an overhanging horizontal eminence on the anteriomedial surface of the calcaneus. It supports the middle articular surface above it and allows plantar vessels and nerves to pass below it. The calcaneal tuberosity posteriorly is bounded by medial and lateral processes.

c. Cuboid—Lies on the lateral aspect of the foot, is grooved by the peroneus longus, and has four facets for articulation with the calcaneus, the lateral cuneiform, and the fourth and fifth metatarsals.

d. Navicular—The most medial tarsal bone; lies between the talus and the cuneiforms. Proximally, the surface is oval and concave for its articulation with the head of the talus. Distally, the navicular has three articular surfaces, one for each of the cuneiforms.

e. Cuneiforms—Medial, intermediate, and lateral, these three bones articulate with the navicular and posterior cuboid (lateral cuneiform) and the first three metatarsals. The intermediate cuneiform does not extend as far distally as the medial cuneiform, allowing the second metatarsal to "key" into place.

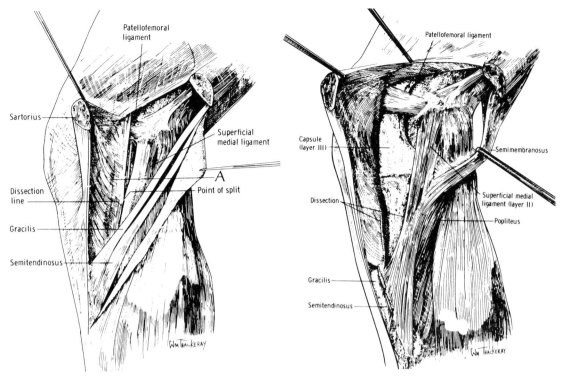

FIGURE 10–55. Medial structures of the knee. (Warren, L.F., and Marshall, J.L.: The supporting structures and layers of the medial side of the knee. J. Bone Joint Surg. [Am.] 61:58, 1979; reprinted by permission.)

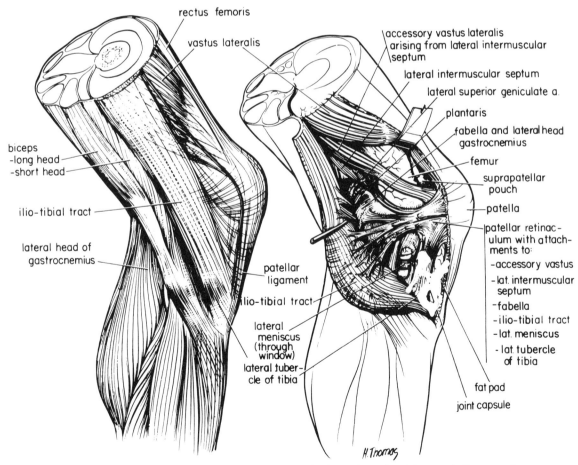

FIGURE 10–56. Lateral structures of the knee. (From Seebacher, J.R., Inglis, A.E., Marshall, J.L., and Warren R.F.: The structure of the posterolateral aspect of the knee. J. Bone Joint Surg. [Am.] 64:533, 1982; reprinted by permission.)

351

2. Metatarsals—Five bones, numbered from medial to lateral, span the distance between the tarsals and the phalanges. In general, they are similar in shape and function to the metacarpals of the hand.

3. Phalanges—Also similar to the hand. The great toe has two phalanges and the remaining digits have three.

4. Ossification—Each tarsus has a single ossification center except the calcaneus, which has a second center posteriorly. The calcaneus, talus, and usually the cuboid are present at birth. The lateral cuneiform appears during the first year, the medial cuneiform in the second year, and the intermediate cuneiform and navicular in the third year. The posterior center for the calcaneus usually appears at the eighth year. The second through fifth metatarsals have two ossification centers, a primary center in the shaft and a secondary center for the head that appears at age 5–8. The phalanges and first metatarsal have secondary centers at their bases that appear in the third or fourth year proximally and sixth to seventh year distally.

B. Arthrology

1. Inferior Tibiofibular Joint—Formed by the medial distal fibula and the notched lateral distal tibia, this joint is supported by four ligaments. The anterior inferior tibiofibular ligament (AITFL) is an oblique band that connects the bones anteriorly. The posterior tibiofibular ligament (PTFL) is smaller but serves a similar function posteriorly. The inferior transverse ligament lies just below the PTFL and provides additional posterior support for the mortise. Finally, an interosseous ligament also connects the two bones.

2. Ankle Joint (Fig. 10–57)—A ginglymus, or hinge, joint is formed by the malleoli and the talus. It is supported by the following ligaments:

LIGAMENT	ORIGIN	INSERTION
Capsule	Tibia	Talus
Deltoid		
Tibionavicular	Med. malleolus	Navicular tuberosity
Tibiocalcaneal	Med. malleolus	Sustentaculum tali
Post. tibiotalar	Med. malleolus	Inner side of talus
Deep	Med. malleolus	Medial surface of talus
ATFL	Lat. malleolus	Transversely to talus anteriorly
PTFL	Lat. malleolus	Transversely to talus posteriorly
Calcaneofibular (CFL)	Lat. malleolus	Obliquely posteriorly to calcaneus

The PTFL is strong and the ATFL is weak; therefore, the ATFL is most commonly injured in ankle sprains.

3. Intertarsal Joints (Fig. 10–58)—Relatively self-explanatory; however, there are several ligamentous structures that deserve highlighting (Table 10–12).

4. Other Joints—Tarsometatarsal joints are gliding joints supported by dorsal, plantar, and interosseous ligaments. The intermetatarsal joints are supported by similar ligaments, and the deep transverse metatarsal ligaments interconnect the metatarsal heads. The MTP joints are supported by plantar and collateral ligaments, and IP joints are supported mainly by their capsules.

C. Muscles (Fig. 10–59)—The arrangement of muscles and tendons in the foot is best considered in layers (Table 10–13). On the plantar surface, intrinsic muscles dominate the first and third layers, while extrinsic tendons are more important in the second and fourth layers. Tendons are arranged about the toe as shown in Figure 10–60.

D. Nerves (Fig. 10–61)—Nerves of the ankle and foot are branches of proximal nerves discussed above.

1. Tibial Nerve—Splits into two branches under the flexor retinaculum, the medial and lateral plantar nerves. Both of these nerves run in the second layer of the foot. The medial plantar nerve runs deep to the abductor hallicus and the lateral plantar nerve runs obliquely under the cover of the quadratus plantae. **The distribution of the sensory and motor branches of the plantar nerves is similar to that in the hand.** The medial plantar nerve (like the median nerve of the hand) supplies plantar sensation to the medial 3½ digits and motor sensation to only a few plantar muscles (FHB, abductor hallucis, FDB, and first lumbrical). The lateral plantar nerve (like the ulnar nerve in the hand) supplies plantar sensation to the lateral 1½ digits and the remaining intrinsic muscles of the foot.

2. Common Peroneal Nerve—Splits into superficial and deep branches in the leg and also has terminal branches in the foot. The lateral terminal branch of the deep peroneal nerve ends in the proximal dorsal foot by supplying the EDB muscle. The medial terminal branch of the deep peroneal nerve supplies sensation to the first web space. The bulk of the remaining sensation to the dorsal foot is supplied by the medial and intermediate dorsal cutaneous nerves of the superficial peroneal nerve.

E. Vessels—Like the nerves that run with them, there are two main arteries that supply the ankle and foot.

TABLE 10–12. LIGAMENTS OF THE INTERTARSAL JOINTS

LIGAMENT	COMMON NAME	ORIGIN	INSERTION
Talocalcanear interosseous	Cervical	Talus	Calcaneous
Calcaneocuboid/Calcaneonavicular	Bifurcate	Calcaneus	Cuboid and navicular
Calcaneocuboid-metatarsal	Long plantar	Calcaneus	Cuboid & 1st–5th metatarsals
Plantar calcaneocuboid	Short plantar	Calcaneus	Cuboid
Plantar calcaneonavicular	Spring	Sustentaculum tali	Navicular
Tarsometatarsal	Lisfranc	Med. cuneiform	2nd metatarsal base

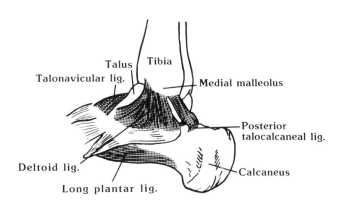

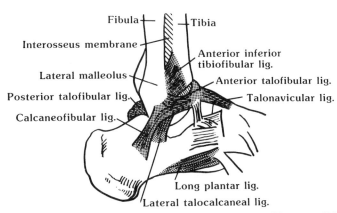

FIGURE 10–57. Ankle ligaments. *A*, Medial. *B*, Lateral. *C*, Posterior. (From Wiessman, B.N., and Sledge, C.B.: Orthopedic Radiology, pp. 593, 594, Philadelphia, W.B. Saunders, 1986; reprinted by permission.)

TABLE 10–13. MUSCLES OF THE ANKLE AND FOOT

MUSCLE	ORIGIN	INSERTION	ACTION	INNERVATION
Dorsal Layer				
Extensor digitorum brevis (EDB)	Superolateral calcaneus	Base of proximal phalanges	Extend	Deep peroneal
First Plantar Layer				
Abductor hallucis	Calcaneal tuberosity	Base of great toe proximal phalanx	Abduct great toe	Med. plantar
Flexor digitorum brevus (FDB)	Calcaneal tuberosity	Distal phalanges of 2nd–5th toes	Flex toes	Med. plantar
Abductor digiti minimi	Calcaneal tuberosity	Base of 5th toe	Abduct small toe	Med. plantar
Second Plantar Layer				
Quadratus plantae	Med. & lat. calcaneus	FDL tendon	Helps flex distal phalanges	Lat. plantar
Lumbricals	FDL tendon	EDL tendons	Flex MTP, extend IP	Med. & lat. plantar
(FDL & FHL)	Tibia/Fibula	Distal phalanges of digits	Flex toes/Invert foot	Tibial
Third Plantar Layer				
Flexor hallucis brevis (FHB)	Cuboid/Lat. cuneiform	Proximal phalanx of great toe	Flex great toe	Med. plantar
Adductor hallucis	Oblique: 2nd–4th metatarsals/Transverse: MTP	Proximal phalanx of great toe lat.	Adduct great toe	Lat. plantar
Flexor digiti minimi brevis (FDMB)	Base of 5th metatarsal head	Proximal phalanx of small toe	Flex small toe	Lat. plantar
Fourth Plantar Layer				
Dorsal interosseous	Metatarsals	Dorsal extensors	Abduct	Lat. plantar
Plantar interosseous	3rd–5th metatarsals	Proximal phalanges medially	Adduct toes	Lat. plantar
(Peroneus longus & tibialis posterior)	Fibula/Tibia	Med. cuneiform/Navicular	Everts/Invert foot	Superficial peroneal/Tibial

Note: For abduction and adduction in the foot, the second toe serves as the reference.

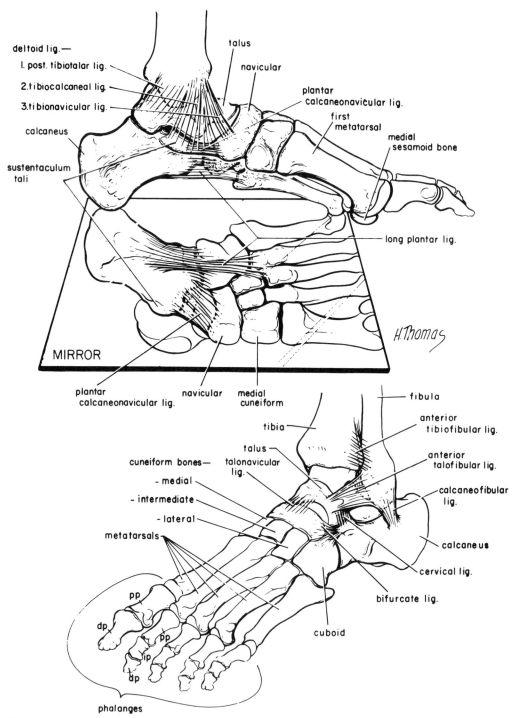

FIGURE 10–58. Ligaments of the foot. (From Jahss, M.H.: Disorders of the Foot, p. 14. Philadelphia, W.B. Saunders, 1982; reprinted by permission.)

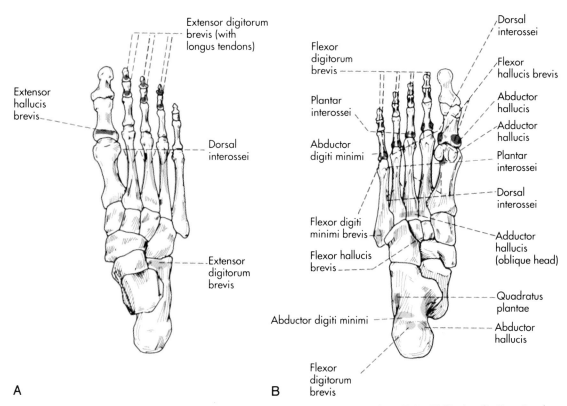

FIGURE 10–59. Origins and insertions of muscles of the foot. (From Jenkins, D.B.: Hollinshead's Functional Anatomy of the Limbs and Back, 6th ed., fig. 20–7. Philadelphia, W.B. Saunders, 1991; reprinted by permission.)

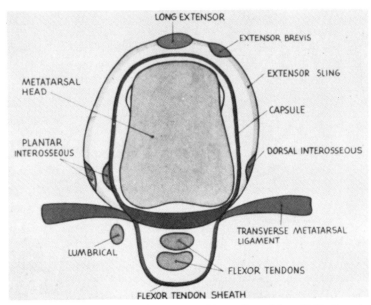

FIGURE 10–60. Cross section of the toe at the metatarsal base. (From Jahss, M.H.: Disorders of the Foot, p. 623. Philadelphia, W.B. Saunders, 1982; reprinted by permission.)

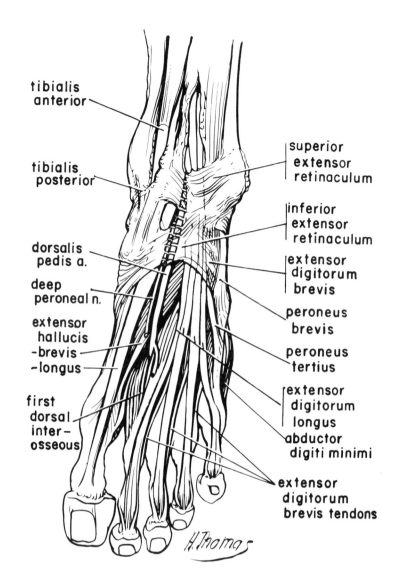

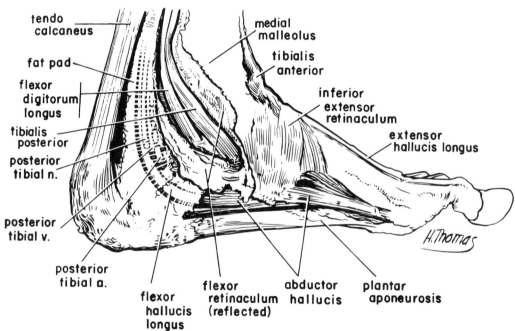

FIGURE 10–61. Muscles and tendons of the foot. (From Jahss, M.H.: Disorders of the Foot, pp. 18–20. Philadelphia, W.B. Saunders, 1982; reprinted by permission.)

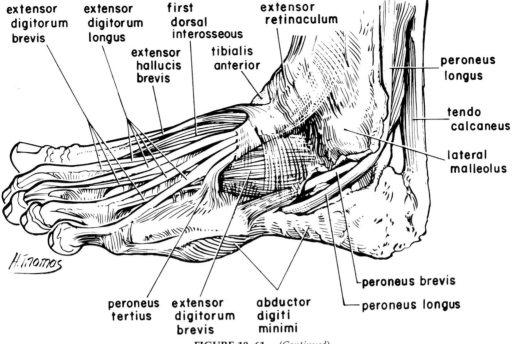

extensor digitorum brevis

extensor digitorum longus

first dorsal interosseous

extensor hallucis brevis

tibialis anterior

extensor retinaculum

peroneus longus

tendo calcaneus

lateral malleolus

peroneus tertius

extensor digitorum brevis

abductor digiti minimi

peroneus brevis

peroneus longus

H. Thomas

FIGURE 10–61. (*Continued*)

1. Dorsalis Pedis Artery—The continuation of the anterior tibial artery of the leg and provides the blood supply to the dorsum of the foot via its lateral tarsal, medial tarsal, arcuate, and first dorsal metatarsal branches. Its largest branch, the deep plantar artery, runs between the first and second metatarsals and contributes to the plantar arch.
2. Posterior Tibial Artery—Divides into medial and lateral plantar branches under the abductor hallucis muscle. The larger lateral branch receives the deep plantar artery and forms the plantar arch in the fourth layer of the plantar foot.

F. Surgical Approaches
   1. Anterior Approach to the Ankle—Used primarily for ankle fusion, this approach utilizes the interval between the EHL and EDL. Before incising the extensor retinaculum, care must be taken to protect the superficial peroneal nerve. The deep peroneal nerve and anterior tibial artery, which lie directly in this interval, must be retracted medially with the EHL.
   2. Approach to the Medial Malleolus—This approach is commonly used for ORIF of ankle fractures. It is superficial, and can be approached anteriorly or posteriorly. The anterior approach jeopardizes the saphenous nerve and the long saphenous vein; the posterior approach places the structures running behind the medial malleolus (tibial artery, FDL, post. tibial artery, vein, and nerve, and FHL) at risk.
   3. Posteromedial Approach to the Ankle/Foot—

Used for clubfoot release in children, this approach begins medial to the Achilles tendon and curves distally along the medial border of the foot. Care must be taken to protect the posterior tibial nerve/artery and their branches. The posterior tibialis tendon is a landmark for the location of the subluxated navicular in the clubfoot.
   4. Lateral Approach to the Ankle—Used for ORIF of distal fibula fractures, this approach is subcutaneous. The sural nerve (posterolateral) and the superficial peroneal nerve (anterior) must be avoided.
   5. Lateral Approach to the Hindfoot—Used for triple arthrodesis, this approach uses the internervous plane between the peroneus tertius (deep peroneal nerve) and peroneal tendons (superficial peroneal nerve). The fat pad covering the sinus tarsi is removed and the EDB is reflected from its origin to expose the joints. The lateral branch of the deep peroneal nerve (which supplies the EDB) must be protected with this approach.
   6. Approach to the midfoot and digits is direct and is not discussed in detail. In general, care must be taken to protect digital nerves/arteries.

XI. Summary

   A. Important anatomical landmarks are summarized in Table 10–1.
   B. Surgical approaches. A summary of key intervenous intervals is summarized in Table 10–2.

Selected Bibliography

Arnoczky, S.P., and Warren, R.F.: Microvasculature of the human meniscus. Am. J. Sports Med. 10(2):90–95, 1982.

Chapman, M.W., ed.: Operative Orthopaedics. Philadelphia, J.B. Lippincott, 1988.

Clemente, C.D. ed.: Gray's Anatomy, 30th Am. ed. Philadelphia, Lea & Febiger, 1985.

Crock, H.V.: An atlas of the arterial supply of the head and neck of the femur in man. Clin. Orthop. 152:17, 1980.

Doyle, J.R.: Anatomy of the finger flexor tendon sheath and pulley system. J. Hand Surg. [Am.] 13:473–484, 1988.

Girgis, F.G., Marshall, J.L., and Monajem, A.R.S.: The cruciate ligaments of the knee joint: Anatomical, functional, and experimental analysis. Clin. Orthop. 106:216–231, 1975.

Harding, K.: The direct lateral approach to the hip. J. Bone Joint Surg. [Br.] 64:17–19, 1982.

Henry, A.K.: Extensive Exposure, 2nd ed. New York, Churchill Livingstone, 1973.

Hollinshead, W.H.: Anatomy for Surgeons, Vol. 3, 2nd ed. New York, Harper & Row, 1969.

Hoppenfield, S., and DeBoer, P. Orthopaedics: The Anatomic Approach. Philadelphia, J.B. Lippincott, 1984.

Jenkins, D.B.: Hollinshead's Functional Anatomy of the Limbs and Back, 6th ed. Philadelphia, W.B. Saunders, 1991.

Kaplan, E.B.: Surgical Approaches to the Neck, Cervical Spine, and Upper Extremity. Philadelphia, W.B. Saunders, 1966.

Ludloff, K.: The open reduction of the congenital hip dislocation by an anterior incision. Am. J. Orthop. Surg. 10:438, 1913.

Morrey, B.F., and An, K.N.: Articular and ligamentous contributions to the stability of the elbow joint. Am. J. Sports Med. 11:315–319, 1983.

Morrey, B.F., and An, K.: Functional anatomy of the ligaments of the elbow. Clin. Orthop. 210:84–90, 1985.

Netter, F.H.: The CIBA Collection of Medical Illustrations, Vol. 8, Musculoskeletal System, Part I. Summit, NJ, CIBA-Geigy, 1987.

Orthopaedic Knowledge Update Home Study Syllabus I, II, and III. Chicago, American Academy of Orthopaedic Surgeons, 1984, 1987, 1990.

Rockwood, C.A., Jr., and Green, D.P., eds.: Fractures in Adults, 3rd ed. Philadelphia, J.B. Lippincott, 1991.

Ruge, D., and Wiltse, L.L., eds.: Spinal Disorders Diagnosis and Treatment. Philadelphia, Lea and Febiger, 1977.

Sarrafian, S.K.: Anatomy of the Foot and Ankle. Philadelphia, J.B. Lippincott, 1983.

Seebacher, J.R., Inglis, A.E., Marshall, J.L., et al.: The structure of the posterolateral aspect of the knee. J. Bone Joint Surg. [Am.] 64:536–541, 1982.

Turkel, S.J., et al.: Stabilizing mechanisms preventing anterior dislocation of the gleno-humeral joint. J. Bone Joint Surg. [Am.] 63:1208–1217, 1981.

Verbiest, H.A.: Lateral approach to the cervical spine: Technique and indications. J. Neurosurg. 28:191–203, 1968.

Warren, I.F., and Marshall, J.L.: The supporting structures and layers on the medial side of the knee. J. Bone Joint Surg. [Am.] 61:56–62, 1979.

Watkins, R.G.: Surgical Approaches to the Spine. New York, Springer-Verlag, 1983.

Index

Note: Page numbers in *italics* refer to illustrations; page numbers followed by t refer to tables.